The
Psychopharmacologists II

Interviews by Dr David Healy

Altman
An imprint of Chapman and Hall
London Weinheim New York Tokyo Melbourne Madras

Published by Chapman & Hall, an imprint of Lippincott-Raven Publishers, 2–6 Boundary Row
London SE1 8HN, UK

Lippincott-Raven Publishers, 227 East Washington Square, Philadelphia, PA 19106-3720, USA

First edition 1998

Copyright (c) 1998 Lippincott-Raven Publishers

Typeset in 11/12 Bembo by Saxon Graphics Ltd

Printed in Great Britain by St Edmundsbury Press, Bury St. Edmunds

ISBN 1 86036 010 6

  Care has been taken to confirm the accuracy of the information presented and to describe generally accepted
practices. However, the authors, editors, publisher, and society [or societies] are not responsible for errors or
omissions or for any consequences from application of the information in this publication and make no warranty,
express or implied, with respect to content.

  The authors, editors, publisher, and society [or societies] have exerted every effort to ensure that drug selection
and dosage set forth in this text are in accordance with current recommendations. The reader is urged to check the
package insert for each drug for any change in indications and dosage and for added warnings and precautions.

  Some drugs and medical devices presented in this publication have FDA clearance for limited use in restricted
research settings. It is the responsibility of the health care provider to ascertain the FDA status of each drug or
device planned for use in their clinical practice.

A catalogue record for this book is available from the British Library

∞ Printed on permanent acid-free text paper, manufactured in
accordance with ANSI/NISO Z39.48-1992 and ANSI/NISO Z39.48-1984
(Permanence of Paper).

Contents

Contributors

Professor Per Bech
Frederiksborg General Hospital, Psychiatric Research Unit, Hiller¾d Sygehus
Dyrenhavevej 48
DK-3400 Hillerød, Denmark

Dr Klaus. P. Bøgesø
Director of Medicinal Chemistry H Lundbeck A/S, Ottiliavej 9, DK-2500
Copenhagen-Valby
Denmark

Professor Joseph. V. Brady
Director, Behavioural Biology Research Centre, Johns Hopkins University
School of Medicine
5510 Nathan Shock Drive, Suite 3000, Baltimore, Maryland 21224, USA

Dr Leonard Cook
6 Radburn Lane, Newark, Delaware 19711–2479, USA

Professor Gerald Curzon
Institute of Neurology, Miriam Marks Department of Neurochemistry,1
Wakefield Street,London,
WC1N 1PJ

Dr Joel Elkes
1516 Pelican Cove Road, Apt GR 243, Pelican Cove, Sarasota, FL34231, USA

Professor Irving I Gottesman
Department of Psychology, Gilmer Hall, University of Virginia, Charlottesville,
VA 22903, USA

Professor Leo E Hollister
The University of Texas Houston, Health Science Centre, Harris County
Psychiatric Centre
2800 South MacGregor Way (77021), PO Box 20249, Houston, Texas
77225–0249, USA

Professor Leslie Iversen
University of Oxford, Department of Pharmacology, University of Oxford, Mansfield Road,Oxford,
OX1 3QT

Dr Paul Janssen
Janssen Pharmaceuticals, Turnhoustseweg 30, B-2340 – Beerse, Belgium

Professor Roland Kuhn
FMH fur Psychiatrie und Psychotherapie, Rebhaldenstrasse 5, CH-8596 Scherzingen, Switzerland

Professor Louis Lasagna
Associate Dean, Tufts Medical School, 136 Harrison Avenue, Boston MA 02111 USA

Dr Paul Leber
Division of Neuropharmacological Drug Products, Food and Drug Administration, 5600 Fisher's Lane, Rockville, Maryland 20857, USA

Professor Thérèse Lempérière
28 Rue de acacias, 75017 Paris, France

Professor Juan Lopez-Ibor Jr
Clinica Lopez Ibor, Nueva Zelande 44, E-28035 Madrid, Spain

Dr Max Lurie
301 J H Professional Building, 3120 Burnet Avenue, Cincinnati, Ohio 45229, USA

Professor Isaac Marks
The Institute of Psychiatry, De Crespigny Park, 101 Denmark Hill, London SE5 8AF

Dr Vagn Pedersen
Divisional Director, Clinical Research & Development, H Lundbeck A/S Ottiliavej 9, DK-2500 Copenhagen-Valby, Denmark

Dr Roger. M. Pinder
International Product Manager CNS NV Organon, PO Box 20, 5340 BH Oss, The Netherlands

Professor Oakley Ray
Executive Secretary ACNP, 320 Centre Building, 2014 Broadway Nashville, TN 37203, USA

Professor Linford Rees
62 Oakwood Avenue, Purley, Surrey, CR8 1AQ

Professor Mogens Schou
The Psychiatric Hospital, 2 Scovagervej DK-8240 Risskov, Denmark

Professor George. M. Simpson
Director of Clinical Research, University of Southern California, School of Medicine LAC-USC Medical Centre, 1937 Hospital Place, Suite 240, Los Angeles, California 90033–1071, USA

Professor Ian Stolerman
Institute of Psychiatry, Department of Psychiatry, Section of Behavioural Pharmacology, De Crespigny
Park, London, SE5 8AF

Professor J.C Watkins
University of Bristol, Department of Pharmacology, School of Medical Sciences, University Walk, Bristol, BS8 1TD

Professor Myrna P. Weissman
Professor of Epidemiology in Psychiatry, College of Physicians & Surgeons of Columbia University, 722 West 168th Street, Unit 14, New York, NY 10032, USA

Dr David Wheatley
69 Broughton Avenue, Richmond, Surrey, TW10 7UL

Preface

This section of the book is about prejudices and biases. Mine. In interviews such as these, the interviewer is the instrument through which the actors in a historical drama, in this case psychopharmacology, reveal themselves. Readers, therefore, need to know how the gain on the instrument they are using has been set – at least in so far as biases have been consciously registered. There may of course be many other distortions which will come to light between this and a sister volume of interviews and The Antidepressant Era[1], where my efforts to assemble the events and personalities of the psychopharmacological era into a narrative have probably also provided a flourishing medium for the growth of biases. While clearly the questions that were asked here owe a great deal to the details of the interviewee's career and concerns, inevitably they owe something also to my agendas. Recognising some of these agendas may make it clear why certain interviews took particular turns. It may even make this clear for the first time to some hitherto puzzled interviewees.

There are many different approaches to history. This comes through perhaps most clearly in the interview with Gerald Curzon, who takes a quantitative approach. Shortly before I interviewed him, I had begun to ask interviewees to think about possible historical vignettes. The historical vignette, of course, is a completely different approach to history from the quantitative one but where the quantitative approach wins hands down against a more qualitative approach in the natural sciences it is not clear that this is necessarily the case in the human sciences and in particular in history. Gerald Curzon, inadvertently perhaps, illustrated the point by producing what is perhaps the best historical vignette in the book. He described attending a case conference at the Institute of Neurology in the early 1960s on Parkinson's disease, at which he raised the fact that he had heard that there had been some claims for a deficiency of dopamine

---

[1] These volumes of interviews are, at present, much more psychopharmacology friendly than historian friendly. To be properly user friendly for a historian from outside the field they should have far more in the line of footnotes to explain points that many inside the field will take for granted. By way of an apology I would like to point to The Antidepressant Era, which is something of a gigantic footnote to the interviews in both volumes of *The Psychopharmacologists*.

in the brain of subjects with Parkinson's disease. The meeting was being chaired by an eminence who clearly thought this idea was preposterous and dismissed it by observing that if Dr Curzon had ever seen the brain of a person with Parkinson's disease he would realise that this could not be a chemical disorder.

This vignette very dramatically brings home the idea of the past being another country. In order to understand the past sometimes it's necessary to learn an almost completely different language or to unlearn the usual usages of contemporary languages. How did people see Parkinson's disease before dopamine was discovered? What did it once mean to see the world as flat? If attention is not drawn to the fact that sometimes key words in the space of a few years can undergo a complete change of meaning and can end up meaning in essence the opposite to what they had meant only 10 years previously, as happened with the word neurosis around 1900, the unsuspecting reader in years following may be significantly misled. The corollary of this is that, at any one point in time, we live in a rather slim cultural envelope and while our aspirations towards understanding may have remained constant over hundreds or thousands of years, particular understandings rarely last a generation.

As these interviews were being conducted, Dolly the sheep was cloned and newspapers and television were full of her story. This story was literally 'news worthy' by virtue of the Shock of the New which it conveyed. Where once we depended on politics and politicians for novelty, science has become an increasingly good hunting ground for newshounds of various sorts because of its capacity to deliver stories with this impact. But in producing the new, science at the same time creates history – older sets of meanings, the world as it was before Dolly, or before chlorpromazine, imipramine or Prozac. The best history should convey this; it should convey the Shock of the Old. As the speed of scientific developments picks up, a good case can be made for the growing importance of a history of science and medicine. Where once we depended on politicians or natural events to transform our understanding of ourselves and in the process make history, scientists and technical developments increasingly rival them, potentially transforming perceptions of where history itself is happening.

The field of receptor studies may illustrate the importance of some of these issues. The notion of a receptor is closely linked to images of locks-and-keys, Magic Bullets and therapeutic specificity. These arguably have been the dominant therapeutic metaphors of our century. They play a part in every exchange between clinician and patient. They drive medical developments. But what notions of receptors did Fridolin Sulser, Sol Snyder or George Ashcroft have before they put forward the first specific receptor hypotheses in psychopharmacology? What models of a receptor were they operating with and how consistent have those models been with subsequent receptor research? The connotations of the word receptor and the implications for drug development of the technical developments that have enabled us to determine receptor numbers all owe a great deal to the work of Snyder, Ashcroft and Sulser and in the process these men have contributed significantly to cultural history as well as to psychopharmacology. The chances are that the shifting understandings that went with their work will die with them unless they are interviewed. Many of these scientists are history. One of the surprising things about interviewing many of them is how little they have been aware that a great deal of history dies with them. In part the fault here lies with both the scientists and the historians who have connived with them in seeing science as something of an a-historical realm.

Again Gerald Curzon brings home some of the key points. While LSD was clearly doing something fairly dramatic to minds in the 1950s and 1960s there was nevertheless, and still is, a bias against thinking that manipulating brain chemicals has anything much to do with our 'real' selves. Millennia of human beliefs in immaterial souls are at stake here. His account of how what he was doing was seen as somewhat scandalous in the early days coincides exactly with my own experience. Herman van Praag, in Volume 1 of this series, describes the death threats he received because of his engagement in this supposedly Satanic work. But yet twenty years later, Prozac has become a common topic of coffee-table conversation and all but a fashion accessory. This is an epochal transformation in our self-understanding. For this alone the history of psychopharmacology deserves a place on the shelves along with Histories of Private Life, of Sexuality and of Death.

The history of psychopharmacology is a new and particularly important discipline. It is a sister discipline to the history of psychiatry and the history of neuroscience. To date the history of psychiatry has been something of a traditional medical history dominated by assessments of great men and the rise and fall of ideas and concepts. While not so dominated by the great man approach, as technical developments play a far greater role in the development of neuroscience than they have hitherto played in psychiatry, the history of neuroscience to date has been about the emergence of concepts. The history of psychopharmacology, in contrast, must necessarily embrace a history of commodities. Commodities such as chlorpromazine, lithium and imipramine. Once these drugs enter the public domain, they have a life that is subject to market forces and the various other vagaries of the marketplace, as the career of Prozac makes abundantly clear. The drugs become cultural events and some of them such as Valium, Prozac and Thalidomide define epochs.

The creation of brands, such as Valium etc. and the effect these have on the scientific process, I would argue is highly relevant to the conduct of modern science. Far from it being something that simply happens in the health marketplace, academia itself, it seems to me, is dominated by brands. Customers buy ideas from firms with reputations for quality products, such as Harvard and Yale, Oxford or Cambridge, almost regardless of the intrinsic merits of what they are buying. The best-selling ideas are also ones that invariably have the snappiest slogans, such as Type 1 and Type 2 or positive and negative schizophrenia or the amine theories of depression. And as Max Lurie, and Gregor Mendel before him, found out discoveries rarely take root unless the marketplace is ready for them.

xii The Psychopharmacologists II

This bears on a question that has been topical within historical circles ever since Marx: does technology drive history? Since the Second World War, it has become increasingly difficult to deny claims that technology plays some important part in driving at least contemporary history forward. The debate, therefore, is between three groups: those who think it is the sole engine of history, those who think it interacts with social and economic culture to produce developments and those who think the most significant historical developments emerge accidentally from technical progress. All too often debates on these issues are conducted on the historical record of the physical sciences or engineering and in terms of late 19th century capitalism. Psychopharmacology provides a marvellous alternative. It came clearly into being within living memory. The drugs, at its core, are discrete instances of technical developments. The resulting interplay between these drugs and in the first instance psychiatric culture and thereafter the larger culture are significantly newsworthy because, unlike other drugs, psychotropic drugs have implications for our ideas of ourselves.

In psychopharmacology, the balance between the historical actor and the background forces of history is of great interest and more than ordinarily accessible to scrutiny. Jean Delay, Len Cook and others were involved in the discovery of chlorpromazine and its actions but once released on the market it set in train a transformation that none of these actors can in any meaningful way be held responsible for. Chlorpromazine, imipramine and lithium are the subjects of this book as much as Kuhn, Schou and Shepherd. But behind the drugs are yet other forces, forces making for corporatism and forces that have been transforming our self-understanding ever since Julien Offray de La Mettrie two centuries ago predicted that once medical developments permitted us to intervene effectively to shape human behaviour, medicine would replace philosophy.

Despite this credo, one wonders whether the scale of current cultural transformations would have surprised La Mettrie. What is clear is that he would not have been surprised by the entrenchment of medical power as represented by the adoption of prescription-only status for modern miracle drugs and a set of related developments that were part and parcel of the 1962 amendments to the Food and Drugs Act in the United States. Prescription-only status has been something of an unnoticed development. I took the issue with me into many of the interviews but it was difficult to get much comment on it. Without prescription-only status, however, the history of psychopharmacology would have been significantly different. Drug companies would not have had to sell depression, panic disorder or schizophrenia to the same extent as they now do. If these drugs had not been sold as magic bullets for disease entities, in the way they have been, clinicians might not be as helpless in the face of Len Cook's key question of them – what do you want this drug to do in order to get your patient well?

I am certain that prescription-only status is a factor of overriding importance in psychopharmacology. One of the reviewers of the previous volume noting the list of prejudices I owned up to at the start of that volume stated that not all had been confirmed. The fact, however, that none of the interviewees may agree with me on the importance of this issue doesn't necessarily discon-firm my hunch. Only time will tell whether I've been unhelpfully prejudiced on this issue or whether this was one of the factors operating outside the awareness of almost all the key actors of the era. The creation of prescription-only status was not a clearcut event shaped by a single actor. It emerged shaped by some of the subterranean forces at work.

I have been arguing that science is of relevance to history; the converse is also true. One of the best examples of the relevance of history to science comes from the field of evolution. Ecological science can examine the interrelation-ships and energy flows between currently existing species and systems but on its own it cannot account for evolution. In order to understand why things are the way they are, a number of extraneous events need to be factored into the equations, such as the impact of meteors. Once one begins to take these into account, the investigator must leave pure ecology and involve themselves in natural history. From this perspective, historical events such as the eruption of the Krakatoa volcano in Java provide marvellous natural experiments, where-by both ecologists and natural historians can see how biodiversity establishes itself on landforms newly risen from the sea.

Chlorpromazine, imipramine, prescription-only status and randomised tri-als have been the meteors and volcanoes in psychiatry. Historians and scientists should be mounting expeditions to see together how the new landform is being colonised. All too often the history of science, medicine or psychiatry has been a history of nineteenth or early twentieth century developments only. This runs the risk of falling foul of Voltaire's jibe that history is a trick that the living play on the dead. In the case of the natural experiment that is psy-chopharmacology, those who were around at the birth of the new species are for the most part still alive and can answer back. This is a challenge that nei-ther the historian nor the scientist should shirk.

One of the things that the colonisation of new land has thrown up in the case of psychopharmacology is a diversity of organisational structure. There is a real question about what this does to issues and personalities. The single-year honorary Presidency system of ACNP, for instance, seems to defuse some of the clashes that have occurred in an organisation like the BAP where the term of office of the President is 2 years and a further 4 years are spent as President-elect or past-President, and candidates for the Presidency to date have been selected by a mixture of a vote of the membership and a fix. The inclusion of interviews covering the origin and functioning of ACNP, ECNP, BAP, WPA, AEP and EBPS in this volume, as well as further interviews chasing the origin of CINP and BAP in Volume 1, may help bring this issue into focus.

The period covered in these interviews has been a period of largely mecha-nistic thinking, despite for instance the example of Joel Elkes in this volume, and Arvid Carlsson in Volume 1, who have perhaps been shifting in the oppo-site direction to the rest of the field during the course of their careers. During the past 30 years the guiding metaphors have been the image of the receptor and the notion of therapeutic specificity. Are we now perhaps on the verge of a new era which will place much more emphasis on ideas of functional management? Is psychiatry likely to move from the all but 'antibacterial' mode it has been in for 30 years now to an approach that resembles more the approach taken in cardiology? A great deal depends on the development and impact of new technologies such as neuro-imaging and whatever new drugs emerge. It depends on whether moves to over-the-counter (OTC) sales of formerly prescription-only agents continue. If the pharmaceutical industry began to sell Functional Management Tools rather than Magic Bullets to either clinicians or the population at large the impact on culture generally would be enormous (see The Antidepressant Era for a fuller exposition of this point). The fact that neither policy-makers nor cultural commentators in general have much feel for this is one indication of how we are failing to feed the historical imagination in these areas and in the process closing down future avenues of development as well as past vistas.

Most of my views about the history of medicine have remained constant across both sets of interviews but one in particular is worth re-emphasising here as a factor to be taken into account when assessing how the interviews went. I believe that scientific views prevail not simply because of their accuracy nor simply because of their place of origin but also because of their potential to generate livelihoods. Views out of which someone can make a living prevail. The medical arena is a very good one in which to see this process happen in that a view out of which someone can make a living translates into the recognition of a disease or condition upon which a particular technique or approach will work. Views about the nature of what is out there are then in turn shaped by the techniques that have become established. In this process the marketing of disease entities or the marketing of the evidence becomes part of the business.

This volume contains six different landfalls of the randomised clinical trial (RCT) on the new landform of psychopharmacology. The RCT has subsequently played an important part in generating marketable evidence more broadly in psychiatry and even in psychotherapy. There is an interview with Louis Lasagna outlining the origins of some of the elements that went into the controlled trial and the establishment of controlled trials in analgesia. Joel Elkes, Linford Rees, Mogens Schou, Michael Shepherd and Leo Hollister then all describe their first stabs at a controlled clinical trial in psychiatry proper. The principles of randomisation etc. have been at the heart of some of the most bitter disputes in the field, as will become clear in some of these interviews. There were two particularly notable sets of disputes: those involving lithium and those involving the panic disorder studies run by Gerald Klerman and colleagues during the 1980s. It will be clear from the views expressed and from the emotions around these disputes that something important was at stake in both cases. Exactly what is a matter of interpretation.

Another feature present in some of the interviews is some indication of how myths can develop. A particularly nice illustration involves Len Cook's views of how Paul Janssen came about haloperidol and vice versa Paul Janssen's views about Len Cook's involvement with chlorpromazine. Both of these views are close to the views of the primary player in the lead scenario but they involve a slightly different take on what happened. Whether the views of the original player are to be accorded any more validity than those of others is perhaps a questionable point but the emergence of a range of overlapping views points to the potential in the drug discovery/development process for myth making.

While these interviews were in progress, Frank Sulloway's *Born to Rebel* was published. The thesis of this work is that scientific developments are often shaped by the place in the birth order occupied by the various protagonists. The eldest child, Sulloway claims, tends to be a conservative upholder of the status quo while revolutionary breakthroughs come from the younger born. Intrigued by this, I checked the birth-order of all those interviewed for both volumes of *The Psychopharmacologists*. Of 54 interviewed (including Gerlad Klerman in the calculations), 36 were first born. Of those 27 were either only children or only sons. There is little support here for Sulloway's thesis. Instead one of the features that emerges is families have got considerably smaller – 35 came from families of only one or two children. The odds on a Darwin emerging as the fifth in a family of six have become progressively smaller. It may be therefore that something that might have held true for 19th century science no longer holds in modern science, just as it seems improbable in the near future that such a heavy preponderance of interviews in a field such as this will come from men.

I owe a great deal to Ned Shorter and Tom Ban, who have greatly encouraged me to chase these interviewees and the various issues raised. Ned Shorter came to interview Roland Kuhn, whose original interview was in German. This was translated by Urzel Luhde-Thompson and Dinah Cattell. Irena Hadaçova organised the French transcription of Thérèse Lempérière's original interview. I also owe a debt to Brian Leonard, Gene Paykel, Tom McMonagle, Tony Roberts, Marie Savage, Richard Tranter and many others who will recognise places where they have influenced me or who have covered my absences, as well as to Paul Hooper of Lundbeck UK and Ian Bruce before him. Finally, the fingers of Jacky Thomas and Bev Evans have been critical to the exercise of putting together these two volumes – between them they have now typed over a million words.

Glossary

CINP – Collegium Internationale Neuropsychopharmacologium. This was founded in 1957 and held its inaugural meeting in 1958. A number of the interviews in the book explore the impulses and the sequence of events that led to its foundation. The origins of CINP can be found in greater detail in:
Ban TA, Ray O (eds) (1996). *A History of CINP.* JM Productions, Brentwood, Tennessee. As well as in interviews with Frank Ayd, Hanns Hippius, Silvio Garattini, Jules Angst and others in *The Psychopharmacologists* Vol I.

ACNP – American College of Neuropsychopharmacology. This was founded in 1961. The proceedings of the foundation meeting are recorded almost verbatim in a fascinating volume entitled *In The Beginning*. A number of the interviews in this book refer to the foundation and subsequent development of ACNP as do interviews with Frank Ayd, Jonathan Cole, Floyd Bloom and Donald Klein in Volume 1.

APA – American Psychiatric Association. In contrast to the ACNP, which is a scientific society whose membership comprises clinicians, a range of neuroscientists and pharmacologists and both clinicians and neuroscientists from within the pharmaceutical industry, the APA is a professional body whose existence is predicated on the interests of the psychiatric profession. The dynamics of both bodies therefore differ.

BAP - British Association for Psychopharmacology. The BAP was only established in 1974 – rather late as national psychopharmacology associations go. One of the reasons for the first interviews in this series was to trace the origins of the BAP. Relevant interviews are those with David Wheatley and Ian Stolerman in this volume and with Merton Sandler and George Beaumont in *The Psychopharmacologists.* My assessment of what happened can be found in the History of British Psychopharmacology in *150 Years of British Psychiatry, Vol 2 (1996).* ed Berrios GE, Freeman H, Athlone Press.

RCP – Royal College of Psychiatrists. The RCP was only founded in 1971 but it had a previous existence in the form of the Royal Medico-Psychological Association, which was established in 1841. The RCP is to the BAP as the APA is to ACNP. A great deal of the history of the RCP/RMPA can be found in Berrios GE, Freeman H (1991). *One Hundred and Fifty Years* *of British Psychiatry*. Gaskell Press, London, Vol 1. Berrios GE, Freeman H (1996). *One Hundred and Fifty Years of British Psychiatry*. Athlone Press, London, Vol. 2.

And interviews with many of the best known names in British psychiatry, including figures relevant to this volume such as Max Hamilton and Michael Shepherd, can be found in Wilkinson G ed. (1993). *Talking about Psychiatry*, Gaskell, London.

AEP – Association of European Psychiatrists. With the development of 'Europe', there have in recent years been moves to develop European-wide scientific forums and professional associations. The AEP is the European equivalent of the APA and the RCP. Its origins are touched on in the interview with Pierre Pichot in Volume 1 as well as several interviews in this volume.

ECNP – European College of Neuropsychopharmacology. The ECNP is to AEP as ACNP is to the APA etc., except that at present ECNP is probably more clinically oriented than ACNP or BAP. The impetus to the development of ECNP came from Per Bech, Alex Delini-Stula and others. The politics of ECNP have been anything but smooth to date. In addition to several interviews in this volume, interviews with Hannah Steinberg and Alex Delini-Stula in Volume 1 touch on this. See also Healy D (1993). One Hundred Years of Psychopharmacology, *Journal of Psychopharmacology*, **7**, 207–214.

Psychiatric Institutions

Quite separate from the APA and the RCP there are psychiatric institutions geared toward research in both America and Britain. The best known of these in America are the National Institute of Mental Health (**NIMH**) and the National Institutes of Health (**NIH**), along with the National Institute on Drug Abuse (**NIDA**) and National Institute on Alcohol Abuse and Alcoholism (**NIAAA**). In Britain, there is the Institute of Psychiatry, which is at the Maudsley Hospital.

The Neurotransmitters

- Monoamines: these include catecholamines and indoleamines.
- Catecholamines: these are noradrenaline, adrenaline and dopamine.
- Indoleamines: serotonin, also called 5-hydroxytryptamine or 5HT.
- Peptides: the brain contains a vast number of peptides, many of which appear to function as neurotransmitters – see interviews with John Hughes and Arvid Carlsson.

The Instruments

- Spectrometer; Fluorimeter; Spectrofluorimeter; Spectrophotofluorimeter – the development of these is covered in Kanigel below.
- Chromatography: of which there are thin-layer forms (TLC) and high-pressure forms (HPLC).
- Radio-labelling: this permits radioautography, radioligand binding or receptor binding and other techniques. Radio-labelled imipramine is sometimes referred to as tritiated imipramine.

- Scanning: available techniques now include computerised axial tomography or CAT scans, positron emission tomography or PET scans, single positron emission tomography or SPECT scans and magnetic resonance imaging or MRI scans.

We live in a golden age of popular science writing. Not only have there, recently, been excellent popularisers of science, but equally this is an age in which clinicians and other scientists have sought to communicate directly with the public. This seems peculiarly apposite for both psychiatry and the neurosciences, in that unlike astrophysics or cosmology, the world that is being investigated is we ourselves, and informing the public not only informs the public but also increases the pool of people who may be able to contribute towards offering solutions to problems.

There are some excellent books from neuroscientists or about neuroscience, which outline more about the role of neurotransmission and the development of instrumentation; these include

- Changeux J-P (1985). *Neuronal Man. The Biology of Mind*. Random House, New York.
- Kanigel R. (1993). *Apprentice to Genius. The making of a scientific dynasty*. Johns Hopkins University Press, Baltimore.
- Levi-Montalcini R (1988). *In Praise of Imperfection*. Basic Books, New York.
- Richter D (1989). *A Life in Research*. A Stuart Phillips Publication, London.
- Rose S (1993). *The Making of Memory. From Molecules to Mind*. Bantam Press, London.

In terms of contributions to drug discovery the seminal volume is

- Ayd F Jr, Blackwell B (1970). *Discoveries in Biological Psychiatry*, Lippincott, Philadelphia PA. This includes pieces by figures mentioned in these pages such as Joel Elkes, Pierre Deniker, Nate Kline, Roland Kuhn, John Cade, Paul Janssen, Frank Berger, Joel Elkes and Roland Kuhn, among others.

Other accounts can be found in

- Shepherd M (1982). *Psychiatrists on Psychiatry*. Cambridge University Press, Cambridge. This includes pieces by Pierre Pichot, Seymour Kety and Eric Strömgren.
- *The Neurosciences. Paths of Discovery*, Vol 1, ed Worden FG, Swazey JP, Adelman G, Birkhauser, Boston
- *The Neurosciences. Paths of Discovery*, Vol 2, ed Samson FE, Adelman G, Birkhauser, Boston

Neuropsychopharmacology
- Ayd FJ (1991). The early history of modern psychopharmacology, **5**, 71–84.
- Lehmann H (1993). Before they called it psychopharmacology, **8**, 291–303. *Journal of Psychopharmacology*, especially vol **4** issue 4.

- Richter D, Healy D (1995). The origins of mental health related neuro-science in Britain. *Human Psychopharmacology*, **9**, 392–397.

There are a number of excellent histories of psychiatry which cover the emergence of the field and the shifting relations between biological, social and psychological camps and the differing views on nosology (the science of what constitutes a disease), and psychopathology (the science of what mechanisms are disturbed to produce the manifest features of mental disturbance). These include

- Berrios GE, Porter R (1995). *A History of Clinical Psychiatry*. Athlone Press, London.
- Pichot P (1983). *A History of Psychiatry*, Editions Roger Da Costa, Paris.
- Shorter E (1996). *A History of Psychiatry. From the Era of the Asylum to the Age of Prozac*. J Wiley & Sons, New York.

In the field of the history of psychopharmacology see:

- Swazey J (1974). *Chlorpromazine*. MIT Press, Boston.
- Johnson FN (1982). *A History of Lithium Therapy*. Macmillan Press, Basingstoke.
- Pernick MS (1985). *A Calculus of Suffering. Pain, Professionalism and Anesthesia in Nineteenth Century America*. Columbia University Press, New York.
- Valenstein ES (1986). *Great and Desperate Cures. The Rise and Decline of Psychosurgery and other Radical Treatments for Mental Illness*. Basic Books, New York.
- Healy D (1987). The structure of psychopharmacological revolutions. *Psychiatric Developments*, **5**, 349–376.
- Healy D (1990). The psychopharmacological era: notes towards a history. *Journal of Psychopharmacology*, **4**, 152–167.
- Smith MC (1991). *A Social History of the Minor Tranquillizers*. Haworth Press, New York.
- Kramer PD (1993). *Listening to Prozac. A psychiatrist explores antidepressant drugs and the remaking of the self.* Viking.
- Olie JP, Ginestel D, Jolles G, Lôo H (1992). *Histoire d'une Découverte en Psychiatrie*, Doins Éditeurs, Paris.
- Healy D (1997). *The Antidepressant Era*. Harvard University Press.
- Wyden P (1997). *Conquering Schizophrenia*. Alfred A Knopf.

The following accounts contain some assessment of the issues facing the pharmaceutical industry:

- Lazell HG (1975). *From Pills to Penicillin. The Beecham Story*. Heinemann London.
- Tausk M (1984). *Organon. The Story of an Unusual Pharmaceutical Enterprise*. Akzo Pharma BV, Netherlands.
- Braithwaite J (1984). *Corporate Crime in the Pharmaceutical Industry*. Routledge & Kegan Paul, London.

- Liebenau J (1987). *Medical Science and Medical Industry. The Formation of the American Pharmaceutical Industry*. Macmillan Press, Basingstoke.
- Swann JP (1988). *Academic Scientists and the Pharmaceutical Industry*. Johns Hopkins University Press, Baltimore.
- Baulieu E-E (1991). *The Abortion Pill*. Simon & Schuster, New York.
- Breggin P (1991). *Toxic Psychiatry*. St Martin's Press, New York.
- Lynn M (1991). *The Billion Dollar Battle. Merck versus Glaxo*. Heinemann, London.
- Mann CC, Plummer ML (1991). *The Aspirin Wars. Money, Medicine and 100 Years of Rampant Competition*. Alfred A Knopf, New York.
- Djerassi C (1992). *The Pill, Pygmy Chimps and Degas' Horse*. Basic Books, New York.
- Healy D, Doogan DP (eds) (1996). *Psychotropic Drug Development. Social, Economic and Pharmacological Aspects*. Chapman & Hall, London.
- Galambos L, Sewell JE (1996). *Networks of Innovation*. Cambridge University Press, Cambridge.
- Cornwell J (1996). *The Power to Harm. Mind, Medicine and Murder on Trial*, Viking Press, London.

Dramatis personae

Thérèse Lempérière (Paris)
Thérèse Lempérière began training psychiatry in Paris in 1949 in the department of Jean Delay before the discovery of chlorpromazine. She trained and researched during the period when chlorpromazine, prochlorperazine, haloperidol and other early neuroleptics were discovered and developed and psychopharmacotherapy took shape. She was also involved in the discovery of the anti-obsessive compulsive action of clomipramine. She later became Professor of Psychiatry in Paris and since retirement has been involved in the development of psychiatric services in Vietnam.

Len Cook (Delaware)
Len Cook did a PhD in pharmacology in Yale, graduating through a programme aimed specifically at training scientists for drug development. He subsequently joined SmithKline & French and did the early laboratory experiments on chlorpromazine that persuaded the company to launch it as Thorazine. He established a series of tests which discriminated between the effects of chlorpromazine and other antipsychotics from those of librium, minor tranquillisers and associated agents and did early work on the effects of psychotropic agents on conditioned responses, drug discrimination and drug self-administration, many of the implications of which have not been followed up in clinical practice. He subsequently worked with Roche and Du Pont, became a president of the American College of Neuropsychopharmacology and now with colleagues has his own drug development company.

Paul Janssen (Beerse)
Paul Janssen established his own pharmaceutical research company in Belgium in the early 1950s. Among the early compounds they created was haloperidol, which became the most widely used antipsychotic in the world. He charts the discovery of haloperidol, its trials and subsequent rise to a position of pre-eminence and work that has been done since on agents such as pipamperone and risperidone, as well as the changing face of drug development. He has been a recipient of many prizes and honours for his role in psychotropic drug development and in shaping psychopharmacology, as well as research on the development of a range of other compounds from analgesics and anaesthetics to antifungals.

Joseph Brady (Baltimore)

Joe Brady qualified as an experimental psychologist in Chicago in the late 1940s. He subsequently moved to the Walter Reed Hospital, where along with Murray Sidman he established a famous behavioural pharmacology laboratory. His early work led to the discovery of the Conditioned Emotional Response, an animal paradigm sensitive to the effects of ECT and subsequently reserpine. This led to further work on the effects of psychotropic drugs on behaviour and an involvement in harnessing the processes of psychotropic drug development to the study of behaviour. He outlines the contributions behavioural pharmacology has made and continues to make to psychiatry in general and to the psychiatry of substance abuse in particular.

Roland Kuhn (Münsterlingen)

Roland Kuhn was born in Switzerland in 1912. He trained in psychiatry before the Second World War with Jacob Klaesi and Ludwig Binswanger in a golden age in Swiss psychiatry. He moved to practise in Münsterlingen Hospital, where in the mid-1950s he was involved in the discovery of imipramine (Tofranil) and subsequently in the development of maprotiline and other antidepressants, agents which have done much to shape modern psychopharmacology. He is an outspoken critic of modern methods of evaluating psychotropic drug effects.

Max Lurie (Cincinnati)

Max Lurie trained in psychiatry in Cincinnati, Chicago and Iowa and subsequently entered private practice in Cincinnati with his father, also a psychiatrist, in the years immediately after the Second World War. Along with Harry Salzer he investigated the effects of isoniazid in depressed patients before the formal discovery of antidepressants. Their work constitutes an unrecognised breakthrough in psychopharmacotherapy, the implications of which have still not been fully explored.

Louis Lasagna (Boston)

Louis Lasagna trained in medicine and pharmacology and subsequently helped establish the discipline of clinical pharmacology. He is commonly referred to as the father of American Clinical Pharmacology. He trained with Harry Beecher in Harvard in Massachusetts General Hospital at a time when the placebo, randomised control trials and the other techniques for evaluation of drug efficacy were being worked out. His work on evaluating the effects of analgesics paved the way for application of similar methods in psychopharmacology. He had a considerable role in shaping the 1962 FDA amendments on the question of evaluation. He has subsequently been President of the American College of Neuropsychopharmacology, Professor of Pharmacology at Johns Hopkins University and more recently Dean at Tuft's University in Boston.

Linford Rees (London)

Linford Rees began training in psychiatry in Cardiff in the mid-1930s. He subsequently moved to the Maudsley Hospital and began a career in research which led to his active involvement in the evaluation of early biological treatments in psychiatry from electronarcosis through to insulin coma, cortisone and chlorpromazine, conducting in the process some of the first controlled trials in psychiatry. He was a founder member of the CINP and subsequently became a president of the Royal College of Psychiatrists and of the British Medical Association as well as Professor of Psychiatry at St Bartholomew's Hospital in London.

Joel Elkes (Florida)

Joel Elkes was born in Lithuania, trained in medicine in London and then established the first Department of Experimental Psychiatry in Birmingham in the early 1950s – significantly before the discovery of chlorpromazine. There he and his wife Charmian conducted one of the first randomised control trials in psychiatry and he and Philip Bradley outlined the first systematic vision of brain functioning in terms of neurotransmitters and receptors. He subsequently moved to the NIMH at St Elizabeth's Hospital in Washington before becoming Professor of Psychiatry at Johns Hopkins University. In both cases, he established departments that recruited and trained many of the subsequent leading figures in the field of psychopharmacology. He was a founder member of the International Brain Research Organisation, International Society of Neurochemistry and a founder member and first President of the American College of Neuropsychopharmacology.

Leo Hollister (Houston)

Working from a background in general medicine in Veteran Administration Hospitals, Leo Hollister ran some of the first controlled trials in psychiatry on reserpine and subsequently chlorpromazine. He established a career as a clinical trialist along with John Overall, the creator of the BPRS. His studies involved large multi-centre trials looking at the effects of a variety of neuroleptics and antidepressants. He was the first to describe withdrawal syndromes to both benzodiazepines and antipsychotics. He later went on to investigate the psychotomimetic effects of a variety of hallucinogenic drugs and has been a leading figure in the field of substance abuse. He became a President of both CINP and ACNP and remains active in the field.

Michael Shepherd (London)

Michael Shepherd trained in the Maudsley Hospital in London from where he organised one of the first randomised control trials in psychiatry looking at the effects of reserpine in depression. He became a founder member of the CINP and Professor of Psychiatric Epidemiology at the Institute of Psychiatry from where he ran the MRC multi-centre comparative trial of antidepressants which reported in 1965. His role in establishing the methodology of systematic evaluation of therapies has been critical to the development of the field. Of equal importance was his role in the development of psychiatric epidemiology, which led to the recognition of depression in primary care. In more recent years he has been critical of an increasingly exclusive focus on specificity in psychopharmacotherapy and of 'Kraepelinism'. He died in August 1995.

Mogens Schou (Aarhus)

Mogens Schou trained in psychiatry and research in Denmark, New York and Norway before moving to Aarhus to work with Eric Strömgren where he subsequently became a Professor of Biological Psychiatry. Early in his career he ran a randomised control trial of lithium in mania demonstrating its efficacy for that condition. Along with Poul Baastrup he outlined the prophylactic effects of lithium in recurrent affective disorders. His career has been closely associated with the development of lithium therapy and the methodologies for evaluating its usefulness, for which he has won numerous prizes including the Anna Monika and Lasker prizes.

George Simpson (Los Angeles)

George Simpson trained in psychiatry in McGill University with Ewen Cameron and subsequently in New York with Nathan Kline, where he participated in the development of psychobiological research at Rockland State Hospital and witnessed the controversies surrounding the discovery of the psychotropic effects of iproniazid. He developed the first instrument for measuring extrapyramidal side-effects of neuroleptic therapy. He has actively promoted the need for controlled assessment of both antidepressant and neuroleptic treatments. He has been President of both ACNP and the American Society for Clinical Psychopharmacology.

Gerald Curzon (London)

Gerald Curzon trained as a biochemist in Leeds before moving to the Institute of Neurology in London in the 1950s, where he has worked on the role of the serotonergic (5HT) system in psychiatric disorders and neurophysiological functions, such as feeding. His career illustrates how the individual brain disciplines came together in neuroscience and psychopharmacology. He is the archivist for the International Society of Neurochemistry and has latterly developed an interest in applying quantitative methods to research on the history of psychopharmacology.

Leslie Iversen (Oxford)

Leslie Iversen trained at Cambridge, the NIH and Harvard before taking up a position in the Medical Research Council Pharmacology Laboratories in Cambridge. He did significant work on reuptake mechanisms, the neurophysiology of GABA and excitatory neuropeptides and the role of the dopamine system in schizophrenia before becoming the Research Director of Merck, Sharp & Dome's United Kingdom CNS research facility at Harlow, where he spent 10 years in the development of neuroprotective and other psychotropic agents, in particular modulators of neuropeptide systems, such as the Substance P and cholecystokinin systems, before returning to a post as Professor of Pharmacology in Oxford.

Jeff Watkins (Bristol)

After graduating in chemistry from Perth, a PhD in Cambridge and post-doctoral research in Yale, Jeff Watkins returned to Australia to Canberra to work in the laboratory of the Nobellist John Eccles where, along with David Curtis, within weeks he discovered the potential neurotransmitter properties of glutamate. It took, however, 20 years before this early work on glutamate won some acceptance and a futher decade before it began to move into the mainstream. In the process, the NMDA receptor was discovered and the action of diverse groups of drugs on this system, offering the possibility of interventions that might be of benefit in neurodegenerative and a range of psychiatric conditions and treatment approaches that might target synaptic plasticity.

Irving Gottesman (Virginia)

Irv Gottesman trained in psychology on the Genetics of Behaviour in the University of Minnesota with Paul Meehl, Sheldon Reed, Starke Hathaway and others in the 1950s. He moved from there to Harvard and subsequently spent time in psychiatric genetic research with Eliot Slater at the Institute of Psychiatry in London in the mid-1960s. His early twin studies done with Slater and James Shields were seminal in re-establishing the field of psychiatric genetics after the Second World War. This and subsequent studies done at the University of Minnesota and at Washington University have shaped the further development of the field. He has made a distinguished contribution to the Danish Genetic and High Risk Studies and subsequently as a consultant to Congress and other bodies on genetic research in mental illness and behaviour.

Juan Lopez-Ibor (Madrid)

Juan Lopez-Ibor is from a distinguished Spanish family who have had numerous members play a leading role in both medicine and psychiatry in Spain. Early in his career he was involved in detecting the anti-obsessive effects of chlorimipramine. This led to an interest in notions of impulsivity in general and personality disorders in particular and the role that 5HT might play in such disorders. Exploring these issues has involved studies in gamblers and bullfighters. He participated in the Cross-National Collaborative Studies on panic disorder. He has had considerable involvement with ECNP, AEP and is now the President Elect for the World Psychiatric Association.

Oakley Ray (Nashville)

Oakley Ray trained in clinical psychology in the late 1950s before moving into experimental psychology in the Veterans Administration System in Pittsburgh. He later moved to the Veterans Administration at Nashville and Vanderbilt University as Professor of Psychology, Pharmacology and Psychiatry and became Chief of the Mental Health Service at a time when psychiatry in Nashville withdrew from service delivery. His experimental interests lie in the field of psychoneuroimmunology and his book *Drugs, Society and Human Behaviour* is a best-seller. He became the Secretary of the American College of Neuropsychopharmacology and has steered it through a successful growth period. He has most recently drawn ACNP attention to the need for an involvement in the history of psychopharmacology.

David Wheatley (London)

David Wheatley began as a general practitioner in London in the 1950s where he formed a general practitioner research group. This led to links with the Psychopharmacology Service Centre and subsequently ACNP. He was a prime mover in the establishment of the British Association for Psychopharmacology in 1974 – a foundation that crystallised many of the tensions of the field and had to involve their resolution. His career spans the development of trials from single investigator experiments to multi-centred, multinational trials on conditions ranging from stress, through depression to Alzheimer's.

Ian Stolerman (London)

Ian Stolerman trained in psychology and pharmacology at the University of London with Hannah Steinberg. This led to an early interest in the phenomena of drug discrimination, drug self-administration and drug combinations. He later worked with Murray Jarvik in New York on the effects of nicotine on learning and memory. He returned to work in the MRC Unit in Birmingham with Philip Bradley and others where he was involved in the foundation of the British Association for Psychopharmacology. He subsequently moved to the Institute of Psychiatry, where his work on substance dependence and drug discrimination has been influential. From there he was a co-founder of the European Behavioural Pharmacology Society.

Per Bech (Riskov)

Per Bech began psychiatric training and research with Ole Rafaelsen in Copenhagen. His early research involved measurement in psychopathology and the development of influential rating scales for both depression and mania. He has subsequently developed a range of instruments for the measurement of aggression, social dysfunction and quality of life. He participated in the Cross-National Collaborative Studies on panic disorder. He stimulated the foundation of the European College of Neuropsychopharmacology and has developed a programme of European Consensus Conferences on Clinical Trial

Methodology. He has also been President of the Association for European Psychiatrists.

Myrna Weissman (New York)

Myrna Weissman came to psychopharmacology from a background in social work. With Gerald Klerman and Gene Paykel, she was involved in influential studies in Yale in the late 1960s and early 1970s that led to the creation of inter-personal therapy and the development of instruments to measure social functioning in depression. She participated with Gerald Klerman in the Cross-National Collaborative Studies on panic disorder and used both these and the Epidemiological Catchment Area Studies to establish psychiatric epidemiology. She married Gerald Klerman and gives an insight into his role in the development of modern diagnostic systems, modern evaluative methods and the Osheroff case.

Isaac Marks (London)

Isaac Marks is one of the foremost behaviour therapists in the world. He is closely associated with the development of exposure therapy and an advocate of its use for phobic and obsessive disorders. This led to his involvement in a series of influential studies in the 1970s and 1980s comparing behaviour therapy and pharmacotherapeutic methods for Obsessive Compulsive Disorder and subsequently Panic Disorder. These studies and the issues they raise are landmarks in the field.

Vagn Pedersen and Klaus Bøgesø (Copenhagen)

Vagn Pedersen and Klaus Bøgesø joined the Lundbeck pharmaceutical company in the late 1960s and early 1970s respectively. Vagn Pedersen has been involved in market development and Klaus Bøgesø in medicinal chemistry. They give a perspective of the origins of the Lundbeck company, the role of PV Pedersen in establishing CNS research in the company with antipsychotics like chlorprothixene and flupenthixol and antidepressants like amitriptyline and nortriptyline. They outline the evolution of depot and acuphase forms of neuroleptic medication as well as the development of Cipramil and Sertindole, the recent specialisation of the company in CNS research and development and the turn to combinatorial chemistry in drug development programmes.

Roger Pinder (Oss)

Roger Pinder trained in medicinal chemistry with the famous Alfred Burger in the University of Virginia. He subsequently worked at the UK Chemical Defence Establishment in Porton Down on hallucinogens before moving to Holland as Scientific Director for CNS Drugs at Organon Pharmaceuticals. There he participated in the development of both mianserin and mirtazapine and was centrally involved from Organon's side in managing the regulatory difficulties that befell both mianserin in the 1980s and the third generation oral contraceptives since – difficulties which illustrate the nature of risk–benefit assessments in pharmaceutical developments.

Paul Leber (Washington)

After training in medicine and pathology in New York and Boston, Paul Leber subsequently changed career and entered psychiatry at a time of upheaval in the United States when the new classificatory system – DSM III – was being developed. He joined the Food and Drug Administration, where he subsequently became head of the CNS section. While there, he was responsible for a renewed emphasis on the importance of a placebo arm in clinical trials, a change of emphasis that had a major impact on drug development programmes. He outlines the realisation of the importance of this as well as the impact of AIDS on the approval process.

Chronology of interviews

Linford Rees – January '94 London
David Wheatley – January '94 London
Michael Shepherd – June '95 London
Isaac Marks – January '96 London
Paul Janssen – March '96 Beerse
Louis Lasagna – May '96 Boston
George Simpson – May '96 New York
Leo Hollister – June '96 Melbourne
Gerald Curzon – July '96 London
Ian Stolerman – July '96 London
Per Bech – July '96 London
Joel Elkes – July '96 Leicester
Roland Kuhn – September '96 Münsterlingen
Juan J Lopez-Ibor – September '96 Amsterdam
Roger Pinder – September '96 Amsterdam
Leslie Iversen – October '96 Oxford
Vagn Pedersen/Klaus Bøgesø – November '96 Copenhagen
Mogens Schou – November '96 Aarhus
Oakley Ray – December '96 Puerto Rico
Len Cook – December '96 Puerto Rico
Joseph Brady – December '96 Puerto Rico
Myrna Weissman – December '96 Puerto Rico
Irving Gottesman – January '97 Cardiff
Paul Leber – January '97 London
Jeff Watkins – March '97 Bristol
Thérèse Lempérière – March '97 Paris
Max Lurie – May '97 Cincinnati

1 Thérèse Lempérière

In the beginning in Paris

When did you join the Department of Psychiatry in Paris?

I began in Sainte Anne in the service of Professor Delay in 1950 as an intern – a resident. It was my first job in psychiatry. I stayed there for a year and after that I went to the Salpêtrière to finish my training in neurology with Alajouanine and Garcin and in child neuropsychiatry with Michaux. During this year in Sainte Anne I had the chance to get to know psychiatry before the arrival of the neuroleptics. At that time we were giving a lot of electroshock and the Insulin Coma treatment of Sakel but if all of that failed one felt very helpless.

Were you with the university department or were you in the hospital?

I was in the service of Professor Delay, which was the only university service of psychiatry in the hospital. I was working with Deniker, who at that time was a young assistant.

How many patients were there in the hospital at the time?

In the service of Professor Delay there were approximately 200 patients. Altogether in Sainte Anne there were approximately 1000 patients. The services were overcrowded and living conditions were very mediocre. The medical heads of departments were competent practitioners but they were working in very difficult conditions with few collaborators. Sainte Anne was the only psychiatric hospital within the boundaries of Paris.

How many patients did you have to look after?

Approximately 50 but this was under the supervision of Deniker. In Delay's service, which was a university service, the number of medical people was much greater than in other services.

There was also Dr Harl. His name is on the first papers about chlorpromazine.

Jean Marie Harl was one of my friends. We had met first in the Faculty of Medicine. He succeeded me as a resident in the service of Delay and it was he who made the first clinical studies of chlorpromazine with Deniker. He was a good clinician and he had an excellent rapport with patients. When his residence came to an end he did not continue with a hospital career. He turned instead to private practice in psychiatry where he was very successful. However, he died young in a climbing accident in the Alps.

When did you become aware of chlorpromazine, because you weren't actually there when they began to give it?

I remained in contact with the service of Professor Delay and I was aware of the studies with chlorpromazine. We were very quickly able to use the product and I can recall that we had already used it during the summer of 1952 when I was the resident in the Salpêtrière in child psychiatry. That service had access to a number of beds for adult patients and the Chief of service, Michaux, was very interested in this new medicine. Very quickly therefore we were able to establish for ourselves the activity of the product for patients with schizophrenia or mania. I can recall that we used to dread phlebitis. There were a number of cases partly perhaps because it was the practice to let patients remain in bed because of hypotension.

When I returned to Sainte Anne in 1953 to Professor Delay's service, Largactil was clearly already in widespread use. Very shortly afterwards reserpine came and we were able to make a comparison between the two medicines. I remained there in that service initially as an assistant and then later as Associate Professor until 1970. Then I left to become head of the university service in a new hospital in the suburbs of Paris: the Hospital Louis Mourier at Colombes. During all this period I participated personally in trials with a number of psychotropic drugs.

Pierre Deniker when he talks about the discovery said that for a while, during 1952 at least, people were not very interested.

In the milieu in which I was, at the Salpêtrière, interest was immediate but this was a university setting. It is true that in general psychiatric settings the first publications on chlorpromazine did not generate a great interest. There was scepticism and a certain reluctance to admit that chlorpromazine was not a simple sedative like chloral or the barbiturates. You must remember that at this time we used to do a great number of sleep cures for the most agitated patients. Delay and Deniker had difficulty in persuading people that chlorpromazine had some antipsychotic specificity. As so often when a new innovation comes along, it was the younger psychiatrists who most quickly appreciated the importance of the new treatment. In many cases it was the residents who introduced chlorpromazine into the services where they worked.

The introduction of the neuroleptics transformed the atmosphere in clinical practice, it greatly reduced the states of agitation, it reduced the number of days that people remained in hospital; these are all things, however, on which I don't need to insist. Psychiatrists generally received it as a major step forward in practice but it didn't lead to a complete change in their way of thinking. They already had the idea that disorders such as schizophrenia or mania had a neurobiological substrate – at that time one didn't talk about brain biochemistry and the fact, therefore, that an antipsychotic treatment had been discovered did-n't come as a huge shock, in contrast to the situation when the effectiveness of the first antidepressants was established – then many psychiatrists were greatly troubled because this did challenge their ideas about what depression was.

I can see what you are saying, but even in the case of people who are depressed there was the example of electroshock treatment which was working and Jean Delay had tried dini-triles and also isoniazid, so obviously he thought something could happen.

Jean Delay had already the idea that mood disorders whether mania or melan-cholia were influenced by a biological disorder. In his book which appeared in 1946 he had already laid out his views on the possible disorders of mood. He had worked a great deal on the biology of electroshock and he was interested, without having any preconceived views, in all agents which were capable of modifying mood.

The majority of French psychiatrists, however, were not particularly inter-ested in biological psychiatry. The dominant trains of thought at the time were psychoanalysis and social psychiatry. Even though they were prepared to admit that electroshock was efficacious in melancholia, many psychiatrists thought that the majority of depressions were neurotic or reactive and were caused either by unconscious conflicts or unfavourable living conditions. They had great difficulty admitting that imipramine could work as well for these kinds of depressions.

Also you must remember that psychiatrists at this time who thought that there might be a biological disorder in depression thought that this would be an endocrine disorder. They suspected that at some point someone would dis-cover an effective hormonal treatment.

Was Jean Delay closely involved with the work? For instance, if we look at the first sympo-sium on haloperidol at which your work was presented, the presidence d'honneur was Divry but he was not involved with any of this work at all – even though his name was on a num-ber of early articles. Was Delay more than a presidence d'honneur in the department?

Jean Delay had great intellectual breadth and he was a very creative spirit. In addition his medical training, and you have to remember he was a professor of medicine before he became a professor of psychiatry, and also his psychologi-cal training, where he was a doctor of philosophy, gave him openings to many different domains of thought. He immediately understood the interest in chlorpromazine and followed this up quickly with other studies undertaken in his service. He was not a hands-on person in the sense that he did not spend time every day at the bedside of the patient but he did make a point of seeing the difficult cases. He was also tremendously stimulating for his co-workers and he clearly indicated to them the direction in which research should go.

In addition to his interests in psychopathology, Jean Delay was also con-cerned about what the advances in psychopharmacology might teach us about the workings of the mind and also about mental illness. As he had done with electroshock, for instance, he used the antidepressants to analyse depressive syndromes. His classification of psychotropic drugs reflects well his psychopathological orientation, which was one that had been inspired by Janet.

How do you weigh the respective contributions of Jean Delay and Pierre Deniker?

Deniker was very involved in both clinical research and in the care of patients. He personally saw many patients and supervised very closely the work of the residents. If we take the case of chlorpromazine he was the one who supervised the clinical trials from day to day. Delay, looking at the developments from a greater distance, immediately understood the importance of the results. He became very quickly convinced, as did Deniker, that this was a product with original properties and that we should pay great attention to it.

Did you know Laborit?

Not very well – it was Deniker and Delay who principally knew him. I met him a few times at meetings, for example at the international congress on chlorpromazine which was held in 1955. This was the first time that I met him.

What did you make of all the fuss about the discovery of chlorpromazine?

I think that Laborit had a very good feeling for the potential interest for psychiatry that chlorpromazine offered. He himself, however, was not a psychiatrist and had never tried the product out in a psychiatric patient. I think that the clinical studies that Delay and Deniker did really were the turning point because they immediately noted the antipsychotic activity and all that it was about this drug that made it original and distinctive compared with other sedatives and tranquillizing agents.

You also must not forget the researchers in Rhône-Poulenc Spécia who already had produced antihistamines before chlorpromazine. In the 10 years before the arrival of chlorpromazine there already had been clinical trials in psychiatry with a number of antihistamines. So this idea was in the air.

The 1955 congress – what can you tell me about the atmosphere of that meeting?

This was the first great international congress to be organised on the subject of psychiatric treatments and it came about because of the development of chemotherapy with chlorpromazine. At the meeting there was also talk about reserpine and sleep therapies. At the meeting the audience were mainly psychiatrists because at the time there were no psychopharmacologists. I can remember very well the atmosphere. I can remember my impressions at seeing people like W Mayer-Gross, Manfred Bleuler or HR Rümke. At that meeting I met for the first time Fritz Freyhan and Heinz Lehmann. The psychiatrists who had been invited to the meeting all had good experience with neuroleptics. Many of them had already treated hundreds of cases. The discussions therefore were very interesting and there was a certain consensus about the effects and side-effects of the neuroleptics. Mayer-Gross was already insisting at this time on the need to move beyond empirical studies to controlled studies.

When you came back from the Salpêtrière to Sainte Anne you got involved in a trial to compare chlorpromazine with reserpine. This came out in 1954 within weeks of Nathan Kline's study but your study is rarely mentioned in terms of the discovery of the psychotropic effects of reserpine. How did it compare to chlorpromazine?

Our publication dated effectively from July of 1954. It was the second in the world. We followed up the studies with reserpine during the succeeding years. The similarity of the antipsychotic effects and side-effects of both it and chlorpromazine led Delay and Deniker to their definitions of neuroleptics as a novel class of therapeutic agent. We considered at the time that the activity of reserpine was possibly superior to that of chlorpromazine for chronic schizophrenics.

Why did it fall out of use?

Well, there were difficult side-effects. It caused drooling, akathisia and cardiovascular difficulties. It was also dangerous to use with electroshock. Furthermore there was a risk of depression. The prescription of reserpine began to fall progressively following the appearance of other neuroleptics and in particular haloperidol.

Did you see people with schizophrenia become depressed when they took reserpine?

No, I don't remember seeing people with schizophrenia who were on reserpine become profoundly depressed – that is to say melancholic. A certain number of them were dysphoric. But I had occasion to treat a number of patients who had become depressed with reserpine for their hypertension.

When some of the early neuroleptics were used, in particular prochlorperazine, people began to describe some surprising – what we now know are extrapyramidal – syndromes.

It was the psychiatrists in Lyon, Broussolle and Dubor, who first drew our attention in August of 1956 to certain atypical psychomotor phenomena in patients taking prochlorperazine: a certain type of spasm, trismus and athetosis.

They described these things as somewhat hysterical manifestations, which seems surprising now.

Not quite. They talked about the hysterical effect of the medicines. In effect they were suggesting that the patients appeared particularly suggestible. They noted that they were able to suspend their crisis, at least partly, if it was asked of them. In the case of others, if a patient in a room had a crisis this appeared to be able to trigger off a crisis in another patient who was also taking prochlorperazine.

Was it akathisia they were describing?

No, these were dyskinetic crises. Akathisia had already been observed with chlorpromazine and in particular with reserpine. We had already in addition remarked on the oculogyric crises.

When were these syndromes first discussed?

It was quickly appreciated that these dyskinetic crises bore similarities to the excitomotor phenomena that were observed in post-encephalitic Parkinsonism. In those conditions also patients appeared to present a particular suggestibility. Furthermore the use of prochlorperazine raised some practical problems. It had been developed as an antiemetic agent because its neuroleptic properties appeared at least in the laboratories to be somewhat weaker – although this was not later borne out entirely. It had been prescribed for both children and pregnant women. The appearance of dyskinetic crises raised diagnostic questions because they did not immediately associate what was happening with the taking of the medication. With children the immediate thought was that they had an encephalitis, for instance. I can also tell you the story of what happened to a secretary of one of my former heads of department who was a neurologist and not a psychiatrist. The young woman who was pregnant was taking prochlorperazine for morning sickness. She presented with paroxysmal contractions and trismus. She was hospitalised immediately in the belief that she had tetanus. The problems, however, cleared up 24 hours after the medication was halted.

How troubled were you by these dyskinetic reactions? Did you think you could be doing a serious injury to the patients?

For patients in psychiatric hospitals this was not a serious problem; the psychiatrists and hospital attendants were well acquainted with dyskinetic crises and were able to reassure the patient. You could give an anti-Parkinsonian injection which would bring the problem to an end very quickly. The principal diagnostic problems occurred at home when a general doctor prescribed a neuroleptic as a tranquilliser or as an antiemetic agent without being fully aware of the possible side-effects.

Was it only later with drugs like haloperidol that these effects became more common?

With haloperidol and thioproperazine these effects were frequent but not more frequent than with prochlorperazine.

One of the reasons to come to interview you was because Paul Janssen has said when he got Jean Delay to use haloperidol that the person he used to contact to find out what was really going on was you. He did not ask Jean Delay or Pierre Pichot as he felt you were the person who really knew what was happening with the drugs.

At this time I was an assistant and was already well acquainted with the first neuroleptics and those that came after, such as levomepromazine, thioproperazine, acepromazine etc. This was in 1959. The experiments with haloperidol were interesting because it was a new family of neuroleptic drugs and we were interested to compare it with the phenothiazines and reserpine. I became very quickly aware that it was a neuroleptic that was extremely potent. Initially there were problems because one had to feel one's way to getting the right dose. There were Parkinsonian syndromes that appeared more quickly and were more severe than with chlorpromazine and we began to use more anti-Parkinsonian drugs. But once we had got through the difficulties at the start in trying to find the dose, the product appeared to us to be very easy to handle.

When you were doing the trial with the haloperidol, did you think that it was an improvement on chlorpromazine?

Yes indeed, it had a quicker onset of action and was more potent in acute psychoses. Clearly there was the question of the dosage but one had the impression that this was a neuroleptic which would in due course, in some areas at least, supplant chlorpromazine.

You described how the secretary of the neurologist you knew took prochlorperazine and had an extrapyramidal crisis. That kind of vignette brings home the reality of what was happening – that people were not expecting these things. Is there anything you can remember with haloperidol that brings home what was different about it? Are there any patients that you can see in your mind's eye who illustrate what haloperidol meant?

One of the things which took us by surprise was its rapidity of action, particularly on hallucinations. For example, I remember one female patient who had been chronically delirious and very hallucinated whose voices disappeared in a few days. She said to us that they had cut the telephone wires. She herself was very surprised at what had happened.

When you had patients who responded like this, did you go back to Pierre Pichot and Jean Delay and sit in their office and ask them to explain to you what was happening?

Yes indeed. We discussed all this frequently. In fact there had been a very famous psychiatrist during the period 1920 to 1930: De Clérambault. He had a view, a very mechanical view, about chronic hallucinatory delusional states and had proposed that their basis lay in certain small cerebral micro lesions – these provided a focus of irritation which gave rise to mental automatisms and hallucinations which were the building blocks of the delusional state. Along with Delay and Pichot we discussed the ideas of De Clérambault precisely because of this hallucinolytic effect of haloperidol and the implications of this for delusional states.

What answers did you come up with – that De Clérambault was right?

I think, given all that has been now uncovered about the biology, biochemistry and neuroanatomy of schizophrenia, that De Clérambault was on the right road. His ideas perhaps appear very simple to us now but in 60 years time I am quite sure that our ideas will appear equally simple.

Who did you discuss these issues with the most?

On the implications for psychopathology I discussed most with Delay and Pichot. We also had in Sainte Anne Thuillier and Nakajima and with them I discussed the questions of biochemistry and psychopharmacology. I also had a chance in the course of daily clinical work to discuss clinical problems with Deniker and with a number of other young psychiatrists such as Ropert and Ginestet.

Was there any feeling that haloperidol was Pichot's drug and he wanted it to do better than chlorpromazine because of a rivalry between himself and Deniker?

No. Pichot was objective and in our publications we only reported that which had been established. Thirty years on you can see that haloperidol is in widespread use. It has become the reference neuroleptic for many control trials. We did a great deal to explore the psychotropic properties of haloperidol, using in particular the rating scales of Wittenborn which enabled us to show that it did not have a particular action against the negative mood states that go with schizophrenia. Pichot was always very interested in both quantitative psychopathology and in psychometrics.

Did you meet Paul Janssen around the period 1959-60? What was he like at that time?

I can remember having already met him at several meetings. I got to know him better when we did our studies with haloperidol and then later with trifluperidol. He is a man with whom it was easy to get on, who was very down to earth and direct. He already had a reputation of a first class researcher. It was his laboratory which had also discovered Palfium. When he suggested to us a clinical trial with haloperidol we thought that since it was he who was proposing it and that he had already made a screening of the drug in his laboratory there was a good chance that this was an active drug.

There is a very French idea, and I don't know who is responsible for it, that the neuroleptics were not all the same that there were sedative neuroleptics and disinhibiting neuroleptics. Do you know who had this idea first?

I think that the first people to talk about a disinhibiting effect were Broussole and Dubor in their first communication on prochlorperazine in 1956. The first classification of neuroleptics was put forward by Lambert in 1960 and Revol. This was a linear classification in the sense that on the left were sedative agents and on the right incisive agents, that is to say antipsychotics.

As far as I can remember French psychiatrists have always had the idea that neuroleptics are not interchangeable. This was already the idea of Delay and Deniker, who put forward a series of increasingly complex classifications. The first one was in 1961. These typologies generally tried to establish a relationship between therapeutic effects and secondary neurovegetative or extrapyramidal effects.

The concept of a chlorpromazine equivalent which was put forward by Davis and Ban always seemed to us to reductionist and was never accepted in France. In the USA, psychiatrists had access to much fewer neuroleptics than we had in France. This may have played a part in leading to a divergence of opinion. The arrival of the benzamides, for example sulpiride, reinforced for us the idea that it was possible to have 'different' neuroleptics. I think the

Americans are now in the process of revising their position because of the atypical neuroleptics such as clozapine.

Do you think that sulpiride is different? Where did it begin to be used? Were you involved with any studies on it?

Sulpiride was marketed in France in 1969. I don't know who did the first clinical studies. It was a product which had a curious career. It had been widely used by general physicians for nervous problems of a functional nature. In psychiatry it did not take long to begin to mark out its distinctive properties. The patients themselves appreciated it a great deal because it was much less sedative than other neuroleptics and did not give them the same locked-in feeling. In an empirical fashion it became clear that it had a particularly interesting effect in schizophrenias with deficit states and this was confirmed during the 1980s by some well-focused studies. The fact that it was a disinhibiting antipsychotic with minimal extrapyramidal effects made it an atypical neuroleptic.

Outside of France everybody has heard of Jean Delay, Pierre Deniker and Pierre Pichot, but not Pierre Lambert. Why?

Pierre Lambert was head of department in the psychiatric hospital Bassens in Haute Savoie. He was not a professor and because of this he had much less influence with international audiences. His publications almost entirely appeared in French reviews and I think that this explains why his work is not known very widely outside of France. He was, however, an extremely good clinical observer with enormous experience in the use of psychotropic agents. He was also a psychoanalyst and he brought a psychodynamic dimension into his thinking about the action of these drugs.

One of the other Rhône-Poulenc compounds that Lambert worked on earlier was trimipramine (Surmontil).

Yes indeed. In France we have always had an interest in therapeutic cocktails whereas in England you are much more likely to use monotherapy. When we had imipramine, for instance, as an antidepressant it was common to use it in conjunction with a sedative neuroleptic such as levomepromazine, with results that appeared very satisfactory to us. From this came the idea of some of the researchers in the laboratories of Rhône-Poulenc Spécia that it would be a good idea to produce a drug, trimipramine, which would have in its molecule the nucleus of imipramine and the side chain of levomepromazine. The psychiatrists in the region of Lyon and in particular Lambert were the ones who made the first studies with this.

Lambert was also involved with sodium valproate?

In France, we have had two very similar products for a long time: the valproate of sodium (Depakine) and valpromide or dipropylacetamide (Depamide). Both of these were antiepileptic but valpromide was also used as a thymoregulator. In addition valpromide was a prodrug, of which 80% was transformed into valproic acid, and the properties both pharmacokinetic and psychotropic of these two products were somewhat different.

Lambert did studies with valpromide as an antiepileptic and observed that in addition to anticonvulsant effects this drug had a beneficial action on some of the character difficulties and mood problems of his epileptic patients. This gave him the idea to study valpromide in mood disorders without epileptic complications. His first publication dates from 1966 but there was an even more important one in 1968. Since then valpromide has been very widely used in France in association with neuroleptics or lithium during episodes of mania but also as a prophylactic treatment in bipolar mood disorders.

In the late 1950s and the early 1960s there was a real idea that drugs which were useful for epilepsy might be useful for psychological disorders too. The whole idea of the interface between epilepsy and psychoses was being explored. Does that seem right?

The idea of a relationship between epilepsy and psychosis is a very old one in both German and French psychopathology. It was drawn from clinical experience and had given rise to a great number of theoretical formulations. The shock therapies with cardiazol or electricity depended initially on the idea of an antagonism between chronic psychoses and epilepsy. In addition a number of people had proposed that there were resemblances between epileptic paroxysms and the paroxysms of acute psychoses and of mood disorders. I think Lambert initially began from clinical observations and knew of the beneficial action on mood of Depamide on epilepsy and went on from there to study this effect in manic depressive patients. I don't know if the Japanese psychiatrists, Takesaki and Okuma, who were the first to investigate the action of carbamazepine in mood disorders around 1970-72 had a theoretical presupposition. After all that then there was the work of Post and the North Americans who became interested in clonazepam and also in valproate.

Can I ask you about Anafranil? What did you think of it and when did you begin to use it first?

I did my first studies with Anafranil with Pichot and our first publication was made at the 4th World Congress of Psychiatry in Madrid in 1966. We had at this stage already treated 50 depressed patients and we had formed a very favourable impression of the product. We have used it a great deal since and our first positive impressions have been confirmed. I can remember advising Geigy to market it in France. I certainly had the impression that it was a good drug.

At the same Congress, Sigwald and Raymondeaud had made a communication on intravenous perfusions with clomipramine in 80 depressed people with good results. In France, the practice of intravenous perfusions with antidepressants was already current at that time. Delay and Deniker had already written an article about this matter in *Encéphale*.

What was it about the product that made you think it was a good one and can you remember anything about why you thought it was so good?

Well, our first work consisted of open studies. I think that the experience of clinicians is extremely important. We had already done studies with medications that had been presented as potential antidepressants but these were either ineffective or were very badly tolerated and were not developed. Furthermore we had had the experience in practice of using imipramine, the MAOIs, and amitriptyline. You could therefore make comparisons. The opinion of the patients was also very important. When you have a good product, patients are more likely to adhere to their prescriptions. When they leave hospital they came back for research to follow up whether they remained well or whether there had been a relapse. Anafranil was not marketed in France until 1967. I was quite sure, however, that it was a good drug.

Did you get the impression that Geigy weren't very interested in this drug?

They already had developed Tofranil. They had both Pertofran and Anafranil in clinical trials. They were not certain that they were going to develop all three. Finally Pertofran was marketed in 1966 and after that Anafranil in 1967.

You described antiobsessional effects of Anafranil but Guyotat from Lyon also did so. Did he talk about these effects first or were you talking about them first?

This is Jean Guyotat and his collaborators. Guyotat was professor of psychiatry at Lyon. In their publication which appeared at the 64th Congress of Psychiatry and Neurology in the French language, which was held in Dijon in July 1967, they insisted that Anafranil had an action in obsessional neurosis. They reported on 12 cases that had been treated, with 10 either good or very good results. They also noted that this effect did not wear off even though certain patients by then had been treated for over a year. They concluded that 'in obsessional neurosis, it is the medication that is most reliably active that we have yet seen on the most troublesome symptoms of this disorder'.

The use of Anafranil in obsessional neurosis spread rapidly in France. In a congress organised by Geigy in 1970 on 'Anafranil in conditions other than depression', which was held in Palma in Majorca, there were a number of communications in French on its use with obsessional patients from Michaux, Gallot, Scherrer and myself. In this period it seemed accepted that Anafranil was more effective than other antidepressants such as imipramine or iproniazid and that its effectiveness did not depend solely on its action on an associated depressive state, that the patients relapse frequently when treatment was halted but that the effects of treatment did not wear off in the long term. I myself had followed up patients for over five years then. When I retired in 1993 I was still looking after patients who have been on clomipramine during this whole period. It had enabled them to live in a reasonable way during almost 30 years. Before this they would have been seriously incapacitated. The appearance of evidence that clomipramine had an antiobsessional activity was very intriguing for the psychoanalysts and a great number of psychodynamic explanations were put forward to account for this. I must also say that during the same years a number of French colleagues were in the habit of treating obsessional neuroses with large doses of pericyazine (Neuleptil), a sedative neuroleptic which had been widely used to reduce the aggression and person-ality disordered manifestations. On the basis of this there were theories that this medicine might have a selective action on the 'sado-anale structure'. Neuleptil, however, did not have a very long career for this indication.

What can you tell me about Buisson and isoniazid?

Jean Francois Buisson was of my generation. We were residents together with Delay. Delay had the idea because of his awareness of the beneficial effects of isoniazid on the mood of patients with tuberculosis who had been treated with this medicine. He proposed to Buisson that he should do his thesis studying the effects of isoniazid on depressed patients. The results were interesting.

But the odd thing is why, with the results they had with isoniazid, did they not say – we have found an antidepressant?

Yes, you would have thought that they might have made more of this.

Why not? In 1952 they had shown it was good for people who were depressed but Pierre Deniker and Jean Delay all say that Roland Kuhn and Nathan Kline discovered the antidepressants six years later.

I think that the results they had were somewhat inconsistent. They were not decisive. It may not have been much superior to other drugs which they were using at the time in asthenic depressions such as the amphetamines. I believe that isoniazid is not a monoamine oxidase inhibitor and that in this sense it is different from iproniazid. Perhaps it is only a psycho-stimulant?

We have mentioned a few other people like Harl, Buisson. Can I ask you about Thuillier? My impression is that he was one of Jean Delay's most important protégés. Then he left. What kind of person was he?

He was a dynamic extroverted individual with whom I got on very well. He had trained both as a pharmacist and as a psychiatrist. He ran a number of studies with animals and worked a great deal with the first neuroleptics. He had lots of ideas but did not have the means to study them all in detail. The laboratory was not very well equipped. I think that he left the service because he didn't have the possibility of a further career in INSERM or at the university. After that he entered a pharmaceutical company laboratory. But at the same time he also did a lot of other things. He occupied himself with a portrait gallery. He also wrote books which had some success, among which was one about Charcot.

Who were the other important people in Sainte Anne, at the time?

With Delay there were a great number of other people who came from very different backgrounds. This was always fascinating. There was an active department of neuropathology under Brion which, during the 1960s, did important work on Pick's disease and Korsakoff's syndrome. These studies are classics. There was also a department of psychotherapy where a great number of reputable psychoanalysts worked. From 1953 through to 1963 Jacques Lacan used to come each week to give a seminar with the presentation of a patient from the service. Because of the reputation of Delay and Deniker following the discovery of chlorpromazine there was also a constant influx of foreign psychiatrists who came to train in psychopharmacology. Many of these eventually became eminent practitioners or academics in their own country.

There was also at that time in Sainte Anne many other psychiatrists who played an important role in the development of ideas and who influenced the younger generation. For instance, Georges Daumezon, who was a head of service in Sainte Anne, was a pioneer in the movement for the reform of psychiatric institutions. This was a very vigorous development in France immediately after the War, which was brought to completion with the progressive establishment of sectorisation. There was also Julian de Ajuriaguerra who, up until his departure to Geneva in 1959, conducted his reseach at the Henri Rousselle, an institution which was included within Sainte Anne. He influenced younger psychiatrists by his innovative teaching in the fields of neuropsychology and developmental psychology. Above all there was Henri Ey, who had a huge influence both nationally and internationally. He was the secretary general for the First World Congress of Psychiatry. He also directed his own society – L'Evolution Psychiatrique – which brought together a number of psychiatrists and psychoanalysts and faced them with issues on which there was a divergence of opinion. Henri Ey was the Head of Department of the hospital at Bonneval, 120 kilometres from Paris. He used to come every Wednesday to Sainte Anne to conduct a seminar. These seminars were very popular with younger psychiatrists. At these he developed his ideas on psychopathology and in particular his theory of 'organo-dynamism', which greatly influenced French psychiatric thinking in the years between 1950 and 1970. The library at Sainte Anne where he gave these seminars is now called the Henry Ey Library.

Was there any hostility to those of you who were working in psychopharmacology?

No, not during the first few years. The chemotherapy of mental patients became established progressively in the practice of psychiatry to some extent throughout all of France. There was no hostility at that point in time. Rather there was an interest although perhaps not a massive conversion to biological psychiatry. Psychoanalysis or social psychiatry remained the major attraction for most psychiatrists. The problems began with the anti-psychiatry movement which culminated in 1968 but it remained influential right through to 1975 and 1980. At that point in time there was rejection of all biological treatments and in particular both shock treatment and the neuroleptics and there were a great number of conflicts in clinical practice. I think this was even the case in Great Britain.

One of the things that must have begun to happen with the new medication was out-patient psychiatry?

In Sainte Anne and in particular with Delay there was already an important consultation service. With the arrival of chemotherapy, the levels of consultations went up enormously. It also became necessary to follow up those who were discharged from hospital and in addition we had to accept a huge influx of new patients who were sent by general physicians who had become aware that it was now possible to help people who were depressed.

When did you begin to realise that you were going to have to educate people, to train them to use these new treatments? Did you have to do much lecturing on how to use the treatments?

It was particularly in the case of depression that it was necessary to make an effort to educate general physicians. Training in psychiatry in the course of medicine at the time was very brief. It was necessary therefore to teach clinicians how to recognise and treat a case of depression. There was a great deal of postgraduate medical education needed. It seems to me that in Great Britain the education of general physicians in this area was better than in France at the time. Perhaps your National Health system was better prepared for this?

When did people begin to be aware that maybe the patient did not have to come into hospital at all? That they could be seen in the clinic, given a prescription and sent home?

I think that these things developed gradually and the demand grew among patients and general physicians following the introduction of the antidepressants. You must not forget that in France private psychiatry developed greatly in the years 1970 through 1980. At the same time there was also put in place a sectorised public psychiatry service with dispensaries which were located in the towns and not in the hospital. As a result, in France the number of psychiatrists is much greater than in Great Britain. In actual fact there are 11,000 of us, of whom more than half work in private practice.

What about the treatment of anxiety with drugs in France?

In France we consume a great number of both anxiolytics and sleeping tablets. In fact it is the country with the highest consumption of benzodiazepines in the world. Although there have been some restrictions on the prescriptions of benzodiazepines for the past few years following directives from the Department of Health, the consumption of these drugs remains at a very high level. We have frequently debated what the reasons for this might be. Generally it can be said that the French consume a great number of medications of any kind, including alcohol. Another point is that medications are not expensive. Finally there is not in public opinion any great campaign against the benzodiazepines. As with a great number of other countries, however, there has been for more than 10 years now an important increase in the prescription of antidepressants but this seems to me to be very reasonable. I think this corresponds to a better assessment of patients who are depressed, of whom a great number to date have not been diagnosed and accordingly not treated appropriately.

Select bibliography

Pichot P, *The Psychopharmacologists*, Vol 1.

2 Len Cook

Pharmacology, behaviour and chlorpromazine

How did you get started in the area?

I graduated from Rutgers in 1948, after being in the Air Force in the 1940s. I was a celestial navigator in the Air Force. After I was discharged from the Service, I went on to college. After I finished college I was wondering what to do next. I was married less than a year. My wife was working in a lab for a pharmacologist, Dr Molinas, while I went to college at night. Dr Molinas had a picnic at his house one day and while we were sitting under a tree, eating salad, he said 'What are you going to do?' I said 'I don't know, I've finished college, I'm not sure what I'm going to do. I'd love to go to grad school in some sort of science but I just don't know.' He said 'Have you ever heard of pharmacology?' I said 'I didn't want to work in a drugstore and make ice-cream sodas.' He said 'No no', and he explained to me what pharmacology really was. I said 'That sounds fascinating.' Would you believe that I had never heard of it before and here I was a college graduate. I said 'Where do I go for training?' and he indicated that one of the best training courses was in Yale. I said 'I'm not going to be able to go to Yale, a poor kid from the inner city' and he said 'Oh no, go and see so and so.' I went and was interviewed by the Chairman, Bill Salter, and by the end of the interview he said 'I'd love to have you here.'

So I went to Yale. They provided a fascinating opportunity for me as it turned out because, quite distinct from offering a conventional course in pharmacology, they were specially training pharmacologists to go into the pharmaceutical industry with specific training in drug discovery. It was the only department before or since, that I am aware of, training people for drug discovery rather than training in terms of certain scientific theories or specific interests. It was great and most of the 15 students who went there at the time became the leaders for drug discovery in the industry for the next 30 years – myself, Irv Tabachnick, Bill Grey and Bernie Rubin. We learned the strategy of drug discovery, which few people learn in more classical departments.

Even then, there was hostility to working in the pharmaceutical industry. At Yale, I was with a Professor Desmond Bonneycastle, a Canadian, an MD PhD. I worked with him on certain aspects of analgesic research for my doctorate thesis. Finally, because the department was set up to train people for the industry, I had six offers without having to leave New Haven. All of the companies knew about this programme and the pharmaceutical industry was getting rolling around then – 1950/1951. It was beginning to become a strong research and discovery business. But my professor thought it was wrong to go into industry when you could spend your career training others who could train others etc. At that stage I had a 4-month-old baby.

SmithKline came up to interview me and after that I received an offer from them. This was in 1951. They offered to pay me $6000 a year – at a time when my professor, Dr Bonneycastle, a full MD, PhD at Yale, was getting $5000. Naively, I said 'Professor Bonneycastle I received a job offer' and I showed him the letter, which as I reflect on it now was a stupid thing to do. He was a brilliant scientist but he had his own ideas about 'prostituting' oneself. I thought he was going to say 'Len I'm so happy for you.' He knew my wife, Rheva, worked upstairs in nutrition and that we had a baby but he was obviously very upset. Next morning he called me in and said 'You know Len, I've been thinking that you really should spend another year here for your own good.' I said 'But Dr Bonneycastle my thesis is just about ready, I've had my primary defence, I've accepted the job, I have a little baby. What do you mean another year? I've not only done every single thing in my proposal but I've done more. Nobody else around here in recent years has ever come close to doing more than 50% of what was in their proposal.' He said 'Well this is for your own good.' I looked at him. Maybe two years in the Air Force helped but I said 'Dr Bonneycastle, if you do this to me, I'm going to see the Dean of the grad school and have a hearing on this thing.' He said 'Okay if you want to be a whore, if you want to prostitute yourself, go ahead.'

I still had the final defence of my thesis ahead. I went down the hall to a friend of mine, Professor Nick Giarman, who was the 'defender' of grad students, and said 'Nick, I'm in trouble' and I told him what had happened. He said 'Don't worry, I'll be there at the defence.' Everything turned out okay even though my own professor let me swing in the wind. Interestingly, I then had another letter from SmithKline saying that my salary was no longer $6000; owing to adjustments it was $6350, a $350 raise without even starting, which I went and showed to Professor Bonneycastle. Subsequently, every time he would see me in Atlantic City at the annual pharmacology meetings, he would say 'Hi moneybags, how are you doing?' Ironically about 7 years later Kapp Clark, the vice-president at SmithKline, called me down and asked me if I knew a Dr Bonneycastle and said he had just applied for a job, even though as Kapp commented 'He doesn't seem to very friendly to the pharmaceutical industry even though he wants a job here.'

There was an enormous hostility among the academic community to young students going into the pharmaceutical industry. Do you know about KK Chen at Lilly? He was the one who brought over *Ma Huang*, ephedrine, and he was head of pharmacology at Lilly. He was thrown out of the Pharmacological Society because he worked in the drug industry. Ironically, he subsequently became president of the society years later. During that period of my career, for the first ten years or so, we were not considered very legitimate by many academicians, even though we were doing as good research as most people in university. I am very proud that I became a member of the Pharmacological Society after only 4 years out, and years later one of the proudest moments of my life was to become a fellow of ACNP. I'm the only person from industry to hold an office in ACNP, first vice-president and then later in 1982 I was voted in as president. This was so exciting – it was on a par with my son being born. That legitimised me in my own mind but it also was a recognition of what was happening in industry. In fact, even in ACNP there was some hostility to industry at the time. I also got the Paul Hoch award, which is one of the highest awards the ACNP hands out. Many people in industry told me that they considered that my experience in this society helped legitimise their own scientific role, which greatly pleased me.

Anyway, at SmithKline in Philadelphia, my first job, my initial research project was on gastrointestinal pharmacology. The head of research, Kapp Clark, later came to me and said 'Len what we would like to do right now is to get into a non-barbiturate sedative programme. The barbiturates have had a bad rap, they're not very safe and there is a real need out there for such sedatives.' Now at that time sedatives were the main CNS modulators – sleep-inducers such as barbiturates along with methylparaphenol and chloral hydrate. That was essentially it. What was available pharmacologically was not behavioural modification as much as behavioural knockout. I said 'That sounds good to me and very interesting but I wonder, how do you measure sedation in animals?'

At that time, if you gave the available CNS depressants or sedatives to animals you didn't see 'sedation'; they got excited and then they'd fall on their backs. You don't see in animals that sub-hypnotic sedative effect you see in humans. Essentially I set up a few laboratory tests. In college I took Psychology 101, which was a six-month course, and I remembered something about conditioned reflexes – Pavlov and all that. One of the things I set up therefore was a conditioned reflex test which ended up being a conditioned avoidance response. The animals were essentially trained to avoid auditory stimuli associated with aversive stimuli such as electric footshock. I tested many of the then available drugs on this approach.

I also had an apparatus to monitor and quantitate spontaneous exploratory motor activity. I did neurologic exams on mice and rats, such as placing reflexes, cross-extensor and other neurologic reflexes – this was something I had learnt at Yale. But when I tested all these compounds, nothing very useful came up, so when Kapp Clark said 'Len how're you doing on the non-sedative research programme?', I said 'Not very well. I think I've got effective test procedures but I don't have any compounds that work the way I project that they should.'

One of the tests people were using in 1951 to identify sedatives was to administer a low dose of a short-acting barbiturate, hexobarbital, and then combine it with the experimental compound. If, instead of sleeping for 20 minutes, the control condition, the mouse slept longer, this was used as an indirect way of measuring sedation. One day, my technician, a young man named Ed Weidley, said

'Gee, Len, the mice are still asleep. I gave them hexobarbital and instead of sleeping for twenty minutes they're still asleep and it's almost an hour.' I said 'They must be dead Ed'. I went over and sure enough the mice were still asleep. The next day I said 'Do it over again' and sure enough it was not only confirmed but there was a dose response to this phenomenon. They were sleeping longer than any single dose of a barbiturate could ever produce without killing them. Most importantly the drug itself was essentially pharmacologically inert – it produced no CNS effect. We subsequently found out that this compound, SKF 525A, interfered with the metabolism of the barbiturate and prolonged the plasma level and this was its mechanism of action.

That was a critical finding in the field of pharmacology. It opened up a new research programme. I went to the president, Mook Boyer – it was a small company at the time – and said that 'If we can get compounds that are innocuous in their own right but which prolong the effects of other drugs that might be a new research area – we could call it the 'drug potentiator' programme. He said 'Go ahead.'

About six months later, I heard about a compound from France, made by Rhône-Poulenc, which they were primarily testing for its enhancing or potentiating effects on other primarily CNS drugs – you may have heard about Laborit's lytic cocktail. I requested a sample and received a gram and tested it in my new 'drug protentiating' programme. Now, whereas my research compound SKF 525A prolonged sleeping time without any obvious overt pharmacology of its own, the French compound, RP4560, chlorpromazine, did the same but even on its own it also made the animals sluggish and heavily sedated. By this time the non-barbiturate sedative programme had significantly slowed down but I thought I'd test the French compound in the tests I had developed for that programme. So we gave it to animals in doses from 1 mg/kg and higher. They became progressively quieter until they became totally immobile. For the first time in pharmacological history they were not moving around although they remained upright on all four feet. I turned them on their side but they righted themselves. I pinched their tail and they pulled it away. I clapped my hands but they didn't move. I tested corneal, pinna and placing reflexes, everything I could. These animals were alert, their motor system was intact, but they were totally impassive to their environment. I had never seen a pharmacologically induced syndrome like this.

In order to chase the CNS profile of this compound further, I set up the conditioned avoidance apparatus again. With the barbiturates in this procedure, whenever I reached a dose where conditioned rats did not respond to the conditioned stimulus – a doorbell – which preceded an electric footshock, I also blocked their ability to escape the effect of a shock. In other words the rats didn't respond to the conditioned stimulus because they couldn't move. Their failure to respond was a physical incapacitation. When I gave RP4560 and rang the bell they also didn't move. Now these were animals who were well trained and when you rang that bell they normally jumped onto the pole immediately. But after treatment they didn't move, unless I subsequently gave them a footshock, which they did escape. Therefore they could still feel the shock and they could still move but they didn't seem to care about the warning – the conditional stimulus – that was my first interpretation. Six months of a psychology course and I didn't even know what words to use in defining this phenomenon.

After that I carried out a full dose–response curve in the conditioned avoidance procedure and in almost every other task I was trained to do in grad school. I reran the barbiturates and everything I had in the CNS armamentarium and what I found was, with most compounds, the dose that blocked the response to the conditioned stimulus also blocked the response to the shock, but with RP4560 you could totally block the response to the bell with no effect on the response to the shock. It was a unique effect. The question was, what was the significance of this effect? Did it have any therapeutic applications?

How big was the company at the time?

Well, I was the first PhD in pharmacology they had ever hired. They did have some technicians and other scientists and a modern laboratory facility. I used to have lunch with the president and director of research at the time. Over lunch one day I said 'This is really really strange, this new drug is making the animal totally impassive to the environment.' The research director said 'What good is that Len? Maybe if you give it to people, they might kill themselves. It may totally inhibit all life-preserving reflexes and warnings.' I pointed out that not all responses were obtunded – it was only an inhibition of responses associated with emotionality, at least that was my first interpretation of the effect.

You must remember that this compound, chlorpromazine, was originally made as an antihelminthic and it had already been touted to seven companies in the United States as an antihistamine. Quite appropriately they had turned it down – it was a strong sedative and everybody wanted an antihistamine that didn't have the strong 'Benadryl-type' sedation. This one certainly had no less. Mook Boyer, the SKF president, said 'These Rhône-Poulenc people were here about 6 months ago trying to sell this compound as an antihistamine.'

Was this before the psychiatric indications had begun to come out?

Rhône-Poulenc were pushing it as an antihistamine before Delay and Deniker had made their claims for its psychiatric utility. Mr Boyer asked me 'Len, on the basis of your findings what do you think?' I said 'I think this is a totally new aspect of pharmacology', so Mook Boyer said 'Let's call these guys from Rhône-Poulenc over and talk to them.' We contacted them and a month or two later they sent over a scientist named Pierre Koetschet, who was their research director. At this time they were still interested in it as a drug potentiator in lytic cocktails. I explained the work I had done on its effects on behaviour and he said 'There are two doctors called Delay and Deniker in Paris who have contacted us and said that they have found very significant effects on abnormal mental states' – we didn't have any better terms then. He went back to Paris and I was left thinking whether this correlated with my data on behaviour in animals. Again the president said 'What do you think Len?' and I said that it still seemed to me that this could be a whole new area of pharmacology. So we had the French back again and by this time Delay and Deniker had studied a few more patients and their effects and my work on conditioned avoidance and other tests seemed to fit ...

Rhône-Poulenc had also done some behavioural work in this area?

Yes, Mme Courvoisier had. I heard about her work after I had carried out mine. After M. Koetschet saw my work, he sent over the brochure of pharmacology but her behavioural work was not really conditioned avoidance behaviour. Her animals were trained to climb up a rope to get food so it was a different thing but it essentially fitted in with what I had seen, which was a decrease in the tendency to respond. She never did many more studies after that. We formed an SK&F/Rhône-Poulenc collaboration and I ended up going over to Paris a great deal – I was only 28 years old at this time.

The companies then signed a deal for chlorpromazine. The rest, as they say, is history. I started our research on Compazine and Stelazine right after that. Mook Boyer and Kapp Clark called me down to their offices one day soon after the deal had been signed and they said 'You know this looks like something interesting.' I said 'I'm glad you said that because from my limited experience I think we're into a whole new field. There's renal pharmacology, there's cardiovascular pharmacology etc. but I think we're into something totally new – I would call it psychopharmacology.'

Did you coin that word then?

As far as I know I did. I know I used it publicly at a seminar in Emory University in 1953 when I started to talk about some of the work.

You said Rhône-Poulenc pushed chlorpromazine first as an antihistamine and then you guys asked them back – did they do a further tour of US companies trying to sell it as an antipsychotic?

No. We at SK&F expressed a strong commitment to chlorpromazine and we were the only US company to get it. My research findings were then very influential with the SK& F people and also in Rhône-Poulenc regarding the use of the drug.

Paul Janssen also tells a story about you saying to SK&F that if chlorpromazine failed to work as an antipsychotic it would be good for nausea?

Well, one of the other things I did at that time was an anti-apomorphine vomiting test in dogs. We used dogs hanging in a sling from the ceiling and I had one technician, Ed Weidley, spending all day pushing the dogs back and forth until they vomited. I did all of the research with chlorpromazine initially with two technicians who were both high-school youngsters. One of the things we had noticed while doing the apomorphine-induced vomiting work was that you would go into the room with a laboratory tray to give the experienced dogs their apomorphine injection and they would vomit. We were using this as a screening test for antiemetic drugs, which one of the vice-presidents felt was a good market. Now one day one of the technicians said to me 'Len its so funny, I give the dogs an injection twice a week and after five or six injections, when I walk in with the tray they start vomiting even before they are injected. I rattle the tray and they start vomiting their heads off' – you see this in humans too, cancer patients for instance. So I said 'Why don't you give them chlorpromazine before you come into the room and see what happens' and he came back to me and said 'None of them are vomiting.' I said 'That's a conditioned reflex. Why don't you go further and give them the drug and see if it blocks the actual apomor-phine-induced vomiting' and he came back and said that none of them were vomiting. We made a new solution of apomorphine and repeated the studies and it really worked. We later did some work with the chemoreceptor trigger zone and the vomiting centre and it was clear that chlorpromazine didn't block drugs which had their effect on the vomiting centre. It specifically blocked agents which stimulated the chemoreceptor trigger zone.

I went to see the president and vice-president and told them about this and they said 'Len you know it looks like we're off and running.' We now had more and more information coming from Paris from Delay and Deniker. Laborit was still demonstrating chlorpromazine's effects in his lytic cocktails. I said to them 'I'd really love to give up the other pharmacology I'm doing, the GI pro-gramme etc. and get into this full-time.' They said 'OK, anything you want, we've got the money, you set up whatever you think you need. What do you need?' I said 'Can I go home and think about it?' They said 'Sure, we'll see you Friday.' I thought about it and I went in Friday and they were both there, very kindly guys who did everything so I wouldn't be intimidated. This was 1952 and I said 'Right now we can go into three things. What I'm doing is psycho-logical research' – I didn't use the word behaviour at the time, it was psychol-ogy as applied to pharmacology. 'Or there's a new field opening up called biochemistry.' They said what's that and I explained that its measuring epinephrine and other biochemicals in the brain. Also I'd been up to Harvard and MIT and spoken to a woman named Mary Brazier who was doing EEG – where I saw a room full of equipment for doing EEG analysis.[1] I had spent a week there learning about electrophysiological signals. When I was in Boston I also went and saw a person called BF Skinner who was doing some work with pigeons pecking and rats pressing levers. I learned something about operant psychology there. I also met Peter Dews and said that I was really interested in what they were doing and asked if they had anyone I could hire to do similar studies in my laboratory. That's where contact with Roger Kelleher came from. He had worked with Charlie Ferster in Florida at Yerkes' lab. I learned most of my behaviour from Kelleher. I later spent at least a month every year learning psychology in Wisconsin and other places looking at what people were doing in the line of experimental behaviour with monkeys and rats etc.

---

[1]See Lasagna L (1997). Back to the Future. *The Psychopharmacologists*, Vol II, p 139.

Anyway I said 'As far as I can see we can do these three things – behaviour, biochemistry and electrophysiology – and I think they are all going to become relevant. However, if I tested a drug – today it costs $100 million to put a drug on the market whereas then it ran about $2–3 million which was a lot of money – and I came to you and said I had biochemical, electrophysiological or behavioural data, which would you go with?' I said 'I'd go with the behaviour because we can see changes in something we want to change in people but we need to have some information on the other aspects as well.' They said 'Why don't you hire whoever you have to?' I already had working in my group a young man named Bob Shuster. Bob had both a BA and an MA I then hired Roger Kelleher from Ferster's department to run the behavioural studies. I hired Keith Killam, who had just got out of Chicago with his PhD, and he ran my neurophysiology lab. Harry Green ran the biochemistry. So essentially we had a little bit of all three areas. I used to go over to Rhône-Poulenc frequently and we had Laborit come to our laboratory to demonstrate the effects of chlorpromazine containing lytic cocktails.

Around 1953, as I understand, both Laborit and Pierre Deniker came to the US and at that time Laborit and his anaesthetic indications were still the front-runner at least in Rhône-Poulenc's eyes.

Laborit's interests were still the lytic cocktail, whose primary objective was to achieve a state of hypothermia for cardiac surgery that would let the surgeons go beyond 2–3 minutes, which was the limit at the time, to 15 minutes. This was a big deal then. I started to do similar hypothermia work in dogs and rats in which we would wrap them in ice-cubes and bring them down to body temperatures that were impossible to sustain without chlorpromazine. Chlorpromazine and Laborit's contribution was twofold here. You could take advantage of its drug potentiation properties so that you only had to use a little bit of each of the various drugs in the lytic cocktail but it also rendered the animal poikilothermic. Essentially they lost body temperature control and you could bring them up or down to body temperature levels you couldn't possibly achieve any other way.

We subsequently went to Maimonides Hospital in Brooklyn to talk to a surgeon, Dr Ribstein, who carried out the first clinical trial with chlorpromazine in the United States – for surgical hypothermia. I used to go up to see him because at that time the preclinical pharmacologist used to personally deal with the clinician – we don't have this interaction very much today but it was so fruitful. We used to learn from each other. He'd say something and I'd go back and test it in the animals or I'd say something about the animals and he'd say 'You know I saw this.' Anyway he was doing cardiovascular surgery, where he would drop the body temperature to allow a longer surgical time. I went up frequently but at one session he said 'Len, something's really weird, when I'm giving this drug' – and it was not the lytic cocktail, we'd narrowed it down to just chlorpromazine – 'when I give that drug people behave real funny.' I said 'What do you mean?' and he said 'It looks like they're amnesic.' That was the only word he could think of. 'They're not with it and I've noticed something else – they don't seem to care.' That was the first clinical observation in the United States, as far as I am aware. Of course I wondered if the conditioned avoidance data meant anything that was relevant to this. It ended up that it was very relevant. But along with the anti-emesis data, the hypothermia angle was another thing that helped drive this compound forward into clinical use.

Through all this I was supported with almost anything I needed. I was riding a crest and I could do no wrong. Support that would be incredible today. We developed many different laboratory test procedures which are still used today that seem to measure relevant and predictive aspects of the pharmacology. Conditioned avoidance is perhaps the most important test. I used to call it conditioned fear but later I realised that was irrelevant, it's not conditioned fear. We looked at all of the CNS drugs that had been developed over the years for schizophrenia and found that their clinical potency correlated 0.99 with their effects on inhibiting the conditioned avoidance task, so it's measuring a pharmacological property that is particularly relevant to therapeutic applications in severe emotional disorders.

The next step was that we had to get to the psychiatrists with chlorpromazine. Now this was a revelation to me. In the early 1950s, Freudian psychotherapy was popular and many people in the field were psychoanalysts. I remember one who later became very famous saying to me 'Len, are you telling me what you've got in this little pill is going to modulate libido and other complex behaviours – how's a chemical going to do what I can do with 6 months of psychoanalysis?' It's hard to relate now, the scepticism that psychiatrists had then, to the concept of an intervention with a drug – they had forgotten what Freud himself had said. Then we went to Paul Hoch in New York and I remember him saying 'That's very interesting, if you want I'll try some.' He tried it and said 'Its great.' We went to Heinz Lehmann, Fritz Freyhan and others for clinical evaluation. We went to Kinross-Wright in Texas, who did a conditioned avoidance response which he had developed using the thumb. It worked and confirmed in humans what I had seen in the rats.

We seemed to be developing the building blocks of a new area of pharmacology and I was very fortunate to be involved. In France everything seemed to stop after Mme Courvoisier did some of the early work. She dropped out of the scene – I think she was ill. So I was the leading scientist all through the 1950s while Compazine, Stelazine and all of the follow-throughs came on line. We developed these on the basis of the pharmacological principles we had set up at SK&F. I began to get super people working for me during this time and I began to build up in SmithKline the best, most advanced lab in psychopharmacology in the world. I remember an advisory board meeting where I gave a presentation and Lou Goodman afterwards said 'In all the research the government has funded, I have never seen a programme as comprehensive, relevant and productive as what you have here.'

My understanding is that SK&F, when they applied to the FDA for a licence for chlor-promazine, did so for an antiemetic. Is this true?

Yes. They were so smart. At that time I was somewhat naive and I didn't understand the marketing strategy. SK&F went to the FDA with chlorpro-mazine as an antiemetic and they got the approval for something that was very conventional pharmacologically – no sweat, no raised eyebrows. They said here's the data we have on the antiemesis, motion-sickness and on the anti-apomorphine test.

I was not privy to all of the business thinking but their strategy was to get it approved as a drug and if somebody wanted to write prescriptions for some-thing else that would expand its therapeutic use that was OK. So they got the drug out there as an antiemetic and then when it was out there they began to broaden the indications. I mean who in the world in 1955 was going to go to the FDA and say we have a drug that will modulate the symptomatology of schizophrenia or modify behaviour or mood? As I recall it that was their strat-egy, there was no question about it.

On the basis of all this I personally started to learn more about experimen-tal behaviour. I said to the vice-president that the basic preclinical research is relatively easy but the clinical people don't seem to understand how to do clin-ical research in this field and I would love to go to medical school so that I could become a clinical psychopharmacologist. I was all set for SK&F to send me to medical school but in the end one administrator killed this plan.

One of things that was particularly at issue in those days was the relevance of what we had seen in animals to the clinic. Even though there were high cor-relations between what we saw and what happened clinically there was still this enormous reluctance based on the idea that people are unique – 'they're not rats'. There also was this concept of dualism – there's a body and a mind and 'I'm in charge of my mind and drugs can't change my mind. They can change my heart and my kidney but they can't change my mind.'

I decided to look further at correlations between animal and human behav-iour regarding responsivity to pharmacological agents. I did this by setting up in one of the prisons a conditioned avoidance procedure with prisoners. You could do it easily then. And I found that when a human being is put in the same exper-imental conditions as an animal, they will show the same pharmacological effect, e.g. specific inhibition of conditioned avoidance behaviour. Chlorpromazine did this just as in the animals and the barbiturates and meprobamate didn't. We pub-lished that data – you couldn't tell by looking at the data if it came from a rat, a mouse or a human, when you controlled the contingencies in the environment in a similar way in each case. This doesn't necessarily prove therapeutic use but it proves that whatever drug–behavioural interaction is seen in animals is not something special that is seen only in animals.

At SmithKline, we also did some nice work with benzodiazepines and con-flict behaviour which has some interesting resemblances to anxiety in humans. What we found was that where the animal was trained in the conditioned avoidance procedure, if you gave a conditioned stimulus that encouraged overt behaviour such as jumping, moving or pushing a lever in order to avoid an unpleasant consequence, chlorpromazine would inhibit that. But if you can arrange for the environment to inhibit a behaviour rather than to produce it, chlorpromazine will never reverse that inhibition. However, certain low-dose barbiturates, benzodiazepines or meprobamate will attenuate environmentally induced suppression, whereas they never selectively inhibit active conditioned avoidance. That's the work that shows that major and minor tranquillisers are not linear in their effects – they are qualitatively different. We published on this in 1960.

In the same way that we showed that human subjects would selectively press a telegraph key to avoid an electric tingle and this could be blocked with chlorpromazine, at Rutgers University Medical School, several years later when I was with Roche, Peter Carlton and I did something similar with benzodiazepines. We got medical students as volunteers. They were selectively trained to make money by pressing a lever when a green light was on. Every once in a while a red warning light would come on and during this time they could make more money but they would also run a high risk of losing all the money they had earned. When the warning light came on they would show severe anxiety as the counter showing how much money they had earned began to sink. When that happened, they started sweating, their operant behaviour slowed down and some of them used language a sailor wouldn't use. Their behaviour was suppressed until the red light went off. When we gave them one 10 mg dose of Valium they would work right through the red light period just like a rat would. Chlorpromazine didn't have this effect. This was exactly what you find in animals. Benzodiazepines inhibit conflict suppressed behaviour but not active conditioned avoidance behaviour.

I also began to realise that what we had were a series of compounds that selectively suppressed certain things in the brain and not just everything. I began wondering, given that we could selectively inhibit certain brain functions, whether we could enhance certain functions as well. At the time we had an advisory board and Lou Goodman, Al Gilman and a number of other very famous people were on it and they kept saying 'Len, where do you think we're going to go in the next ten years?' I said 'Well, I think the future may be in enhancing certain brain functions' and they said 'What do you mean?' I showed them some slides that certain compounds made the animal learn more and learn it faster and I said 'It's not that the animal did it faster but he did it better and remembered longer.' The drugs were nicotine and strychnine. Nicotine works in more different types of learning tests than any other drug I tested. I developed Skinnerian test procedures with monkeys where they had to remember over 10, 20 or 30 seconds what they had to remember for appropriate reinforcement and I gave strychnine. At very low doses the animals learned better. I said these are not the specific drugs that will have a future but they prove the feasibility of enhancing learning and memory. We started a programme for learning and memory drugs in the late 1950s and early 1960s and we found that drugs like imipramine, nicotine and strychnine, in the right dose, improved cognitive function.

Another research area which I felt was very important started one night when I was doing some paperwork in my office at home. I was nervous and I wondered what was I nervous about – everything's fine at work, the kids are OK, everything seems to be fine, why am I nervous? And I suddenly realised I'm nervous because my heart is going fast and because my stomach is a little queasy and because of noticing the tachycardia and queasiness I'm nervous – that is really interesting. So I went into the lab the next day and I set up a type of Pavlovian test procedure. I put very fine catheters into a dog's vein and I trained the animal to lift its paw to terminate an electric shock. Then I went ahead and injected a low dose of epinephrine and whenever the monitor showed that blood pressure began to rise, which was an indication that it was just beginning to have a physiological effect, a shock was presented to the dog's leg. It was just like an exteroceptive conditioned stimulus but I was now using an interoceptive conditioned stimulus. After a while I found that just as soon as a small dose of epinephrine was administered, the dog would lift his leg and avoid the shock. The next step in another dog was to use two catheters in the same vein to give the lowest physiological dose of acetylcholine and the lowest dose of epinephrine and reinforce only one of the drugs. The dog learned to discriminate the effects of one drug from the other and this could be reversed. Not only that but what I found was that once you trained an animal on a conditioned avoidance paradigm to an external stimulus you could extinguish this in about 20 trials. If you don't reinforce it they lose it. But once you develop a behaviour that is controlled by an autonomic system response you never ever extinguish it. Then I began to realise that much of our behaviour is interacting with our internal physiology and our internal physiology can essentially control some of our behaviour. Chlorpromazine, incidentally, inhibited both exteroceptive and interoceptive controlled avoidance behaviour.

I went to Kapp Clark and said 'Kapp, I got a big one to request. I want to go to Russia. All of Russia is very heavy into conditioned physiological responses and I want to learn what they know. The available literature is terrible.' He said OK. It took me almost a year to set up. I went with an interpreter to Leningrad and visited Pavlov's old lab with a Dr Ariapetsyanse. I visited the biggest primate lab in the world on the Black Sea, Sukumi, and I went to Moscow. I gave several lectures. They referred to me as the American Pavlov, which was a great title. I presented my findings on conditioned physiological responses and they said 'Oh yes, Dr Bikov did that 50 years ago' – and he did. That was very interesting. I went back and said to Kapp Clark that one of these days we would be testing for drugs that would have effects on psychophysiological disorders. Nothing much happened in this area, however.

Around then we heard about Milltown – meprobamate. This was put out by Frank Berger originally to compete with Thorazine. We tested it to see if it had effects in the conditioned avoidance test like chlorpromazine and it didn't have the specific chlorpromazine effect. Subsequently, Librium was put out by Roche and they also originally put that out as a competitor to Thorazine, until they discovered that it had other unique effects of its own.

They were all seen as tranquillisers in those days weren't they?

Yes, the word tranquilliser was an all-encompassing term. I don't know how it was coined.

There was a guy called Yonkman from Ciba who took some credit for it and there is some suggestion that Nate Kline may have coined it.

I don't know if Yonkman did but Nate Kline didn't.

Another thing I did at this time was that I went to Kapp Clark and said, here I am a scientist looking for drugs to modify behaviour and I don't know anything about psychiatric syndromes. If I were a kidney pharmacologist I would know the kidney like the back of my hand. On the basis of this I went to the University of Penn and saw Karl Rickels, who was young at the time, and made an arrangement that twice a month I would make the rounds with him. I did this for a few years and I saw depressed and schizophrenic patients. I may have been one of the few preclinical scientists that ever did that. What I saw was that a depressed patient is not somebody just hanging over the bed limply, these guys have a lot of anxiety. They're depressed but they're not emotionally blank. I met schizophrenics and after a while I swear I could spot many schizophrenics – some by their odour.

This is not an uncommon claim.

I said this to Karl and he laughed at me but he also said that a lot of people say this. We would walk through the yard of the mental hospital and I would say 'He's a schizophrenic, isn't he? – from his walk, from his body build etc.' So I began to learn a little about what the diseases looked like, what the symptom complexes we were dealing with were and what actions a drug might have to modify the syndrome. It was clear that you didn't want to give a stimulant to a depressed person because he already is somewhat uptight.

Talking about giving stimulants to depressed people, wasn't tranylcypromine an SK&F drug?

Tranylcypromine didn't originally come out of a programme looking for an antidepressant. We were not only looking for drugs which would be useful for schizophrenia, we were looking for sleep-inducers, we were looking for stimulants which would be different from amphetamine.

The concept of an antidepressant can't have been there at that time – stimulant yes.

That's correct, it wasn't. You know the story – it was Nate Kline at the tuberculous hospital and they had the insight that these people weren't feeling better just because they got rid of their tuberculosis – that was a great contribution. So they and others began to work on the pharmacological treatment of depression and this made us aware of the possibility of drugs that might be antidepressant. We did a lot of work and eventually came up with tranylcypromine and went into the clinic with it. I have to tell you it worked very effectively. However, the side-effects were more than we anticipated which, as you know, restricted its use.

Did you have much contact with Alfred Burger – he was the one who made it wasn't he?

Burger was a consultant to our medical chemistry department. He was located in the University of Virginia. A nice person and very capable. Whenever he came in to consult with medicinal chemistry he came into my lab because I was doing the testing of the compounds he advised them to make. He made tranylcypromine. We had carried out some work on it and said 'Well, this looks like a very different agent. We couldn't pick up much on it behaviourally. It was inert on the motor activity tests, on the Skinnerian tests – the fixed intervals, the DRLs etc. But what it did was it worked in the drug interaction tests that essentially identified enhanced biogenic amines. It wasn't until we went clinically and it was tried in depressed patients that we began to realise that it worked well as an antidepressant. We eventually got FDA approval for it but then the cheese and pickled herring interactions began to appear.

My impression is that when the interactions began to appear SK&F stuck with the drug in a way that Roche didn't stick with iproniazid.

Not entirely. When SK&F began to get these reports the reaction was we had to restrict its use. We were broken-hearted when management said we should stop work on this because when you work in a research lab and you find drugs, these are like your children. They pulled the drug off quickly instead of waiting to see how it could be used more carefully. It was later reintroduced for very limited uses. It may have been used more widely but now when I look back I accept that if you have a drug out there you can't be assured that all physicians are going to use it properly. You are going to get problems and people may get injured or worse so I think they did right. Later on management felt it had been premature to pull it entirely off the market and to tell us to forget the antidepressant programme, which is what they did.

However, we were riding high at this point. We had done critical work with the phenothiazines, we were starting a new programme in learning and memory, we had done work on meprobamate and shown it was different from the phenothiazines but then something strange happened in the company. The head of chemistry, Glenn Ullyot, who was a terrific guy, said at one of the meetings 'I think we've got all the drugs we're going to get in this field, I think we should drop the phenothiazine programme.' I said 'What ! – we're just scratching the surface, we're on the edge of new frontier.' 'No', he said 'we've got Thorazine, Compazine, Stelazine, who needs more?' I said 'Don't do this, there are other chemical classes besides the phenothiazines and besides there will always be a competitor in the field, why don't we come up with our own competitive drug, why let other people do it?' For the time they agreed to keep going but ...

I had another interesting insight at the time. Looking through the range of drugs at the time, the only drug that blocked the conditioned avoidance test selectively the way the phenothiazines did was morphine. I got the group to run Demerol, methadone etc. and we found that all of the opiates and powerful analgesics worked like chlorpromazine. I started thinking about whether there was a drug that could do what demerol did but was not also a pain-threshold elevater. It would be out of the class of analgesics but maybe it maintained the behavioural effect of morphine, codeine and Demerol even though it was not analgesic. I went to a meeting and spoke to Paul Janssen about this, who was very interested in the idea. Subsequently haloperidol appeared. I'm almost sure that haloperidol came out of that concept and conversation. Paul is brilliant. He was a happy combination – someone who owned a lab and was both the chief chemist and a brilliant biologist. He could move quickly and efficiently.

Much of the field, you know, came out of the enormous opportunity that industry provided to young people like myself and allowed them to follow their noses. But that era has changed in the pharmaceutical industry. All of the companies now have followed what the Harvard Business School say, which is 'focus, focus, focus'. You can't have what I used to have which was maybe a dozen projects going at any one time, never knowing what was going to pop up in any one of them. Now they say *a priori* you pick your best two or three projects and you put everything into it. Well, as much as the advantage may be to maximising your effort, what you lose is all of the other happenstance, serendipity, the cross-fertilisation. You couldn't today easily follow a lead from a non-sedative barbiturate programme to drug potentiators to chlorpromazine and anti-psychotics. Now there is very little room in the industry for the unexpected. I don't mean to imply for a minute that you should carry out only non-directive research hoping that something might happen, but equally you shouldn't limit or overly restrict the imagination and latitude of young scientists.

SmithKline got into strategic planning very early. They had been ahead of the other companies by ten years in almost everything. The gist of strategic planning was to quantify and analyse and programme the entire process of drug discovery to try to make it more efficient. But they lost in the process those special elements that are required for discovery – intuitiveness, and opportunities for serendipity. Most everything was prescribed and it had to be approved by scientific boards. Very often the essence of research boards that approve programmes is that people are covering their backsides and playing safe. There are good elements to the idea of research planning but they tend to lose something. I recall people asking me how many compounds does it take to discover a muscle relaxant – 'I don't know' – 'guess' – 'maybe 2000' – 'OK, and how long does that take' – 'maybe 30 months'. Then in 30 months or 2000 compounds later they call you in and ask what have you found and you say we've got a couple of leads and they say well if you haven't found the breakthrough by now forget it – the programme is terminated.

Were the people in charge in SmithKline in the early 1950s still in charge in the late 1960s when all of this began to come in?

No, there had been a change at the top. The people who gave the scientists the opportunities to make discoveries were gone and those who came in had little feel for science themselves and they attempted to overly programme the elements of the discovery process. It was an interesting phenomenon, I must say, but it wasn't for me and this is what made Roche's offer to be Director of Pharmacology attractive when it came in 1969.

There are two ways of doing strategic planning: one is that you let your own staff carry it out with guidance from someone. We did it this way first in Du Pont and we ended up with recommendations for the same programmes we had beforehand. 'What are you doing?' they said, 'you're doing the same thing as you were doing before.' I said we evaluated all the factors and we think what we are doing is good. It wasn't just my group that did this – all the groups did this and came up with recommendations to continue what they were doing. So then they called in an outside group to force change. I said change for what reason and they said we need change, change in itself is good, it's the future. Then we realised management were doing it to cover their backsides. They could say whatever we're doing was carefully analysed: 'We've called in hot-shots from New York and Harvard and this is the programme they suggest, so if it falls on its face its not our fault.' It was a security blanket for management. They wouldn't have to put their own necks on the block and say 'Yes, I was in charge and I let these guys do it because I believed in it.' You cannot argue with the process but the process can run away with itself.

What about GLP Good Laboratory Practice and all the things the FDA imposed on the industry, how much impact did all of that have?

I don't think that Good Laboratory Practice or Good Manufacturing Practice had much inhibiting impact on our research. In fact in some ways it helped to improve many aspects of pharmaceutical businesses.

So it's what the companies did to themselves?

Yes. I don't think this was a result of government intervention or pressure at all. There are two kinds of people in an organisation, let's say a drug-house. There are the risk takers and they are generally the scientists and then there are people who are covering their backsides. They know that nine out of ten things you do in the lab are going to fail so if you say no 10 times you're going to be right nine times.

Why did you leave SK&F in the end and move to Roche?

I had the golden era of the pharmaceutical business in the 1950s and 1960s. If I wanted to go to a meeting in Rome and drop off in Milan to see Silvio Garattini that was OK. It was a wonderful time. You could do any different studies you wanted to regarding drug development such as modifying learning and memory or modifying autonomic physiology. The strategic planners changed all this. Things began to get nasty and disruptive in research and decisions were not always made by the people who are the most knowledgeable in the field.

At that time I got a call from John Burns, vice-president for research at Roche, a giant in the field. The director of pharmacology was just about to retire and he said he had been talking to Lou Goodman and asked him who was the best person to take over the department when the former director retired and Lou said Len Cook. I talked to my wife and I thought about the changes at SK&F. However, even when you become a little bit unhappy or dissatisfied, you don't throw away something so quickly when you have invested 18 years of your life in it. Burns called me every Sunday night for a while and then gave me a written offer over a meal at a meeting in Pittsburgh. It was a more than satisfactory offer. It was the best job in pharmacology in the country but leaving a department I had built from nothing that was then over 100 people wasn't easy.

Had Roche begun to go in under a cloud at that stage? They came in for an awful lot of stick during the 1970s because of the benzos.

The harried housewife syndrome. That didn't bother me. I knew that Valium and Librium were legitimate and effective drugs. I had published more on the benzodiazepines than the scientists at Roche had. No, head of pharmacology at Roche at the time was as good a job as there was in the industry but still leaving SmithKline was like breaking up a marriage. However, everything was changing and I felt I wanted a change and I went to Roche and we started a whole new CNS operation in Nutley and in Basel.

Did you meet Willy Haefely in Basel?

Yes, he was an outstanding guy. He was very aggressive but also a very sweet man. He should have been headed for greatness but he was not handled well by Basel. He began to lose ground. He was given a new boss who changed things around without knowing the field as well as Willy. Willy was an extraordinary man whom it was an honour to work with. Moise da Prada was the head of chemistry and Alfred Pletscher was also there but he became more academic. Pletscher had been to NIH and worked with Brodie on the reserpine research.

Did you guys do any of the work looking at the behavioural activation caused by the combination of iproniazid and reserpine which Pletscher and Brodie were involved with?

No, but I can tell you something about reserpine – this guy who brought reserpine over came to us at SK&F before he went to Ciba. He had a gunny sack and said he had some roots. We were highly involved with chlorpromazine at the time – it was early in the 1950s. I got a call: 'Len, there's some guy coming tomorrow with some roots gathered from the foothills of the Himalayas or something like that, would you talk to him?' I said 'Do I have to?'. Anyway this man came with his gunny sack and said 'These are the roots.' I said 'What does it do?' and he said 'It's good for colic, it's good for hypertension, it's good for people with mental disease, it's good to drop body temperature, it's great for sleep' and I said 'Ah-ha, ah-ha!' One of the executives said 'Len, buy him a lunch and get him the hell out of here.' So I bought him a lunch and he later went to Ciba and lo and behold it was reserpine. After that any guy who said he had roots was immediately offered $50,000 for the privilege of testing it. They put him up in a hotel and bought dinner, not just lunch. I remember that because the claims sounded absurd. It was inconceivable that a compound could do all of those things but it did everything he said it would do. If you think about chlorpromazine though, if somebody had said to you it will drop blood pressure, it will drop body temperature, it will help schizophrenia, it's good for nausea and vomiting, it enhances the effects of other drugs – you'd have said 'Right!' and raised an eyebrow.

Roche in the 1960s and 1970s ended up being almost only into anxiolytics – why was that?

I went to Roche in 1969 and John Burns called me down to his office, where I asked him what plans he had in mind. He said 'You know, Len, we've been working with the benzodiazepines for a while and we're getting flak because of the drug dependency issue, so even though we're doing a billion a year, there's so much negative publicity that I'd like you to start a non-benzodiazepine programme. Find a Valium that's not a benzodiazepine.'

So we started a programme in the non-benzodiazepine area but Hoffman-la-Roche was a strange organisation. Basel Switzerland never stopped trying to control Nutley. John Burns was a power in himself so they couldn't do it fully. But they had the most critical control of all, the head of chemistry was a Swiss, who even though he reported to John Burns kept primary contact with Switzerland. I could never get him or the medicinal chemistry people in Roche to make compounds that were not benzodiazepines. They kept flooding my department with benzodiazepines. Burns was getting frustrated and so was I.

You see, medicinal chemists are a strange lot. One issue with them is that when they have an active chemical series they will never leave it. They get patents out of it every week and they aren't going to leave it because to find an active series may take a lifetime. They hate to let go. So I had to deal with them while their leader in chemistry was saying don't you listen to this guy Cook, I want more patents out of this series. Chemists, you see, were evaluated for their annual bonus in terms of their number of patents – so are they crazy? Are they going to leave this series, all the compounds of which are active? That led to a serious problem for the company. The medicinal chemists at many pharmaceutical companies control the research direction. They make the compounds, all I can do is test them. Even though I can identify active compounds, I'm not going to discover anything that they haven't made. So that was a very serious problem at Roche. I don't remember a week going by without some emergency clinical reaction reported to the company with the benzodiazepines and yet, even John Burns, as powerful as he was, couldn't get the chemists to leave the benzos because of the Swiss control network.

Why did you move from Roche to Du Pont?

When I first got to Roche it was a lot of fun but then after about 14 years they also called in the Harvard Business School types, who said you can't have 20 projects going at the same time. You have to focus. Basel decided to move CNS research to Switzerland and I began to lose projects to the Swiss labs. Although Basel owned Nutley we had a very strong protector in John Burns.

When he retired the Swiss moved in and that was when Roche started doing strategic planning and I increasingly saw what I felt were really good projects being pushed aside. Then a friend of mine, Bob Taber, moved from Schering to Du Pont as research director and he offered me a job taking over CNS research. They could afford me, it looked like fun and it was nearer to my family, who were in the Philadelphia area. So I had 18 years at SmithKline, 15 at Roche and 12 at Du Pont.

Behavioural pharmacology of the type you have done has contributed a huge amount to the drug abuse field. Where has that got to?

At present, one of the things I do is to act as a scientific adviser for NIDA on drug abuse. They are looking for medications to intervene in cocaine and heroin abuse. There are two main directions at the moment. One is focusing on cocaine, which is a big issue at present. One option here is to look for agonists, just like methadone for morphine, which will be synthetic, cheaper, produce fewer side-effects and will hopefully get the person out of crime and give them more stability. There is also the antagonist approach like naloxone for morphine. But all of this presumes that the addict wants to get off. With some addicts you have some degree of coercion but unless the person is highly motivated to get off the drug staying off is tough and so the focus is now turning to the issue of craving, in the hope that drug-induced craving can be reduced without decreasing craving for food or other life-sustaining cravings. You need to prevent relapse. You can get someone motivated to stop taking drugs but preventing relapse is the big one. Now relapse occurs in response to stimuli like a glass or syringe causing all kind of secondary things going on internally. Its almost like ...

...Hypnosis almost or autopilot.

Yes, the stimulus precipitates everything, the stimulus causes all the internal longings, cravings etc. If you could get a drug that would block this process and block whatever autonomic effects have been conditioned, that would be great. Behavioural research can best address these issues, so one of the things that have been recommended to NIDA is to focus their research in this area. I think it's feasible to do but getting a good strong programme going using different animal models isn't easy. Right now the problems are getting support to follow all the various approaches because many people still think of drug and alcohol abuse is a loss of will-power, a socially weak personality, when in fact it's a disease, at times an uncontrollable disease.

The recent work on naltrexone and alcohol I think is very impressive and that seems to work on a process related to craving. I was at Du Pont, who sell naltrexone, when the first reports on this came through from Valpocelli and Chuck O'Brien of the University of Pennsylvania and I can remember initially thinking this doesn't make sense. I was asked by the company if it made sense to me and I said that given what I knew, then, it didn't because naltrexone has nothing to do with what alcohol works on but the more I read about the work the more sense their ideas about the mechanism of action made. One of the pieces of research that I came across was that alcoholics have a very low baseline level of beta-endorphins and when they drink alcohol they increase this. In alcoholics there is an even greater increase than occurs in normals so there is a greater contrast effect and this is what they may be getting their kick out of. There's a big literature on this and one of the things that has been shown is that the children of alcoholics who are not drinkers also have low beta-endorphin levels. When you look at the University of Pennsylvania data and the Yale data from O'Malley the results are almost identical – what you find is that people don't totally stop drinking and nobody went cold-turkey but the amount they drink and the frequency of their drinking are down by about 50%. Coming back to the point about the internal stimuli, when they asked them about their drinking they said that they didn't get the buzz from drinking that they used to get.

I think there's a lot of pharmacology that can be done in this whole area of heroin, cocaine, alcohol and smoking. I used to be a heavy smoker years ago – when I would get a cocktail in my hand I had to have a cigarette in the other one. You develop these behavioural patterns. Everytime a knock would come to the door of the office I'd light a cigarette, everytime the phone would ring I'd light a cigarette, after dinner etc. I realised that I probably enjoyed no more than three or four cigarettes a day and the rest were strictly conditioning – I wouldn't even remember lighting up. I wish now I had the opportunity and resources to look at some of these things. I don't think that molecular biology, as valuable as it is, is really going to answer these things.

Who've been the other behavioural pharmacologists who count?

Peter Dews, Roger Kelleher, Joe Brady, Bill Morse, Larry Stein, Jerry Sepinwall, Arnie Davidson, Ed Boff and Charles Shuster. Skinner's significant contribution was that he laid the basis of the field. I used to hire experimental psychologists and teach them pharmacology and I'm probably one of the few pharmacologists who learned the behaviour. Joe Brady did a lot of important work with his executive monkeys, which was relevant to this whole area of the autonomic nervous system coming into play.

Behaviour and drug–behaviour interactions reached its peak in the 1950s and 1960s and maybe the 1970s. Now you don't see that type of elegant drug–behaviour interaction study. People have gone back to very simple, mundane behaviours. The work we did in the 1950s, 1960s and 1970s offered the opportunity to study how drugs fine-tune or modulate behaviour particularly in the area of anxiety. There's still a lot to be done but with the swing of the field to molecular biology, which is also needed, there's not nearly enough *in vivo* behavioural pharmacology being done.

Who were the clinicians you think counted? You mentioned Paul Hoch earlier.

He was a giant. He understood immediately, it seemed to me, what I was talking about when I first discussed chlorpromazine with him. He understood what a drug like that might be able to do and he accepted that this was an effective approach in psychiatry. He knew exactly what dependent variables to look at in terms of a patient population, what the most relevant criteria in drug evaluation clinically might be. There were others: Heinz Lehmann, Fritz Freyhan, who was a friend of Heinz, Nate Kline who came in a little later, Joel Elkes, Jonathan Cole and Seymour Kety who was also a member of our scientific advisory board at SK&F.

Why don't we seem to make the same breakthroughs anymore?

I remember giving a talk here in the Caribe Hilton over 20 years ago and I told the audience, which was composed then mostly of psychiatrists, that the problem in the field and the greatest barrier to the development of drugs that will have applicability in mental disease is a lack of description of the patient population and symptomatology in terms that can be used in animal research. If we were in the cardiovascular area, I would go to a clinician and ask him 'What is it you want a drug to do?' and he would say 'I want you to hit pulse pressure or reduce blood pressure' etc. They would specify things they want the drug to do that I could take back to the lab and try to find. But if I tell psychiatrists that I have a magic wand and I can produce a drug that will do anything that they tell me they want it to do provided they don't just say make the patient well, they must tell me specifically what they want the drug to do in order to make the patient well, they couldn't do it.

I said that at the end of 1960s and then a few years ago I gave a talk again to ACNP and told the audience about the earlier talk and asked them – have you guys settled it yet? Everybody laughed. But you see psychiatry is still a mostly descriptive science of symptomatology and the greatest barrier in psychopharmacology today is the lack of specification in terms that can be applied in the lab. It could be in terms of biochemistry or in terms of the EEG, whatever you want, but not in terms of simply getting the patient well.

In the 1950s, most of all the great discoveries were made by chance in the clinic but not because of any prior specification of what kind of drug was needed. We then used these drugs as standards to develop our test procedures to find similar but better and cleaner drugs. Now in the area of Alzheimer's, for example, if a clinician were to say I've found a truly effective drug, I'd say thank God, we can now go ahead and develop animal models that are sensitive to the effects of this drug. But for now we have to develop tests that have face validity. Molecular biology has a long way to go in this field because many of its approaches are presumptive in terms of their relevance.

I personally believe we should have more pure clinical research. I have proposed to Du Pont and NIDA that we should be doing far more conceptual clinical testing. For example, take a sigma receptor blocker or other compounds which have any possibility of working for any rational reason: once they have been shown to be safe we should put them in the clinic for conceptual clinical testing using good experimentally minded clinicians to see just what they do. Then we could go back to basic research and work it up further and develop meaningful and better preclinical studies.

Forget the impact on the illness, look for the impact on behaviour.

Yes, but it's not happening. If a medical school would accept me today, I would try to get a programme like that going, a programme to carefully study behavioural and emotional changes produced by many different compounds with various kinds of mechanisms. There are so many things that are not being examined that would only take a short-term investment to realise. But today everything is molecular biology. This is the future but it should not happen at a cost to more conventional pharmacology.

3 Paul Janssen

From haloperidol to risperidone

You've written a number of accounts of the way haloperidol came to be discovered. The account in Discoveries in Biological Psychiatry, following the meeting that Frank Ayd put together in 1970, was one of the first. In this you said that when you came to write the piece it was hard to know whether to give an outline of the principles involved in the actual discovery or to give the emotional feel for what happened. I think in that account you looked more at the principles. Perhaps we could look at the discovery more from the emotional feel of what happened?

The whole story probably starts with a friend of mine by the name of Arnold Beckett of Chelsea Polytechnic. He told me something that later on turned out to be wrong but anyway he claimed that pethidine itself was not active but that it entered the CNS and was then demethylated to norpethidine and that this was the active analgesic.

This was something he believed in and he made me believe it for a while so I came home and said if this is true then it should be possible to increase the potency of pethidine easily by putting a Mannich base tail on it.

The new compound, R951, is called a propiophenone. We lengthened the carbon chain by reacting the ketone, acetophenone, with formaldehyde to form R951. And indeed when injected into mice it turned out to be a few hun-

PETHIDINE   R951

dred times more potent than pethidine. Now why did I anticipate this high potency? Simply because chemically speaking the older compound pethidine is more stable than this new compound R951, which is also much more lipophilic. In those days we were still believers in the theory that lipophilic compounds somehow had an easier time entering the brain than hydrophilic compounds, which again is wrong but anyway that is what was believed then.

It's curious how things can move forward even though all the ideas behind them are wrong, isn't it?

Yes, the theory was wrong but in those days we were simply synthesising new compounds, which we injected into animals and asked the question: What kind of a compound is this? What does it do? Does it act like morphine, does it act like atropine? We had a small battery of screening tests. But one of the ideas that we had been working on – no more than a dream – was to find one day an amphetamine antagonist. You know the story behind that probably.

There are a few different stories.

Well, I had seen a number of cyclists who, hoping to enhance their performance, had taken very large doses of amphetamine and was told by a friend that their amphetamine-induced symptoms were indistinguishable from those of paranoid schizophrenia. I knew very little about psychiatry but these cyclists were hallucinating, they were stereotyped in their behaviour, they had delusions and, when asked a question, they would always give the same stereotyped nonsensical answer. They were more or less excited. Clinically the syndrome was reminiscent of an acute attack of paranoid schizophrenia. So the idea was: let us try to find an antagonist of amphetamine – it would certainly be of help for the treatment of amphetamine intoxication and with some luck it might even work in the real disease. So we started to look systematically for amphetamine antagonists.

1953/54 was extremely early to be thinking that a drug that could be used to antagonise amphetamine might be useful for schizophrenia. The whole idea of the amphetamine model had not been born at that time.

No, this was so-called original but it was simply the direct consequence of this observation in the cyclists. But the fact that amphetamine poisoning resembled paranoid schizophrenia was not completely unknown even then. To me it became very obvious and my friend, Fries Claes, had seen many such cases because in those days cyclists in Europe were swallowing very large doses of amphetamine. Subsequently in the chemistry lab we started modifying the structure of R951 and one of the modifications was simply a lengthened side chain with one extra CH_2 group, giving a butyrophenone.

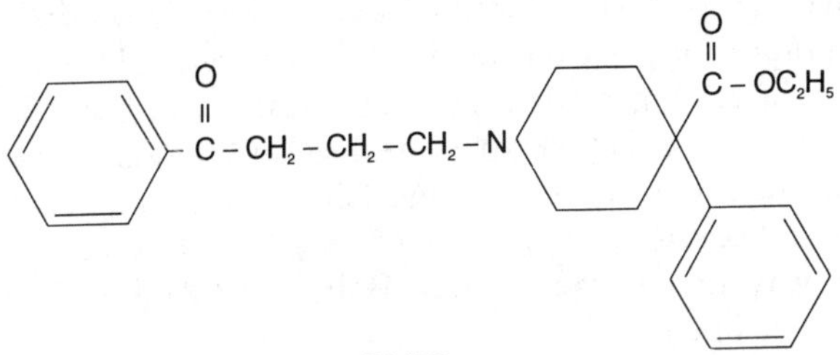

R1187

When this compound, which we called R1187, was injected into animals something strange happened. The first effect seemed to be morphine-like but relatively short lived. This was followed by an effect resembling the effect of chlorpromazine. In those days chlorpromazine was new and its pharmacology was mysterious but sedation, or what we called catalepsy, was a prominent feature of this butyrophenone. We tested it as an amphetamine antagonist and, sure enough, it showed amphetamine antagonistic properties – for the first time.

What we then did was to chemically modify this structure (R1187), trying to increase the antiamphetamine effect and to get rid of the morphine-like effects. This was achieved by putting an extra fluorine group on the phenyl group, leaving the rest of the molecule intact and then replacing the ethylester moiety with a tertiary alcohol group – all very simple, straightforward chemistry. In order to make it long acting we put an extra chlorine group in the *para* position. The product was called R1625.

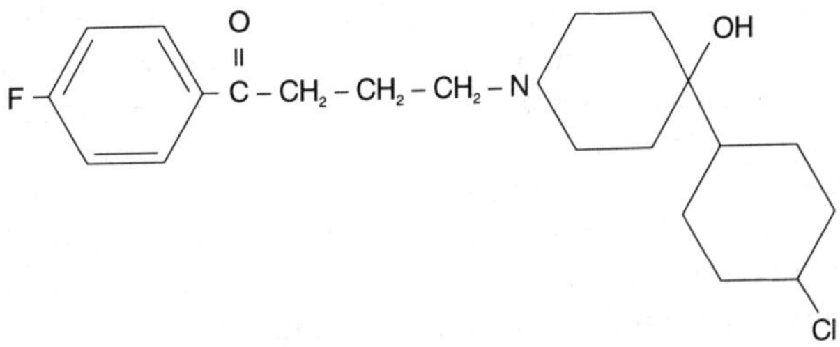

R1625

The difference between R1625 and R951 gives you an idea of the number of compounds that had to be synthesised because each time we tested a new compound it was given the next number. R1625 was then given the generic name haloperidol. When injected into mice and rats, it was very potent as an amphetamine antagonist. We fiddled around a little bit but this was the best we could achieve.

Then we approached a few psychiatrists – one of them was Jean Bobon in Liège – trying to convince them to test my hypothesis in man – which they did but rather reluctantly. For six months they left the ampoules on the shelf. But in the middle of one night Andre Pinchard, one of the assistants in Liège, didn't have much to do and when a son of a local practitioner was brought in at night with symptoms of what appeared to be acute paranoid schizophrenia and severe agitation, he gave him 10 mgs of haloperidol i.v., around 3 o'clock in the morning. That had the effect we know well today. He was very impressed and phoned me, urging me to come to Liège. When I arrived around 9 o'clock the next morning, all I could see was a young boy asleep. His father, a local general practitioner, was there as well as Jean Bobon and Andre Pinchard. We discussed what had happened.

Jean Bobon decided to test the effect of 5 mg i.v. of haloperidol in approximately 50 acutely agitated patients – agitation of any origin, schizophrenia, mania even delirium tremens. His first paper describes the effect of haloperidol on psychomotor agitation, not on schizophrenia. It simply states that the intravenous administration of 5 mg of haloperidol is quite active in calming down acutely agitated patients – that's all. Because even then he had not really tested the new compound in schizophrenia or by the oral route. This was done by Paquay, who was a psychiatrist working in Namur.

The first patient, the young man, treated by Andre Pinchard, was studying architecture. He had never previously had symptoms. His acute attack was completely unexpected. When he woke up the next day he was completely normal as far as one could tell. And then we started talking about what to do next – to continue treatment or what? A compromise was reached which was: 10 mg is a heck of a dose, let us try a much smaller oral daily dose. The patient was given 1 mg in drops in his coffee, I believe, or his tea which he drank daily.

He completed his studies, married and had two children. He had no psychiatric symptoms. Every year I was invited by the father, with Bobon and Pinchard, to discuss the case and the question was always the same: was this really an attack of paranoid schizophrenia or was it maybe what French psychiatrists refer to as 'bouffée delirante' because he had no symptoms, and therefore shall we continue treatment or stop it? For six or eight years the treatment was continued because there were absolutely no side-effects and no symptoms. In the meantime what is today called biological psychiatry had been born. I was of the opinion that it was safer to continue treatment than to interrupt it, because there was obviously no harm done. It could have been paranoid schizophrenia and of course if the 1 mg was really doing what it appeared to do then interruption could lead to relapse.

After about 7 years it was unfortunately decided to advise the boy to stop taking the drug. He did and lo and behold, three weeks later, in the middle of the night, he was brought back to the ward with exactly the same symptoms of paranoid schizophrenia. This came as a shock to the whole family and to the patient because he had studied and had a family and he was not convinced that he was suffering from schizophrenia – this ugly word – and neither was the family. But now with the second attack, the diagnosis was obvious and it ruined his life. After his relapse the dose had to be increased to 3 mg daily and he became more difficult to manage because compliance became a problem.

Paquay, knowing of this case, said – well, haloperidol is obviously very potent against hallucinations and delusions – I am going to try it in chronic cases. He tried low doses – 1–7 mg daily. The objective was very clear – to make the hallucinations and delusions disappear, to control the agitation if necessary and to re-establish normal human contact. These were considered the core symptoms of paranoid schizophrenia.

Haloperidol was not seriously tested in the other types of schizophrenia like hebephrenia, which I always thought was a different disease – it did not resemble amphetamine intoxication. We only tested it in patients that looked like amphetamine abusers – for want of a better word we called it paranoid schizophrenia. The closer the clinical picture was to amphetamine poisoning the more interesting was the patient. This is the reason why hebephrenia was not seriously considered. And even today I still believe that hebephrenia has a completely different aetiology.

Paquay's success rate was very high. His main objective was not to produce side-effects. Patients who would not respond to 1–7 mg daily were considered non-responders. He thought that extrapyramidal side-effects were awful: patients hate them and become very poor at compliance. Paquay was careful and patient and I believe that what he concluded in his first article on haloperidol is still true. It was much later that, under the influence of American psychiatrists in particular, very high doses of haloperidol were given in therapy-resistant patients.

Do you not think the dopamine hypotheses of schizophrenia had some part to play in the fact that people went up to extremely high doses? The idea that if dopamine is abnormal in schizophrenia then if they fail to get well the answer is to increase the dose?

Well, the dopamine theory was not the same then as it is today. Again the whole thing started with amphetamine. I always thought that phenethylamine was the endogenous amphetamine and still believe that. Pharmacologically these compounds have similar properties and chemically the only difference between the two is the extra methyl group in amphetamine.

AMPHETAMINE

PHENYLETHYLAMINE
(PHENETHYLAMINE)

Phenethylamine, like amphetamine, releases dopamine from the vesicular dopamine storage proteins. When phenethylamine or amphetamine is injected into the brain, dopamine is released from these proteins and this is why dopamine concentration increases locally. Now phenethylamine is a normal constituent of the brain. So even today I believe that the story of paranoid schizophrenia is relatively straightforward. My preferred theory is that for some queer reason, in certain regions of the brain, there is increased enzyme activity converting phenylalanine to phenethylamine or decreased MAO activity. This leads to an increase of phenethylamine concentrations and thus increased dopamine release. The rest is really the classical story. Neuroleptics are active against some symptoms of what is called paranoid schizophrenia but also in mania as well and mania and schizophrenia are certainly two different diseases.

But they can also be used for people who are anxious.

There is a problem with anxiety because the English word anxiety is untranslatable. There is the French word anxieté but anxieté doesn't mean anxiety. It is a difficult linguistic problem.

Later on we realised that there were two big problems with haloperidol. One was the problem of compliance and the most obvious reason for lack of compliance was forgetfulness. Another reason was the fact that patients on too high a dose experienced side-effects and actually spit out their pills. And this is why haloperidol decanoate was eventually developed: to improve compliance. When properly used Haldol decanoate gives better results in terms of control of symptoms and certainly in terms of relapse rate reduction.

We then made numerous haloperidol-like butyrophenones and diphenylbutylpiperidines and other neuroleptics, literally thousands of them, and many were tested in schizophrenic patients – always pursuing the same obsessive idea. Most of them were rejected, not because they were inferior but because they were not superior or significantly different. An important exception was R3345, which we tested a long time ago because it was such a powerful drug in the tryptamine test.

After the success of this antiamphetamine story, it occurred to me that amphetamine is not the only compound producing symptoms that resemble schizophrenia. There is also LSD, which was thought to be a serotonin-like agonist. So we started looking for an LSD antagonist hoping that it would somehow complement the amphetamine story. But this was not an easy task. It was even difficult to set up a screening test that would mimic LSD. The best we found was the tryptamine test in rats.

We screened compound after compound after compound until R3345 emerged, which is dipiperone or pipamperone. Pipamperone turned out in the clinic to be very well tolerated and free of side-effects. It resembles Risperdal. The problem was the Americans didn't like it. Not the psychiatrists but the marketing people. They thought that haloperidol was enough – that it could take care of everything – in spite of the fact that in America, certainly at the beginning, there was a very strong and long-lasting anti-haloperidol period.

This was a direct consequence of the first publication on haloperidol in the *American Journal of Psychiatry*, by Herman Denber, which you will have trouble believing.

Denber is a fairly famous name in the early history CINP etc.

But he did something unbelievable. He was responsible for research work in Manhattan State Hospital where he had 60 beds. But he did not get along well with his colleagues, who tended to give him the most untreatable patients. So his whole research ward was full of what we call chronic hebephrenics and they are resistant to whatever. Anyway he spent all his time touring the world looking for new compounds to be tested in his patients because his ambition was to be the first to publish on new compounds in America.

He came to see me after having visited Jean Bobon in Liège to see what haloperidol was doing in patients there. He came to see me asking for samples. I was very pleased because I had never seen an American psychiatrist before. Being very honoured, I gave him all the samples he wanted. He went back home but what he did then was to give the samples to one of his nurses by the name of Mrs Kauffman. And Mrs Kauffman was instructed by Denber to give the new compound to 10 patients in increasing doses to see what would happen. Denber went on another trip probably. He actually never saw the patients. He came back and he asked Mrs Kauffman what was her experience with haloperidol and she said it didn't do anything at all. It was like water. It did not even induce side-effects. So he took his pen and he wrote a paper which basically says that haloperidol is a very effective drug in Europeans but, for genetic reasons, completely inactive in Americans.

I jumped on a plane and I went to see his 10 chronic hebephrenic patients and to my amazement two or three or them were black, two or three were Hispanics, one came from Russia, the other from Germany. Ridiculous! But he had never seen these patients. He must have been as surprised as I was. But it was published. The other Americans including the managing director of McNeil, a sister company supposed to sell haloperidol, said: well haloperidol is a dead fish. It will never make it. Look at Denber, who says it doesn't work in Americans, it only works in Europeans. As a result from 1960 to 1964, I believe, nobody gave even one dose of haloperidol in the States. In the meantime, the drug became generally available in Europe and in Japan. It was a real horror story – until in 1964, a psychiatrist of Italian extraction published an open study on haloperidol in about 250 patients treated in a state hospital in California describing 'European' results in American patients. It didn't bring anything new because it was simply an open study and it confirmed well-known observations. But in America this had an effect because it showed that after all haloperidol was doing something. The doses he gave were small doses. He was dosing his patients like Paquay more or less, so the side-effect profile was OK. This is how interest in haloperidol in America emerged in 1965 approximately. Then eventually it was marketed and today it is the most widely used neuroleptic in America and elsewhere.

Then dipiperone was put on the market in Europe. With hindsight you could say dipiperone is interesting because it is the first D2/S2 antagonist. In those days the serotonin story was completely unknown. There is one publication by an American psychiatrist, Sugerman, on dipiperone which is like reading a paper on risperidone. It is almost the same story. Sugerman was very satisfied but McNeil did not want it. Therefore the 'world' never heard of it. It is a pity because if McNeil had marketed dipiperone, I believe that what is called biological psychiatry would have changed completely. Today the serotonin story is a relatively new story. But it is true that dipiperone was not particularly potent. The doses to be given were high 60–240 mg per day, but well tolerated and effective. Ever since, therefore, we have tried to find a more potent and 'better' dipiperone and for me risperidone is just that – a better dipiperone.

Risperidone is not an atypical neuroleptic. It is a typical neuroleptic but it has very strong effect on S2 receptors, which probably explains the fact that many people who take it sleep better and because they sleep better they are probably less depressed. In recent years I have been interviewing lots of patients and my impression is that a patient who responds better to risperidone than to haloperidol is a typical schizophrenic who over and above his schizophrenic symptoms is rather depressed and claims not to sleep well. This patient is likely to respond better simply because of this obvious effect on deep sleep. I don't like the claims that are being made about negative symptoms. I don't really know what they mean but I know what it means not to sleep well. That I can understand easily – to feel lousy in the morning because you have not slept well. This effect on sleep is probably the additional benefit in my opinion of risperidone plus the fact that fortunately enough from the very first the recommended doses were low and therefore EPS occurs only in a minority of patients, but EPS can be induced with risperidone as with all other neuroleptics if the daily dose is increased.

You had the first meeting on haloperidol here in Belgium, in 1959, a year after it had been launched. At this there were 17 papers describing the full range of uses for the drug. Its usefulness for tic disorders and other conditions had been picked up even then. This all seems extraordinarily rapid.

Well, it took six months. The story is as follows. I knew very little about psychiatry. I had no contacts with psychiatrists whatsoever. And I was very sceptical. My father, who was an MD, told me to beware of psychiatrists. He was convinced that most of what they had to say was simply not true – that they were very good at inventing all kinds of fancy stories. But my father was too sceptical. It took him quite some time to believe that penicillin was doing what it was doing.

Thinking about the problem and feeling convinced that haloperidol was indeed effective – on the basis of very few patients actually and without double-blind evidence at all but based on the notion of obviousness – a recognition of what was obviously effective. In those days the notion of obviousness still existed and was accepted. Like in anaesthesiology, the intravenous use of an opiate is obviously effective. Nobody ever asked me to prove it in a double-blind test.

What I did, with the help of friends, was to find eight of the best-known psychiatrists in Europe. Jean Delay was quite helpful and we became very good friends. I was very young and he took an interest in what I was doing and helped me as much as he could. He told me I should go to Professor so and so – Lopez-Ibor in Spain, for instance, and a few others in Germany and so on. We asked all eight to test haloperidol, on an open basis. They didn't know that they were a group of eight. They all thought that they were the only ones who were doing it and there were no contacts between them. Six months later, we asked them to come to Beerse and to give us their impressions, which we published (references). What really convinced me was that all eight had exactly the same clinical impressions. This is quite clear from the book. I said well, it is statistically highly improbable that eight completely independent psychiatrists, who had not been influenced at all, living in completely different environments, using different languages, customs and even concepts of psychiatry, would arrive at exactly the same opinion in the course of six months. So it must be true and that was the end of clinical investigations. Practically all we know about haloperidol can be found in that first publication.

The fact that people picked up its usefulness for tic disorders so early was quite striking.

Well, this was based on an observation by Jean Bobon, I believe. Simply in a mental a schizophrenic patient with tics, probably a case of Gilles de la Tourette's disease. He responded very well to low doses of haloperidol and other patients with tics were then treated with small doses and in general the effects were quite obvious and published.

Out of that you could deduce potentially the idea that some of the delusions in haloperidol-responsive forms of schizophrenia are mental tics.

Well, yes. This is the stereotypy hypothesis which is in my opinion more than a hypothesis – it's obvious.

On that point, one of the arguments you get from someone like Tom Ban is that 40 years ago what we ought to have done when we found that drugs like chlorpromazine and haloperidol worked was to have defined much more clearly which were the groups of people that they worked for and tried to work out the psychopathological consequences of that. Instead the industry hurled compound after compound at us and we have never had a chance to actually take stock.

We tried very hard using all kinds of tricks and internally it worked very well. One of my pet ideas has always been that schizophrenics for whom haloperidol works well are stereotyped in their movements and their thinking and in their behaviour. As if they have no internal inhibition in the Pavlovian sense of the word. As if they cannot shift from one idea to another very easily. This is a feature of amphetamine poisoning too.

I remember the construction of a small gadget with 10 knobs numbered 1–10. Volunteers in the laboratory were asked to push these knobs at random following the rhythm of a metronome 200 times consecutively and this was then analysed statistically for randomness. These volunteers were able to maintain randomness but if a schizophrenic was asked then he could only do it for a short period of time. After five or six times or so, he would push three and then four, three-four, three-four, three-four. He couldn't do it but if you give him a neuroleptic his performance improved.

I also remember playing around with stimulating the pupil of individuals with invisible light but light of sufficient intensity to create measurable miosis. If you do that there is rapid extinction – in other words the first stimulus produces miosis, the second less, the third even less and after four or five stimuli there is no miosis anymore – except in schizophrenics. In schizophrenics the miotic response continues without extinction. They don't seem to be able to distinguish between what is relevant and what is irrelevant. They seem to be unable to extinguish irrelevant stimuli. In this sense it is the opposite of Parkinsonism. When I talk to Parkinson's patients about their movements, they all claim the same thing, which is that there is a considerable delay between the decision to start the movement and the actual start of the movement. It takes a long time for a Parkinson's patient to actually start doing what is intended. It seems to me that with the untreated schizophrenic it is exactly the opposite – that he cannot but respond to every stimulus and of course being forced to respond it is no wonder that his response is stereotyped. This is the way I see it.

This is probably the reason why the striatum plays such an important role in the mechanism of action of neuroleptics. Because it is in the striatum that internal inhibition is creacted – not in the cortex. This is why I have always believed that the real therapeutic effect of a neuroleptic is indeed a neurological effect. If you do it right internal inhibition is restored. If you overdo it you get something that resembles Parkinson's disease.

What was Jean Delay like?

Jean Delay was a very famous psychiatrist but he was really more interested in literature and in the French academy than he was in psychiatry. He was in charge of the Department of Psychiatry at Hôpital Sainte Anne in Paris but in fact he delegated a lot to Deniker and Pichot.

Did he see patients?

That was far below his dignity. He spent most of his time writing books on Andre Gide and attending meetings of the French Academy. His main interest was the French language. He was really an academician above all. Not only did he not like psychiatry, he actually disliked it. It was not easy to come in contact with Jean Delay.

So he is not then the person who actually discovered chlorpromazine?

The way it happened as far as I can figure out is that Rhône-Poulenc synthesised chlorpromazine as an extension of the antihistamine series; I suppose everybody knows that story. When the pharmacology was done and published by Mlle

Courvoisier it was obvious that this was something completely new. Mlle Courvoisier was thinking of a possible application in anaesthesiology because the compound was first given to an anaesthesiologist by the name of Henri Laborit, who tested it in patients and noticed, because he was a good observer, that they became indifferent. That was the main effect he observed – the fact that it made people indifferent. He had a brilliant idea which was simply that this could conceivably be beneficial in the treatment of certain psychiatric disorders. So he convinced Rhône-Poulenc that it would be a good idea to test it in psychiatry. But in those days, the idea of treating psychosis was considered ridiculous, because psychosis by definition was an incurable disease. When I was young one of the definitions of psychosis included incurability. If the psychosis disappeared, this was indicative of a misdiagnosis. The idea that it could be cured with a pill was ridiculed as simply too childish an idea.

I really do not know how Rhône-Poulenc established contact with Jean Delay but he must have somehow accepted the idea of having this compound tested. His contribution was to coin the word neuroleptic, a very nice word in my opinion with a very clear meaning implying a compound inducing striatal effects. This was, as far as I can tell, Jean Delay's main contribution to the field because he delegated the clinical investigation of chlorpromazine to one of his two principal assistants.

He had two assistants: Deniker and Pichot; Deniker got chlorpromazine. This created, of course, problems within his own service because Pichot was not very pleased. Deniker was somewhat older than Pichot and that is probably why it went to him. Deniker, of course, didn't test chlorpromazine himself but he had another psychiatrist working for him who then reported to him and this is probably how the whole picture emerged. The haloperidol part of the story is, of course, better known to me because I was a witness. Haloperidol, a little bit later, was given to Pichot, Deniker's rival in a certain sense.

Did Pichot actually see the patients or...

Pichot saw patients but not very many. Fortunately he had a very good assistant, a woman by the name of Mlle Lempérière. She was really a very good observer and she took care of the patients and reported back to Pichot. Most of the actual work and the observations were done by Mlle Lempérière as far as I can figure out. When I wanted to know something about the clinical effects of haloperidol, after a very short period of time I realised that the most effective way of knowing was to talk to Mme Lempérière.

I have always been convinced that the quality of the observation in psychiatry in particular is much more important than the quantity. The Goldstein double-blind test work on chlorpromazine versus placebo convinced me of this.

How was that?

Well, briefly one of the first double-blind studies published in the American literature was a study by a psychiatrist working in Miami called Goldstein. He compared 4 g of chlorpromazine per day with placebo in what he called chronic schizophrenic patients. And the conclusion was that there was no difference in efficacy – not even in side-effects.

I went to see him because we ran into similar problems with haloperidol, where American patients apparently were said to be very different from European patients. I said well, this is strange, what on earth is going on on the other side of the ocean? So I went to Miami. I saw Dr Goldstein for the first time sitting behind a large beautiful mahogany desk on one side of the street. On the other side, there was a State Hospital and a large building filled with computers. This was in the 1960s: huge computers with punch cards and lots of girls punching cards and filling boxes.

I asked Dr Goldstein to show me the patients because I could not believe that there were patients who could tolerate 4 g of chlorpromazine without side-effects more serious than those observed with placebo. I simply could not believe the story. There was something wrong. Goldstein when he entered the State Hospital did not even know how to open the doors and it was obvious that he did not know his observers. It also became evident that he had hardly ever seen the patients. He had a small army of paid observers who were walking around the wards from morning to evening, filling in cards and rating the patients. But they could hardly read or write and they were obviously quite indifferent – they could not care less. They hardly knew what they were doing and it was very monotonous to rate patients – always the same patients, always the same ratings. I had the impression that they filled in the cards practically at random because they knew that it was all blind and that the quality of their work was impossible to control. Then the raw data sheets went from the observers to the girls who punched the cards and of course it became very clear this was 'garbage in and garbage out'. It was so crude and unreliable that even a difference between 4 g of chlorpromazine and placebo was not detected.

From that day on I have always been very sceptical when it comes to double-blind trials because the same risk exists everywhere. I don't know of any learned professor or any very good observer who takes the trouble of doing what the protocols require in terms of observing. Certainly not in psychiatry. But what is the reliability of a psychiatric observation if it is done by somebody who does not know anything about psychiatry? I am not talking about theoretical psychiatry, I am talking about someone who knows how to observe psychiatric patients.

Did the Goldstein study have much impact at the time?

Well, chlorpromazine was first approved in the United States by the Food and Drug Administration as an antiemetic. Even SmithKline & French, who had the rights to sell it under a licence agreement with Rhône-Poulenc, did not believe in its activity in psychiatric patients. They thought that this was an invention of some queer French psychiatrist. It was only after the compound was marketed as an antiemetic that it was used more and more by psychiatrists. A few years later it was officially approved for that use in the United States. But even then as far as I can remember, there was no double-blind evidence for its use in psychiatry. In order to get something approved double-blind tests were not always required as they are today. I presume, but I am not sure, that the FDA approved chlorpromazine because they were pressured by family members and various pressure groups. We had pimozide approved in the States for Gilles de la Tourette's disease for the same reason, not because we had so much double-blind evidence but because the associations of parents of patients were actually pushing very hard on the basis that in some patients the effect was so obvious, they claimed, that they could not do without it.

Was the Goldstein study then picked up by the psychotherapists as evidence that neuroleptics did not work as they had always said?

When Rhône-Poulenc asked Deniker to go to the States and promote chlorpromazine for the first time, he was ridiculed by the psychoanalysts because psychiatry in the States in those days was dominated particularly in the large cities by very expensive psychoanalysts and the idea that a simple pill without psychoanalysis could actually be beneficial to patients with delusions and with hallucinations was ridiculed. So much so that Deniker came back completely exasperated after about 2 weeks.

But wasn't there something similar to some extent from psychiatrists here? Divry, Bobon's boss, was never convinced that haloperidol was effective despite the evidence?

Well Divry was the Professor of Psychiatry in Liège and he was super-sceptical. He would practically never use the word schizophrenia. I remember that he once told me: don't believe Bobon; I am telling you, young man, nobody will ever cure schizophrenia. What he really meant was chronic hebephrenia because only patients with a very low IQ who were chronically ill were in his opinion probably suffering from schizophrenia. All the others were doubtful and he was not interested. He was constantly looking at slides of brains and he was more interested in the shape of the brain of a human being than in psychiatry. He was a strange man and he played no role at all in the development of haloperidol.

But Jean Bobon, who was his first assistant, was eager of course to get Divry's job because Divry was approaching retirement. He was very eager to publish something because he had never published and that played a role. I had never been in contact with psychiatrists and I was very pleased that there was at least somebody who was willing to look at haloperidol.

You had problems with your licensing in the States...

With Searle, yes. Searle was a large company in Skokie, Illinois, run by its founder, Jack Searle, who described himself as a glorified book-keeper. They were doing very well and they were good licensees for one of our antidiarrhoeals – Lomotil. That was doing very well and we got substantial royalty income from them. But we had signed a contract and under the contract Searle had the right of first refusal on anything that came out of our research laboratory.

The day came when Jack Searle had to make up his mind whether or not to exercise his right of first refusal for haloperidol in the United States. His decision was negative. His argument was: I am only a glorified book-keeper but we have tried twice to launch a psychotropic drug in the States and we failed twice – first with Dartal and then with Mornidine. Dartal, chemically speaking, was simply acetylated perphenazine or Trilafon. Trilafon has a terminal -OH group which can be acetylated and when you do this you get Dartal. Its main metabolite is Trilafon so there is absolutely no difference between the two. Trilafon had been on the market for a long time and was relatively successful and sold by Schering. Searle with their new compound had nothing to add and they didn't know the field and therefore they didn't sell much.

Mornidine was also a phenothiazine and antiemetic. But it had a very powerful alpha-blocking action and therefore orthostatic hypotension was a common side-effect. This is the main reason why it failed. So Searle said he was not going to make the same mistake three times. In England, in Australia, in South Africa, in Japan, all right, but not with Searle in the States. And this is why haloperidol is still sold by Searle in part of the world under the trade name Serenace but not in the US.

This refusal to me was like Searle planning to kill my brainchild in a certain sense. I said: anything you want but not that. So we discontinued our relationship with Searle and as a result we eventually merged with Johnson & Johnson a few years later. That shows how important one seemingly minor misjudgement can be. Otherwise we would probably have merged with Searle. It is very strange. The fact that Denber had published these negative articles of course strengthened Searle's hand because Jack Searle was led to believe that Americans reacted differently to haloperidol than Europeans did. It is unbelievable but true and I could not really convince him, unfortunately.

From all you have said one could draw the conclusion that you believe that the escalation of doses that we had during the 1960s and 1970s and 1980s has been one of the great crimes. Why did it happen?

Yes, it did a lot of harm. It happened under the influence of American psychiatrists, some of whom I know, who thought that drug-resistant schizophrenics were not given sufficient doses and that more must be better. This, of course, was not resisted by marketing people because the more they sell the better. So this was in a certain sense a conspiracy between psychiatrists who expected to see better results with higher doses of haloperidol and the marketing people, particularly at McNeil, who were pushing the use of these high doses in order to sell as much as possible, in my opinion. This is something that should never have happened because first of all the results were not better except maybe in a few cases. And secondly the whole world became scared of so-called tardive dyskinesia and all kinds of other irreversible extrapyramidal side-effects or EPS.

Could one argue, as well, that to some extent the drugs have been used punitively almost in that they have been used as a means of behavioural control at times in, perhaps, wards where say the ratio of nurses to patients is not all that it should be?

I have always been a strong believer in the fact that in order to get good results with neuroleptics one had to determine what I call the optimal dose, because the difference between a low ineffective dose and a high overdose is small. The optimal dose concept is rather crucial in my opinion. If a patient needs 3 mg don't give him 5. If he only needs 1 mg don't give him 3. I have always been a strong believer in the usefulness of the handwriting test as described by the German psychiatrist, HJ Haase, more than three decades ago.

Hanns Hippius put it to me that yourself and Jean Delay and Haase between you were the people who came up with the idea that in order to have a neuroleptic you have to have a compound that produces extrapyramidal side-effects, while he held out for the possibility of a non-neuroleptic antipsychotic – like clozapine.

I think I know the clozapine story from the beginning to the end. It is not a very nice story. Clozapine was synthesised for the first time by a chemist working for the Swiss company Wander. Stille did the pharmacology and he realised that it was a weak sedative neuroleptic but in his opinion not interesting enough to be tested clinically, so it was shelved. Then Wander was bought by Sandoz, who hoped to find lots of interesting new compounds at Wander but didn't find anything. They started scratching and scratching and found compounds that had been shelved like clozapine. They asked Stille – who later became a good friend – why on earth didn't he test this compound clinically and he answered that it was not interesting enough in his opinion. Sandoz said: well, we have paid a lot of money for Wander and we need something out of it and as marketing people we know that if we can make the world believe that this compound is maybe not as potent as chlorpromazine or haloperidol but free of EPS, then some psychiatrists at least will prescribe it. Because in these days EPS was already something that people were very afraid of.

Psychologically they were right. They approached people like Hippius and convinced him to test clozapine clinically and to start spreading the gospel that this was an atypical neuroleptic free of EPS. It is true that tolerated doses are virtually free of EPS side-effects. It is a neuroleptic in the sense of Delay but only at very high doses. It is above all a very potent alpha blocker. It is a relatively weak S2 antagonist.

Hanns Hippius is a very good friend of mine. His photograph is over there but if he were sitting here I would tell you exactly the same story. Actually I met him in Munich some months ago and we discussed this very openly. He did not contradict my story. Hanns was working in a famous clinic in Munich in charge of the administration and patients were seen as a rule by assistants – Herr Professor did not see many patients. But he went to all congresses you can think of trying to spread the gospel that clozapine actually was an atypical neuroleptic and had no effect on the striatal system and was free of EPS. It was completely different and not a neuroleptic but very potent. Sandoz then marketed the compound until it was found to produce agranulocytosis and then it was withdrawn from the market.

That, I thought, was the end of clozapine. Then, several years later, under the influence of Meltzer, the same story was spread all over again in the States. When Meltzer talks, he pronounces the word clozapine at least once in every sentence, if not twice. He tries to make the whole world believe that it is in the patient's benefit to be treated with clozapine in spite of the fact that his blood has to be monitored every week.

But it does seem to do something for some patients that some of the others ...

It sedates. In my opinion this is all. I would very much like to see these fantastic patients that they are always referring to. I have been looking for them but I have never seen them. It all depends on what we want and what we are talking about. In my opinion a good compound for the treatment of patients with symptoms resembling amphetamine poisoning are drugs that will have a very clear-cut effect on hallucinations, delusions, improve human contact and are active if necessary against psychomotor agitation without side-effects. This is what we should be looking for and this is not at all the case with clozapine. It is practically impossible to treat acute cases with clozapine without running into terrible problems with alpha blockade, for instance. Most of the clozapine patients I have seen are severely sedated. This is not what we want. But it is understandable that if patients are troublesome in a hospital setting and if they are being treated with heavily sedating neuroleptics the nurses have an easier time and are satisfied. Well, if this is the criterion, then yes. I may be exaggerating a little but in my opinion this whole field of the so-called 'atypical neuroleptic' is a pure invention. I would not know how to define an atypical neuroleptic; what on earth does that mean? The word neuroleptic, as coined by Jean Delay, has a very specific meaning. It is by definition a compound that can induce extrapyramidal side-effects.

So can you have an antipsychotic that is not a neuroleptic?

This is what we have been looking for for 50 years now. We and others have never found it. I don't like the word antipsychotic. What are the drugs that we know to be of interest in the treatment of severely diseased psychiatric patients? – the typical neuroleptics and reserpine. What else? I don't know of anything else. Everybody and his brother has tried to find drugs devoid of neuroleptic activity but active in the clinic but each time we have tested such compounds in the clinic we have failed – like everybody else unfortunately. If the dopamine story is correct then we should not be surprised.

If it is correct why do we need the $5HT_2$ input?

Well, what always struck me was that so many chronic schizophrenics not only hallucinate and have delusions and difficulty to establish human contact but they also complain of sleep disturbances and if we actually objectively measure their EEG it is very abnormal. Many of them even sleep during the day and walk around at night or wake up repeatedly. And many of them claim to feel rotten because they have not slept well. This is very common. There is the same symptomatology in dysthymic patients. You don't have to be a schizophrenic to have these symptoms.

When we started looking for pure centrally active serotonin antagonists, the first compound we discovered was ritanserin, which is not on the market. We did not really have the slightest idea of what a serotonin antagonist would do

– except of course antagonise some of the effects of LSD. To our enormous surprise the most obvious effect of this compound, in animals at least, was an effect on sleep. In man it doubled deep sleep – phase 3 and 4 sleep – from 2 hours a night to 4 hours. In these days we had a sleep lab in England with Chris Idzikowski doing most of the work. We studied this compound in normal volunteers and in dysthymic patients – most of these dysthymic patients are seen by GP's, not by psychiatrists. Ian Oswald in Edinburgh looked at this and he became convinced that this compound was very active in the treatment of what the Americans called neurotic depression but what many others prefer to call dysthymia – basically patients who claim not to sleep well. They are not able to have deep sleep – stages 3 and 4 – and when they wake up in the morning they feel lousy. If this goes on for a while, they get depressed. If you make these people sleep better with ritanserin, objectively deep sleep reappears and their complaints disappear. They stop claiming that they have not slept well and they start feeling fit in the morning. They are less depressed, life becomes more bearable and even pleasurable. This is very unusual for these patients because typical dysthymic patients in my experience have forgotten what pleasure really is. Many of them even end up committing suicide.

So for reasons that are not clear to me, dysthymia in schizophrenic patients is very common. Typical dopamine receptor blockers like haloperidol have virtually no effect on sleep. Sleep does not get better or worse: one of the shortcomings of typical neuroleptics. And I believe we have learned that sleep disturbances can be improved with at least some S2 antagonists like ritanserin. But instead of launching ritanserin plus haloperidol, we tried to find a drug which has the two properties, hoping to have less trouble with compliance. With hindsight, this was probably a mistake because we had done studies with patients who were receiving Haldol decanoate optimum dose plus ritanserin and the effects were the same as with risperidone.

In the meantime, I have learned that patients with sleep disturbances when treated with S2 blockers, like ritanserin or risperidone, fairly often feel very much better. They actually like these drugs. This to me is new because as you know many schizophrenics when treated with Haldol don't like it at all. I actually have rarely seen a patient saying I like to take your haloperidol but I have seen many patients and I have received even more letters from patients and their family members about risperidone saying: I feel so very much better, this is changing my life and thank you very much for having discovered it. So there must be something new and this has nothing to do with the schizophrenia itself but with the fact, in my view, that these patients simply sleep better and as a result feel much better, can cope much better and can be more easily reintegrated into society.

Would the market conditions have been as good for Risperdal as they have if clozapine had not been reinvented? It helped to push out the D2-S2 story.

Well I simply expect clozapine to completely disappear and I am very surprised it hasn't disappeared already, because to test the patient's blood every week is not very pleasant. An incidence of agranulocytosis of 1% is not to be taken lightly. To me the word agranulocytosis is more frightening than EPS. Maybe I am blind but when I compare patients treated with Risperdal to those who are treated with clozapine the difference is so huge that even a blind psychiatrist must see it. That is one reason. The second is simply an economic reason. The treatment of patients with clozapine is very much more expensive. So these are two reasons and then purely from a scientific point of view I would like this confusing story to disappear.

Up until about 1988 people seemed to be proceeding down the lines of producing more specific compounds, more specific D2 blockers in particular, and that has all been thrown open now. Was clozapine not responsible for that?

I have never been influenced by clozapine. Clozapine has created an enormous amount of confusion – enormous. It has set psychiatry back, I believe, for a decade or two. All I am saying is only what I am convinced of, by the way. I hope it is right.

Let me hop back to 1957. At the time you seem to have been interested to enter the psychiatric market, which was unusual because companies then weren't terribly interested in psychiatry. It took someone like Jean Delay to force Rhône-Poulenc to develop chlorpromazine for mental illness. Without him they would not have been interested, it seems to me. So why were you open to the idea?

Don't forget in those days we were not a pharmaceutical company, we were a research company. In 1953, my objective was not to create an international pharmaceutical company but to create an independent research company. Marketing did not even enter the field. I knew nothing about marketing. We were not selling anything. Everything was sold under licence by others. McNeil, for instance, was our licensee but before that SmithKline & French was our first licensee, second was Searle with Lomotil and the third was McNeil and in Japan we have had lots of licensees. So marketing considerations did not play a role.

For instance, when we started looking for these very potent morphine-like drugs this was not because of marketing considerations. On the contrary, everybody was saying: what are you going to do with these things? After we had found them, we discovered that they were useful in anaesthesiology. Today they are very widely used and we have a kind of monopoly because marketing-wise they are not very profitable. One of our compounds, Sufentanyl, a very potent morphine-like compound, is used in at least 80% of all cases of cardiac surgery worldwide. Without it, I don't believe that cardiac surgery would have achieved what it has done. So these were considerations that did not even enter my mind – fortunately, because otherwise we wouldn't have done it.

Or, take synthetic antidiarrhoeals: we have a kind of monopoly in this field. They are morphine-like drugs that do not enter the CNS and so are better than codeine because they produce absolutely no CNS effects and their abuse liability is zero. All of this came out of our morphine research but this was not anticipated. We were trying to find active compounds and after having found active compounds we tried to answer the question: what could they be used for? – not the other way around. Not first a marketing consideration and then research but first research and then marketing considerations.

I always thought from the very first day when we started this research company in 1953 that somebody who would be better than anybody else in finding novel and better compounds would have an easy time – would practically automatically become rich. This was true because today we have approximately 34 Janssen companies all over the world selling most of the compounds we discovered on a large scale. Until very recently we still were a research-oriented company where research was really calling the shots and marketing was simply doing what research suggested.

Research can be looked upon as a goal or as a means. I have always considered research as a goal in itself – like playing chess or any other game. And I have always tried to be the world champion in a certain field. Today more and more people in the pharmaceutical industry are looking at research just as a means to make more money, literally speaking. This usually doesn't work and I have no sympathy for it. I believe drug research only makes sense when it benefits patients. To put it in other words I am not ashamed to make a lot of money but only when the drugs we have discovered offer great benefits to patients – it is only reasonable that these patients should pay some money for what we are doing for them. It is like a medical doctor asking for a fee. I am not ashamed of that but I would really be ashamed of selling clozapine, for instance. I would never do that never.

There is a feeling you get from some people who work within the industry these days that there has been a change within the pharmaceutical industry. Whereas before people who were researchers or clinical people headed up the companies, now it is the MBAs and this is not helpful development.

What is paralysing the industry in general as far as I can tell are these regulations called good laboratory practices, good manufacturing practices, good clinical practices etc. In other words everything seems to be based on the assumption that we are all cheating and lying and we have to prove almost daily that we are not. Unfortunately some people are cheating and lying and therefore it's understandable. But today, people in industry are complaining that they are spending more and more time filling in all kinds of forms and protocols and they have less and less time to do research. This is true because if you really have to follow good clinical practice, for instance, then you have to fill in I don't know how many pages per patient.

Is there more than just that though? For instance, I can see the role that GCP plays in all this, but take a company like Ciba-Geigy who in the early 1970s had a string of compounds in the pipeline: early SSRIs, interesting neuroleptics and a whole range of other compounds but none of them ever came to the market. There seems to have been some corporate failure there.

The case of Ciba-Geigy I can explain because Ciba-Geigy is one of our best licensees in the field of plant protection. In the field of plant protection we have always done research, and other companies the selling, until recently. We have been very successful in finding the most widely used antimycotics, for instance, in plant protection and Ciba-Geigy has always been one of our licensees. Now what was wrong with Ciba-Geigy? What was wrong is that the bureaucracy was even worse than here. They had one big tower called research, another tower called development, a third tower called sales, another tower called production and there was too little contact between these towers. The man who was in charge of the development of plant protection was the late Professor Franz Schwinn, who became a very good friend after a while. He was frustrated because he didn't get anything of interest out of research, and if development doesn't get anything interesting out of research what can it hope to do? Management, of course, was constantly complaining that Franz Schwinn wasn't doing a good job.

He learned that there were some azoles available here in Beerse that, in his opinion and in ours of course, were promising drugs for the treatment of fungal diseases in plants. So when we met, he asked whether we would be willing to work with him. He 'jumped' at our azoles and developed them like nobody else ever did. He was very good at it and in a certain sense saved Ciba-Geigy. Now what was his motivation? His motivation was to show that there was nothing wrong with his development group but that there was everything wrong with the research group at Ciba-Geigy. We were both happy of course. We were happy because he was doing such a wonderful job with the compounds we had discovered and he was happy because he saved Ciba-Geigy. Unfortunately the management of Ciba-Geigy is flying so high in the sky, the story as I am telling it to you is probably even today not generally acknowledged.

Then there is something else that I am seeing more and more and that is that it seems to have become fashionable these days to 'manage by fear' – to manage by saying: if you are not going to do what I tell you to do I am going to fire and replace you. It is brutal, it is stupid and it doesn't work. But that is what is going on in the world. It is terrible. I have always tried to convince people – to follow the philosophy that good people need to be convinced and by definition don't need to be controlled.

I always believed that in order to be successful, certainly in a large company, decentralised management is essential. To decentralise and to delegate is very simple if you have good people because good people by definition don't need to be controlled. But today everything is being controlled all the time. Good laboratory practices actually demand that everything should be controlled all the time. Good people don't like to be controlled. I certainly don't. It demotivates. So the system itself I believe is rotten.

But the system is there because of the individuals who, as you say, have cheated.

Yes, criminals should be put in jail but unfortunately we cannot prevent crime. Cheating cannot be prevented. In my opinion it is very stupid to cheat: it is much more clever to be honest. The advantages of virtue are so obvious that people should practise virtue out of self-interest. People who cheat are simply being stupid and will be caught sooner or later. They will lose their credibility and they should be severely punished in my opinion. But the idea behind these good laboratory practices is to prevent cheating and that is impossible.

I don't know whether you know the story of Mr Poggiolini in Italy. He is now in jail but he used to be the head of the Italian food and drug administration. He was called Mr 10%. Being the oldest of all of his colleagues in Europe, at one point in time he eventually became number one in Europe. Today he is in prison in Naples and he is telling his story. This was the man who called the shots – who had to control the industry, yet he was a cheat. Who was controlling him? Maybe I am getting too old ...

One of the other people who began with a very successful drug during the 1950s and his own company to some extent but who didn't develop in the same way as you was Frank Berger.

I have known Frank Berger quite well and was even present, by pure coincidence, when the word tranquilliser was born. Do you know who the inventor of the word was? Nathan Kline. Frank Berger had invented Miltown, as you know, and he was about to launch it as a modern sedative. He was a friend of mine and we were having dinner in a restaurant in New York with Nathan Kline, who had done some clinical studies with Miltown, seeing sedative effects but nothing very pronounced. Berger was talking about his ideas of how to launch this product. He already had his trade name, Miltown. But he was going to call it a sedative and Nathan Kline said: you are out of your mind. The world doesn't need new sedatives. What the world really needs is a 'tranquilliser'. The world needs tranquillity. Why don't you call this a tranquilliser? You will sell ten times more. Frank Berger was not a fool and he followed the advice of Nathan Kline, called meprobamate a tranquilliser and was quite successful for a while.

Very successful.

Yes, until Roche took the market over with Librium. Randall, who did the pharmacology, was a good friend and he compared all the new compounds with Miltown, which was the enemy to be beaten. Miltown was only active at high doses and Librium was quickly seen by the whole world as being a big leap in the right direction and now we have the other benzodiazepines and God knows what else.

This is important because when we tried in the United States to introduce the word neuroleptic the Americans did not want to hear the word neuroleptic. It was unknown to them, this invention by a strange Frenchman, Jean Delay. Rather than use the word neuroleptic they preferred to call neuroleptics 'major tranquillisers'. Minor and major tranquillisers! I have done my utmost to change this but the word tranquilliser, although invented for promotional purposes by Nathan Kline and although it had nothing to do with neuroleptics, was used in the American literature for a few decades. It is only recently that words like neuroleptics and antipsychotics are replacing it.

What did you make of Nathan Kline?

I liked him. He was funny. He was also one of the first investigators of haloperidol in the States. He wrote me a letter saying: your compound is worthless – I have treated 10 patients, giving them 1 mg the first day, 2 mg the second, 4 mg the next, 8 mg the next , 16 the next. He doubled the dose every day and he said he had to stop treatment in all cases because of side-effects. He was a clown. I liked his jokes and I liked the way he told his stories, like how he invented iproniazid, for instance. I never knew what was true and not true. We met rather regularly. He used to play a very important role in what was called biological psychiatry.

What was the role?

Well, it was very dangerous to contradict him. He was a good speaker, very out-spoken and he was opinionated. To contradict Nathan Kline was politically very dangerous. People were afraid of him and certainly by the end of his life he behaved like a kind of a Pope. At the end he had this habit of coming to con-gresses with a small dog on his lap and patting it all the time and attracting attention whilst smiling to the speaker. And he liked to ridicule.

There were a few famous psychiatrists at that time who actually never did anything. Max Hamilton, for instance, was even more incredible. He was Professor in Leeds and his only contribution, except for a rating scale, was that each time somebody had something to say Max would stand up and say 'My dear friend, it's not as simple as you seem to believe. It is much more compli-cated. You are naive.' And he would then sit down. He would actually never make a positive remark. Everybody was very afraid when Max was in the room because he knew how to ridicule people.

During both the 1960s and 1970s psychiatry and the emerging neurosciences seemed to work quite closely together. Recently things seem to have changed. When you go to the large meetings like the CINP or ACNP, it seems to me that there is an increasing gulf between the two. Neuroscience has become so large, so technical – perhaps too large to be constrained within the clinical domain anymore. It seems to me that there are increasing strains in groups like the ACNP where you get the clinical people unable to see the relevance in all of this. Do we need to be going along to meetings where there is so much esoteric neuro-science? Do you think there is a problem?

It seems to me – this may be a biased view – that the famous gap between clini-cians and biochemists or biologists is, if anything, increasing and the role of slo-gans is increasing – slogans in the general sense of the word. When, for instance, I try to explain to our pharmacologists who have never seen patients, how a schizophrenic patient looks I have the greatest trouble. I try to tell them that schizophrenia is a word invented by Bleuler half a century ago – not a disease but a word. In my way of thinking it is very difficult to accept that this particular word invented by Bleuler can be one disease entity. This is important because we are constantly bombarded with the question: what is the aetiology of schizo-phrenia. And my answer is that the aetiology of schizophrenia is Dr Bleuler.

I am personally very influenced by the fact that in biochemical genetics it becomes more and more obvious that diseases which look like a homogeneous entity, when the chips are down are far from homogeneous. A good example is retinitis pigmentosa. I always thought it was was one inherited disease. But at the moment there are at least 80 different mutations known, all 80 leading to what looks clinically like one disease. So if this is true for retinitis pigmentosa, what odds schizophrenia being one disease?

But can I put it to you that one of the forces holding schizophrenia together at the moment as just one entity isn't just Bleuler and the grin of the Cheshire Cat that was left behind after he died but the industry. They have got to have a big schizophrenia in order to be able to market compounds. If schizophrenia were to fragment so that the target populations were not as big, industry's interest in developing drugs for any of these smaller groups would be much less.

That is true. We have very often been confronted with the problem of how to promote new drugs and all I can tell you is that if we were to do it using purely scientific language then not a single box would be sold. So in a certain sense the industry is practically forced to use simple language. I call that slogans. Slogans in the sense of hypersimplifications of the truth. It is probably human nature that most people are more interested in slogans than in dry scientific facts.

But the interest of the industry in the treatment of schizophrenia is relatively new. For instance, haloperidol was very difficult to sell in a country like Italy for purely economical reasons. To sell drugs to hospitals in Italy used to be a terrible idea because the inflation was very high and these hospitals would not pay. So there was nobody really interested. In the early 1960s in the United States there was practically nobody interested. Rhône-Poulenc, for instance, had a difficult job to find an interested partner in the United States for chlorpromazine.

Rhône-Poulenc was of course one of the largest pharmaceutical companies in Europe and in those days from a research point of view probably the best. After Laborit had done his work and then Delay and Deniker, Deniker was sent by Rhône-Poulenc to the United States to try to sell the idea of a pill being able to make voices and delusions disappear. In those days psychiatry in the States was dominated by psychoanalysts. They ridiculed Deniker, whose English was poor, and rather than stay a month in the States he came back after two weeks, and after five conferences rather than the scheduled 20 or 30, completely exhausted and completely disgusted because they systematically ridiculed this 'silly Frenchman' with psychotherapeutic arguments. Nobody seemed to believe him.

At the same time Rhône-Poulenc approached the large pharmaceutical companies in the States – Upjohn, Parke-Davis, Eli Lilly and quite a number of others – but chlorpromazine was turned down by all of them – because they didn't believe it and because they couldn't see a market. Schizophrenia was completely unknown to them. Don't forget marketing people working in the pharmaceutical industry know nothing about medicine. They know something about existing markets. They have books and there is a market for this and a market for that but in those days there was no market for schizophrenia. They opened their book looking for a schizophrenia market, reported back to management that there was no such market and that was the end of the story. What really saved Rhône-Poulenc was SmithKline and French.

SK&F in those days was a small company in Philadelphia exclusively selling amphetamine as Dexedrine. They had a pharmacologist working for them by the name of Leonard Cook. In desperation Rhône-Poulenc had offered chlorpromazine to SK&F, being unable to find a big company. A sample was given to Cook, who repeated a few experiments described by Mlle Courvoisier. One of these was an antiemetic experiment with apomorphine in dogs and he showed what Mlle Courvoisier claimed in her first publication, namely that chlorpromazine is a very powerful antiemetic. Cook reported to management – because the company was so small a pharmacologist still had access to the top – and he said: well, the strange stories these funny psychiatrists are telling may not be true but I can assure you this is a damn potent antiemetic. So the management of SK&F took the decision to develop chlorpromazine as an antiemetic. They simply forgot psychiatry. For this reason chlorpromazine was first approved as an antiemetic by the FDA. No psychiatric studies had been conducted – only antiemetic studies. Officially psychiatrists were not supposed to prescribe chlorpromazine but under the influence of probably European colleagues they started prescribing it and eventually they started to realise that Delay and Deniker were not hallucinating and they slowly started to believe it.

This is where the major tranquilliser story comes in because commercially speaking they could see the success of tranquillisers but they were still not convinced that there was a market in the treatment of schizophrenia. This is why they started calling chlorpromazine 'a major tranquilliser', hoping that it could somehow be used not only in schizophrenia but in as many psychiatric patients as possible. They were even hoping that it would compete with meprobamate, Librium and Valium and other 'tranquillisers'. The implication of the expression major tranquilliser is that it is better than a minor tranquilliser. So these were two slogans invented by some people at SK&F and taken over by the psychiatric community and by textbooks, even Goodman and Gillman – everybody.

I was blowing my trumpet, saying 'This is nonsense' but nobody was listening. It is obvious both pharmacologically and clinically that Librium has absolutely nothing to do with chlorpromazine. If you call the one a minor tranquilliser and the other a major tranquilliser you are only spreading confusion. These are all funny stories – all of these details of course are not very well known.

Why did your company not get into the antidepressant arena?

That's my fault. First of all because I had a very hard time – even today I have a very hard time – to accurately define depression. As far as I am concerned there are hundreds of different types of depression. The only disease that I know of that in my opinion deserves the name depression is endogenous depression, in other words a psychosis, or the depressive phase of a manic-depressive illness. That is clearly a depression as far as I can see. But in general practice the common type of depression which is so often seen and which is treated by tricyclics, first of all doesn't respond very well to these tricyclics. I really don't know whether they are not doing more harm than good. Secondly, we don't have any animal model to work with. Third, many forms of depression, like for instance dysthymia, are seen by general practitioners, not by psychiatrists, and unfortunately the results of clinical work we are doing with general practitioners these days are no longer believed. Dysthymia, or neurotic depression, is probably the most common form of 'depression' in my opinion.

You actually made a good case for dysthymia being seen as a disease entity as well with the altered sleep stages.

Dysthymia as I define it is something that many general practitioners see every day and usually these patients are treated with benzodiazepines and that usually makes it worse. There is no treatment for dysthymia that I know of except ritanserin. But I am really puzzled with the obvious clinical efficacy of lithium, for instance. There is no animal experiment that would make me predict that lithium would be effective in the treatment of endogenous depression but it is often very effective.

So it is my fault in the sense that in the literature and in our laboratory I have always fought the idea of some of the old pharmacologists who claimed to be interested in making antidepressants – my question has always been: what is an antidepressant? Because the best treatments that I know of for endogenous depression are electoconvulsive therapy and lithium. It may be a biased opinion but for me these two modes of treatment are clinically far more obviously effective than imipramine-like tricyclics.

Imipramine to me is a mysterious drug. I know Kuhn, who was the first to test it in the clinic, and I know Angst, who did I don't know how many double-blind studies with it. To the best of my knowledge there are now and then depressed patients who respond well to imipramine but they are the exception rather than the rule. In classical double-blind tests, for instance, comparing antidepressant A with antidepressant B, a man like Angst was never able to show a difference between groups treated with A versus with B. Many years ago he told me: well, here is what I get with imipramine and here is what I get with this new compound and there is never an obvious therapeutic difference except in side-effect liability. For instance, Prozac is better tolerated than most tricyclics but efficacy-wise it is about the same, not very impressive. Angst never got the permission from the ethical committee to compare imipramine with placebo and he became more and more convinced that to distinguish imipramine from placebo with his protocol was impossible. Not because the compound is inactive but because the percentage of good responders is too low.

I have often put the following question to many psychiatrists: 'How satisfied are you really with whatever you have in the treatment of what you call non-endogenous depression?' And the answer was usually 'Well, I'm satisfied with approximately half of my patients after about 5 weeks.' It's far from obvious therefore. I made a mistake also by believing that it would probably be best to no longer use the word depression because it was so confusing but to use more understandable words like dysthymia and to concentrate on certain types of depression that are more easily understood than other types of depression.

But again the problem will be that if you restrict it and say let's have a drug for melancholia, the response from the marketing division within the company would be: well, this is too small an entity for us to develop drugs for.

Well, the marketing divisions in such companies are doing much more harm than good then. They kill too many good ideas. One could write a book on it. It usually has to do with the fact that when they hear the first rumours about something completely new, they are scared to death. Because there is no such market, they have never seen such patients and they are completely misled by their own slogans.

For instance, one of the areas this laboratory has great success is in the area of mycology. We started doing research in mycology in 1960 when the Belgian Congo had just become independent. I remember very well that everybody told me in 1961 that this was sheer stupidity because all problems that had something to do with mycology could easily be solved with amphotericin B, with potassium iodine or with griseofulvin. Somebody doing research in this field was out of his mind. Incredible but true. This came from some marketing departments. Fortunately in those days we did not have a marketing department. I was simply listening to doctors and veterinarians and people in plant protection who were trying to solve mycological problems without success, and they told me that most problems related to mycological agents could not be adequately solved with what was available. Fortunately, unlike many other people, I was not forced in those days to listen to marketing people, otherwise we probably would not have started.

McNeil, a sister company, was selling griseofulvin – they were promoting it and one of their slogans was 'If you have a mycological problem, griseofulvin will solve it.' They believed that as marketing people tend to believe in their own slogans. They first invent a slogan and they repeat it so often that they believe it even when it is a gross exaggeration, as is usually the case. They are salesmen – they try to promote drugs just like car salesmen – any argument is good as long as it sells.

Drugs like haloperidol were brought out almost 40 years ago now and their cost is now virtually nil. Is that getting in the way of being able to develop new compounds?

Oh yes, of course. In 1953 the cost of research and development of a new chemical entity was a few tens of thousands of dollars approximately. Fortunately for me because that is all I had. In the case of haloperidol probably even less – maybe $20,000–$30,000, everything included, which in those days was considered an enormous amount of money. Today the official estimate is something like $250–$300 million. In my opinion it is much more than that. Johnson & Johnson is spending $1.6 billion in 1996 on what is called

R&D and I don't know how many new chemical entities will come out per year for this tremendous amount of money – only time will tell.

The reason why this tremendous increase occurred has not much to do with research but practically everything with development. I will give you a simple example. In the 1950s and 1960s I was so afraid of being misled by clinicians that I refused to work with clinicians who were asking for money. If they were not interested scientifically, I told them to forget it. But in those days, it was relatively simple to find clinicians who were willing to do whatever was required simply for the sake of their patients and because they were interested. Jean Delay or Jean Bobon, for instance, never asked me for a dime. What was not uncommon was that you would then do clinical investigators a favour after they had done their job. That was a question of being polite and grateful. But to discuss money was simply not done, it was even considered very impolite. Jean Delay I am sure would have been angry if somebody had raised the subject with him.

Today I am not exaggerating when I say that it is simply impossible to do clinical research without discussing money first. And with enough money almost anything can be done apparently. The world has completely changed. As a result of these changes clinical research, or what is called research and development, particularly development, is becoming so incredibly expensive that in my opinion in a few years time it will no longer be justifiable to do it.

Unless it would happen in the Third World?

Theoretically yes, but in practice no. Take the example of malaria, one of the most important diseases of the Third World. Technically with the artemisin derivatives and so on, there are quite a few new drugs that should urgently be investigated clinically because they are, in all probability, very potent. But for reasons that are not clear even the Vietnamese or Chinese, where the disease is very common, are not doing enough. Is this because they don't know how to do it or is this because we ignore what they are doing? Is this because they are publishing in journals that we don't read? Is this because we are not interested in malaria anymore? I don't know. The last antimalarials were discovered and developed for use in the American army during the Second World War as a direct consequence of strategical considerations. Most of the work was done in America. Hundreds of thousands of compounds were synthesised and screened at Walter Reed. Walter Reed now has a very interesting research programme and they have published on an impressive series of drugs that, on paper at least, should be very potent but as far as testing is concerned apparently nothing is happening. Is this because the chronic toxicity requirements are so enormous that even Walter Reed finds it too expensive? Is this because there are too many ethical committees who make it impossible? I don't really know.

As well, in actual practice, for instance, in order to convince the US Food and Drug Administration you have to have US data. They claim that they will accept UK data, for instance, but this is not true. And vice versa. So you have to repeat clinical studies in every important country. That makes it very expensive. Chinese data, for instance, or Vietnamese data in this field are useless because nobody believes them anyway. So it is in a certain sense a loss of time. Again this question of suspicion.

Can you foresee a day when the cost element will actually bring the production of novel compounds to a halt within an area like the neuroleptic area? What about Alzheimer's, where you could bring in new drugs that cost a lot on which you will be able to recoup the cost because you are not constrained by the fact that there are cheaper drugs there?

Well Alzheimer's in the scientific sense of the word is a type of dementia which is inherited. There at least four different types of inherited Alzheimer's. It has become fashionable to use the word Alzheimer's instead of dementia but most demented patients are not suffering from Alzheimer's. Furthermore Alzheimer's is a postmortem diagnosis. So to use drugs specifically for the treatment of Alzheimer's is impossible. But this is a slogan that captures the imagination of practically everybody in the industry – they are all dreaming of selling a drug for Alzheimer's because if the FDA would only allow such a drug to be sold they would make a fortune.

You know better than I do that the treatment of dementia is impossible. The treatment of real Alzheimer's disease is certainly impossible. Patients who don't yet have the lesions would have to swallow pills before the onset of the first symptoms and for the rest of their lives. There is a compliance problem there. This is utopia, I think. It is a dream of sales people that has nothing much to do with real medicine in my opinion nor with 'patient benefit'...

Talking about real medicine why, just when we have become able to produce effective medicines, are people getting so alienated from medicine and turning to alternative methods?

I don't really know but it is a fact, with the only exception of Prozac. My wife and some others tell me that it is becoming fashionable among women to claim to be taking Prozac – that is the only exception I know of. Most so-called intelligent people I meet take pleasure in saying that they never take drugs – only homeopathic medicine or plant extracts. And they are supposed to be intelligent people. I cannot understand that. Except when one assumes that 99% of the complaints of people disappear spontaneously anyway, whether they take something or not. Then of course it is not so difficult to see that almost anything taken with great conviction can have a very strong psychotherapeutic beneficial effect. So that is maybe the reason. Most complaints these people are talking about are of course complaints of self-limiting diseases. Even these people say that for serious disease like cancer or diabetes alternative medicines don't work. They only 'work' for the symptoms like headache or migraine. As a psychiatrist you should be in a better position than I am to explain it. I find it regrettable but it is a fact. I hope I am wrong but I am convinced that the attitude of the world is not only not helping medicine but actually blocking its progress.

Which attitude?

The attitude which takes heed of rumours about negative side-effects of a new drug. Everybody believes these rumours without scrutinising them, without asking questions. People can be made to believe almost anything negative which is scary. The world is becoming more and more sceptical when it comes to accepting positive messages – except when these positive messages are in the form of slogans. A very good example is Taxol, the anticancer drug given to us by 'mother nature', coming from these very rare and expensive tropical forests – three trees per treatment yet it is a simple cytotoxic agent. But if the message can be brought with a slogan that has something to do with 'mother nature' or when a slogan starts with bio, then people are ready to listen. But to listen to so-called dry scientific or rational arguments is the exception rather than the rule.

I don't know, could it be that we are so influenced by modern propaganda that we only tend to pay attention to slogans and to nothing else anymore? When I say we I mean, statistically speaking, mankind in the Western world. We are bombarded by television messages, by slogans not just for soap but for cars and even for drugs apparently. This is something I feel even in the laboratory, where slogans often catch more attention than facts.

It is possible that 50 years ago side-effects were underestimated. When chloroform was killing 1% of patients this was, I wouldn't say accepted, it was certainly regretted, but it didn't stop physicians from using chloroform and I never heard of legal consequences when somebody was killed by it. Today for the slightest thing going wrong patients go and see a lawyer. It seems to me that the population at large is expecting almost miracles from the medical profession and if they don't get these miracles they are dissatisfied. All drugs must work 100% of the time, they must be completely free of side-effects, they must be easy to take and cost virtually nothing. That is what people are led to expect these days.

Talking about side-effects prompts me to ask you about the handwriting test. Who was Haase and when did he come up with the test?

HJ Haase was a psychiatrist in Bonn who did research on gross and fine movements. His handwriting and tapping tests resolved questions in Parkinson's disease but they also first defined the neuroleptic threshold in patients treated with chlorpromazine. That work was impressive and obviously important for haloperidol, so I sent him a message and his reply was enthusiastic.

When we talk about the optimal dose in pharmacology we talk in statistical terms. We talk in terms of an ED_{50} for dogs or rats or mice. This leads to a kind of irrational conviction that there must be something like an optimal dose for everybody of a new drug. The idea that the drugs have to be titrated patient by patient is only accepted for old-fashioned drugs like digitoxin or insulin but not for neuroleptics, for instance. I have the greatest trouble trying to make the point that most neuroleptics have a narrow safety margin of less than 2. It is very easy to overdose or underdose them, and to find the individual optimal dose is not easy. This is not a popular idea. Pharmacologists in general and clinicians prefer to think and talk about the optimal dose for a certain disease.

In the case of Risperdal, for instance, I have seen the results of extensive studies performed in Germany and the lowest optimal dose in a minority of patients was 1mg per day and the highest was 6 mg with the median about 4 mg. This shows that Risperdal is a very potent neuroleptic and not at all an atypical neuroleptic. It does in the handwriting test exactly what typical neuroleptics do. The reason why psychiatrists are so satisfied with Risperdal is because fortunately we have been stressing the point that the dose of 6 mg per day should not be exceeded. At 6 mg per day the number of patients reacting with EPS is low but not zero. We have done that because over and above 6 mg you get into problems with EPS, sedation and with orthostatic hypotension. Also if a patient's response is not good with 6 mg, the probability that it will be better with a higher dose is low.

I have always been convinced that 1 mg of haloperidol is active in some patients. We took 1 mg ourselves here. In those days I was rather nervous and I could easily tell the difference between 1 mg of haloperidol and placebo simply because the neuroleptic made me less nervous. I had to guess eight times and I guessed right eight times out of eight, which carries a probability of one chance in 256. One of my collaborators was a rather phlegmatic individual who was far from nervous but he was also right eight times out of eight. Do you know why? – because it made him lazy. He could feel it all right but for completely different reasons. So there was an obvious correlation between personality and effect.

There do seem to be some people who are made very demotivated by a neuroleptic and others who are not. These areas are unexplored really, aren't they?

In recent years virtually nothing has been done – because this is typically a type of experiment that is no longer allowed by ethical committees. There is no potential clinical benefit expected and therefore we are no longer allowed to do these things. It is a bit strange but there is in my view a great need to do these simple experiments.

I sense you have a certain scepticism about the history of psychopharmacology. Do you think there is anything we can do in the area of history other than compile lists of who was voted onto which committee and who was at which conference? Can we get beyond those supposedly objective facts?

In my opinion, no. The best you can hope for is to come up with a plausible story. Do you remember a Japanese movie called *Rashomon*? From time to time we have been asking ourselves questions that have to do with the history of our company and the various witnesses have different memories. They remember different things and sometimes we really don't know ourselves who is right and who is wrong. There are no obvious reasons for saying a, b or c often. We simply don't know.

There is a small booklet on the history of our company. We tried to keep to the facts as they are remembered by everybody and it was very surprising because we really had to leave out a number of 'facts' because we could not reach a consensus. But it is very difficult to write a book not containing statements that are contradicted by one or another witness – and there are 10 or so remaining witnesses, not more. People remember things differently like in *Rashomon*. So therefore, answering your question, I believe, if you can come up with a plausible story not contradicted by known facts or by witnesses that is the maximum a historian can hope for.

Yes, but that is going beyond the simple list of people. Once you have come up with the plausible story that is not contradicted by the facts – the witness thing is tricky – I think you have got to bring the question of judgement in there. You obviously can't come up with a story that the majority of witnesses don't agree with but I don't think you can have a criterion which says all the witnesses agree.

Well, for this book we have been very strict. There was fortunately complete agreement on the essential facts and we therefore did not really have major problems. But the less important 'facts' are, the more difficult it is to reach agreement. For instance, one of the questions would be: what is it that motivated the founders of the CINP? Everybody probably has his own opinion of the subject but these are guesses. I don't know for sure. I don't know what went on in the mind of the others. So I will probably never know.

Can we not go beyond the details to try and get a hold of what are the forces that shaped the field? Sometimes the clash of personalities and things like that can be interesting because of what it reveals of the underlying forces. Obviously one of the big issues has to be something in the area of: why have we had this huge change from people being so happy to take risks to the current state where people just are not prepared to take any risks at all? Can this not be traced through the perceptions of people as to what are the important events...

For instance, I made a few rather strong statements about the attitude of what I call the American psychiatrists to the neuroleptics and I realise that these are strong statements and they are not entirely correct. There are exceptions but anyway this is what I generally believe. But the really interesting question would be what was actually going on in the minds of these sceptics who were ridiculing Deniker. He was a good psychiatrist and his interpretation was that they felt threatened. That they were all treating rich widows – talking with them on a couch and charging fortunes. Without much therapeutic success but anyway this is how they made a living. Deniker strongly believes that when he came with his simple story these inexpensive pills threatened their source of income. Who am I to question that? Would it be useful to ask that question to these sceptics? I don't think so because they would probably not give you the right answer.

Why is it that in general terms the US was about 10 years behind Europe in this field, except for purely commercial products, like Librium or Valium? As far as I am concerned Librium and Valium cannot be described as major advances in therapy but they had obvious commercial potential and Roche made a fortune selling Librium and Valium in the States. As for the neuroleptics, in my opinion the sales people there were dominating the scene and could not really care less about patients. They probably didn't even believe the true story and they certainly did not believe that there was a market potential. I know that this was true for Jack Searle and for Harry McNey at McNeil because I have seen it and I have heard the same story told by people from SK&F. I was befriended by quite a number of them.

I don't know why chlorpromazine was turned down by the big companies, because I was not a witness. It would probably not even be written down in archives. We have no archives containing information on this subject. Most discussions on new compounds are verbal discussions between two or three people and aren't written down. Maybe these days but I never did.

Select bibliography

Denber HC, Rajotte P, Kauffman D (1960). Problems in evaluation of R-1625. *American Journal of Psychiatry*, **116**, 356–357.

Denber HC, Florio D, Rajotte P (1962). Third evaluation of haloperidol. *American Journal of Psychiatry*, **119**, 172–173.

Janssen PAJ (1970). The butyrophenone story, in *Discoveries in Biological Psychiatry* ed Ayd FJ, Blackwell B. Lippincott, Philadelphia, PA, 165–179

Sugerman AA (1964). A pilot study of floropipamide (Dipiperon). *Diseases of the Nervous System*, **25**, 355–358.

Symposium International sur le Haloperidol (1960). *Acta Medica Belgica*.

4 Joe Brady

The evolution of behavioural pharmacology

In 1956, when the Psychopharmacology Service Center organised the first Conference for the Evaluation of Psychotropic Drugs you were there as the lead person representing the potential input from or stake of behavioural pharmacology in this new world. How did you get into that position?

I was working with Murray Sidman in the laboratories at Walter Reed at the time, when the first of the tranquillisers appeared, which as I recall was reserpine. Around 1950/1951 I had looked at an animal model for affective performances, emotional responses – the conditioned emotional response, in which reserpine had some effects. In this animals were taught to perform a lever pressing response for food or water. They were put on a schedule so that they got paid off intermittently for a performance. In the middle of the performance you would turn on an auditory stimulus – in those days we used a clicking noise – and this would continue for three minutes. Contiguous with the end of the clicking noise, the animal received a footshock through the grid floor. Initially the clicker has no effect upon the performance – the animal goes right on pressing the lever – but depending upon the intensity of the shock, after a single trial many animals, the second time they heard that clicker, after they'd been shocked on its termination, showed complete suppression. That's an unusual case: in most cases you see an early approximate response but as you continue to run trials with the pairing of clicker and shock you get complete suppression.

Now how did I come to this? Before I came back to the University of Chicago, I had been in Germany for three years, in the early part of which I was one of the people who made the world safe for democracy. I had been in the infantry and I stayed in the army of occupation for a year or two more but under rather strange conditions. There was a practice at the time to send people back home in relationship to the amount of time they had been there. You got points for each month. I had been a late arriver and therefore had relatively few points for repatriation. But I was picked up at the headquarters in Frankfurt at the time and sent to the 317th station hospital as the chief clinical psychologist of the European command. Now only the military can rationalise a move of that sort. They went through my record and found that I had taken a course in psychology once as an undergraduate and said oh well, obviously this is the chief clinical psychologist of the European command. I spent two years there with four psychiatrists, who knew about as much about psychiatry as I knew about psychology. Three of them had a medical degree and an internship and they had spent 3 months at Fort Sam Houston where they learnt all about hebephrenic and paranoid schizophrenia. The chief of psychiatry at that time, on the other hand, was a major who had had a one year residency. I remember him well. He was well known for telling his patients when they would tell him what their problems were that that was a sin and they should stop doing it.

I remember checking into this assignment with my infantry badge on. The military used to assign speciality numbers to you – I was a 2285. I checked in with the chief of the hospital, Colonel Boyle, who looked at my record and said 'oh you're a 2285, I've always wanted one of those – what do you do?' He had no idea. As an indication to the extent of the confusion, within 3 weeks I found myself on a roster one weekend for medical officer of the day. So I spent a weekend on call. I had one phone-call from a woman, a dependant, who was in pain because she had a tooth removed and she wanted to know if she should take an aspirin. I told her to take two and call somebody else in the morning.

The important thing about this was that when I went to see the chief of service he said 'My God am I glad you're here, I've got a major general up on the 2nd floor who's just been brought in. I've got to get a Rorschach on him right away'. Now I had this image of somebody holding up card 5 in an undergraduate course with a butterfly on it and telling me that that was the Rorschach – that was the extent of my knowledge. But when you have just come from the infantry and you're a first lieutenant and a major tells you something, there's only one answer – Yes Sir! So I rushed into the hospital library and as luck would have it I found a book by a man named Klopfer on the Rorschach and I read that book that night as though it was an army field manual. I memorised it and came back the next day and gave the first of approximately 500 Rorschachs over the next two years – I became the greatest living expert on the Rorschach in Wiesbaden, Germany.

This group of psychiatrists that I worked with and I, as I say, were out there all by ourselves, so we would give ourselves courses. We'd read something and then we'd meet on Tuesday and Thursday nights – the blind leading the blind. The relevance of this is that this was a German hospital. Remember this was the mid-1940s, where the availability of treatments was extremely limited. There was a big room full of tubs for hydrotherapy. You could put somebody in these tubs and run warm water over them, which was not bad. We used to do this ourselves – it felt pretty good. We also had electroconvulsive shock. And when you were admitted to this service, along with your bathrobe and slippers came your electrodes because this was a very popular procedure.

I was impressed with one very effective procedure. In those days there were a large number of people diagnosed with what was called reactive depression, which was one of those disorders which was largely environmentally deter-

mined, I gather, as opposed to endogenous depression. If you let them sit quietly for 2–3 weeks, it goes away but if you plug them into the light circuit and
give them electric shock it goes away in 2–3 days. It's very dramatic. There
were lots of proposed theories as to why this occurs. I ultimately did a dissertation using electroconvulsive shock and in the process of writing the dissertation, of course, I was required to cover the literature and I found a paper in *The
Military Surgeon* and the title was 'Seventy-Five Theories on Electro-convulsive
Shock & Why it is Effective'. The one I found most engaging theorised that
'shock becomes the Mother'!

*That was in the late 1940s, so it had only been introduced a few years before but even then
they had 75 theories.*

Exactly. I only remember one, which was shock becomes the 'Mother' theory
and indeed it was a mother in the current sense of that word. I think a perfectly
plausible hypothesis is the reason that it worked so fast in these reactive
depression cases is that you can easily come to the conclusion that if you don't
get out of there these guys are going to electrocute you! Levity aside, there is
clearly an effective physiological process involved here.

I remained in the military but they sent me back to Chicago. What happened was that at the end of the war the surgeon general in Washington hired
a consultant from the Meninger Clinic in Kansas, who was sent around to
evaluate the facilities that the military was supporting. He came to Wiesbaden,
Germany to the neuropsychiatric centre of the European command and he
couldn't believe what he found there. He told the surgeon general that he
either had to get these people trained or get out of the business. So in typical
military fashion, they picked this up and sent us back to school. They sent me
back to graduate school in Chicago. One of the psychiatrists went back to there
with me to do a residency at the medical school.

There were big things happening in Chicago at that time. They had just gotten a new departmental chairman, James G. Miller, who was an MD/PhD
from Harvard University and he came in with fresh ideas on how to train
graduate students in psychology and the behavioural sciences. One of the
brightest of his ideas was that there would be a complete review of the field
within your first 9 months. You came in in September and in May of the following year you took comprehensive exams over the whole field and those
were the qualifying exams to get you into advanced training. This was quite a
chore. For everyone of the faculty you would do something. Miller did medical psychology for which the textbook was *Cecil's Textbook of Medicine* – this
was a large volume. Even in the early 1950s it was a substantial body of knowledge. I still have that book in my library. I read *Cecil's Textbook of Medicine* in 2
weeks and memorised it. Subsequently I discovered that if I got myself a *Merck
Manual* along with *Cecil's Textbook* I could practise medicine. I can't actually lay
on hands but not many of these guys here can fool me.

In any event, there was another condition – in order to take the qualifying
exam you had to have selected an experiment from the literature and replicated

it. That sounds like a reasonable requirement, but have you ever tried to replicate an experiment that's in the psychological literature? Believe me it's a formidable task. They're unreplicable. The experiment I selected was one by Estes and Skinner on conditioned anxiety which was published in 1942. This was the procedure I described earlier. The publication was in the *Journal of Experimental Psychology* and it was represented in cumulative records. The interesting thing about it is that in order to see what I have just decribed to you, the animals in the Estes–Skinner experiment were trained on a fixed interval schedule rather than a variable interval schedule and, in this case, in order to see the 'perturbation' that occurred as a result of this condition superimposing a 'Pavlovian' procedure on an operant baseline, you had to hold the reprint up and sight along the curve which tells you it wasn't a big change.

As I got to know Fred Skinner better, this was one of the eras in his life when he fell under the influence of someone by the name of Heron in the Unniversity of Minnesota. Heron was a big mechanical apparatus person and Heron and Skinner devised a device where a group of animals would run concurrently on a lever-pressing procedure and all the responses would feed into a single stepping switch which drew a cumulative record for the group. When you do group statistics you get a group average which is not typical of any animal. He obviously became disenchanted with that but it's an interesting note on his evolution into a single organism approach to biology. In this experiment what he published was average data which over the years no one in the world would ever accuse him of.

That was the experiment I decided I could replicate. I was working with Howard Hunt and we had just built two rat boxes and we were learning how to get animals to press the levers – it was wonderful. I took these two boxes and I had four animals, I remember very well, and I trained them to press levers, only we used a variable rather than a fixed interval, which was close enough, and then we superimposed the clicker and the shock and got complete suppression. Actually, to start with I got nothing and then I discovered you had to crank the shock level up a bit. Then the first thing you know, every one of those animals when they heard the clicker they didn't just slow down a little, they stopped cold, they defecated, they had piloerection – I had produced real anxiety in these animals. The name of the game was the shock level. Increase the shock level and you didn't have to worry about these 'perturbations', you got complete suppression of behaviour.

Anyway that satisfied the requirements for my exam, which I passed in May. Now I had these four animals available who were completely trained and I had a summer when I was relatively free. I was in clinical psychology and I was enrolled the following fall with Carl Rogers. I became a non-directive therapist and I spent a year learning how to out-non-direct people. But anyway during the summer I remembered my old days at Wiesbaden and I said to myself, I wonder what would happen if we plugged these animals into the light circuit and gave them electoconvulsive shock.

There was a literature on ECS in small animals. I found a paper by someone who had developed an electroconvulsive shock machine for rats. This was late 1940s. You used alligator clips wrapped in gauze soaked in saline on their ears and it was hooked up to a timer and a shocking device which delivered 50 mA of current for 2/10 of a second. That was all it took. That produces a full-blown tonic-clonic convulsion in the laboratory rat and within 60 seconds the animal stands up, shakes its head and walks away and I would defy you or anyone else to tell the difference between an animal who has just had one of these convulsions and a normal or a control animal – which I also did. Two of the four animals were controls and I did everything with them including putting on the clips, except that I didn't pass the current – I even threw the switch on the box except that there was no current.

I remember going through this. I took a week or two taking baselines to make sure we had good suppression. By that time we had other graduate students using the apparatus and since I was finished with my experiment the only time I had on the apparatus was from midnight to 2 a.m. I ran these four animals at midnight every night and I gave them ECS. The reason for selecting the values I used was completely fortuitous – there was no literature. But three times a day for seven days I gave them a convulsion. I remember it was 2 a.m. one morning when I ran the four animals in the box post-treatment and an experience like that is an experience that says you will never do anything else in your life. It was an incredible reinforcer. The two rats that had the control procedure continued to show complete suppression, piloerection and defecation but the two animals who had had the treatment, when the clicker came on they worked right through it without any piloerection or defecation. I had completely cured them.

You hadn't just caused them amnesia?

It is amnesia but it's a very selective amnesia. They went right back in there and went to work but when the clicker came on they paid no attention to it. Plus we did all sorts of other controls. We hadn't knocked out their hearing, for instance. Anyway that was sufficient for my dissertation. Here I was 3 months after I finished my qualifying exam, I had my dissertation done and I was ready to leave. But while I was working by day in the counselling centre, I continued running experiments at night. One of the ones I did was a parametric study on the number of electric shocks. What would happen if you did this once a day for 7 days as opposed to 15 times a day for 7 days, what do you think turns out to be the optimal number?

The one you picked?

Three times a day for 7 days. You don't get it if you do one shock a day for 7 days and you don't get it if you do all 21 shocks in 1 day. There is this temporal distribution which is rather critical. At any rate that was the history that I came to Walter Reed with.

Can you tell me something about Howard Hunt?

He and I were about the same age. He was in the Navy but he had gotten his degree before he went into the military whereas I had not. He and I arrived at the University of Chicago at the same time but he came as an assistant professor. He had gotten his degree at the University of Minnesota, where he trained with Stark Hathaway. Howard was big on the Minnesota Multiphasic Personality Inventory and he was trained in clinical psychology but he aspired to be an experimentalist and that was how we got into building the rat boxes together. I guess one of the important influences on his career was that he was a classmate of and shared and office with Bill Estes. Estes had been Skinner's first PhD in Minnesota.

Why did so much of this come out of Minnesota? The movie Fargo wouldn't suggest to you that a lot would come out of Minnesota.

I think in large part Skinner is the responsible agent for the basic experimental part of that. Although it is a remarkable place. When I came to Washingon at Walter Reed, I took an appointment at the University of Maryland and I started the first 'psychopharmacology' lab there. My first post-doc there was Travis Thompson, who got his PhD at Minnesota with Gordon Heistad, who was one of my contemporaries at Chicago and was also trained by Howard Hunt before going back to Minnesota. Travis Thompson's programme after he returned to Minnesota of course became the focus of psychopharmacology training in the United States. Most of my lab at Hopkins is now staffed by Travis' students from Minnesota. They come extremely well trained – George Bigelow, Roland Griffiths, Maxine Stitzer. I don't have any account of why this should be.

Nothing to do with any German influence?

No, but they have a reputation for being highly inbred, they keep rehiring their best people, plus Paul Meehl and Ken McCorkadale are intellectual giants and they have only about one decent day of summer a year as far as I can make out. Whatever it is it is interesting. I attribute much of it to BF Skinner. His influence on Howard was second-hand but still potent.

When I was still a graduate student I remember I gave my first paper at the American Psychological Association meeting at Penn State. This was the late 1940s/ early 1950s when only about 250 people would come to an APA meeting. They met at universities at the end of the summer so they could use the student rooms. I was due to give this paper and I had taken a movie with an 8 mm movie camera showing the conditioned emotional rats defecating, and freezing as well as their cure with electroconvulsive shock. The papers began at 8.00 a.m., so I came early to set up the movie camera. Leonard Carmichael was the session Chair and when he called the session to order for the first paper, which was by a man named Bugelski, at Buffalo, there were three people in the room: Leonard Carmichael, Bugelski and me – and I was only there to set up my camera but I obviously was obligated to stay. And I heard a historic paper that everybody has completely forgotten by now. Bugelski discovered Sidman avoidance but nobody knows it. The moral of the story is try to avoid giving your paper at 8 in the morning.

Bugelski reported a study in the late 1940s of a rat jumping back and forth over a barrier without an exteroceptive stimulus because he timed the shock. The animal had ten seconds to jump over to one side without being shocked and if he wasn't out of there in ten seconds he got a shock. This is Sidman avoidance, where the shocks are based every 20 seconds except a lever response resets the timer. This didn't appear in the literature until the early 1950s. I've often told Murray about this but he had never heard of Bugelski's experiment because it was never published. But I swear that was the report he gave at this meeting, and look how famous Sidman avoidance has become since then. Bugelski missed the boat. As I've said to my students repeatedly, if you don't write it up and publish you didn't do it. I heard it and pretty soon I'll be gone and nobody will remember Bugelski's experiment at all. He was chairman of the Department of Psychology at Buffalo and he wrote a textbook on psychology but to the best of my knowledge he never published this experiment, whereas Murray of course published his paper in *Science* and it has become a classic.

At any event when my paper came on at 10 a.m., guess who was sitting in the front row – B Fred Skinner. Howard, who knew him, arranged for us to have lunch and I had lunch with Skinner, Howard Hunt and Skinner's wife Eva. That was the greatest moment of my life. This turned out to be true of Fred Skinner right to the end of his life. When he came to a meeting he was parked up front listening to papers, he wasn't out politicking. Fred and I developed a rather close relationship over the next 30 years. He and I were on the President's Science Advisory Commision during the Kennedy administration. We were convinced we could save the world but nobody cared, as usual.

What about Bill Estes, did you know him then?

No, not at that time. I knew him by his publications. I subsequently got to know him but not well – nobody knew Bill Estes well. He was a very quiet, retiring individual. Howard on the other hand was a very articulate person, who expressed himself well and continuously. One root then of the behavioural pharmacology tree came from this group in Chicago and Minnesota.

I did another experiment there which had something of the beginnings of psychopharmacology in it. One of the controls we were interested in for the electroconvulsive shock study was the extent to which the electricity was the critical variable and the extent to which the convulsion was the critical variable. My somewhat less than successful entrée into behavioural pharmacology came with an attempt to produce convulsions chemically, which of course can be done if you know what you're doing, but I had no idea what I was doing. I did read a lot and I discovered that both strychnine and Metrazol would produce convulsions. Strychnine is a spinal cord convulsant whereas metrazol gives a more general CNS convulsion. I trained up all the animals but the problem was the lethal dose and the convulsant dose of both strychnine and Metrazol are very close – I killed an awful lot of animals. I finally ended up doing the experiment with audiogenic seizures.

This was in the transition between Chicago and Walter Reed and we did a few collaborative things. We tried nitrous oxide and a few other things, which began the behavioural pharmacology emphasis at Chicago. Subsequently Howard developed a relationship with the pharmacology department. Len Seiden is still there in both the psychology and pharmacology departments. Over the years Bob Shuster and Lynda Dykstra, among others, staffed the laboratories there so the behavioural pharmacology tradition persisted at Chicago after these early experiments.

Given a normal distribution of laboratory rats, 50–60% of them are subject to audiogenic seizures. What I did was to get a garbage can and a set of keys and I put the rats in the can and shook the keys around the outside. They start with a running fit and then they have a full-blown tonic-clonic convulsion. This was very nice because it gave you a control group as well at the same time. It was very clear that the convulsion was the critical element. The animals who had the convulsion showed an attenuation of the conditioned suppression and the animals who had the keys jingled over them but had no convulsion showed no attenuation of the conditioned suppression. This was the setting into which the reserpine experiment came. When you have a hammer everything looks like a nail!

The trick is then to find a few nail-like things. Where did reserpine actually come from? Did you approach Ciba or did they approach you?

It had nothing to do with Ciba. It came from the clinical side of the house. There were all these reports about reserpine as an effective tranquilliser. This was in 1953 and 1954. So I decided, let's see if it works in the laboratory and that's when I did the experiment with reserpine and saline controls. I have no good rationale for saying why I did this experiment the way I did it except that when we gave reserpine its acute effect was a heavy-duty suppression of all behaviour. You can't argue about differential effects if you wipe all behaviour – it's like curing mental disease with decapitation; it works like a charm. That was initially the way I looked at reserpine – you can hardly say that this is a cure if I'm knocking you cold.

That was when I decided that maybe the thing to do was to give the drug after the run each day and to do it the way I did the electroconvulsive shock study. This way they had a 23-hour period during which they 'recovered' from the acute effects of the drug. I did this for 7 days for no good reason except that it seemed like a good idea. Sure enough, gradually what happened was that although reserpine suppressed the overall rate of lever pressing, it clearly elevated the rate in the presence of the clicker and reduced the defecation and so on. On the other hand, with amphetamine, which was one of our controls, the overall baseline rate was elevated but in the presence of the clicker whatever residual behaviour was there beforehand there was no behaviour at all now – one could argue that there was an increase in their anxiety response, if you will.

Murray Sidman and I were so enthralled with that clear effect, which we replicated several times, that we decided to give every animal in the lab reserpine, including for instance a bunch of animals Murray had on Sidman avoidance. This turned out not to be a smart move. We learned subsequently that reserpine does dramatic things to serotonin and we never recovered the baseline in many of those animals. Reserpine has certain shortcomings that we are now well aware of but in those days if you had something with such dramatic effects, there was the temptation to 'see what it does'. What it did was to ruin the lab for all practical purposes. Having a good baseline and being able to recover it was critical to all the research we were doing at the time: A-B-A designs.

Did it have any effect on Sidman avoidance?

Well we didn't do it the way we did the CER studies. We only looked at acute effects and we didn't go back and do it because Murray was a little discouraged – he wasn't going to have any more of his animals ruined. And we moved on to chlorpromazine.

What can you tell me about Murray?

I can tell you that Murray Sidman was the discoverer of Sidman avoidance! Like me he did this as a graduate student. Avoidance procedures were long-standing in our business. They are always done where you get a warning stimulus – a tone or a light – and you say if you don't press this lever you're going to get a shock or if you press the lever you can avoid the shock. What he showed was that it could be done without the need for the exteroceptive stimulus by just shocking the animal every 30 seconds – the animals learned that beautifully, even as me and thee would learn it I suspect.

After I'd come to Walter Reed the division of neuropsychiatry was just starting. We had the advantage of being there first. This is a great advantage when you're establishing laboratories and doing things – you don't have to buy anyone else's problems. I had to go out and recruit people and the first thing I did was to call up my friends and relatives at Columbia – Nat Schoenfeld and Fred Kelleher. They lined up some people for me to talk to. I talked to three or four, one of whom was Murray, and it was clear I wanted him. This was in 1951–52; we offered him the grand sum of $6000 a year and he jumped at it. A lot of money – it was a government job at the GS-9 level as I recall.

He came to Walter Reed. We developed our families together in Washington at that time. He wrote a classic text while he was with us – *Tactics of Scientific Research*, which I think of as the 20th-century equivalent of Claude Bernard's *Treatise on Experimental Medicine*. When Claude Bernard wrote *Experimental Medicine* nobody paid any heed to it – it was a hundred years ahead of its time. The vital force was still alive and well in physiology. Murray's *Tactics of Scientific Research* in my view is to the behavioural sciences what Bernard's book was to the physiological sciences. I had read Claude Bernard and while Murray was writing his book I asked him if he was aware of Claude Bernard's work but he had never even seen the book. So it wasn't plagiarism, which was something I might have done – you may know of Tom Lehrer from Harvard who wrote satirical songs such as 'Shooting Pigeons in the Park' but there was also one about a Russian mathematician Lobatchevsky who plagiarised, which had the line 'Let nobody else's work evade your eyes'. You end up plagiarising yourself after a while which is OK – that's when you become original.

While he was writing the book he had an inviolate period from 9.00 to 11.00 in the morning, when he was undisturbable. I remember our boss Dave Rioch came by one morning at 10.00 and Murray's door was closed. He opened the sliding door quietly and said 'Murray'. Murray didn't answer. This was his boss but he went right on writing and Dave stood there for a while. I was outside handling some rats and I could observe this whole thing. Dave Rioch was a psychiatrist and a very sophisticated man. Eventually he quietly turned around and tiptoed out and walked away. Murray never budged. He knew damn well who it was. That I regarded as a testimony to both of them. But that's Murray Sidman. He is still very much involved in the business, writing very creatively these days on second and third order derived phenomena of stimulus events and he's got a firm handle on the thinking problem.

What relationship if any does the CER bear to learned helplessness?

Well, Howard and I did another experiment which bears on this. If you make a slight modification of our procedure – when the clicker comes on, instead of the shock occurring contiguously with the turning off of the clicker, the shock is contingent on a lever response, this is what you would characterise as a discriminative punishment procedure. If they make a response in the presence of the clicker they get a shock. Topographically those two performances look identical. On the cumulative record you see a 3-minute period during which the animal is not responding. However, reserpine has no effect on the punishment performance but it did on the conditioned anxiety. Subsequently Irv Geller, who was with me in the lab before he went to Wyeth, took that procedure which he called a conflict procedure because you have a hungry animal who is constrained from pressing to get food, and he demonstrated that if you titrate the intensity of the shock they will work through that but at a lesser rate. But if you gave librium to that animal you could get an elevation of the rate and this became a screening procedure for minor tranquillisers.

In that sense you can characterise the CER as a form of learned helplessness. What differentiates it is that it does not seem to be generalisable. It's confined to that clicker. Learned helplessness, as I understand Seligman's work, generalises, and the procedures for generating these responses are different. In learned helplessness all behaviour is punished. The CER is very discriminative – it's clear what you are going to get hit for.

The one thing all these procedures, including conditioned avoidance, have in common is aversive control. What we are talking about here are various ways of attenuating the effects of aversive controls. The complexity of the matter is contributed to by the multiple procedural variables on the behavioural side as well as the multiple chemical variables on the pharmacological side and it is the dedication to sorting out all of that which defines behavioural pharmacology. I think it is a reasonable parcelling out to talk about those events that are under aversive control and those that are under appetitive control. The big rage these days is more away from the aversive side and it's on to 'cognitive enhancers'. We even have people who call themselves cognitive behaviourists, which is the oxymoron of the decade.

Anyway the fact that we were in there doing all this drug stuff in the early 1950s came to light in a number of ways – one was the publication of the *Science* paper on reserpine. Science is a medium that is looked at across the pharmacological sciences – at least it was in those days. That experiment was the one that brought the drug houses to the door. I did not solicit them. The other thing was a visit by a neurophysiologist by the name of Irwin Slater who came from Eli Lilly where KK Chen was the director of research. Irwin Slater came to visit Bob Galambos, an electrophysiologist, in the lab with us at Walter Reed. He turned right when he should have turned left as he came down the hall. Murray and I, at the time, were working in a huge shielded room which made it look as though we must have been doing something like electrophysiology. Actually what we were doing was protecting Galambos who was across the hall. He had complained about our work because in those days we were not solid state – we were using stepping switches and relays and there were sparks flying around the place which were driving him crazy across the hall with his electronic recording equipment. So we ended up shielding him in and shielding us out.

Of course, Slater ended up in our middle control room, where we had all the relays and recorders and saw all this and asked what it was. I said it was an animal behaviour lab and he asked where the hell the animals were – if you're in an animal behaviour lab you expect to see animals behaving. They were in four smaller rooms on each side and I explained to him what we were doing, that we had some two-way mirrors, that we had a couple of monkeys and that we had done the reserpine studies but that they weren't quite published yet.

Anyway he asked me whether I'd be willing to come out to Indianapolis and tell them about some of the work we were doing. I thought it was one of those cocktail party type invitations, the next time you're in town why don't you give me a call. But within the week I had a call from KK Chen wanting to know whether I would come out to one of their weekly research seminars and give a talk on the things we had been doing on drugs and behaviour and these new procedures. I'm talking about the early 1950s, when if someone offered me a captive audience I would have crawled out there on my hands and knees but I hoped they were going to pay my way. I was making maybe $6500–$7000 a year and I had five kids. He said, well of course we'll pay your expenses and I breathed a deep sigh of relief, and then he got very apologetic and said unfortunately they were coming toward the end of the fiscal year and they could only offer me a $200 honorarium. Nobody had ever offered me a $200 honorarium before that. When I picked myself up off the floor, I mumbled that that would be all right, as though I would get one of those every day. He said, of course you can answer questions at the end of your talk or not as you choose.

This was a man who knew what he was doing. They put me up at the Indianapolis Athletic Club. They invited me at the time of the Indianapolis Decoration Day. They have this big car race out there and they took me to it. Drug companies knew how to treat you in those days. I gave my talk and answered a few questions. Then he invited me into his office and asked me what I thought it would cost for them to set up a laboratory of the type I had described. I assured him it was prohibitively expensive, probably $40–50,000. He said 'Do you have any idea what it costs us to get a drug to the market, in terms of the preclinical work and clinical trials and so on? $10 million. That was what it cost in the early 1950s, so $40–50,000 was a drop in the bucket. Ten million dollars is still a lot of money but in those days it was an incredible amount.

About a year ago I did a job for Pfizer in which I was invited to chair a workshop on a new compound which they had taken through the preclinical stages and they had to make a decision whether to go into clinical trials with it. They had gathered a large group of clinicians and scientists. The only issue had nothing to do with efficacy, which was about the same as the comparator, but it had fewer side-effects – a mild attenuation of side-effects was what had recommended it. They had already put $20 million into the preclinical stages and they were facing a total expenditure of $200 million if they went ahead. So the decision was, do we stop here or do we put the other $180 million to get this to the market?

The bottom line was that Eli Lilly and every other company in the country in the 1950s and 1960s had literally hundreds of compounds on the shelf without any way to screen them for these unique 'behavioural' effects that had appeared with reserpine and chlorpromazine. Chlorpromazine when it came on the market grossed $75 million in its first year on the market. That's a drop in the bucket these days but in the 1950s that set the stage for every other drug company in the business to pursue their 'me too' programmes.

Frank Ayd was saying to me recently that in Maryland alone there were three state asylums each with a population of 8–9000 patients and in 1955, perhaps a bit like you with reserpine and the rats, every single one of those patients just about was getting chlorpromazine – so in those terms this was clearly a substantial market.

That's exactly right. The issue here was me-too drugs. SKF made $75 million the first year on the market. Every other drug company had to have one of these compounds. They all had them on the shelf – but how do we know? This is where behavioural pharmacology in the drug houses came from. Of course when the word got out that Eli Lilly had gone this way ... The other issue was staffing.

Len Cook's lab would have been going at this stage.

Yes but that was pharmacology. I also was invited to give a talk at Merck. Paul Beyer was the head of pharmacology at Merck and he invited me. They also decided they had to get into this.

Apropos the issue of where do you find the people, an interesting comment was made after my talk at Merck. Beyer asked why they couldn't send somebody, one of their pharmacologists, down to our lab to be trained and then have them come back to work in the Merck programme. Ciba asked the same question. I said yes, they could do that and it would certainly be better than not doing anything at all, but the problem was that while that pharmacologist was on the way back on the train a new development might come about on the behavioural side – in other words they wouldn't be able to keep up with the field. Actually Skinner also suggested this but I disagreed with him – I thought the field would get away from them very quickly – if in fact the critical parameter was the behavioural methodology. They didn't have to worry about the pharmacology but what they needed was someone who was professionally competent on the behavioural side and would keep in touch with that science community. So I ended up sending people to companies. Tom Verhave was the first one – he got the job at Eli Lilly. They weren't pharmacologists at all but they were good behavioural people and I figured they could learn pharmacology or they had enough pharmacological support and enough models to work out what would be appropriate for screening purposes, which is what they were wanted for – to screen drugs.

Many of these people came from Walter Reed because we had a recruiting system at Walter Reed you can't beat – the Korean War – and there was the draft. We drafted in all these guys and had a whole lab full of PhDs at Walter Reed. Larry Stein was one of them, John Boren, George Heise, Irv Geller, Dick Herrnstein – guys who had to do military service. We would get calls from all over the country from medical schools about physicians, for instance, who hadn't even taken internship but had gone straight into research – Dave Whitlock, Ed Perl and folks like that who were MDs but they never had any clinical training. The army didn't bother making those fine distinctions. If you were an MD you were fair game for assignment to a battalion aid station putting on band-aids and giving aspirin. I used to get these calls and we would go out of our way through the surgeon general to get them assigned and we always felt we were doing a great service – not only for the scientific community but for the patients who might have been at risk under the circumstances. So we got these guys assigned to Walter Reed and later sent them off to academic and industrial jobs.

An interesting background feature was that we had people from Harvard and Columbia, who were the better trained group. They had good academic training but at Walter Reed we were into all sorts of applications and they then went off to the drug-houses. Some never even came through Walter Reed because the demand became so great that I ended up dealing directly with the universities looking for someone who had a degree in this area.

You mentioned reserpine but what about chlorpromazine, which had also appeared at this point?

Yes, we were also moving from rats to monkeys at this stage. We did similar type studies with chlorpromazine in the monkey and we were able to demonstrate its effects on the CER and avoidance behaviour in the monkey. The screening techniques we set up at Merck ended up capitalising on Sidman avoidance. I remember them training large numbers of small animals. The interesting thing about Sidman avoidance and the way we came to look at the behavioural effects of drugs, we made it possible for an organism to learn something that they never learned otherwise. If you have an animal on a 30-second RS interval in a Sidman avoidance, the rate at which he is pressing that lever to keep the shocks away is faster than one every 30 seconds. He is probably doing it once every 5–10 seconds. There is excess behaviour, in other words, to make sure they don't get shocked. Now if you give them a drug like chlorpromazine what we discovered early on was that the rate got suppressed but not necessarily in a manner that produced an increase in shock. They may be pressing slower but still fast enough to avoid all the shocks and when you took the drug away they had 'learnt' something and they would continue to press at a more moderate rate and still avoid the shocks.

That's interesting. Is there a therapeutic application for that?

Well, the use of certain therapeutic drugs is based on the ability of the drug to bring the organism into contact with the contingencies in the environment, which for whatever other extraneous reason they haven't been very good at. Nonetheless the suppression of avoidance turned out to be a very effective way to screen certain tranquillising drugs and that was the standard procedure at Merck. Of course, the other thing was that the influence of many behaviourists who went into the industry spread far beyond screening for drugs. Tom Verhave would be a classic case. In some instances this was not to their advantage. Tom developed a technique where he trained pigeons to do quality control over pills. The pill would normally come down a chute and women would stand there and pick out the defective ones. He trained pigeons to discriminate anything that was different and he had this working beautifully but he got into trouble with the unions.

The presence of behavioural pharmacologists in industry peaked and then dwindled off. But there are still people in there. The new breed are guys like Jim Barrett. The University of Maryland lab turned out to be a source of training for behavioural pharmacology and as a result when I left there to go to Hopkins it was taken over by people like Jim Barrett and we in turn hired Nancy Atour, who is a Jim Barrett product. Receptor dynamics had become a big thing. They are now very much concerned about the relationship between a specific receptor site and behavioural expression. These are now much more sophisticated, much more basic behavioural pharmacology than we were looking at when we were just taking hundreds of compounds off the shelf and seeing if they had an effect that might be interesting. It's a more rational approach now to designing drugs for specific behavioural effects. Jim Barrett is a good example of the new look even though he came from the old school.

What was the influence of Peter Dews?

He and I are exactly the same age. Peter had a history that goes back to Cambridge and the pharmacological route. While in Cambridge, he was given a jar full of hashish and had to find out if it had any behavioural effects. He saw how limited the relevant procedures they were using were. Obviously these kinds of beginnings were important because they alerted him to the fact that there is an important field here that has to do with establishing the effects of these compounds across a range of phenomena, including behavioural ones. When he came to the United States, he took the initiative of going over and hanging out in Skinner's pigeon lab. Its probably that kind of history that led Skinner to recommend to the pharmaceutical industry people to send – people who he could train and send back. Given someone like Peter Dews, that would be obviously the right way to go but they weren't all going to be like Peter who would then take off and become a real devotee of the field. It was through Peter that the whole Harvard group, Charlie Catania, Charlie Ferster, Roger Kelleher, Larry Bird, Bill Moss and people like that, got into behavioural pharmacology. As near as I can tell, with the group at Harvard, the pigeon lab had very little interest in pharmacology until Peter got there.

Even though Skinner himself had done some work with caffeine and things like that in the 1940s?

That was in the 'Behaviour of Organisms' that Skinner published 50 or 60 years ago. There was of course very little that Skinner hadn't done but in terms of a more sophisticated interest in the field, Peter was responsible for that. It wasn't the casual 'let me see what these guys have to offer', he really got himself into it. His appointment at the Harvard Medical School is as a Professor of Psychobiology in the Psychiatry Department. Bill Morris, Roger Kelleher and that whole crowd were clearly out of the Dews tradition. They had less of an immediate influence on the drug house development than the group that came out of Walter Reed and Columbia. There were also second generation influences. Len Cook had an assistant by the name of Bob Shuster, who I took as a graduate student. When Bob left that lab Len replaced him with Roger Kelleher and Charlie Catania, who came from the Harvard lab.

What about the drugs of abuse field? This is an area where it seems to me the behavioural pharmacology input has been very sophisticated.

That's where all the money has been for the past two decades. I think that came out of the Maryland lab from the behavioural side. As often happens, there were two things that happened concurrently without the people who were doing them even knowing about one other. Weeks did a rat experiment at Upjohn in the early 1960s and at the same time Bob Shuster, who was a graduate student with me, and Travis Thompson, who was my first post-doc, started looking at whether or not monkeys would do drug self-administration. Their early work in that regard provided more impetus to the behavioural community to get into this area than the Weeks work – Weeks was a pharmacologist.

Bob's dissertation was the beginning of the drug discrimination field. An animal was trained to get food only if a certain substance was injected into a cannula and they learned to discriminate the difference between a drug and saline. In the paper, this was characterised as interoceptive conditioning, which was very big in the Soviet Union. Gregory Razran, who was a professor at City College in New York, was fluent in Russian and very well connected in the Soviet Union, convinced Bob and me that we should submit that paper for publication to the *Pavlovian Journal of Higher Nervous Activity*. We did. Years went by without us hearing a word from them. About three years later we got a reprint in Russian of that paper. I still have it. Its completely unintelligible. Because of their different alphabet we couldn't even recognise our names. We found someone at Walter Reed at the time, a military-intelligence type, to translate it back but it was completely unintelligible. We didn't know whether the problem was in the translation from English to Russian or from Russian to English but the whole thing was a garbled mess.

Bob and Travis, when they had the cannula in and had done their interoceptive conditioning experiment, asked what would happen if we gave the monkey a lever and let him inject the drug himself, and that's where the primate drug self-administration study was first done. That was published in *Science*. I think the major conceptual influence the animal drug self-administration observations has had on the field of substance abuse is that it changed the way we looked at these performances from being controlled primarily by antecedent events. The prevailing view was that people are driven to be drunks or substance abusers by the environment, by having a mother-in-law that drives you crazy. Well the monkeys had no mothers-in-law. One of my favourite quotations is by WC Fields: 'It was a woman who drove me to drink and I never got a chance to thank her.' That was how one presumably got to be an alcohol and/or drug abuser but animal self-administration calls attention critically to the consequences of drug intake. The relationship between performance and its consequences, I think, is the critical one and that study opened up a whole new way of looking at drug abuse. It was the start of new therapies such as the contingency management field. What Steve Higgins is doing in New Hampshire with cocaine abusers is clearly part of this.

You've moved into therapy yourself – you have a mobile drug treatment programme in Baltimore.

I have a mobile drug abuse treatment programme which came out of human work I had been doing for some years in controlled environments. We did get into looking at drug effects in a programmed environment and this was an extension into a larger unprogrammed environment.

Are any of the behavioural principles paying off in this?

Well, I can give you the classic example of approximation. This mobile drug abuse programme clearly had its origins in a problem in the city of Baltimore.

We have 50,000 i.v. drug abusers in the city. The proportion who are positive for AIDS is larger in the city of Baltimore than in any other city in the United States. We have 5000 treatment slots. By the same token there hasn't been a new drug abuse treatment programme in the city for 25 years. It's the NIMBY problem; everyone wants to go to heaven but nobody wants to die, everybody wants drug abuse treated but not in their backyard, even though all the abusers are in their backyard. The logic of this escapes me but its not a logical issue. Never was.

I got this idea about a mobile drug abuse programme. It turns out that what the communities object to is fixed site programmes because the drug abusers hang around there. So I said, suppose we just come in for a few hours, provide the medication, do some counselling and then we're out of there. I talked to the Mayor of Baltimore, who is very progressive, and he said 'It's a great idea, now here's who you need to talk to.' I talked to everyone of the city council members who all said 'Great idea, now here's who I want you to talk to.' I spent a year talking to people and was making very slow progress. Baltimore is a very community-oriented city – all sorts of ethnic groups who all have community associations and I had to go and talk to each one and they listened to me and said 'It's a great idea, why don't you park it over there?' They didn't want the bus to stop on their corner.

Then I finally stumbled upon the answer, which if I had thought of it a year earlier I'd have been in business a lot faster – the local clergy. In the city of Baltimore, when one of the church pastors says this is how it's going to be – that's how it's going to be. I talked to a few clergymen and told them we were having trouble finding sites where we could park the vehicle but that we had a few dollars in the grant that could be put towards something if one or another of the parishioners could help us find us a place to park. The people who turned out to be the most helpful were the clergymen themselves, suggesting that we use the church parking lot but never on Sunday. A dynamite idea. We lined up three or four churches and started.

Carrying off this demonstration research project involved some logistics and this is where the behavioural principles come in. When you run a medication-based drug abuse treatment programme, you can't just go out and medicate people. The community is not delighted with this approach, sometimes seeing it as another trick to get folks on a drug that you control like methadone or another opiate. The FDA requires that you do counselling and so forth. So when I got a 5-year demonstration grant from NIDA, I had to get self-propelled medication vans to deliver the medication and trailers in which we did the counselling. The medication vans had to meet all sorts of requirements from the Drug Enforcement Agency. When I went to see the head of the DEA in Baltimore and told him about this great plan, he said – 'You're going to do what? You mean like a Good Humor truck?' (an ice-cream van). I said 'No bells, we're just going to go out there quietly and do our thing and get out.' He said that they required that each one of the medication vans have a bullet-proof nurse's station, with the very thick bullet-proof glass you have in banks, behind which the medication was dispensed. We had to have an armed guard on board, a safe for the medication and an alarm system that alerted the whole East Coast of the United States, if anyone looked crooked at one of these vehicles.

We only did counselling once a week whereas we had to do the medication every day, so we had to work out a plan whereby the medication van tows the trailer and goes to site A on Monday, for example, where it drops the trailer all day for counselling, while the medication van went on and did the other sites. On Tuesday it drops the trailer at site B etc. Well, one day while I was out there getting all this going right, I noticed that on the outside of one of the churches, close to the door, was an external AC plug. Now remember when you run a mobile programme everything has to be self-sufficient. Each one of these trailers has a generator on it, mobile phones etc. Anyway I asked the pastor of the church whether we could use the AC plug because in that way we could stop using the generator on the trailer and then maybe we could help out with the church's electric bills. A few days later, I noticed that just inside the door there was a modular telephone jack, I said these mobile phones are very expensive, if we could use the jack we could help out with the church's phone bill. The bottom line is that for the past two years we haven't brought the trailers out at all. We've been doing the counselling in the churches and are near to consolidating the entire programme in a church.

We had been doing everthing except the medication in the churches because of the requirements for the safe etc. A short while ago one of the pastors asked me why we didn't just leave the drugs there and I said, well we need a security man with a gun and an 800 lb safe. He then showed me that in a corner of their church, which was split level on a whole block, they used to have a cheque cashing place, which had big thick cinderblock walls and big thick glass. Its a perfect place to put a medication site, so we're now working on rezoning a church as a drug abuse treatment programme.

If you think that's an easy task you should try it sometime. There's a good reason why Baltimore hasn't had a new drug abuse treatment programme in 25 years. First you have to have three members of the city council introduce a bill, which has to have three readings at the city council over a 3-month period. Between the readings you have to come up with approvals from the housing department, the planning commission, the medical department etc. – everybody has to sign off on this. You have to hold three public hearings, where anybody from the city of Baltimore can come and say why we don't want this. You have to advertise in two separate newspapers for a month at a time and then you have to post signs all over the city giving the address of where you're going to do the rezoning. Is it any wonder we haven't had a new programme. No one in his right mind would go to this trouble but the pastor of the church said not to worry. He produced three council members who were part of his parish and we put the signs up and we got to the housing department etc. The day before I came here, we appeared before the planning commission, who had to ask why we want to do this and what the neighbours think etc. The pastor did the introduction and this was really inspired. He said he came there to talk to them about his substance abuse treatment and rehabilitation *ministry*. By the time he got done, the head of the commission stood up and said that he wanted to compliment him on this great work. These are people who wouldn't normally let you rezone anything. That's approximation. It proved absolutely invaluable in this case.

However, this has not been fast – it has taken 3 years to move from a little outside AC plug. But this really is the answer to the drug abuse problem in a place like this. We have demonstrated that we can gain entry into a community and we have published data on the 3–4 years we have been running the programme. We have compared our programme to six other fixed-site programmes in Baltimore. The average length of stay in our programme is 18 months. In fixed-site methadone treatment programmes normally the turnover is absolutely drastic. Within the first 30–60 days you have usually lost 40–60% of your patients. One of the reasons is that these are programmes where they have to show up every day to get your medication. Now if you have to take two trolley-cars and a bus, which most of the people in this kind of a programme have to because they can't afford automobiles or taxi-cabs, this gets onerous very quickly. The behaviour gets weak and there's a man on the corner who will supply you a lot faster – that's where the mobile treatment programme comes in. The rationale was a response–cost rationale. I thought that's the reason why you have such a large drop-out but if we bring the mountain to Mohammed, retention shoud be better. The single most important factor to success of treatment is retention. Now we have demonstated that we can keep them in treatment and my plan is that we can now use this method to get a community that was completely against this approach to accept it and to be more effective in the treatment. This may not be the final step of behavioural pharmacology in the drug abuse business but I never expected to be participating in a ministry when I undertook this initiative.

Apotheosis is hard to beat.

It's going to be about as far as I'm going to go. It's been an all-consuming business. The grant money ran out and we're hoping to run it as a private programme. NIDA gave us 5 years of money to do this, which was very generous, but the whole point behind a demonstration programme is to show that it works and then it should be taken over by the city or the state or somebody. The trouble is that drug abuse treatment is off the screen. It's not high on anybody's agenda. The state and the city are completely out of money and they're cutting down on the programmes, so we have had no support from any of these people. I decided that we should see if we can't go on our own as a private programme.

You might have serious questions as to whether the population I had been treating would have the money to pay. My view was that the new lick in this age is that those who profit most from a service should pay for it – sounds like a Republican, I'm sure, but it's very popular in this country right now. So we told the clients we're out of planning here – we can't keep treating if we can't start charging and the charge is $75 a week. I heard the counsellor with some of the first patients who were exclaiming '$75 a week!' and she asked 'Well, how much do you pay the "man?" They pay the 'man' $30–40 a day and to get that they have to steal or commit other acts of violence. So she was able to sell a deal for $75 a week and they've been coming up with it. It reminds me of another Tom Lehrer song when he alluded to the fact that one of his relatives was selling what they used to give away! We've got 125 patients now paying for their own treatment and I have to tell you that they are different from the group we used to treat for free. They get better a lot faster, they get their urines clean a lot more easily. When they ask to get off, we detox them. And it turns out there's a population out there willing to pay.

The behavioural pharmacology of substance abuse has really capitalised on the behavioural developments in a dramatic way – from drug discrimination and drug self-administration work and animal psychophysics. As regards psychophysics, my first assistant at Walter Reed in the early 1950s was a young man by the name of Bill Stebbins, who ultimately wrote the book on animal psychophysics. I now have one of his students running the shop for me at Hopkins. It's an extremely effective way to do behavioural toxicity – to look at not only the extent that a drug has reinforcing functions, or the extent to which it has discriminative functions but the price the organism is willing to pay and we ultimately pay for the toxic effects.

Behavioural toxicity was something you talked about a lot in the 1956 meeting but it still hasn't taken off. It hasn't become an FDA requirement.

Well, drug self-administration is required by the FDA but in my view this is something that is not restricted to drugs of abuse. We've been running psychiatric drugs like the benzodiazepines, for instance, and there are clear effects on auditory and visual thresholds at therapeutic doses so there are people driving around in cars whose eyeballs and ears aren't working at full capacity. But you're right, it hasn't caught on as a critical part of the assessment. We continue to do it and I argue that it is critical because simply determining if a substance is discriminable and whether it is reinforcing is not a sufficient condition for making it abusable – if that was the case popcorn and Hershey bars would be schedule 1. Abuse liability is determined in large part by toxicity. Scott Lucas and I published a little book on screening drugs and I made the point in there that there are some drugs that are not very reinforcing but their toxicity is so great that they are regarded as highly abusable drugs. It's the behavioural consequences that make LSD what it is and this is so as well with the amphetamines and the opiates.

Can you remember how you were asked to participate in the 1956 meeting – did the invite come from Jonathan Cole or Ralph Gerard or Seymour Kety? What can you remember of the flavour of the meeting or the process of putting it together?

I think it was Seymour Kety, with whom we had most contact at Walter Reed, who invited my input, the flavour of which, as I recall, was very upbeat in considering the prospects for new pharmacological approaches to psychiatric and behavioural problems.

You hinted that there has been a dwindling of behavioural pharmacology input to indus-try – is this because companies have gone down a molecular biology route and have lost interest in in vivo pharmacology or is it that the 'cognitive' revolution stemming from learned helplessness, for instance, has in part distracted the field and diverted attention to areas that are just not pharmacologically friendly ?

I think behavioural pharmacology has had and continues to have relations with industry that are somewhat cyclical. The initial enthusiastic embrace of behav-ioural pharmacology by industry lost some of its passion when new discover-ies did not come fast enough or often enough to affect the 'bottom line'. But I think that behavioural pharmacology may be coming into its own again in industry via the neuroscience route, drug discrimination, receptor dynamics, 'designer drugs' and the like.

Select bibliography

Hunt HF, Brady JV (1951). Some effects of electroconvulsive shock on a conditioned emotional response ('anxiety'). *Journal of Comparative Physiological Psychology*, **44**, 88–98.

Brady JV, Hunt HF (1955). An experimental approach to the analysis of emotional behaviour. *Journal of Psychology*, **40**, 313–324.

Brady JV (1956). Assessment of drug effects on emotional behaviour. *Science*, **123**, 1033–1034.

Brady JV (1956). A comparative approach to the evaluation of drug effects upon affec-tive behaviour. *Annals of the New York Academy of Science*, **64**, 632–643.

Brady JV (1959). In *Psychopharmacology. Problems in Evaluation* (JO Cole, RW Gerard, eds). National Academy of Sciences, public no. 583, Washington DC.

Brady JV, Lucas SE (1984). *Testing Drugs for Physical Dependence Potential and Abuse Liability*. National Institute on Drug Abuse Research Monograph #52, DHHS Publication no (ADM) 84-1332. US Government Printing Office, Washington DC.

Brady JV (1993). The origins and development of behavioral pharmacology. *European Behavioural Pharmacology Society*, Newsletter 7, September 1993, pp 2–11.

Brady JV (1996). Drug policy and the enhancement of access to treatment, in *Drug Policy and Human Nature* (WK Bickel, DJ DeGrandpre, eds). Plenum Press, New York, pp 155–174.

5 Roland Kuhn

From imipramine to levoprotiline: the discovery of antidepressants

What led you into psychiatry?

Accident. Not totally but partially. It was a second love. What I really wanted after my finals was an assistant's placement in surgery. I had an appointment with a professor with whom I was friendly and who was very good but shortly before my final exams he told me he was retiring and he had no use for me. So then I had no placement and that was one of the reasons. I had to find a new position. My colleagues had already all been placed and the best positions had gone. Another reason to think of psychiatry was that I had done my dissertation on iodine metabolism in cretinism and because of this I had become aware that the neurovegetative nervous system and the psyche have a great influence on the endocrine system. So I thought why not do a year in psychiatry, maybe I would be able to get a position there. I thought I would try it for a year and then I would also have time to look for a good place and change. So I went to Professor Klaesi and he was immediately very enthusiastic and welcoming. Of course I could come!

Where was Professor Klaesi at that time?

In Berne. I've studied in Berne and Paris – I was one semester in Paris. So I went to Berne. In the beginning I was a ward doctor and I had a ward of one hundred beds, all men, with five hundred admissions alone in a year. You had to work till evening and half the night and in the night you had to get up, of course. As a result I had so little time that it was impossible to look for another place. So instead of one year I stayed another year. That was in the Waldau. After two years, even before I was finished I was asked whether I would be interested in becoming consultant here in Münsterlingen.

I made inquiries and I heard that a new director, Doctor Zolliker had come to the clinic. I also inquired about the possibility for scientific work there and it happened that the clinic had an excellent scientific library. That was one reason I came. Also not five kilometres away was Ludwig Binswanger. Binswanger was one of the most important Swiss psychiatrists at that time, no doubt about it, and I was told that if I went to Münsterlingen I would surely have contact with him and would be able to learn a lot. So it came about: I came here for what I thought was two years. I thought then I would go travelling but that was in the year 1939 and the war came and there was no possibility to travel. So I stayed. In time I saw that it was a great advantage to stay in one place in psychiatry and I lost my interest to do surgery. I decided to remain a psychiatrist and essentially I have never regretted it.

When I came into psychiatry, in Berne we were already doing sleep therapy with Klaesi and also cardiazol shock treatment and insulin therapy. By the time I came to Münsterlingen we also did it here. So in this way I learned biological psychiatry very early in my career. In Berne there were two consultants who were both psychoanalysts – Arnold Weber and Otto Briner, who was trained in psychoanalysis in Berlin. From these two I learned psychoanalysis. I also learned to hypnotise – at that time we still used hypnosis. That was a terrific business. I got acquainted with the Rorschach test from Weber. He was an analyst with Rorschach and he had been taught by Rorschach himself. Weber was also psychopathologically excellent. He also had a child observation ward where I learned child psychiatry. There was also Jacob Wyrsch, who was a general clinical consultant who was absolutly brilliant in psychopathology – not in this modern psychopathology as we have it today but in the psychopathology of that time. He was an immediate pupil of Eugen Bleuler. He was very good at exploring patients and he showed us how to do this. He was Director of the Polyclinic. So by the time I came here I had a complete overview of contemporary psychiatry, which I had got in a very short time – in two years – and all from people with excellent credentials.

Then there was Max Müller who was in Münzingen; he arranged seminar evenings there. There was also Walter Morgenthaler, the man who had the case of Wölfli, the artist who painted these famous pictures – that along with Prinzhorn was the start of the dealing with art of the insane. Max Müller invited Walter Morgenthaler, who talked about education in psychiatry, and Storch, who was interested in philosophical psychiatry. I was also made aware of the modern philosophical psychiatry, of course, because of Ludwig Binswanger, who was the foremost figure in philosophical psychiatry. At Binswanger's I met Kurt Goldstein and got to know him personally, as well as Gebsattel, Heidegger and numerous other people, with some of whom I corresponded.

So when I joined this establishment, I did mainly biological psychology in the clinic and philosophical psychiatry with Binswanger. I started at the same time to do psychotherapy with Binswanger checking my therapy. It was an absolutely unique education. I knew Kretschmer through Klaesi and I also heard a lot from Viktor von Weizsäcker.

But he was never in Switzerland?

No, Weizsäcker was not; that is, I never knew him personally, but I had the first edition of the *Gestalt Circle*, that is, when the edition first appeared I got it within the first half year. As part of my training I was told I had to read it. Every two weeks also I went to Binswanger for dinner in the evening and afterwards there was a demonstration of a Rorschach protocol and I had to interpret the protocol. After that the consultant presented the case history and Binswanger with his knowledge of the case produced a synthesis.

A psychoanalytical interpretation?

Yes, an interpretation. He was already then producing his Daseins-analysis. So here, then, the Daseins-analysis originated. It took decades to evolve.In this fashion I always got to know new people who came to our clinic. I have to mention something here. Binswanger as the owner of a private clinic had an unrivalled grasp of depression and manic depressive illness. He was treating very severe cases in famous people. He regularly had professors and heads of departments as patients – these highly intelligent people with their depressions. He also had alcoholics and drug dependence – everything in psychiatry and of course we got to know these cases.

Were these patients presented to your seminar?

Not the patients but the case history along with the Rorschach test and maybe other psychological tests. We discussed all this and in this way we learned an incredible amount and we gained enormous experience. These meetings took from 7.30 p.m. till 11.00 o'clock at night. Additionally Binswanger visited us now and then in the clinic here and we presented cases to him and he gave us his opinion. In this way I learned a great amount. I also had contact with Hans Binder, who was professor in Basel and Director of the Rheinau clinic. He was an excellent psychopathologist.

You mentioned some of the treatments that were being used when you came to Münsterlingen; were there any drug treatments being used and what were the prospects for drug treatment?

Drug treatment was the treatment of choice with sedatives, morphium and scopolamine and sleep therapy as Klaesi did it modified by Cloetta. Very early on we used Trional, which was taught to us by Ernst Grünthal, who came from Reichhart in Würzburg – he was an anatomical brain neurologist and psychiatrist. So we did Trional sleep therapy, that was wonderful. It lasted 6 weeks. One gave Trional up to a certain dose and then came down, like with opium. Very early on, as soon as I joined, we did malaria treatment. It was very difficult during the war because we couldn't get malaria from the tropical institute in Hamburg, where we used to obtain it. So we cultured our malaria base in chronic schizophrenics, so that we were able, during the war, to provide the whole of Switzerland with malaria blood. By the way, this developed from the experience of its effects on chronic stuperous catatonics, where it helped a lot. Malaria treatment really helps these people. I would say they got better; not completely well, but they got better.

I thought these malaria treatments were only used for paralysis?

Well, it's possible that nobody else did this. This idea arose out of necessity.

Where did the idea of introducing Trional treatments come from?

It came from the Würzburg Clinic and Grünthal brought it from there. He had the expertise of how much to give, up to a certain maximum dose. It was a good preparation to pacify some of the raging women on the open wards who simply screamed for 24 hours a day. In this way we managed to significantly improve the atmosphere in the clinic. Also we used electroshock treatment and Cardiazol shock treatment. At that time, I gave the treatment three times a week between 10 and 12 to between eight and twelve cases with cardiazol shock.

Why did you prefer these to insulin shock?

Insulin shock was much less effective. Insulin treatments helped in those cases when a spontaneous epileptic fit occurred – then one would say 'all right, then it will help'. Following this idea we treated people with an additional Cardiazol shock when there was no epileptic fit when they were in the insulin coma. But of course the disadvantage was that after about eight shocks you got a psycho-organic syndrome, which was the beginning of the relapse. After three months these psycho-organic syndromes stopped and the psychotic experiences reappeared.

In 1949 Geigy produced G22150 – the forerunner of imipramine. What do you understand they were hoping to treat when they first produced it?

The true beginning was that I had a connection with the Waldau clinic, where Grünthal was. He had a Brain Anatomical Institute which Klaesi had founded and he had contact with Geigy and had tested an anti-parkinsonian drug for them. He wished to expand the trials and asked me whether I was willing to take part. This is how I came in contact with Geigy.

Which year was that?

That was around 1949. Geigy had at that stage a brilliant pharmacologist, Domenjoz. He later went to Saarbrücken and became professor of pharmacology and did some highly interesting work there. It is incomprehensible that nobody took much notice of this work. Anyway, Domenjoz came to me and said I have a new sleeping pill, would I try it out? I told him I would be interested to try it.

Did he ask anyone else?

Yes, there were other people. Exactly who, I cannot remember – not at least concerning this specific drug. Afterwards I told him: 'This is no sleeping pill, but this substance has curious effects on chronic schizophrenics – not on their sleeping pattern, but on their schizophrenic symptoms.'

At the time when Rhône-Poulenc produced chlorpromazine, they had no idea what the pill would do and they gave it to respiratory physicians and cardiovascular physicians as well. Do you think Geigy also gave this to respiratory and cardiovascular physicians?

No, no. Geigy's drug had the structural formulation of an anti-parkinsonian drug. The anti-parkinsonian drug they had introduced together with Grünthal was Parpanit and it was from this family of drugs that the suspected sleeping pill came from. It had a formula already similar to Tofranil, with a seven-molecule central ring. I had tried Parpanit out with people suffering with Parkinson's but we had very few Parkinson's cases and there were no new ones. The ones we had all originated from the epidemic of encephalitis lethargica. The Waldau also had a few but we were always looking for more cases. That is how this whole thing developed. At this point I already realised that these anti-parkinsonian drugs work better if you give iron. I observed that during treatment where I did a blood analysis all the patients developed a slight anaemia. So I thought to myself I would treat these patients with iron and I realised that if you add iron the neurological symptoms improved, more than if you didn't. When I looked into this, I learned that the nucleus niger is the most iron rich in the whole brain. From then on I've never treated Parkinson's disease without iron. I've always said this but even today nobody believes me. I've always been concerned with such metabolic phenomena.

Anyway then I wrote to Geigy, to Domenjoz, to ask whether he would make available more of this trial drug, because I had an idea to try it on patients with schizophrenia, who had had psychosurgery. At that moment Geigy thought it was clear Kuhn had gone mad, he was not quite right in the head. Now, he wants to treat schizophrenics, whereas we only want to treat Parkinson's. So they sent me these little bottles with tablets and I said this is stupid – that I had to have more and so I gave up.

Did Geigy come round to the idea that it might be useful for schizophrenia after Paul Kielholz had held a meeting in Basel in 1953?

The first meeting of the Swiss Society for Psychiatry did not take place in Basel – it was in Biel. It was the spring meeting, where Kielholz reported for the first time on Largactil. At that point in time I said to myself that I had seen what he was reporting two or three years before with the preparations from Geigy. It was immediately clear to me and I still remember where it happened – I remember where I sat and I remember how he spoke about it and how I thought, it is exactly that which I have seen 2–3 years ago.

Following that meeting we got Largactil gratis – for half a year – and the whole clinic was swallowing Largactil, as one could imagine. Then one day a company rep came and said 'The trial phase is over, now you will have to pay for the Largactil.' Well, we were a poor county; these were poor people and we only had a pharmacy budget of 6000 SFr a year, which we needed first and foremost to buy morphium and scopolamine. You couldn't get much for it and we needed it in great amounts. So we had no money and we couldn't buy Largactil. This was when I said to my boss 'You know I've seen all this with a drug from Geigy. I will write to Geigy and tell them that I know their drug has the same effect.' This is how I went into business with Geigy and they sent me huge bottles!

So I tested it for a whole year and showed that it was truly a neuroleptic, but that it had a lot of unpleasant side-effects and that it was not as good as Largactil. So then the question was 'How does the formula differ from

Largactil?' Because in those days one thought if the formula is fairly similar it should have the same effect. I said that it obviously depended on this side chain, which was different in G22350, that they should use the same side chain as Largactil. As it turned out the substance already existed – it had been synthesised. When I told Domenjoz about my idea in a meeting in a Zurich hotel, he spread out his samples and I said 'That is the substance which has the side chain of Largactil, that is the one I want.' He was immediately agreeable.

They also gave this compound G22355 to lots of other people to try, and you were the only person to pick up the antidepressant effect?

They wanted a neuroleptic. The problem was that I was also looking for a neuroleptic as similar as possible to Largactil. I wanted a formula which was as close as possible to Largactil, so the most obvious thing was to look for the compound with the same side chain, and I tried the compound as a neuroleptic and observed that it was not so good, that it didn't work as well. But I saw that it was different, so then I used it with depression and in particular with clearly endogenous depression.

There were also reports that not only was it not awfully good for schizophrenia but it actually seemed to be unhelpful for some people. You said in your essay in the Pongratz volume that it had a disinhibitory effect on schizophrenics, that people got almost manic.

Yes in any case it didn't do the schizophrenics much good, that was very evident. It was certain that it was no replacment for chlorpromazine.

Where did the idea that it might be useful for treating people who were depressed come from? Was it from hints that one or two people, who were on the study for schizophrenia, went 'high'?

Yes, yes. It is like that. Tofranil affects schizophrenics and the reason is, in my opinion, that schizophrenics often start with a depression, we may be dealing with an Einheits-psychose. Many schizophrenics have depressive symptoms and with these it worked, of course, but at this time I didn't understand how it worked.

At that time you were of the opinion that you were dealing with two separate illnesses.

That was the other thing. I knew what depressions were and that you could heal them with electricshock. So I reasoned that depression is not reactive, that it has to have an organic basis because otherwise electricshock would not work. That was clear. So in principle there had to exist a drug against depression. There were other pointers to the same realisation ... it would lead too far here, to explain this now, it has to do with the psychopathology. In 'vital' depression the most important fact is that the depression is worse in the morning and better in the evenings. Healthy people who work are tired in the evening and fresh in the morning, but if somebody who does not work is tired in the morning and fresh in the evening then this can only be explained on biological grounds. It cannot be psychogenic; there has to be something biological at work.

I know that you have a different philosophy of drug discovery from the currently prevailing one. Can I ask you to expand on the methods of clinical observation you used to discover the antidepressant effects of imipramine?

Given that there has been no discovery of more efficient drugs than imipramine in the last 40 years, I am impelled to ask how I was able to discover these effects and later was in a position to offer to Ciba a modification of the chemical formula of a substance synthesised in its laboratories which was later called maprotiline. My methods were entirely different from those which are nowadays applied in clinical research. I have never used 'controlled double-blind studies' with 'placebos', 'standardised rating scales' or the statistical treatment of records of large numbers of patients.

Instead I examined each patient individually even every day, often on several occasions, and questioned him or her again and again. Many of the patients were also under the observation of my assistants and nursing staff and I always regarded their proposals and criticism seriously and their observations and considerations were also recorded.

Thus, in 1957, I published the results of treating 40 patients for at least 1½ years. Some years later the outstanding Belgian psychiatrist, Bobon, said to me 'The results of your research are surprising. Even more surprising, however, is the fact that in your first publication you discussed 95% of everything there is to be said in essence about imipramine.' Even today, at the most only a small modification would have to be made to the original text.

The essential result of the first publication can be expressed in the following quotation: 'A particularly good effect is achieved with typically endogenous depressions ... as far as they present symptoms of vital depression.' Furthermore, at that time I pointed out that reactive depressions also respond to antidepressant medications.

But it has turned out that most psychiatrists did not know what is meant by the term vital depression. It is a syndrome which consists of tiredness, often combined with disturbed sleep, psychomotor retardation and difficulties with thinking, deciding and acting. Patients have physical and psychological sensations of oppression and narrowness and they have lost the ability to experience joy. But the most important feature is that all of these symptoms are much more marked in the morning than in the evening.

One needs to realise that the symptoms of vital depression are often not spontaneously mentioned by patients and cannot be found easily through questioning. They are often concealed by other symptoms which may seem to be more severe. They may not come to the patient's mind even with questionning. Patients admit to these symptoms only as the links of an integral whole in a dialogue that is free and comprehensible. Isolated questions of a standardised scheme cannot be understood by many patients. He or she may be unable to make any connections between them and his or her former experiences and as a consequence may answer 'no'.

Nowadays you can read in ICD-10 that 'it is acknowledged that the symptoms referred to here as "somatic" could also have been called melancholic, vital, biological or endogenomorphic but that the scientific status of this syndrome is somewhat questionable. The classification is arranged so that this somatic syndrome can be recorded by those who so wish but can also be ignored without loss of any other information.' That is exactly the opposite of what I wrote in 1957 and have stated again and again ever since. Vital depression is based on a correct observation and it can be very often found in almost any psychiatric disorder. But to conclude that this symptomatology is to be considered as a non-specific syndrome which has no meaning is a fundamental error. In any psychiatric disorder which includes vital depression, this syndrome responds to treatment with an antidepressive medication, whatever the other psychopathological diagnosis may be. It may be interesting to note that this comes close to an observation made by the Belgian psychiatrist Guislain 150 years ago, who put forward the idea of a unitary psychosis which always began with a state of depression. I pointed out in 1964 that some support for such views has been shown by the generally acknowledged fact that many patients with obsessional disorders respond to antidepressants.

I have never been urged to change my methods or the interpretation of my results. I have continued to practise and to research as I did before and have obtained significant results. However, they have not received much notice. As long as there is no willingness to understand that psychiatric illnesses, especially affective disorders which form the basis for states of depression, cannot be reduced to mathematics, nothing is going to change.

In the future the researcher needs to turn away from computers. In clinical research, most of the statistics are useless and reliance on them can be severely limiting. It is necessary to turn toward our patients, examine them as individuals, study them and then begin to draw some conclusions based on solid clinical experience. Negative results can prove to be as fruitful as positive ones and can point to the discovery of new facts. The discoverer does not need to go to congresses in order to gain information but does need to examine every patient individually, to talk to them in familiar surroundings and not just in the doctor's office. The doctor has to have a free and open, not preconstructed conversation with the patient, adapted to their situation in a manner that can be easily understood by them. It is necessary for the doctor to continue in that way until the necessary and important information has been obtained, and this work has to be done by the researcher himself and not left to assistants.

You mentioned that you always depended on the observations as well of ward staff and the other people working with you. Now it is quite clear in one sense that the response that you describe to imipramine is something that the ward staff couldn't have fully appreciated – in a sense that what you actually described was the response of a vital depression to this treatment, and they wouldn't have been trained to appreciate concepts such as vital depression – but what role did the observations of the ward staff play in alerting you to what was going on?

I have to explain something at this point. In Münsterlingen we had an outpatients department in the general hospital and the consultants in surgery and gastroenterology, gynaecology and obstetrics were well disposed towards us and sent us cases which were ambiguous and even those which did not show obvious psychological disorder. Every Wednesday we went to the general hospital together with an assistant. We then had to examine six to twelve patients, and decide whether the psychiatrist could have anything to offer to these cases. And often we could. These were average hospital patients who came to hospital with everyday kinds of physical complaints and did not come because of psychological reasons.

Why were these patients referred to a psychiatric outpatients department?

Because the consultants of the departments, when they received a patient who complained about stomach pains and nothing was found during the examination, said 'Let's see whether the psychiatrist can find something.' And what did the psychiatrist find? Mainly there were two diagnoses which we came up with: the first was alcoholism which had been missed by the physicians and the second was vital depressive mood disorder. Here I learned to ask questions which are decisive in finding the underlying vital depressive mood disorder.

I can see this but how much did the people under your supervision, other personnel, nurses for instance, understand this and help with their own observations?

Well, what I learned in the hospital I did not keep to myself. I showed the assistants who came on the rounds with me. They would show me their patients when they couldn't find anything, or else found something very odd and then I would explain to them: 'This women has a depression and that is why she is in hospital.' This is how the assistants learned from me. In the same way I taught the nursing staff how they have to observe the patients in order to see vital depressive mood disorder. It happened for years like this. The discovery dates from the year 1957 and I came here in 1939, so I had worked on this for 18 years before I made the discovery.

So these insights came from you to others and obviously not the other way round?

Yes, and when these people noticed a response to treatment, of course, they then told me 'You were right.' Even my boss, the director who, of course, also got to hear about it, observed the same thing.

How much was the actual discovery of this drug at this time an accident of history in the sense that if you were to give Tofranil to people who were being treated today for being depressed, it possibly couldn't be shown to work as well, maybe because community cases of the kind we have today are milder cases, while on the other hand if you look at the drugs that are used today for people who are depressed, the SSRIs, they mightn't have worked as well for the more severe cases you had in the 1950s in hospital?

It is certain at that time of course that we had a different kind of patient from today. They were people with a more severe depression. Today the depressive comes for treatment only after their general practitioner has already done everything possible with them. The cases then were much better suited for trials because those today who are suitable for trials don't come anymore to the psychiatrist and even less into clinic. The clinical picture has completely changed because of treatment.

The second remark reaches very far and it is very complicated. It's because of the fact that catecholinergic as well as serotoninergic active drugs work as antidepressants. In my opinion, the number of people who are affected by catecholinergic drugs only is larger than those on which serotoninergic drugs work only. There is a third group that is affected by both. Purely catecholinergic-responsive cases are probably a quarter of all cases, at a guess, purely serotonergic are probably 10–20% and the others are mixed, and the composition is not always the same. During treatment the effectiveness of one or the other drug may change. Under certain circumstances you can get a pure catecholinergic effect in the beginning, with Ludiomil, but after a while you have to add something else or vice versa. There are probably 10% of all cases where the catecholinergic drugs don't work at all (Ludiomil), who respond very well to serotoninergic agents. That doesn't mean that after half a year it is still like this – it might be that you have to add Ludiomil after half a year in order to maintain the good effect because the inner dynamic is changing all the time. This has to do with the fact that the serotoninergic and the catecholinergic systems are most intimately connected with each other. So you see the serotoninergic system can induce a reaction in the catecholinergic cells. And the opposite is possibly also true.

Now, you actually discovered the antidepressant effects of the drug at the end of 1955?

No. It is absolutely clear, the date is fixed – it is one day and that I can tell you. I have here a copy of the case history of the first patient.

'On 12 January 1956 the treatment has begun with 100 mg of Tofranil. On 14 January there was an acute symptom of delusion... Ah here, 21 January 1956: For three days the patients is a totally changed person. So since the 18 January, six days from the beginning of the treatment (I added that afterwards), all her manic behaviour and restlessness has disappeared. The day before yesterday, she remarked herself, that she had been terribly confused and as stupid as she had ever been before and she didn't know where it had come from but she was only glad that she was better now.' – That was the 18 January 1956.

OK, but why this long interval between your first report of antidepressant effects to Geigy and the final marketing of the drug? Why did the company hesitate so long?

That is another story. In January 1956 I made the discovery and shortly afterwards sent a report to Geigy. After this report, Geigy sent the compound to ten Swiss clinics. Of these ten clinics, I think six replied. All six said that the drug was completely useless. Following that, Geigy said that they would not proceed and that I didn't know a thing. But then there was a very prominent person at Geigy, Robert Böhringer, – who was also a shareholder at Geigy. He had some influence in the running of Geigy. He was known as the 'grey eminence'. He constantly moved around in the company, opened every door, and asked everybody what they were doing. He had an office employing two secretaries who wrote reports for the attention of the management. Now a relative of Robert Böhringer became depressed and he had heard that there was something about that might help and he asked whether he could try the drug. So Robert Böhringer went with Tofranil in his pocket back to Geneva and gave it to his relative. After five days she was actually healed and he came back to Basel and said Kuhn is right – it is an antidepressive. So then the firm introduced the preparation. But this is not publicised anywhere.

Extraordinary.

This is absolutely authentic because Böhringer himself told me. At that time there did not exist any government departments who concerned themselves with these things. Anybody could put onto the market what he wanted without asking a soul but Geigy still thought it was not true. So they said 'OK, we will introduce it but only in Switzerland and only for psychiatric clinics.' Then Kielholz, who was working at the psychiatric clinic in Basel, said how wonderfully well it worked and after that other people said how excellent it was – for instance Lieser, in Haar, near Munich, where there is still a big clinic.

But on the other hand there was also somebody else, for instance, who summoned me after about a year, who told me it was terribly painful for him to have to inform me that everything I had said about Tofranil treatments of depression was untrue. It was all incorrect. He had made trials with his colleagues and he found that it was all untrue. I said, 'I have to ask you, what kind of patients did you test it on?' He replied patients, of course, with unambiguous depression – depression with melancholic delusions. I answered that 'I have never claimed that it would work with these kinds of depressions but I have always said that the important part was the vital depression.' To which he replied that this was such an ambiguous expression that he didn't know what to make of it. So, I explained to him what I understand vital depression to be. He said that now it was clear to him and I told him, 'Now go and please do not treat that other kind of patient because the drug will not help there. You have to use it with the right kind of patient. If the patients are manic you have to also give a neuroleptic.' Today everybody knows these things.

Was another reason for the hold-up the fact that the effects of the drug were counter-intuitive, in the sense that everyone expected an antidepressant, if there was such a thing, to be something of a stimulant but here you were proposing that a sedative drug was antidepressant?

That again is a very complicated question. The idea of stimulus and inhibition, these opposite activities, of course is a scientific idea which has been carried into the debate artificially. It is much too simplistic in order to explain what happens. One needs a very intricate exploration in order to know exactly what is happening.

Certainly, but from a naïve point of view, people within the company would have thought that if there was a drug that was going to be antidepressant, that it would be more likely to be a stimulant. Within Geigy were there other reasons to hold back apart from the reason that many other clinicians did not believe in it?

That I do not know. Of course nobody at Geigy knew what a depression was. Now the whole world talks of depression but then depression, as an illness, was predominantly only known of in specialist medical circles. Everything I said sounded to these people highly curious.

Was it seen as a rare disease at this time?

Yes, there were the great melancholias with delusions, with suicidal ideas, with stupor, with agitation, with food refusal, the classical great melancholia which was then, as today, a rather rare presentation, while vital depression, as I have described it, is the most common illness over all although at the same time it is the least well known – exactly because it occurs together with hypochondria, with obsessive-compulsive disorders, hysterical manifestations, manic behaviour etc. And then people only treat these symptoms, nobody thinks to look beneath it.

Were you aware that they called in other experts to help them assess the drug? People like Frank Ayd were asked in.

That is true, when it got around, of course everybody came to Basel.

But not before?

No, before there was nobody. Before there were only these ten Swiss clinics which were asked and all of them were told it was a new neuroleptic, the same as Largactil, and they were to try it out. Six replied it was totally useless, there were only side-effects.

All tried it as a neuroleptic and nobody tried it for depression?

But nobody thought that they could use it for depression, nobody thought of it, of course.

But by then your report was with Geigy saying that it helped against depression?

Geigy didn't notice that there was anything new within this report. Geigy was only looking for a neuroleptic, they only wanted a competitor to Largactil. They said to themselves, those French are earning big money with Largactil and we want to have a share of the money.

They only realised after Böhringer?

Well, even then they didn't fully. Only very few believed it at that time. But it was the case that Böhringer could prevent them from telling me to terminate the trials.

That was the key moment then?

What Böhringer said was the most important factor at Geigy, at least this is how Böhringer presented it to me. Böhringer was a poet from the Stefan George Circle. He was an extraordinarily educated man. He owned one of the few original marble images of Plato. I do not know how he was paid by Geigy, but one day Geigy gave him a painting by a very famous Renaissance painter, Montegna, in order to reward his services to the company. He was an amazing personality. And he was the one without whom Geigy would have let the whole thing drop and nobody would have ever known about it.

Some additional evidence for what you are saying comes from the fact that in 1958 Geigy produced G34568, which was later clomipramine and they gave it, as I understand it, to Walter Pöldinger first and asked him to try it out in schizophrenia. They still weren't looking for a compound for depression.

I tested clomipramine and also dichlorimipramine – Geigy had a compound dichlorimipramine where both phenyl rings had a chlorine atom. This preparation was also effective. The specific effect of clomipramine on obsessive compulsive behaviour I saw in 1964 when I said that you could use this compound to heal OCD. In 1964 I wrote to Geigy about this but it is the case that I also only realised later that clomipramine has a specific effectiveness in OCD.

How does this link with the idea of a unitary psychosis?

The same thing applies to hysterical manifestations. Only that with hysterical manifestations, even more than with others, in addition to the manic-depressive constitution, a paroxysmal symptom of the epileptic kind is present as well. This is why women with hysterical manifestations – of the notorious kind – have to be treated with additional Tegretol. In these kinds of cases I give Tofranil, Ludiomil or Anafranil, and depending on how big a part the obsessional behaviour plays, I give Tegretol. I had very good successes but you cannot leave it out.

To come back to 1957 and Geigy's dilemma about whether to market this compound as an antidepressant: Did the fact that Nathan Kline, in 1957, came out and said I have an antidepressant and there is a big market out there for that kind of compound, make any difference to the way they thought?

I do not know how much that played a role. I came to America in 1958 to the American Congress in San Francisco, when there was a great deal of news about Nathan Kline and Marsilid. It was printed in the American daily papers that the congress commission had interviewed Kline and that Kline told them that the Russians with their Sputnik were way ahead of the Americans in the Arms Race. Now it was important that America should get ahead of the Russians and they could only do it by increasing the psychic abilities of the American researchers. So he said that everybody should take Marsilid, in order to help with their psychic powers, so that America could catch up with the Russians in the space programme. And this was printed in the newspapers in May 1958 at the time when we were in America.

Was Kline's name known in Basel?

Yes, yes, Kline was known in Basel. Kline was widely known, he himself saw to it that he was well known ... And at this congress in San Francisco, he made a big show and tried to impress everybody. Hoffmann La Roche were also there with Pletscher, who stated that the benzodiazepine compound, Librium, would do exactly the same as Kline had promised. He gave a major lecture on the point that if one was to change this or that on the benzodiazepine molecule and I don't know what else ... that then there was a prospect that you would find a wonder drug as well. This lecture by Pletscher I heard myself. I guess that there are records from this congress – it was in May 1958.

I also had to give a lecture on Tofranil, which I did but I had very few listeners, just like in Zürich. In Zürich there were fewer than a dozen people, when I gave that lecture at the World Psychiatric Congress in September of 1957. But it was published in the *Swiss Medical Weekly*. That was the original publication. The Russians, who were there, read that and they went home and declared through diplomatic channels that they had to obtain this compound immediately. They got it through diplomatic channels and in Moscow the pharmacology of the compound was reproduced and I had the impression that it ended better than when Geigy produced it. Basel was then 2–3 years behind in the work of their pharmacologists.

Later I went to Russia and talked to the relevant pharmacologist and he told me the whole story. It was a very embarrassing one. When the congress in Zürich took place the Russians had recently invaded Hungary. Following that the Swiss Society of Psychiatry cancelled the invitation to the whole Russian delegation. So then the Russians took the issues of the *Swiss Medical Weekly* where everything was published. They read it and instantaneously translated it. Then they realised that of everything that was in the issue about new developments that were being debated at the congress, the most interesting was the publication of Tofranil. Which was true! And they immediately – the pharmacologists told me this for sure – switched a whole institute to the analysis of the pharmacology of the substance. The original compound from Basel was bought through the embasssy in Berne in large amounts and went to Russia. And there they realised its importance, long before America realised it ... that also is part of this story. Psychoanalysis was very influential in American.

When you gave your talk at the World Psychiatric Association Meeting in Zürich in 1957 this was the first public talk on the use of imipramine for people who were depressed. Why were there so few people in the audience? Why do you think there was so little interest?

Because it was one of several hundred presentations, you see. And that was for 20 minutes. And there were a lot of other people who spoke. I was myself the chairman of this session, because it was of such little interest. Nobody thought that it was of any importance to us. One of the psychiatrists, he was the professor in Lausanne, knew it. He himself treated depressed patients and he had had Tofranil before it was on the market, I sent him the medicine, and he was cured in five days. There were some people who noticed but it was a very small percentage of the many people who were there.

Why was the level of interest so low?

Because nobody believed that there could be a drug against depression. One drug rep from Geigy told me he had been to see one of the heads of department in Germany. He had wanted to introduce Tofranil and the professor listened for a while to him and then said 'Well, my dear colleague, we are clear about something here – depression is a reactive illness and nothing else and you can go with your drug back to where you came from, it doesn't interest me.' This was a famous German professor.

When did it come on the market here in Switzerland?

I believe 1 November 1957.

Were you at the CINP meeting in 1958 in Rome – you're not listed as one of the speakers?

I was there. There was a meeting one morning with I think eight papers. I did not speak – I was not invited to speak – but the meeting was a singular triumph for Tofranil.

Why weren't you invited?

That I don't know. I thought it was curious but Geigy obviously still did not believe that I was right.

That's strange.

Yes, it was like this. I was not invited by Geigy to speak but I was invited in order to help write for the journal in which the congress proceedings were reported. So then I wrote the papers on depression. They are mine. I've got copies of this paper if you are interested and if I can find them you can have one.

It is curious that you did not take the stage – others gave talks on imipramine. Did you talk to Geigy about it?

I thought it was strange but that simply is how it was. It may have been connected to ... I can't remember who chaired the meeting, I would have to look it up, but I suppose that the chairperson of the meeting had to organise the symposium for the congress management and he did not know me. He only invited famous people instead. And there were very famous people there. For one there was Hoff from Vienna amongst the audience and then Jean Delay from Paris.

Jean Delay came up to me after the lectures. I knew Jean Delay and he knew me. I had worked several times at his clinic and I was friendly with his EEG specialist. He made me explain why I had gone ahead with this, without letting him and his clinic know. I said that I was very sorry but his consultant Deniker had been in the possession of the drug for a year and had up till now refused to test it. When he heard this Jean Delay challenged Deniker and made a huge scene in public in Rome.

I had been previously introduced to Hoff in the Engelsburg but he took no notice at all of me. But after the lecture, which he had been present at, he suddenly came towards me and greeted me and told me how highly interesting it was. I had to come to Vienna and give a talk. That same year (or the year after) he invited me to a meeting of the Austrian Society in Graz. We were late, because the train was late, so we just crept into the lecture theatre, where Hoff, who chaired the meeting, interrupted the proceedings, greeted me with all his Viennese charm and politeness and spoke of 'his dear colleague whom he'd been intimately connected with for many years'. But I have to say that he was very nice to me. He invited me several times to his clinic in Vienna, where I stayed in his private quarters. In the morning a sister came with an enormous breakfast, and I came and went into his clinic as if I were at home. He then showed me the clinic, introduced me to the patients and so on and was very, very nice to me. He planned at one point to make me his successor – he once approached me. Nothing came of it – I didn't really actively pursue the matter. He then approached Kielholz but Kielholz did not go. I presume that Hoff thought I would not go.

Were you at the CINP meetings in Basel in 1960 or the USA in 1962? You are not listed as actually being a speaker. Why I ask is, that one of the odd things about the whole story is why there was no prize for the discovery of the antidepressants. Do you have to go to conferences and be seen in order to be proposed for prizes?

I don't know. I always say in psychiatry you get a prize not for the biggest successes but for the biggest disasters. It is just like that but why this is so I cannot tell you, you probably know better. I never got a prize – I did once get a prize as a fresh young man. I got 300 SFr from the Lucerna Foundation for my work on the interpretation of the Rorschach test. Otherwise, I never got a penny. I am an Honorary Doctor of the University of Löwen (Louvain) for Medicine, and Honorary Doctor for Medicine at the University of Basel – I received this one two or three years ago. It was Pöldinger's doing. Also I am an Honorary Doctor of Philosophy at the Sorbonne in Paris for my work on the Daseins-analytical philosophy. Not for medicine. I go in a yellow gown of the philosophy faculty rather than the red one of the medical faculty.

How do you account for that?

Well. Envy plays a very big role. That is certain. I am convinced. Constantly people say that I have only made these discoveries by accident. And this I deny. It was not an accident. It was an accident that I happened upon this compound but I did choose it.

If you hadn't had the insight about vital depression then you wouldn't have been using it on these patients.

I wouldn't have found it. That was no accident. It was the result of a long historical development. The fact that nobody will accept this is inconceivable.

Everybody thinks 'It's a pity that this accident didn't happen to me.' Everybody thinks it could have happened to him just as well. I'll tell you a good anecdote about this. There is a Frenchman who wrote about the history of this, Thuillier, who put it like this: 'Un petit psychiatrie de campagne, foutu dans ses montagnes, a fait par hazard le decouverte de Tofranil.' The point is nobody gives a prize to someone like this.

But even before that weren't you involved in introducing the EEG into Switzerland?

No. It was introduced in Waldau. If I hadn't come to Münsterlingen, then I might have been the first, because Klaesi offered me an EEG apparatus from Tönnis. This was before the war – it was a machine with three connections. Incomprehensibly I did not follow this career and went to Münsterlingen. But after the Waldau, mine was the second psychiatric clinic in Switzerland which had an EEG in June 1950.

How did you get involved in the maprotiline story?

Yes, the maprotiline story went like this. After Tofranil was a success, there were several pharmaceutical companies who turned to me with the idea that if they gave me a compound, then something would come of it. This was the case also with Ciba. Ciba offered me a compound and I told them that I was agreeable to try it. The thing was, Ciba wanted a competitor to the benzodiazepines. They had a compound which acted as a muscle relaxant and they suggested to me that I should try this compound. I tested it and said it was slightly anxiety reducing and slightly sedative. But for clinical usage in psychiatry it was much too weak. They then introduced this compound anyway, and it was a flop. So I said to Ciba the ring system was in my opinion very interesting, but one should alter it, and give it the side chain of Tofranil, which is the same as in Largactil. They should attach this to the ring system and they might have a useful psychopharmacological drug.

The pharmacologist said Kuhn should try our compounds and not suggest compounds. But later, after the first meeting where we talked about this, I got very friendly with this pharmacologist – Hugo Bein. Then he told his chemist – who was Wilhelm – to create this substance which had not been already produced. So then Wilhelm had to obey Bein although he was highly appalled that a psychiatrist would suggest to a chemist what kind of substance he had to produce! And that compound was maprotiline.

You are responsible for it. But you do not participate in the profits?

Well, I have received something. It wasn't riches. I had a share in the turnover for 12 years. It wasn't a great deal but never the less ... Of course the compound would never have been produced if I hadn't told them.

When you looked at maprotiline clinically you looked at it in the same way as you describe Tofranil: you looked at it in depth with a large number of patients. At the same time the company was beginning to do clinical trials with placebo controls. That was fine then, but the interesting story comes about later on with levoprotiline. Can you fill us in on that story?

How did the idea come about first of all that it might be an antidepressant. What did you discover when you used it and what in your opinion went wrong in the company?

This is a complicated history. The complication lies in the fact that levoprotiline was produced as a racemate. It was found that one of the compounds was biochemically active and the other inactive in all the usual tests. They decided to separate the two isomers, which you can do, with the intention of using the inactive substance as placebo whilst testing the other one. But it was evident that the placebo was more effective than the actual substance which was on trial.

The thing was this: levoprotiline had been given to half the world to try. I also received it and I started levoprotiline in a large investigation with over 100 cases. I produced a study which was ripe for publication but still today is a manuscript that has never been published. Then Ciba gave America levoprotiline. From America came a damning report, which was as expected. This experts' report I have never seen. It was explicity denied to me. But a friend of mine, a very good psychiatrist and pharmacologist in Germany, a man of good renown, saw the report and he told me it was completely unqualified, absolutely. Without asking me, or telling me anything, Ciba decided not to pursue the matter any further and the last stocks of the compound which had been synthesized were burnt last year.

Why has your manuscript never been published?

Ciba did not want to keep the analysis; they wouldn't know what would become of it and so on. Germany was very interested in it and insisted on importing it. I said one should license it because it is a compound that has no effect on either the serotonin or catecholamine systems but it is an antihistamine. I had an interesting case with a lady professor, the wife of a very wealthy Swiss gentleman, who told me how treatment with an antidepressant I was giving her had diminished her extreme allergy. She called me to tell me that her cat allergy had gone. One can surmise that the biochemistry of depression and the antidepressants and the histamines and the antihistamine drugs affect each other. That is very probable but nobody is interested in it, even though it is extremely interesting that a substance that is active on neither the catecholamine nor serotonergic systems is without a doubt antidepressive.

You are sure of that?

Yes, yes, absolutely. It is less active than Tofranil and less active than Anafranil or Ludiomil but it is almost the same as lithium and without a doubt specifically an antidepressant, without a doubt.

You were very angry with the company? And with the FDA? I've heard you say that we have got to resist the regulators.

Yes, it is terrible. The reason why levoprotiline was not licensed is this: the drug was not shown to be effective in a placebo-controlled trial and the FDA implied it was just sugar, so it could not be licensed. It was impossible. But Astra in Sweden wanted to buy it. Three representatives from Astra came to

Switzerland to talk to me. I had a long conversation with them, explaining the situation, and they refused it in the end because it could not be tested under any of today's methods.

Was that before or after the catastrophe with zimelidine?

It was after. The zimelidine catastrophe was another chapter – I tried zimelidine as well.

What can you tell us about it?

I can tell you the following. I was given zimelidine to try out, and I tried it but I didn't see any effect. Then I was invited to Stockholm to take part in the launching of zimelidine. I listened to the whole thing. They had a very good biochemist who gave a very good introduction, then there was a good bio-pharmacologist. But after that there was a disastrous clinical report, totally unsatisfactory. The longest trial lasted four weeks – well, I cannot say anything after four weeks. I reckoned they would find out even less than I. In any case I was of the opinion that one couldn't be responsible for recommending this drug for licence, on the grounds of the clinical trials which had been done. It was impossible to judge whether it could be licensed. That is the proof for the total inefficiency of bureaucratic regulation. I thought if they are lucky they will get it through but they have to have undeserved luck. And they did not have the luck.

There is a drug you have here for a condition you have or have had here – and we have neither the drug nor the condition in the Anglo-Saxon world. The drug is Opipramol-Insidon and the condition vegetative dystonia. What is this condition and what is the difference between it and vital depression and between opipramol and an antidepressant drug?

Opipramol is in fact a very good antidepressant. It is weaker than Tofranil, that is clear. It is given usually in doses of 50 mg and not 25 mg, which is the normal dosage. It is very well suited for menopausal women, especially when they experience sleeplessness. If there is depression with sleep disorder then Insidon is an excellent drug. It is, for instance, excellent for reactive depression also with severe bereavement reaction after a death in the family. Excellent. The bereavement reaction is not interfered with but the ability to overcome the mourning process is enhanced. It is an excellent compound against anxiety and has practically no side-effects with normal dosage. We still use Insidon with certain cases and, then, it is a very good drug. But Ciba Geigy never advertised it at all, they never went to anybody to ask them to test the drug with a larger trial base. It is mainly a drug for outpatient usage, it is not a drug for severe psychotic depression. For primary care it is ideal. It is really very good and somebody should speak up for this preparation. One should do the proper tests but Ciba Geigy doesn't contribute a cent for any such trial.

And vegetative dystonia?

This refers to an abnormal frailty of the vegetative nervous system; that is, people whose pulse increases quickly, people who very quickly collapse, who easily break out into sweats, who, because of this vegetative instability, tend towards panic attacks. They also become depressed quickly, because depression goes hand in hand with the whole neuro-vegetative condition. Many depressions are neuro-vegetatively stigmatised. These people have a vegetative nervous system which is less adaptable, it gets out of balance and has little tendency to get back into balance. They suffer from severe dizziness, for instance vertigo, and often in old age they suffer badly from travel sickness so that if they are not at the wheel themselves they get extremely sick, very dizzy etc. It is simply a very generalised instability and a relatively poor performance of the vegetative system which should equip man for the demands of the world.

How do you explain the fact that it seems to be only a Middle European disease – it's not found in the Anglo-Saxon world?

I don't know. What I know is, there is such a thing. I've seen it. In America drugs are given as a matter of course in doses that would kill somebody in Switzerland. Here in Switzerland if we give benzodiazepines, Valium, we give one milligram or two – in America you give 100. I don't know why. I personally think that one can kill off the vegetative nervous system, roughly speaking, so that it does not function anymore and I guess that in America, with such abuse of high dosages of very powerful drugs, the neuro-vegetative reaction in these people is practically non existent. The cause of this are not only the drugs but also for example noise – that plays a big role – constant stimulation, criminality, also the hectic way of life, etc. so that the neuro-vegetative system just cannot keep up. You can get the same thing with caffeine and there are such large doses of caffeine given with drugs in the States which I would think would give people pulse rates of up to 200 and put them at risk of dying!

So many medicines which are given in America ordinarily are clearly poisonous here. I do not know what else causes this or whether this really is the cause – but I have always explained it to myself like this. Of course there is more. Alcohol is drunk there to such an extent which we never see here. I have once seen a statistic on death from acute alcohol poisoning in England – which cannot be compared to here – I have maybe seen two or three in my whole life. I have only actually met one person who really died from alcoholic coma. When I saw these figures from England, I was terribly shocked that there is drunkenness to an extent which we do not usually find here. Another big role is played by smoking. I mean if somebody consumes four packets a day he kills himself, or at least he kills his vegetative nervous system and then you can do anything with him. This is my explanation but I cannot prove it. I can't help you any further.

When there is only one drug in a class of drugs it can often take a while for that drug to have an impact. But when there are two drugs then it can make more of a difference. How much difference did amitriptyline make to imipramine, in the sense in the late 1950s there were lots of MAOIs and only one tricyclic? Then amitriptyline came along and then there were two and the tricyclics became more prominent after that.

Amitriptyline was first produced by Hoffmann La Roche. When the president of Hoffmann La Roche saw the pharmacology he said – I was not present at this but I have heard it said – 'Such nonsense we can't bring it onto the market.' Amitriptyline has very probably a stronger sedative, hypnotic effect than Tofranil and more side-effects than Tofranil or partially different ones.

But did its existence ease the acceptance of Tofranil and the acceptance of this whole class of drugs? If you have two drugs in one class it often helps.

That is one possibility. The other one is that it pushed Tofranil into the background because the advertising campaign of Roche and Merck was much more aggressive than Geigy's. The sedative effect has always been an advantage over the stimulating effect of Tofranil. You can combine Tofranil and amitriptyline – you can give Tofranil in the morning and in the evening amitriptyline. Then there is another unpleasant property of amitriptyline: it loses its antidepressant effect in about six weeks to three months. The sedative effect lingers; this is why people take amitriptyline as a sleeping pill because of its sedative effect, but with regard to the antidepressant effect people get more tolerant, more indifferent.

There is something else to say here which is that everybody in pharmacology compares the antidepressant effect of a new drug not with Tofranil but with amitriptyline. Why – because amitriptyline is less effective than Tofranil and because of this a small effect of the test substance in comparison with amitriptyline has a bigger chance than if you were to compare it with Tofranil. From this you can indirectly conclude that it is true what I say.

In the early 1960s, I think there was some recognition in the company, not all these compounds were the same, that imipramine wasn't quite the same kind of compound as clomipramine and they were quite different from MAOIs, but yet the logic of the marketplace for the companies seemed to be that all these things had to be the same, they had to be antidepressants and there was to be no particular distinction made among the antidepressants. What role do you think marketplace logic played in development of the field?

The differentiation is difficult from a clinical point of view. It is much easier to have everything the same. Everything is antidepressive, and it is of course, the drug reps tell me that general practitioners don't want specific medicines – they want medicines which they can give three times a day, which work, and that is it.

Sure, but also the logic for the companies is they have got to say this pill will treat X million people, they don't want to be in the business to develop compounds for smaller indications.

The companies will say my drug works faster than the competitors'. Secondly my drug has fewer side-effects than the competitors'. Thirdly my drug is just as good as the competitors'. These are three factors. But after maybe four or five years nobody hears of it anymore that it works faster than all others – it doesn't. Secondly nobody says that it has fewer side effects, because it hasn't, and thirdly nobody says anymore that it is just as good as the others because it has been discovered that it is not as good! There is none that is better than Tofranil, Anaframil, Ludiomil and Insidon – nobody has discovered a better drug yet.

In your opinion is this also true for fluoxetine?

Yes, with fluoxetine and paroxetine and the other new ones, they are effective in about 50% of cases – that is proven – while under the same conditions, with the same trial base Anafranil is 50–60% effective. All this comes from statistics, I have seen it many times, and Tofranil (if they include it) is even better. This is the situation. Now, concerning fluoxetine I have read that in the USA about a year ago, two million people are dependent on it. Well I don't know but one reads more and more that fluoxetine is addictive. Why it should be addictive is a riddle to me, because Anafranil I'm pretty sure is not addictive. What the position is with the other drugs I do not know. Fluoxetine of course has been pushed much more and so it has been used much more and indeed it is main-ly used by people who are not depressed but who use it as a pure stimulant. What the consequences will be nobody knows at the moment. We might know in ten years time, when people cannot come off it.

In any case I have used fluoxetine before this was known. I have seen that it has exactly the same irritating side-effects as Anafranil; that is, namely impotence with men and frigidity in women. You read everywhere and in every publication that this is the case only in 3% of patients and if you pur-sue the matter in the literature you will find they must have missed a digit. It is more like 35%. With my patients I find that almost every second one to whom the drug was given ends up with dysfunction in this area. Of course you have to take into account what age you are dealing with: if you give it to a 20-year-old it does not crucially diminish his potency but if you give it to a 50-year-old who is not quite so potent anymore, he will be much affected by this. A statistic about such matters which does not take into account the age of these patients, you can throw away. It tells you nothing. First of all you have to know the age, then you have to know how many men and how many women there are – impotence will be reported more than frigidity, that is well known. Then you have to know whether the patients have been inter-viewed about this. Most of them will not have been explicitly questioned so that only those who complain are included in the statistics and so on. The literature in my opinion is totally worthless. You can throw it all into the waste paper bin, you can light a fire with it and science would be not one iota the poorer.

When you published your paper in 1957 on Tofranil, you said you had people in treat-ment even then for a year and a half. And in 1958 when you published your paper in the American Journal of Psychiatry you said you had people in treatment for two years at that stage. Where did we get the idea that you only need to treat depression for 4–6 weeks? Somewhere in the early 1960s it seems, people got the idea that treatment with an anti-depressant was like treatment with an antibiotic, it could be a short course of treatment.

Of course, one has to know what is important. You can ask specific questions if it is as it is described here that after six days the effect is there, then I do not need to wait two years. It is true that the more experience you have the better you can judge it, but in the beginning I had to have lots of time. I did not treat all 40 cases for 1½ years. There were cases which I had treated for six weeks. I was in America in the spring of 1958, that was nearly one year after the first publication. Then I already had patients whom I had in treatment during two years, who were included before in the first group, who then afterwards were added, and then continued to be treated. I've got patients who have taken Tofranil over 15 years ...

Why has it taken the field 30 years almost to rediscover that a number of people would have to be treated for months or years?

It is like this: chronic depression exists. Chronic depression has always existed. That is one thing. Secondly, cyclical depression which becomes more frequent leads into a permanent depressive state. These are facts that are known since Kraepelin – it was written in the Psychiatry of Kraepelin in 1908. This is well-known classical psychiatry. That nobody talks about this anymore is purely based on the fact that psychiatrists don't know the old psychiatry anymore. Today the psychiatrist who researches reads literature of the previous five years! Because of this we get discoveries today which have been known much better, and described much more beautifully a hundred years ago. And everybody thinks it highly interesting what Mr X has discovered, when all along in the old literature it had been wonderfully illustrated – much nicer, much better. That is so. That is the so-called modern psychiatry of which the psychiatrists of today are so incredibly proud.

Can I ask you, though, if people have to stay on treatment for two years or more, in some sense the disease has not been cured. What is the treatment then treating?

Well, this is a problem. After a while these compounds use up substances which are necessary in order to function. Amongst these substances are iron, copper, zinc, magnesium and chromium. When you have to treat for a long time then you have to supplement with these trace elements. If you don't do it, it will become worse and worse in spite of treatment with drugs. This is because tyrosine hydroxylase is obligatorily dependent on iron. If it cannot be activated because there is not enough iron then the metabolism doesn't change the tyrosine to dopamine but it goes instead from tyrosine to parahydroxyphenylacetic acid. You can prove this because if you give many of these patients iron the parahydroxyphenylacetic acid will disappear from their urine. In addition noradrenaline is produced from dopamine. This process needs dopamine-beta-hydroxylase, which is dependent on copper. And you can check in the urine whether this is working by looking at the ratio of dopamine to noradrenaline metabolites and if the proportion is not right you have to give copper. If you don't, what happens? – after 2–3 days we have a relapse, pure and simple. But to think about that is for the contemporary psychiatrist much too difficult and is rejected as humbug.

The case is very straightforward but it seems these are thoughts which neither the psychiatrist nor seemingly the biochemist thinks. When I told this to the people from Ciba, they said that I was ranting – that I do not understand anything about all this. The strange thing is that these obtuse ideas which I have work very well in the clinic!

Have you publicised your own ideas on this theme?

Partially, partially not. The other day I gave a lecture and in the break I heard two young psychiatrists say 'What Kuhn tells us here is nonsense.'

You worked on librium. Do you want to tell us some more about that?

Yes, I can simply say that I have used librium with a morphine-addicted father-in-law of a very high-up employee of Hoffmann La Roche, before librium was on the market anywhere in the world, and after 14 days this man was as addicted to librium as he had been to morphine. This was the first time that I ever came into contact with this compound, which then had no name – I only knew that it was a benzodiazepine. I realised that this compound is addictive and so I have never used it in my practice again. I have only prescribed Valium for the treatment of status epilepticus, where you can end up in a court case if you don't.

How do you treat panic attacks then?

With carbamazepine mainly. With panic attacks you have to make sure whether the attack is the result of a paroxysm, a manic-depressive illness or a schizophrenic disorder. That is the first thing. If a schizophrenic breakdown is imminent then of course you give a neuroleptic first of all. If you can detect vital depression behind it then you give antidepressants. Often there is also a paroxysmal component where there is a burgeoning of emotions which are suddenly discharged, then you give carbamazepine.

The great days of Swiss psychiatry seem over. The big names like Bleuler and Klaesi haven't been succeeded today. Why has the golden era come to an end?

All golden eras come to an end! Just like those of the important poets, the great musicians or the great painters. Remember in the Renaissance we had all at the same time Raphael, Michelangelo, Leonardo, Montegna, and now ...

Many professors today would not have obtained a position at the clinic of Eugen Bleuler. You have to know how things were with Bleuler. There are many anecdotes about Eugen Bleuler. A foreign doctor came to the clinic as an assistant, announced his arrival to the porter etc. and then somebody came along in a grey coat, took the suitcase of the assistant, and said 'Here is your room, tomorrow morning at 9.00 is ward round, you come to the so and so room,' and then he went. The next morning the assistant realised that the porter of yesterday was Eugen Bleuler, the Professor himself.

Was he a modest person?

Yes, that he was. He had in his pockets a little notebook into which he wrote all his reports. He would sit in some corner of the ward and write what patient X had said and so on. This is how it happened ... And then there was Kurt Goldstein from Berlin. He appeared at 2 o'clock in the morning on the ward, waking the patient in order to give him a neurological investigation in order to ascertain whether something which had occurred to him during his sleepless night made sense: if this patient with this particular type of functional disorder did this or that. He would go into the clinic and try it out to see whether he was correct.

Why is the industry not so interested in the CNS area any more, particularly the psychiatric area? Did Kielholz have any role here?

Professor Kielholz played a foremost role in pharmacology in Switzerland – much more important in this respect than Angst. Kielholz himself was very clever in the employment of psychopharmaceuticals. But psychiatry was not developed enough to lead the industry in the very difficult area of psychopharmacology. That is the problem.

Kielholz was a clever practitioner. Lately I talked to one of his consultants who said about him that with regard to the practical employment of pharmaceuticals, she had never seen anybody who could have done better. But he stayed completely in the realms of classical psychopharmacology. He also gave benzodiazepines for example, which I have never done, and he never understood that iron deficiency plays a role. When I said, 'Listen, you have to give people iron' he said ' I'll look into it.' What did he do? Every morning he sent round a phlebotomist to take blood and get the values for iron. He didn't know of course that the iron concentration is lowest in the evening and highest in the morning. This may have something to do with muscle metabolism. But he never noticed this and in his study only one patient of a hundred patients suffered from iron deficiency. So he would say 'It is not true.' Today we do it differently: we analyse hair, you get the average value for iron in the organ, for the last three months, you take three centimetres of hair, and then you can properly show whether the patient has iron deficiency or not. You even see whether he has too much, so that you must not give iron.

Further you have to know that magnesium is reabsorbed by the body only up to 45 years of age. Then you have to give magnesium as magnesium orotate and not as magnesium chloride or hydroxide, or sulphate. You have to know all this if you give such treatment – you have to know how the preparations are to be given so that they are absorbed and that they enter the cells, so that they can fulfil their functions. Today nobody learns this in psychiatry. A few pupils still come to me sometimes in the evening – they might learn it. Last Wednesday we had two assistants from Würzburg who drove for four hours here in their car. They were here at eight o'clock at night and they left at ten, driving home because they had to be in clinic next morning. Another one comes from Limburg. People say they can learn something here which they can't learn anywhere else.

Select bibliography

Kuhn R (1957). Uber die Behandlung depressives Zustande mit einem iminodibenzylderivat (G22355). *Schweizer Medizinische Wochenschrift*, **87**, 1135–1140.

Kuhn R (1958). The treatment of depressive states with G22355 (imipramine hydrochloride). *American Journal of Psychiatry*, **115**, 495–464.

Kuhn R (1970). The Discovery of Imipramine, in *The Discoveries of Biological Psychiatry* (FJ Blackwell, ed). Lippincott, Philadelphia, pp 205–217.

Kuhn R (1977). In *Psychiatrie in Selbstdarstellungen*, (LJ Pongratz, ed). Verlag Hans Huber, Bern, pp 219–257.

Kuhn R (1987). Some questions and consequences following the discovery of specific antidepressant drugs for scientific research and practical use, in *Thirty Years after Imipramine*. (BE Leonard, P Turner, eds). Rapid Comm, Oxford.

Kuhn R (1990). Artistic Imagination and the discovery of antidepressants. *Journal of Psychopharmacology*, **4**, 127–130.

Kuhn R (1996). The discovery of the tricyclic antidepressants and the history of their use in the early years, in *A History of the CINP* (TA Ban, OS Ray, eds). JM Productions, Tennessee, pp 425–435.

Kuhn R (1996). The first patient treated with imipramine, in *A History of the CINP* ed (TA Ban, OS Ray, eds). JM Productions, Tennessee, p 436.

See also Interviews with Frank Ayd and Alan Broadhurst in Volume I.

6 Max Lurie

The enigma of isoniazid

(The conventional history of the antidepressants relegates everything that happened before Roland Kuhn and Nathan Kline to outer darkness; this applies particularly to early work on the antitubercular agent isoniazid. I accepted this for almost a decade and only changed my mind when I went back to look at some of the primary sources. When one does so, it becomes clear that the work of Lurie and Salzer was an unrecognised breakthrough rather than simply an early fumbling. I was impressed enough to try and track down Max Lurie. My sister Miriam Healy, Herb Meltzer and George Simpson all came up with his phone number and address for me in the same week. I wrote and subsequently posted a draft of Chapter 2 of The Antidepressant Era to him, which he commented on. We talked on the phone. He was reluctant to be interviewed. A year later he changed his mind.)

Can we start with your father, who was also a psychiatrist and I presume therefore one of the reasons you went into psychiatry?

My father was Louis A Lurie. He immigrated from Lithuania to the United States and to Cincinnati around 1900. He graduated from the University of Cincinnati. During his undergraduate work, he became interested in psychology and wound up teaching psychology at the university, while going to medical school at the same time. After completing his medical studies, he went into general practice, which he continued until entering the Army Medical Corps during World War I. In the service, as I guess was the case throughout medicine at the time, psychology and psychiatry sounded very much the same to the average physician and so he was sent to Ann Arbor, Michigan for psychiatric training and then continued to practise psychiatry in the army. After being discharged, he trained further at the Boston Psychopathic Hospital for almost two years before returning to Cincinnati, where he went directly into the practice of psychiatry. I believe there were only about five men practising psychiatry in Cincinnati at that time. He became particularly interested in child psychiatry and in 1920 founded a residential treatment centre for children known at first as the Psychopathic Institute and then as the Child Guidance Home, which later became the Children's Psychiatric Center. He served as its Director until 1949 and thereafter as consultant to the Director.

That was pretty early. Who influenced him to go into this area?

Yes, it was early. I don't know who influenced him to go into this area. His primary interest seemed to be child psychiatry although he actively practised general adult psychiatry. At the Child Guidance Home, he and a paediatrician, J Victor Greenebaum, worked closely with the Jewish Hospital, the social agencies and with the public school – always seeking a possible physical basis for the child's abnormal behaviour. They did extensive work-ups on them, often keeping them in residence for many months. They attended a nearby school. While doing this, he did a tremendous amount of writing and research on all aspects of psychiatry and orthopsychiatry.

In later years, he became interested in whooping cough and what are now recognised as the encephalitides that can develop from that – the changes in personality that can occur. He was particularly interested in pancreatitis and the development of depression in pancreatitis. His work was some of the first work to emphasise this connection. Yet another major area of interest was endocrinology. He began to study the children's endocrine development to explain their retardation or advancement, their physical growth or the lack of it. This led to research with pituitary hormones. Other areas of interest and research included pernicious anaemia, hypertension and the behaviour disorders generally. These were all parallel interests. There was always research going on in one area or another. At the same time, the child guidance work was expanded.

I came into the office with my father in 1948 and became involved in some of the research and some of the papers. Actually, the first one in which I was involved was back in 1943 and concerned the determination of bone age in children by studying X-rays of their epiphyses.

Well, now that we have moved on to you, why did you opt to go into psychiatry? Was it because of your father?

We have to go back one step and ask why I went into medicine. As far back as I can remember, it was a foregone conclusion. It was taken for granted by my immediate family, by my parents, by the relatives of the family that I would go into medicine. There was never any question about it. As I grew up and went through medicine, I was fascinated with seeing what he was doing in his practice. I got to know the other men who were active in psychiatry in the city and was accepted by them. It became what I wanted to do. I had no particular motive or goal, but I was very much interested in psychiatry.

The interest was intensified while working under the supervision of John Romano during my internship at the Cincinnati General Hospital, now the University Hospital. It became clinched while a resident at the Illinois Neuropsychiatric Institute in Chicago, Illinois. John Romano was eclectic but his successor, Murray Levine, was a dedicated psychoanalyst. Everyone in his department was encouraged to commute to Chicago, to the analytical institute there to be psychoanalysed. Drug research or anything pertaining to physical therapies was minimised. This, of course, became an important factor later if we consider why the isoniazid research didn't generate more impact locally. We were in a hotbed of psychoanalytical orientation.

In Chicago it was an extremely interesting year under the aegis of Francis Gerty, Hugh Carmichael and Virginia Tarlow. Strangely, the Institute there was not as psychoanalytically oriented as the area here, even though we had seminars with Franz Alexander and other famous figures from the analytic group. In addition, there was much influence from the neurologists, including LJ Meduna, and that kept things in balance. Medication and electric shock therapy were utilised. It was a neuropsychiatric institute that was symbolised by the shape of the building – two large towers which were connected only in the lobby and the cafeteria on the ground floor. The dichotomy was emphasised for a long time but there was great training there.

Unfortunately, being wartime, I couldn't get a deferment for a second year there, but it was possible to arrange for it with their close associates at the Psychopathic Institute in Iowa city, Iowa under Wilbur Miller, Jack Gottlieb and Paul Huston. They were much less interested in the psychodynamic school and much more interested in the physical therapies, even though there had been some interest in these in Chicago. Both hospitals were interested in electric shock therapy. It fell to our lot as residents to give the treatments. We started very early on – 1944. Cerletti had first tried ECT in 1938. The equipment was primitive and difficult to work with. There were no medications with which to pretreat people. We had to develop techniques to keep the anxiety levels down, how to safely hold people, etc. When I got to Iowa they were doing a lot of shock therapy and insulin coma therapy. There was some psychotherapy but the system in the hospital was such that people were only there briefly so you didn't get a chance to get to know them. There was an interest in drug therapy starting up about that time – mainly using sedatives. I went into the service then and I was lucky enough to be detailed to the psychiatric service. There were a variety of people from different schools there, but we again gave a lot of electroshock therapy. I was stationed in Germany after the war at the 317th station hospital in Wiesbaden.

By the time I came back here there had been an improvement in electroshock therapy. Insulin therapy was also being used, as were sedatives. My father, having grown up in general practice, used a lot of sedatives. He taught me how to use bromides and bromides mixed with hyoscine to smooth out the effect of the bromides. The bad taste was part of the therapy. Phenobarbital wasn't available at first – it was just beginning to come in. This was followed by Donnatal – a combination of hyoscine and barbiturate. That was useful but relatively minor compared to the introduction of Thorazine. However, these were all sedatives. There was very little in the way of treatment for depression other than electroshock treatment and a modification of insulin coma treatment. We also gave sub-coma doses which had more of a tranquillising effect. It certainly wasn't very antidepressant. Hydrotherapy was another useful modality.

Now by this stage you must have met Harry Salzer. What's his background?

Harry Salzer had been practising here in Cincinnati for years. He was a good deal older than myself. He was Professor of Neurology, but he was moving over from neurology toward psychiatry. This is an important subject – the history of neurology. Neurology started out as an independent field. The knowledge base was, however, limited in scope. Harry was recognised for his expertise in neurology but, little by little, as there was less neurology and the psychiatric pastures were looking greener he began moving over into psychiatry. At about the same time, psychiatry began to engulf neurology and a lot of my training was in neurology. I started out with the anticonvulsants and working from that base we got interested in each other. There were relatively few neurologists, psychiatrists or neurosurgeons and we all functioned as one group to some extent. We affiliated as members of the Cincinnati Society of Neurology and Psychiatry.

Harry himself was an invalid. His health was failing when I came into the picture. When he was ill, I would cover for him. He was interested in electroshock therapy. I would give the treatments for him and the friendship grew from there. It became natural to work together.

He was a fairly rigid man. He was a very strong believer in electroshock therapy – the more the merrier. I could not always give treatments the way he would. He would give multiple consecutive treatments. The net result was periods of intense confusion afterwards, which to my mind were absolutely horrendous but that was what he was seeking. It was his theory that by producing all that confusion and memory loss you blotted out all the conflicts and problems that troubled the individual and then you could nurse them back to a better state.

A bit like what Ewen Cameron was doing several years later?

Yes. It may be that this is one of the ways in which electroshock works, although, as the years went by, the trick became to minimise the confusion and the memory loss because we came to realise that some of the organic changes could be irreversible. In some cases, memory never did come back fully and that obviously was undesirable rather than desirable as was thought at first. That is where the spacing of treatments came in. When I was treating a manic patient, for instance, I might treat him every day for two or three days and then move to every other day and then three times a week, twice a week, once a week, etc. My practice had been to taper off, especially with depressed patients – finally giving one every few weeks. This led to what we later called interval treatment, which seemed to help with a lot of chronic or recurring depressions. By agreement we would treat them once every 4 to 6 weeks regardless of how well they were and that seemed to maintain them. Eventually it stopped with the advent of antidepressants. We were always on the lookout, however, for some other way to treat these patients, some equivalent to the way the sedatives seemed to treat the anxious patients. That's where isoniazid came into the picture.

How did you come up with the idea of trying isoniazid?

I was reading an article on tuberculosis by Robitzek and colleagues. I cannot in all honesty say why I was reading it. But what caught my eye was that these authors were complaining that a significant problem with treating tuberculosis with isoniazid was that, unlike other treatments which were usually uncomfortable or even depressing, their patients were getting euphoric. That's where the idea came to my head – 'Hey, is this something that could specifically treat depression?' I talked to Harry about it and we decided to try using it. You must bear in mind that in those days the boundaries of many of the psychiatric syndromes were very fuzzy. They still are today, but it was worse then. In retrospect, many of the so-called hebephrenics would more properly be called schizoaffective, depressed type now. We both had patients in hospital and we started working with them and with office patients using isoniazid. There was one individual who clearly responded to parenteral isoniazid who hadn't responded to the oral dose, but apart from that one patient, I can't particularly remember a difference between the two modes of delivery.

Looking back at our original paper in 1953, there is something else in there that seems very topical today. We've been hearing a great deal in recent months about withdrawal effects from antidepressants, especially the SSRIs. The thinking now is you should taper them off and not stop abruptly. Now in our study we had this in mind. We tapered people very slowly. We just didn't know if there would be a problem.

Do any of the early cases stand out in your mind? Did any early responses persuade you both to continue with this line of investigation?

Yes, the early responses influenced us, but even looking back over the case histories in the paper I still cannot specifically recall any of the patients. What I do remember is the intense thrill of seeing a number of these people getting better. Not necessarily getting well, but getting significantly better. That was extremely gratifying. We were seeing faster results than we had seen with anything else. We were seeing results from a treatment that was so much easier to administer than sub-coma insulin or electroshock therapy. It was always worrisome to me if they hadn't responded to 6, 8, 10 or 12 treatments, or even if they had, when you saw some of them relapse. You must bear in mind here the manner in which the treatment was given in those days. It was totally different to today. At first there were no sedatives and there were no muscle relaxants. We traded on their retrograde amnesia. The individual could remember being brought into the room and being placed on the table. Some could remember the electrodes being put on their head, but nobody ever remembered more than that. It was a big step when Anectine was introduced and after that the use of anaesthesia. These agents had their own difficulties because a muscle relaxant could affect their breathing and that could be very frightening. It was very hard on those of us giving the treatment. It was a cold callous treatment so when an antidepressant came along and you could give a pill by mouth, it was more gratifying.

When you had the first series together you gave a talk at the American Medical Association in 1953. How did the audience respond? Was there anybody there who thought the treatment of depression might be of any interest?

There was, in retrospect, an interested group from the Section on Nervous and Mental Diseases. They weren't beating down the doors, but there were psychiatrists there whom I knew from the Central Neuropsychiatric Association. One man from the audience cut me down during the question and answer period. He said this is all very interesting but 'I hope the authors will treat as many people as possible as quickly as possible before the effect wears off.'

That's a standard way to put down new developments – Nolan Lewis used it a lot. But apart from that, were there any arguments put up as to why you weren't really seeing what you claimed you were seeing?

No. The main point I think was that he just wasn't convinced that it would work en masse. There was scepticism everywhere. We received a better reception outside Cincinnati. For example, the psychiatrists at Ohio State University were much more interested.

Did any other groups use it?

Not groups, but some other psychiatrists locally did indeed use it and obtained comparable effects. Why it faded out was, I think, owing to the relative potency of isoniazid compared to iproniazid and imipramine when they came along.

As compared to the potency of the action of these drugs or the potency of the sales action of the companies or the figures who were pushing these other therapies – Kline, after all, was very flamboyant and well placed to bring iproniazid to public attention.

Yes, your point is well taken. It was important then, as now, for a drug house to really push it. Probably the problem was that there wasn't big money to be made for Eli Lilly in isoniazid.

Can you remember who you approached in the company?

I cannot recall, but I did maintain a relationship with the company and later did some work for them on Aventyl.

Did the fact that isoniazid was produced by Lilly and Roche and Squibb make any difference and perhaps the fact that, at least for the first series of patients, you got the supplies of the drug from both Lilly and Squibb?

That certainly lent credence to the possibility that they did not anticipate any potentially substantial profits from isoniazid. These companies are highly competitive and very profit oriented.

When Thorazine appeared and had the impact it did, I know Eli Lilly, among other companies, went back to their shelves to see what they might have there that had a psychotropic effect.

True, but don't forget reserpine. This played a part, too, in stimulating them to look for other new compounds. It was an interesting decade. The psychoactive drugs were just burgeoning in psychiatry compared with what we'd had before. Thorazine, reserpine and imipramine were the three that I think had the biggest push. And the same thing was happening in the rest of medicine. A lot of conditions were being delineated that hadn't been sorted out before. Drugs were coming out hand over fist. You might say it was part of an information explosion in medicine. These things made isoniazid small peanuts.

But in 1952, the fact remains there was nothing else. We had no comparative antidepressant drug we could use as a baseline standard against which to compare isoniazid. You can argue about the criteria we used. Nobody gave much thought as to whether the subjects should all be hospitalised patients because hospitalised patients are more severely ill or whether they should all be outpatients because they're milder. Should you exclude anyone who has had more than one episode and treat only first episodes? I touched on all of these points in the paper.

Well, you reported results that are the results you would expect from any antidepressant now – two-thirds of people responding and taking 2–3 weeks to respond. The papers are a lot more persuasive than the early reports produced by Kuhn or particularly by Kline. The first patient Kuhn reports on responded after only 5 or 6 days, while Kline's patient samples seem to have been an unholy mess and it's very difficult to get an idea now from his papers as to what actually was going on. Were there any other forums you took the results to?

The next one was a follow-up study presented to the Ohio Psychiatric Association in 1954. As the name implies, this was a branch of the American Psychiatric Association. There were psychiatrists from all over the state with varied backgrounds and training including psychodynamically oriented therapists, psychotherapists who incorporated the physical therapies as well as psychoactive drugs in their armamentaria as well as psychoanalysts. The paper was well received. How many more tried it after that, I don't know. The paper was delivered in 1954 but it was a while before it appeared in print – in 1955 – and, by that time, we were entering into the Thorazine era. Attention was dramatically drawn away from the antidepressants toward the tranquillisers. 'Let's give Thorazine or reserpine' is what you heard – 'this is going to cure depression.' Thorazine was brought out with a great fanfare and the business people could see big money in it. The detail men began to come around to promoting it.

Probably the two biggest things that acted against isoniazid was the fact that we were working in a hotbed of psychoanalytic therapy, and the university department here, which might have otherwise supported us, didn't help promote it and the lack of push from the drug houses along with their interest in chlorpromazine instead. We were just a little bit ahead of our time, not in terms of what we thought we were doing, but in terms of what we found. As I look back at the methods we were using, in many ways they were more organised than the early protocol that was being used, for instance by SmithKline & French when they were developing Parnate. Ten of us went up to Philadelphia in 1959 to talk about our experiences with Parnate and I don't think that there was as much organised protocol in that series of studies as we had in our two articles.

You say Thorazine came on stream and the companies went after schizophrenia because they could see big bucks coming from the fact that there were a lot of visible patients around with schizophrenia, but did any of the lack of interest in an antidepressant stem from the fact that people didn't think there was that much depression around the place?

Part of the issue was the fuzzy borders and overlap between agitated depression and anxious depression. The thinking was that if Thorazine is this good a drug, maybe we can use it in anxious depressions as well – give it in a graded dose. This is what permeated the scene and it took some of the impetus away from developing antidepressants as such.

I'm sure you're right but another problem, which may have been more a European one, because there was much less office practice in Europe, was that the drug companies over there, when they thought about depression, thought about melancholic depression and there's not much of that. Besides which ECT was already a pretty good treatment for it. They didn't see the anxious depressions as depression, they saw anxiety and said, well we've got anxiolytics for that. Did you have that over here?

In those years, depression was not their primary thrust or interest.

Did you at any point go to Eli Lilly and say, look you've got a treatment for depression?

I'm sure they were shown the results of our research and had copies of our papers, but we didn't go to them in any aggressive way. Nor did we ask them if they had any similar drugs in their pipelines which we might study in depressed patients. We talked up isoniazid wherever we could and obviously continued to use it.

Until when?

Until imipramine came along. Iproniazid concerned us. I didn't know just what bothered us, but something about it made us hesitant. Then Tofranil came along and that was great.

Why did you switch? Was it more potent?

Yes, it seemed to be. But then, too, you must go with the flow. The referring doctors had heard about Tofranil, whereas they hadn't heard much about isoniazid. It's the same reason why we use any new drug. We tend to try out and use the latest medications that the pharmaceutical companies bring to us.

There's a good point here in that we have switched en masse to SSRIs even though some evidence now points to the fact that the older drugs were more potent for severe depressions anyway and in my experience at least one of the SSRI companies knew this even as they brought the compounds out, so I'm sure a lot of our impressions have to do with the marketing that gets done. Can I chase you a bit further on the other people who were using isoniazid? In your list of references for the 1955 paper you've got William Turner listed under personal communication. Did he ever publish that?

Not that I'm aware of. I think he must have known Harry and presumably the communication was to him.

The interesting thing is that he came from New York. Now the relevance of this is when Nate Kline came to do his work on iproniazid he doesn't refer to any of this and you might have thought that if someone else was doing this sort of work in the New York area, Kline should have known about it.

Your point is well taken, but I've tried to remember and I can't come up with anything.

Were you aware of the French use of isoniazid, not in terms of being influenced by them because they weren't doing it any earlier than you, but their findings confirm your own. Kline held a meeting in 1958 to celebrate Marsilid and Jean Delay was there saying that he was very excited at the developments with iproniazid but he would like to point out that he and Buisson had got similar results in 1952–53 with isoniazid.

No, I was unaware of that interesting and important fact. I must own up to a lack of sophistication.

I don't think that it's anything to do with a lack of sophistication. For some reason the iso-niazid story didn't take off. You've alluded to a few possible reasons but Delay was one of the most famous names in world psychiatry at the time and even in his hands isoniazid didn't make it.

There are other interesting aspects to this story. Today you often find that if patients respond to one drug but then discontinue it, they may not respond as well if they later relapse and the drug is restarted or else you may have to use a higher dose. In our studies, we reported some people who stopped isoniazid because they felt they were doing very well but they later relapsed. They responded again, however, to the same dose and just as well the second time around.

My first reaction to that is that it was probably because you were dealing with a treatment-naive group but they weren't were they? Your paper makes it clear that many of then had been tried on a range of other things and a third of them had had ECT before.

Yes, many of our subjects had a fairly severe depression and many of them were experiencing recurrent depressions. Another thing in retrospect, not only was isoniazid having an antidepressant action, but it was having it without any of the horrendous side-effect profile we've come to expect from other antidepressants and even from some of the newer ones. It had very few side-effects. One man in the 85 patients we gave it to had to stop because of what we described as a thyroid-like effect – in other words, a stimulant-like effect. One patient developed a rash. Some of our patients developed a hyperreflexia, but this didn't require them to stop treatment. The side-effects in general were mild and they were reversible. In particular, the drug wasn't plagued by the horrendous side-effects seen in the monoamine oxidase inhibitor group. At first there was some question as to whether isoniazid was an MAOI, but it's not.

What does that do to the whole theory about how the antidepressants work? Do you know anything about the biochemistry that might indicate how it works?

It proves that here is something else for the neurobiologists to figure out – it's beyond my capacity. All this biochemistry has surfaced well after I finished medical school. I had no training along those lines. I try to keep up with the literature, but it's not enough to really be able to answer your question.

Well, I pose the question from an emperor-has-no-clothes perspective. I think most of the biochemistry is biomythology really that is good marketing copy rather than good science. But if isoniazid had registered maybe we wouldn't have had fluoxetine, for instance, because all these drugs in some sense came out of the idea that MAOIs increase brain amines and depression is about having low amines. Isoniazid must do something else completely and arguably there is something else completely that all of the other antidepressants do that we've been neglecting all these years which we mightn't have done if more people had paid heed to isoniazid.

Would we have been better off or worse off?

Who knows? How did you or Harry Salzer feel when people like Nate Kline then went on to be recognised as the discoverers of the antidepressants?

It's hard to say how I felt. Disappointed, of course. Truthfully, it was sometime before I fully appreciated the real import for the future of the concept of antidepressant medications.

Those were exciting years – then and subsequently. I have always found myself more interested in the psychopharmacological approach to the treatment of mental illness than purely in the psychodynamic. My interest in psychopharmacology continued and I continued to do research studies on subsequent antidepressant agents.

Before we leave isoniazid, just one more thing. You say you were actually trying to find an antidepressant rather than just a pill to improve sleep in people who were depressed. You were clear on that even though no one else had ever found one – something that would work fairly directly on mood rather than indirectly.

That's right. What we were seeking was something that would work on the mood which we saw as the core of the depression. By definition, such a substance was an antidepressant.

But did the word antidepressant actually exist in 1952? The stimulants, as you said earlier, were being used to treat depression but they weren't called antidepressants and Nate Kline a few years later was calling iproniazid a psychic energiser rather than an antidepressant. Even Tofranil was called a thymoleptic for a while rather than an anti-depressant – so was there such a word before your 1953 paper where much more clearly than anyone else at the time you called isoniazid an antidepressant? Where did you get the term from?

We called it an antidepressant because we wanted something that would work specifically against depression – therefore it would be an antidepressant. Isoniazid seemed to fill that requirement. I don't think popularly it was known as, or looked upon, as an antidepressant but we were calling it that as opposed to an antianxiety agent.

Let me push you further on this. Did you actually coin the term? I think you may have because I'm not sure there is an earlier use in the literature.

That's for someone other than me to determine. I don't think we were looking to make up a word or term. On the other hand, I don't remember anyone else using it. It wasn't like naming a baby – we didn't go through a phase of debating what should we call this agent, but this effect was definitely what we were seeking. Therefore, we referred to isoniazid as an antidepressant.

Before we turned the tape on, you said that the group in Ohio State University in Columbus got you involved in the early trials on Parnate – tranylcypromine – can you tell me anything about that work?

The Psychiatric Department at Ohio State University was quite interested in psychopharmacological research and treatment. Because of my work on isoniazid, I was approached at a Central Neuropsychiatric meeting in Columbus, Ohio in regard to an antidepressant drug, SKF 385, which was being studied. They asked whether I knew anything about it and when I said no, they asked me whether I would be interested in working on it. I was. The prospect was exciting. I became involved in the study and began to use it. I worked with SmithKline & French and went to a meeting in Philadelphia in 1959 when they were reviewing the results. There were 12 of us in attendance. That's when I got to know Frank Ayd. I already knew Howard Fabing from Cincinnati, who was also there. Everybody at the round table presented their impressions of the drug. They weren't prepared papers as such. Each of us gave a summary of what we were doing, our observations and experiences. What strikes me going back now and rereading the proceedings of the meeting was the seeming looseness of the research project. The parameters of the project were not rigidly defined – what group of patients should be treated, whether they should be hospitalised or office-based or even the dosage of the drug that should be used. The dosage given was quite variable. At that point, no one was comparing SKF 385 to imipramine or to any other drug – imipramine hadn't yet been accepted as a baseline or comparative treatment agent.

What was the feeling in the company about the compound at that time?

They were excited about it despite the fact that there were indications that it had more side-effects. The nasty one, of course, was the very severe, devastating headaches which turned out to be hypertensive crises. I had a man – an attorney, no less! – on it and he developed one of these headaches. We brought him through it. He knew it was a research drug. The bottom line was that the drug was very helpful to him and he continued to use it. At this early meeting, some of us had seen the problem of headaches and some of us hadn't. Dr Roebuck had encountered the problem of headaches in two subjects. We had talked about the problem before the meeting, and in his presentation he expressed it as relating to a heavy meal – that was the conclusion we had come to at that time. We had pinned it down to food and we thought it had to do with a heavy meal. The advice that went out from that meeting was to avoid excessively large meals. Although it was just a hunch, it was a good start.

Did you meet Alfred Burger, the discoverer of the drug at this meeting?

No. That would have been a thrill.

What impression did Frank Ayd make on you?

He came across as a brilliant researcher. He was very positive in his approach to things. If he had an idea, he tried to follow through on it. He was a very determined person and very successful. He did a tremendous amount of research. I later sent several patients to him for consultation and he delivered a lecture to the psychiatric group here in Cincinnati.

Fritz Freyhan was also there. He was one of the really big names in the early days. How did he come over?

He, too, was an impressive researcher. However, I didn't have an opportunity to get to know him.

You have told me before that people like you who were working in private office practice got forced out of clinical trial work because of insurance problems. Can you tell me about what happened?

That was a hurtful turn of events. When the thalidomide scare occurred, the insurance companies became frightened and began to alter their rules and coverage. We were quietly told to be careful what we got involved with because though they presumably would cover you if you gave a drug to someone and got into trouble, thereafter you might find it very difficult and expensive to get further insurance coverage. I went both to SmithKline & French and to Eli Lilly – I was working on Aventyl at the time. I said to them, look, the way it stands now is if I give your product to a patient and some irreversible side-effect happens, I'll get covered for that case but from then on I'm persona non grata. It was a frightening situation.

I wanted to continue doing research work so I asked the companies to provide liability insurance coverage, pointing out that if the drug is successful, I do not get a nickel but if it's successful you make a fortune, so why don't they insure me? Apparently a lot of people were saying that to them, but they refused to supply liability insurance coverage. Some people were later able to organise themselves into research groups and get coverage that way – through hospitals, etc. I couldn't see how to get it and where I had two youngsters at the time, I couldn't afford to take the chance. The financial risks were too great. I could have been wiped out so I backed off.

How many people were forced out of clinical trials because of this?

I think that a majority of the individual investigators were forced out by this change. For individuals who were studying drugs in private practice, the whole liability factor became too frightening. Malpractice rates went up astronomically high. Individual drug research was one of the risks that were specifically frowned upon. I dropped out of the Aventyl research in the middle of it. It didn't make sense for me to continue.

When you stopped doing clinical trial work in the 1960s what sort of research did you get into after that?

I became involved with our oesophagus centre, studying associated psychiatric problems and personality traits demonstrated by some of the patients with dysphagia. This included a group of subjects who required oesophageal reconstruction surgery. We elicited some striking and not readily explainable findings, especially in those subjects with a background of functional dysphagia. A number of them revealed some dare-devil, aggressive personalities, habits and hobbies – such as hang-gliding. One man comes to mind. He used to watch railroad crossings and when he saw a train coming, he would time himself and race it to the crossing. For a variety of reasons, we did not pursue these observations with a formal study.

Other interests have included involvement in forensic psychiatric work and especially in psychiatric problems stemming from industrial accidents. As the various new psychopharmacological drugs such as the SSRIs and antipsychotic agents have been introduced, I have eagerly tried working with them in my private practice. In recent years, I have become more involved in geriatric psychiatry and the treatment of individuals in their late 80s and 90s. This has included the use of the newer psychoactive drugs, including the atypical antipsychotic drugs, but using individually titrated and significantly reduced dosages. Overall, their response has been quite gratifying. However, I am not involved in any formal research study at this time.

I notice on your wall a plaque saying that you were the president of the Central Neuropsychiatric Association in 1980/81. This has come up in the conversation before – what was this group?

The Central Neuropsychiatric Association was founded in 1922 as a unique association of neurologists, neurosurgeons and psychiatrists selected for membership by invitation. The purpose was to promote interest in their related fields. Membership was limited to physicians who had already reached a position of prominence or who demonstrated some success and promise in their respective speciality. A further purpose was to promote the acquaintance and relationship of the members with each other. This philosophy soon expanded to include the spouses and to foster a relationship amongst them. As the members moved, the territorial boundaries gradually spread from the original central states to include the entire United States.

At first, all of the presentations were given by the members themselves, describing their current studies and research, and with part of the programme devoted to each of the specialties. In more recent years, outside speakers were brought in and the papers were directed towards a central theme. I was elected to membership in 1954 after attending the required two annual meetings to become known. Since then, I have presented several papers to the organisation and have been on the Executive council for almost 20 years. I was President from 1981 to 1982.

Select bibliobraphy

Salzer HM, Lurie M (1953). Anxiety and depressive states treated with isonicotinyl hydrazide (Isoniazid). *Archives of Neurology and Psychiatry*, **70**, 317–324.
Salzer HM, Lurie M (1955). Depressive states treated with isonicotinyl hydrazide (Isoniazid): a follow–up study. *Ohio State Medical Journal*, **51**, 437–441.
Delay J, Buisson J-F (1958). Psychic action of isoniazid in the treatment of depressive states. *Journal of Clinical and Experimental Psychopathology and Quarterly Review of Psychiatry and Neurology*, **19**, 2 (supplement), 51–55.

Ad Sitsen, Professor of Clinical Pharmacology in the Medical Faculty at Utrecht University and Head of Clinical Projects – Depression in N.V. Organon was asked to comment on this interview and also to answer a number of questions.

First of all let me say how interesting the interview with Max Lurie was. I also enjoyed reading his papers on the antidepressant effects of isoniazid. The discovery of psychotropic drugs – and for that matter many other drugs – was and usually still is a serendipitous process as evidenced by the way chlorpromazine, imipramine, lithium and iproniazid were discovered. It is important to note that astute clinical observation of patients treated with experimental drugs played a major role in these discoveries. The antidepressant action of isoniazid is just such an astute observation that until now has escaped the attention of historians. Fortunately and rightfully this almost unknown action of isoniazid has now been brought to the surface again. Why was it buried for so long? Lurie himself gives some ideas in his interview. At the time isoniazid was marketed by several pharmaceutical companies and there was probably insufficient commercial push further to pursue its use as an antidepressant. In addition, iproniazid came along and a great deal of attention and scientific interest went on this new compound.

With the benefit of hindsight can the antidepressant action of isoniazid be explained with today's psychopharmacological knowledge?

Zeller in 1983 recounts that 'when the two antitubercular drugs iproniazid (Marsilid, Hoffmann-LaRoche) and isoniazid became available in 1952 they were immediately accepted as promising tools for our investigations [on

MAO]. Isoniazid, as expected, exhibited DAO [diamine oxidase]-inhibitory action while at the same concentration it was without noticeable effects on MAO. In contrast, iproniazid turned out to be a much stronger MAO inhibitor than ever seen before.' Nevertheless, isolated cases of the 'cheese reaction' and other interactions have been published and Robinson *et al.* in 1968 described that at therapeutic doses isoniazid inhibits *plasma* monoamine oxidase. Thus it seems that isoniazid, at clinical doses used for the treatment of tuberculosis, possesses at least some monoamine oxidase inhibiting properties. This may be particularly relevant in patients who are slow acetylators. Like moclobemide, isoniazid inhibits mainly monoamine oxidase-A, which may explain the rare occurrence of the cheese reaction. To what extent this property explains its antidepressant action right now is unclear but merits further investigation. It is conceivable that isoniazid is a kind of moclobemide 'avant la lettre'.

Another interesting pharmacological property is its inhibition of glutamic acid decarboxylase, which reduces the brain concentration of GABA and may result in seizures. It does this by inhibiting the enzyme pyridoxyl kinase, which catalyses the formation of pyridoxyl-5-phosphate, a cofactor for glutamic acid decarboxylase. In pharmacological experiments, isoniazid is used as a convulsive agent and convulsions are a side-effect in man, in particular in patients with seizure disorders. Overdoses with isoniazid may also result in seizures for which pyridoxine is the antidote. It shares this epileptogenic property with most if not all currently available antidepressants but relating this to its antidepressant action is difficult.

For the sake of completeness, it is worth mentioning that the mechanism of its antibacterial action is not well understood either. Effects on lipids, nucleic acid synthesis and glycolysis have all been proposed. An inhibitory action on the synthesis of mycolic acids would explain the high degree of selectivity of its antimicrobial activity because mycolic acids are important constituents of the mycobacterial cell wall.

Would an earlier appreciation of isoniazid's antidepressant effects have changed the course of antidepressant drug development?

Who knows, but it is interesting to speculate. Isoniazid inhibits DAO particularly for which histamine is an important substrate. Histamine is an important neurotransmitter in the brain with an effect on sleep patterns and pursuing the mechanism of action of isoniazid may have shed light on the role of histamine in various psychopharmacological processes earlier. In addition to a role in sleep, H-3 heteroreceptors found on central catecholamine, indoleamine and acetylcholine nerve endings could inhibit or increase the release of these neurotransmitters. Polyamines are another important substrate for DAO and these are currently vigorously being investigated. Affective disorders are associated with maladaptive responses to stressful life events. Based on the observation that rapid but transient changes in brain polyamine metabolism are a characteristic response to stressful stimuli, it has been hypothesised that a maladaptive polyamine stress response system is involved in the pathophysiology of the affective disorders. Because of their involvement in the functional states of a variety of receptors and their multiple role in cellular metabolism, it has been suggested that the polyamines deserve special attention, although at present the evidence in favour of their specific involvement in neuropsychiatric disorders is scarce. Would other antidepressants have been discovered by focusing on histamine and polyamines further? It is a possibility I would not exclude.

Another aspect that should not be neglected is isoniazid's inhibition of GABA biosynthesis. GABA is the major inhibitory neurotransmitter in the brain and GABAergic neurons are widespread through the brain. The hypothesis that GABA might be involved in the aetiology of mood disorders emerged following clinical observations that valproic acid was effective in the treatment of bipolar mood disorders. This increases brain GABA and GABA also interacts with other amine systems. GABA function is also related to anxiety and facilitating GABA neurotransmission is associated with a reduction of anxiety in animal models. The benzodiazepines in part exert their anxiolytic action this way. Interestingly, Salzer and Lurie already noted the anxiolytic effects of isoniazid.

In addition, carbamazepine, another anticonvulsant, is thought to act in limbic structures through an interaction with GABA-B receptors and this has psychotropic effects and is used in mania. Vigabatrin, another anticonvulsant with GABA-agonist properties, has recently been reported to induce psychoses and affective disorders. But in view of the still somewhat unclear 'mood-stabilising' effects of GABAergic compounds, I doubt whether investigations on the involvement of GABA in affective disorders would have provided insights that would have altered antidepressant drug development.

In summary, I had no idea that this compound had such a complex pharmacology. It is a pity that the early opportunity for research on psychopharmacological aspects of isoniazid and on the development of antidepressant drugs that was provided by the early clinical observations of Lurie and Salzer were not followed up.

A list of 18 references supporting the points made here can be obtained on request from Ad Sitsen.

7 *Louis Lasagna*

Back to the future: evaluation and drug development 1948–1998

Can we learn anything from the past?

One hopes that there are some lessons. At a meeting several years ago at the ACNP, a man responsible for CNS drug development at Merck bemoaned the fact that animal models were not terribly helpful in predicting what a drug was going to be good for and he couldn't afford to do endless randomised controlled clinical trials, so what should he do? Some of us old timers said 'Well, is it possible that you could do what they used to do in the old days, which was to go to some skilled psychiatrists and say here's a drug – we think it may be good for this or that but we don't know for sure. Try it out and see what you find'. And he said 'Oh no, we have been led up so many false paths with unbridled enthusiasm etc.' I'm not sure that he is right because to me what he was describing was a philosophy of despair – we don't know where the hell we're going, we don't know how to pick drugs and then we are stuck with spending a lot of money doing things that may turn out to be negative but falsely negative just because we have studied the wrong patients.

My own contributions to the field were really mostly in the field of analgesics, although I watched other drugs develop and was responsible for selling, in the early 1950s, the concept of controlled clinical trials which had started with Bradford Hill and the streptomycin study back in the 1940s but which took a little while to be transferred over here. There was a double problem with selling people the notion of controlled trials. One problem was selling people on a seemingly artificial way of studying drugs – different at least from what they had been doing for years. The other was convincing them that subjective responses could be studied in a valid fashion.

When the analgesic work first started, people said you can't find out whether people are in pain or not – I mean, this is within their head. How can you ever get any insight into it? And the answer was, well, if you structure your questions in a certain way or use visual analogue scales or whatever and do it properly with attempts to eliminate bias and use controls and so forth, by God it can make sense and one can get dose–response curves and so forth. So the analgesic research in a way opened up the whole field of subjective responses and brought into the tent of science, if you will, the measurement of anxiety and depression.

When was all this – when did Beecher and Gold start?

Beecher started, I would have guessed, in 1950 or thereabouts as far as his clinical trials were concerned. He made the observation during the war on the Anzio beachhead that soldiers suffering wounds at least as grievous as those suffered by civilians seemed not to demand as much in the way of analgesic medication as did the civilian patients with whom he had had experience prior to the war, and he concluded that this was because there was a neurophysiological component to pain and then an emotional response to the stimuli being perceived which allowed the meaning of pain, if you will, to get into the act. His suggestion for the difference that he observed was that in civilian life grievous wounds were ordinarily a tragedy but on a battlefield it might be a blessing because it got you at least away from the front lines to a base hospital and maybe out of the war completely. Who knows whether that was the correct explanation or not but that is what got him started.

When exactly the analgesic research started I don't know, except I joined him in 1952 and it had been going for a couple of years before that. He had an internist with him called Jane Denton and a man named Arthur Keats who had been a classmate of mine in high school and college. I first got into it by meeting Keats on the Atlantic City boardwalk at one of the so-called clinical meetings and having him tell me about this new research they were doing. And it sounded so exciting to me that when the time came for me to pay my time back to the armed forces for having paid for part of my way through medical school, I eagerly acceded to Beecher's request to come and join him.

He pulled strings. I had been in the Navy and then was transferred to the Public Health Service. I actually got paid by the US Army because Beecher had an army grant to study psychotomimetic drugs. He came back from a trip to Europe with this lurid story about how the Russians were building not one but two factories beyond the Ural Mountains to make LSD, which they would drop into the drinks of diplomats or generals to get secrets from them and so forth. So he got me assigned to work on this top secret project. I had to be screened for top secret level believability and so did Beecher. We passed that. A psychologist of the name of von Felsinger with whom I worked refused to go through this because he thought this was McCarthyism, and Beecher's secretary who typed all the reports refused to be screened – so we had this mixed security. The reports would go back to the Pentagon by an armed courier with a briefcase manacled to his wrist. And I know at least once they called up and wanted another copy and Beecher said, well, you told us to destroy everything after we sent it to you, what happened to the first one? The answer was – it's lost in the Pentagon somewhere.

After I left Beecher and came back to Johns Hopkins to start the first division of clinical pharmacology, I couldn't help but be interested in the new developments that were occurring in this field and couldn't help but be impressed by the fact that indeed most of the early discoveries were serendipitous. They weren't science marching down a pathway in a straight line but lucky observations by people in studies where the controls were really historical controls and not randomised controlled trials. Meprobamate came along that way, as did the benzodiazepines, imipramine, chlorpromazine and the monoamine oxidase inhibitors. So here I was on the one hand saying, well, once you identify a compound, if you want to persuade people that it works you really ought to do controlled trials but having to face the fact that the breakthroughs were not achieved in that way. So it is interesting that so much of that was serendipitous and maybe will continue to be that way.

In the field of analgesics, for example, we are a lot better at identifying new receptors than we are at figuring out what to do with them. My major contribution in terms of drug discovery, I would say, was the discovery that nalorphine, which was given to us as a pure antagonist, was in fact a mixed agonist/antagonist. The way we stumbled on that again was serendipitous. Beecher and I had this funny idea that if we combined in some magical ratio nalorphine, allegedly a pure antagonist, plus morphine we might get rid of some of the bad things that morphine did. We were willing to settle for whatever God sent our way in the way of losses of bad things – less nausea, less vomiting, less constipation, less addiction, whatever. So we had a couple of ratios and I, in my obsessive-compulsive way, said well, we really ought to have a nalorphine control just for the hell of it and to our surprise it turned out to be effective as an analgesic. So that opened up pharmaceutical research which was pursued in part by Arthur Keats, whom I mentioned earlier who had left Beecher to go to a chair in anaesthesia in Texas but mostly by the Sterling-Winthrop company. They looked and looked and ultimately a number of mixed agonist/antagonists made it to the market but not nalorphine because they thought it had too many hallucinatory potentials. I'm not sure that any of them has been a major contribution to the search that started in the 1930s to come up with a non-addictive substitute for morphine.

My training was as a physician internist. Then I had a postdoctoral experience in the pharmacology department at the Johns Hopkins School of Medicine where I did primarily laboratory work and published several papers. Beecher sold me to the army as someone who was uniquely qualified to pursue these problems – he couldn't imagine anyone in the world better than me to do this. It was hilarious to me at the time. In addition to the episode I told you about the lost Pentagon paper, I got a call from a General from a base in the United States asking me whether I would be willing to work on this top secret project. I said, well, I would love to go to the Massachusett's General Hospital to do it but what is the project? He said, I can't tell you, it's too secret. So I took it feeling fairly certain that whatever else I did there for the army I would be doing something interesting and I did the first controlled trial on hypnotic drugs whilst I was there.

Which ones were they?

Chloral hydrate and a barbiturate. What we did was to study several hypnotic drugs and we had a placebo group. It was the only trial that I have ever done that had a no-nothing group – a group that got neither placebo nor an active drug. I often refer to that because it is the only trial I've ever done where I could with some certainty decide how much of the placebo response was due to suggestibility and how much was due to spontaneous change. Using a very crude endpoint – of falling asleep in less than an hour as success – 65% of the placebo group did so but the no-nothing group was also about 65%, so we were just studying the relative ease with which people admitted for elective surgery fell asleep. I had thought they would have a terrible time being anxious about the next day. This is the only time I ever did that and I doubt that many people have done it – the end result is that you get a lot of crazy talk about placebo responsiveness.

Beecher, by the way, was responsible for people going around for years – to this day – saying that about a third of people respond to a placebo. He took a bunch of published articles ranging all over the place and he averaged them up, and the average was about 35% or so. But the average, as usual, hid a lot of variability and to this day some people still refer to the magic third but more sophisticated people realise that if you ask a stupid question like 'Will a placebo prevent you from dying from the common cold?' you get a 100% success rate which has nothing to do with the placebo talking you out of dying.

One of my contributions was convincing people that you can study sleep. This was prior to the sleep lab days when people moved over from just the subjective responses or the evaluation of night nurses or technicians trying to see whether people were awake or asleep to using electroencephalograms. In a way I think it is a pity that so much stress is placed on the sleep lab and so little on clinical studies because the sleep lab is a highly artificial hot-house – wires on your head and so on.

Can I ask you some more about Harry Beecher? Who was he, where did he come from?

He was a very complicated man. His name probably wasn't Beecher. He was born in Kansas and if you look at some of his early publications and some of the books that he had in his library, you saw two middle initials, K and U – Henry KU Beecher. The U as far as I was able to tell stood for Unangst.

An appropriate name.

Exactly. My guess is, if anything, maybe his mother was a Beecher. He later took great pride in attending Beecher family reunions and so on but I have a feeling that his paternal name was probably Unangst. He went to school in Kansas but then came to Harvard Medical School, started off to be a surgeon, went off to work with a Nobellist called Krogh and I think while there they asked him whether he would like to come back and be Professor of Anesthesia in the Massachusetts General Hospital. I forget what he did to train himself as an anaesthesiologist but he came back and chaired this department. He always spent a lot of time travelling, around Europe especially, recruiting a lot of very talented Europeans to come to work at the Mass General for a year or two.

He was a very dramatic figure in many ways. I always dreaded writing papers with him because he would always insist on the introduction referring to the previous stuff from his lab and then ending with rather more dramatic conclusions than I would have wanted. He engaged in a number of controversies. He did a study on curare, for instance, implicating it as a bad performer in anaesthesia. People who thought it was perfectly safe to use it if you used it properly took umbrage at that report. But he was clearly a leader in American anaesthesiology and maybe beyond America; he was well known in Europe. He had a very good clinical department. He supported investigators who were not anaesthesiologists, like me for example. He had a woman named Mary Brazier, a Brit, who was an EEG person and he supported her research. He had a couple of young men who were neuropharmacologists or neurophysiologists, I guess you could call them. He let people do whatever they wanted to. He was very supportive but a complicated man. Very few people felt neutral about him – they either liked him a lot or disliked him a lot.

He wanted me to stay on and succeed him as Professor of Anesthesia. I said, Harry there are two problems with that: one is that I don't really want to be an anaesthesiologist and the second is what makes you think you will be able to pick your successor – it's not exactly a hereditary post. I enjoyed thoroughly my two years with him. It was a lot of fun. He enjoyed the fact that von Felsinger and I were interested in the placebo response.

We published a paper in which we attempted to see what predisposed people to respond positively to placebo. In retrospect it was a bit naive because while I do believe that some people are more suggestible than others and more influenced by their feelings about the medical profession and pharmaceutical substances, there are so many things that specifically will affect the placebo response given the situation, person, the physician and so forth that it is probably silly to think about placebo reactors and placebo non-reactors. Probably none of us are consistently placebo reactors or non-reactors.

Is there any way then to evaluate the placebo response? Is it in essence the question about how do you evaluate psychotherapy?

There was a paper published by my two of my colleagues at Hopkins: Park and Covi. They took a small number of neurotic outpatients and they said 'We are going to give you a placebo. Do you know what a placebo is? A placebo is a non-active medication but it helps some people or it has been known to help.' To their great surprise many of these people said it was wonderful; some said it was the best thing they had ever had; some of them disbelieved that it was really lacking in medication. They published it as an example of how for some people their attitude towards medications or physician gestures, which I guess the placebo is, make it impossible to eliminate suggestibility and anticipation of a good effect. Obviously you could also anticipate a bad effect. You could be a sort of negative placebo reactor, dislike doctors or nurses and hospitals and so forth or be fearful of medication.

Today, I think if you do a crossover trial where patients are given both the active treatment and the placebo, then in fact those patients unable to distinguish between a placebo and an active treatment are useless and the only differentials that come out of it are in those patients who respond to one treatment and not the other.

These days the placebo is being clobbered by certain bio-ethicists who believe that the Helsinki Declaration doesn't allow placebos. In fact it doesn't but it doesn't allow a lot of other things. It was put out in the 1970s and modified once or twice. One of the modifications says that every patient in the trial including those in the control group should be guaranteed access to the best treatment available. Now that means that not only will you have trouble doing a placebo control but how would you ever study a new medication unless you were treating a disease for which nothing existed? I think the Helsinki Declaration was written by people who really didn't understand what research was about.

I'm not saying there aren't ethical problems. The FDA in this country really insists most of the time on placebo controls. The reason they do is that they know that at least with some therapeutic areas it is quite possible to do a study comparing say a standard antidepressant with placebo and have the two come out no different because the population just couldn't discriminate – depression being a remitting disease you can see why that would happen. So in a sort of statistical morality sense FDA staff feel that if the FDA lets a compound get on the market because there has been no difference demonstrated between it and the standard drug in a couple of trials, it may be doing terrible harm to thousands and thousands of patients by subjecting them to something that really is ineffective or poorly effective, which you would find out if you really studied the right population.

My own view is that one can defend that although I think there are other ways to handle the problem. For example, in the analgesic game we do dose–response relationships with the standard drug and the new drug and if you get those then you come up with a therapeutic ratio for the two preparations and pretty reliable conclusions about how many milligrams of this is equivalent to 10 mg of morphine. So I think in situations like that or situations where you are comparing a mixture of two or three drugs against individual drugs, if the mixture turns out to be better than any of the individual drugs I can't understand why you need a placebo arm.

Do you think trial design possibly by virtue of the 1962 amendments of the Food and Drugs Act has become a very rigid thing? There are other things that we could do like a multiple-baseline design where you could in essence give all the people involved an active drug but you begin at the point at which they begin the active compound in a staggered way.

A man named Walter Modell and I were really responsible for the demand for well-controlled trials being in those amendments. The reason we did it was because in the bad old days, while occasionally physicians would come to the truth – morphine, digitalis, aspirin – there were also other medicines which were ineffective but were used for years. So I still believe that the randomised controlled trial is a hell of a good way of persuading people that you have something. But in contrast to my role in the 1950s, which was trying to convince people to do controlled trials, now I find myself telling people that it's not the only way to truth.

My favourite quotation was taken from Austin Bradford Hill's Heberden Lecture. This was probably 30 years ago, and in it he said, 'If one came to the conclusion that the only way to find out the truth about a medication was to use a controlled clinical trial, it would mean not that the pendulum had swung too far but that it had come completely off its hook.' And this is from someone who might be called the father of the controlled trial. In another part of the paper he comes up with something else that I have been trying to sell to people, with not an awful lot of luck. What he said was that a controlled trial does not tell the physician what he would like to know, which is how do I know in advance without engaging in trial and error which antidepressant is better for Mr Jones or Mrs Smith? That's what doctors and patients would like to know. We don't do that.

To get a drug on the market in the United States and in the most other jurisdictions all you need to do is show that on average when a group of people are untreated they would do less well than a group of people that are treated. That is enough to get a drug on the market. And if you look back at your trials retrospectively saying it looks like left-handed Lithuanian women did better or middle-aged Mexicans did worse you are accused of data dredging. It's really silly because any scientist worth a damn would look at his or her data to see what clues are there, not necessarily convincing you because we know that occasionally by chance you come up with correlations that are meaningless. For instance, Richard Peto had a trial that shows that people born under a certain zodiac sign did a lot worse than everybody else. But why shouldn't one be looking at whether Ashkenazi Jews get more agranulocytosis on clozapine or not? If one had been able to predict who is going to get agranulocytosis from clozapine, it would have made the marketing in this country completely different. Clozapine would have got on the market a lot sooner, would not have had requirements for doing white blood cell counts periodically and so forth.

Some people won't even buy the fact that you can do case control studies or pharmaco-epidemiological studies to get some feeling for what is really there. I think that's a pity because the controlled trial world is really a very hot-house world. Not every patient qualifies and you tend to have patients that are not complicated. It's a pity that we have got so rigid about it.

Another craziness, which used to be just an American disease but is spreading like a virus to other parts of the world, is the so-called intent to treat analysis. The notion that even if people don't take a drug they ought to be counted as if they had is bizarre. I can understand people saying you have got to watch these scurvy knaves in the pharmaceutical industry, they'll discard patients that fail, to make the drug look good and that is a problem. I remember one time talking to an anaesthesiologist and he said you know it's not true that morphine's effect peaks in about an hour, it peaks much later and it lasts for a long time. I said 'Really?' Then he showed me his data – what he had done was eliminate everybody that dropped by the wayside so by the time he got to the

12th hour all the failures had disappeared. He was only counting the happy subjects who have gotten pain relief and that's it. You can't do that. So yes you can't ignore drop-outs and the best thing to do with drop-outs is not to have them. You can't ignore them but while it is perfectly legitimate to ask the question if I took 100 people and told them to take the drug this way and some of them took it this way and some of them didn't and some didn't take it at all, what would happen? – not a bad question to ask; a real life question – but it's different from 'What would happen if 100 people took the drug as told?' They are two completely different questions and why one shouldn't be interested in compliance as a determinant of effect I don't know, especially these days where we don't have to rely just on pill counts or an occasional blood or urine specimen, which have been shown to be not very good because people can throw pills away and a specimen about once a month tells you something about what has been going on in the recent past but not for the whole month. Now there are these little electronic monitors where you can at least see whether the patient opened the container or not. If the container has been unopened for a month you can be relatively certain that anything that is happening to the patient, either benefit or harm, is not due to the medicine. It is a pity that we get so bogged down in these rigid, inflexible ways of doing things.

Is one of the other things that has come out of the controlled trial the idea that there is a single right dose for a drug? It seems to me that before we went down the RCT road, with drugs like digitalis, for instance, you would titrate the dose for each person but in order to run trials you had to have a fixed dose. What comes out of the trial then is the recommendation that if you want to treat people who are depressed this is the dose you should give – a dose that may be great in the mean but extremely poor for some people and too high for others.

In the psychotropic area you have trials that sometimes do involve titration – antidepressants that start low and work their way up. One trouble with that approach is that it's wonderful for coming up with a false U-shaped dose–response curve because the ones that are doomed never to respond, maybe because they don't have the disease you are studying, are going to be in the group that got the highest doses. Sometimes there is a legitimate U-shaped curve as is true with certain antidepressants and certain antipsychotic drugs, but the only way you can pick that up reliably is to do a standard fixed dose for each subject with some people getting one dose and some getting another, and then if a high dose produces a less good response than an intermediate dose you can argue that there is a therapeutic window and that is important.

Yes, but it seems to me that the problem is we don't actually go back to the patient – and this is perhaps true more for the neuroleptics than the antidepressants – and ask their verdict of whether they are on the right dose. We aren't prepared to begin low and work our way slowly in a particular person after the drug has been licensed.

You know another consequence of ignoring compliance is that you end up with doses that are too high for the obsessive-compulsive patient that follows directions. You conclude that 60 mg is the best dose because you get as good an effect as you are ever going to get benefit-wise with little toxicity but that is only because some of your patients are taking less than 60 and maybe the best dose is really 40 mg. So if you are marketing it at 60, the obsessive-compulsive patient who takes the drug religiously will not be at this nice point on the dose–response curve. They will be getting more toxicity than they need.

The dose–response relationship is the only thing that differentiates pharmacology from the other basic sciences. Its very hard to think of many things that are just pharmacology's domain and it's amazing how little attempt is made to be sophisticated about that.

In the cardiovascular area, for example, in the treatment of hypertension the original approved dose for hydrochlorthiazide was 200 mg. If you look at the standard textbook on hypertension, this is what you find in the first edition. Second edition it's 100 mg. Third edition it's 50 mg. Fourth edition it's 25 mg. And the last one I think was 12.5 mg. Now it's shameful to have been that wrong in recommending the optimal dose. You can see how it happens. If you're a pharmaceutical company spending a lot of money on these trials you're not going to try and shave it so close to an ineffective dose that you have a good chance of coming up with a negative result. But that's for convincing everybody that you have got a drug, the fine tuning which is what seems to be the ultimate goal for medicine shouldn't then be ignored. This is too bad.

Did Harry Beecher know or have any contact with Harry Gold at all, because he was also using placebos ...

Gold as far as I can tell probably coined the term double-blind. I tried to pin him down on this one time and he more or less said he thinks he was responsible. He was doing studies on ether, as I remember. He did believe in controls and in placebos. And actually he used to edit a series called the Cornell Conferences on Therapy. That is where I first got turned on to both pharmacology and placebos. He would have a session on placebos and would tape what people said and then edit it and publish it in a book. Harry Gold probably deserves credit for the concept, but when exactly he did that I'm not sure – it was probably in the 1940s.

Who was Harry Gold?

He was a cardiologist in practice in Manhattan, on the staff of the Cornell Medical College but never a fully legitimate academic because he was in practice earning money. He earned quite a bit of money because he was a very good cardiologist and had a wealthy clientele. I met him on a few occasions and liked him. He was an interesting figure. He never got academic recognition because he was not a full-time academic. But he was very interested in how to study drugs properly and very interested in studying humans as opposed to animals, although he did do some animal work too as I remember. He had a bio-assay for standardising the potency of digitalis glycosides that utilised EKG changes.

Beecher did know Gold but not terribly well I think. He met him on one or two occasions and he may have corresponded with him but I don't think they were bosom buddies.

So they both came to their ideas very much independently of each other. Was there anything else back behind them? Were there any other figures before either Gold or Beecher?

Bradford Hill, but I'm pretty sure the original streptomycin trials didn't employ placebo. They thought it was unethical to stick people on placebo. As far as placebos go, I think Gold probably deserves credit for being the first man in the territory.

You pick Bradford Hill as the person who actually created the RCT. What was the chain of events that led from Bradford Hill to here?

I'm guessing because I can't trace it with certain accuracy but the streptomycin trial got a lot of play over here, plus Harry Gold had begun to plant the idea of the controlled trial. Then Beecher came along and there was an increasing awareness of placebo effect and the ability of physicians in the past to be misled about medications by reason of not having done proper controlled trials. I guess that is the way it happened. I am not really sure exactly what raised the level of attention. I'm trying to think what was the first trial. Some of the things that came along about that time were deemed to be effective without the need for randomised controls. I'm thinking of penicillin for subacute bacterial endocarditis and so forth. In the case of the blood pressure-lowering agents, they weren't satisfied with surrogates for those until finally somebody came along to do the first controlled trials showing that there were benefits in terms of prevention of cardiovascular catatastrophies of one sort or another. Maybe there was no big leap, maybe it was a trickle down thing because you know at those hearings of Kefauver's, Walter Modell and I were the only people who addressed the clinical trial issue. Other people talked about prices and profits and generic labelling and so forth. Kefauver's original orientation was an economic one, it wasn't the quality of research etc.

This was in 1959/60?

It started in December of 1959 and it went through until 1962. So it was about two years' worth of hearings in the House under a man named Blatnik and in the Senate under Kefauver. No one expected it to happen because Kefauver had a history of looking into things and then no legislation appearing so the pharmaceutical industry were not too worried because they thought this would fail too. And were it not for thalidomide the legislation would have failed.

The hearing was more about excess profitability. An economist would get up and say, now 20 mg cost how much to make and the box costs 2 pennies, ignoring the investment that had produced these, the sort of thing that one hears today also. And then there was a flap about medical advertising being unmonitored and unvetted.

The idea that if articles were inimical to a company's interest they might pull the advertising out of the journals ...

There were those threats. I don't know if they were real. I testified in a weird way. I was a consultant to the committee but one day they had a man named Mark Nickerson who was supposed to testify. He had been in Michigan but he was living in Canada and during one of the breaks one of the staff people of Kefauver's committee asked, did I think he was going to be a good witness? I said jokingly that he should be because he had appeared before the House Un-American Activities Committee. For what? He was and may still be a card-carrying Communist, I said. Well that was all they needed to hear. They whisked him out immediately lest that come out and the testimony would be tarnished by this anti-capitalist tone and in a moment of madness I agreed to go on unprepared as a witness in his place. That is how I got to testify.

Originally I was just there to answer questions like, what does this term mean and what does that term mean? I tried to help them on medical advertising. The man after whom this building is named, Arthur Sackler, was the inventor of the multiple-page, multiple-colour spread ad in medical journals and Kefauver wanted to subpoena him to testify. I said, if you want real information from Sackler why don't you meet him in camera? You may get more that way than if you have him on the stand and he refuses to answer questions because it is embarrassing. To my great surprise Kefauver did this and they got along splendidly. But nevertheless all of that would have gone down the tubes if thalidomide hadn't come along. While it had nothing to do with the bill as it was written, it nevertheless turned the Congress's attitude around and we have been living with it ever since, both the good and the bad effects.

At a Congressional committee meeting earlier this year I was asked by the chairman of one sub-committee why we couldn't pass a law that you only had to study 84 patients to get a drug on the market. I thought, oh my god, how am I going to communicate to him that this isn't really the way to do it? But then even worse than that was his saying 'Why can't we go back to before 1962, make sure that safety isn't an issue and let the marketplace decide if the drug is effective or not?' I had to disagree with him because I don't really think anybody wants that. If I were the Commissioner and I was told that I no longer had the authority to approve a drug when I was convinced on the basis of the evidence available at that point that if the drug were used as labelled it would do a hell of a lot more good than harm I would resign. You should handle it differently if you are dealing with a life-saving drug for a disease for which nothing exists as opposed to the 45th clone of an anti-inflammatory. So one hears of occasional Luddites willing to take us back to before 1962 but I am sure that isn't going to happen.

To chase the placebo further, Michael Shepherd was one of the people who took the controlled trial furthest, at least in the mental health arena, but he ended up it seems to me deriving the conclusion from it that the placebo was almost the thing that was actually discovered by the RCT in a sense. Obviously when people got well on things before the RCT, which we now know weren't effective? there must have been a placebo component to it. But what the RCT did quite clearly was to dissect out a specific placebo in a sense – a placebo that was totally different to anything that ever went before.

When I was referring earlier to certain bioethicist complaints about placebo, another reason they object to approving a drug on the basis of superiority over placebo is that they quite rightly point out that for the practising physician and for the patient you really want to know how a new drug stacks up against what is already available. That is really more important than, is it better than sug- gestibility or spontaneous change?

It has gotten so complicated in some areas. I am interested in obesity man- agement. In the old days, trials would compare an appetite suppressant against a placebo but today it is an appetite suppressant against dietary advice, exercise advice and sometimes behaviour modification therapy. Now those things are hardly suggestibility controls. They really put it to you to top off what is per- fectly fine medical practice but it is such a far cry from what used to be the placebo. The placebo in the old days was just giving people a tablet and really seeing whether the appetite suppressant worked better than that.

This is the point that interested Michael Shepherd. When they did the NIMH studies of placebo versus cognitive therapy versus inter-personal therapy versus antidepressant they figured that they could not have a no-nothing kind of placebo. They had to have the best possible clinical management to compare with the other so-called specific treatments. And it turned out to be extremely powerful in its own right.

You know when you finally get a drug on the market the benefit it provides is obviously a combination of the placebo effect plus whatever pharmaco-thera- peutic benefit is derived and in a way it is strange to compare it against a place- bo tablet or capsule because in real life, unless you prescribe something, you don't get that therapeutic gesture, if you will, with whatever it connotes because doctors don't these days, at least in the United States, often prescribe placebos purposely. They may be prescribing drugs which are ineffective, like giving vit- amin B12 for weakness or something like that. That is a therapeutic gesture made by the physician who is hoping that it will work but at the very least there is going to be a demonstration of his intent to do something for the patient.

I don't take care of the sick any more but when I used to I invariably was able to think of something that might help the complaints of a patient that I was seeing, although I couldn't guarantee it. I never prescribed placebos and I think most doctors don't. In order to capture the placebo benefits you have got to write a prescription for something. That is what I think doctors do. With all the criticisms about doctors maltreating patients it is unfair to accuse them of often purposely giving patients placebos just to cater to their whims.

I suppose you could say that if you are giving penicillin for a sore throat you feel pretty sure isn't streptococcal in origin, that's giving a placebo. But I think most physicians would probably say they are doing it not because if they don't do so the individual will go down the street to see another physician but because it is damned hard to be sure that it's not streptococcal and penicillin is cheap, it's pretty damned safe and if it's streptococcal it's important to give it. It's interesting that with the so-called abuse of antibiotics over the last 40 years, there has been a decline in rheumatic fever and rheumatic heart disease, which I think is probably most easily explained by the promiscuous prescribing of penicillin to a lot of people who didn't need it but to some who did.

In 1969 you had an article that has always appealed to me, where you gave volunteers some instructions on the side-effects of a drug they were scheduled to take and found that many of them were unwilling to, on the basis of side-effects, take what later turned out to be aspirin. At the same time what they now knew about aspirin didn't affect their willingness to take it outside the experimental setting. So much for informed consent!

I serve on a local institutional review board, what you would call an ethics committee, and I keep pointing out to them that first of all we should pay attention to the language that we use, and I am not just talking about saying baldness instead of alopecia. A lot of patients don't understand some other language like maybe they don't know what a protocol is. And there are some shocking misinterpretations of words like 'orally' in New Haven, which was described by many people as meaning how often you would take it – not that you would take it by mouth. Whether they were hearing it as hourly I don't know. The second problem is if you are obsessive-compulsive about putting everything in, then you should face up to the possibility of information overload and should ask whether you are getting the major messages across. What our study showed was that if you had the same information but more and more embroidery you will get fewer subjects and some of the ones that you do get will miss very important information.

What was also interesting, I thought, was the fact that they were told about all the risks of this drug and said no, we are not going to have it, but when they went home they had it. It is a completely different thing between risks that are ones you know how to live with and risks you are having to process cognitively but you have not had to live with as it were. It is curious, isn't it?

It is the fear of the unknown. We once studied obstetrical pain experiences and I was convinced at the end that for women who have never had a baby before but whose exposure to the procedure was in movies, where invariably the woman was having a dreadful time, this was hardly conducive to peace and tranquillity as you were awaiting the experience yourself. Once you had it you were sort of prepared for the next one, however bad it had been. By the way, in that study you might be amused that we asked the women who delivered babies and their obstetricians how effective the control of pain had been. About 20% of the time they agreed pretty well but 80% of the time they disagreed. Almost invariably these women said they had had a harder time of it than their physicians said they had had. It is easy to explain why that might be. First of all physicians don't like to think they are doing a bad job of controlling pain but also the typical experience in the United States is for the obstetrician to come in, and using a baseball term, signal for a fair catch but not having been there during the hours that the woman was groaning and moaning and asking for help.

I delivered two of my own babies in our car because we didn't make it to the Johns Hopkins Hospital in time. The first time it happened was the first time that I had ever seen a baby born of an unmedicated mother. In the old days they used a lot of medication, including opioids. Out came this baby, ready to go. I had only seen sleepy babies and I thought that the normal status for a newborn was to be sleepy, not realising until that moment that it was because I had never seen a baby born from an unsedated mother. I think one of the reasons that doctors decided to make the procedure less unpleasant for the patient was that these patients would then go to their friends and say, oh you ought to go and see Dr so and so if you are pregnant. These days they have a different attitude about the hazards of doing this and the desire of many women and their spouses to be together going through the process and not expecting it is going to be dreadful.

Whilst I was at Hopkins we had some Australian midwives training there and they were the most popular health practitioners because they spent a lot of time with the women during their visits prior to the delivery, explaining to them and diminishing their fears and anxieties to a certain degree, being with them throughout the whole delivery, rubbing their backs and answering the questions that were often not answered by nurses in other situations.

Let me take you to the 1956 conference which was organised on the back of the monies that Nate Kline and others got out of Congress to fund the evaluation of psychotropic agents. It seems awfully curious for a start that the key people behind it were yourself, Ralph Gerard, Seymour Kety, Joe Brady – hardly a single psychiatrist there. It was a bunch of non-psychiatrists who put this thing together which...

Well, you know I can't remember the organisation of that meeting. Nate Kline was of course always angry that academia did not give him the credits that he thought he deserved for his role in the monoamine oxidase story.

He pitches it in the press as being that he did not want to get tied down with professorial jobs – he wanted to be a free spirit. He doesn't pitch it in terms of being disappointed.

He won any number of awards for his contribution to the field. He created an institute, he had battles with some of his colleagues. He was a complicated man. But Heinz Lehmann and Fritz Freyhan also did a lot of the seminal work on neuroleptics and they never got academic recognition. Working in Montreal the Royal Victoria was the most elegant place to be and Heinz was at the Verdun Protestant. Freyhan was at the Delaware Hospital in Maryland. So you have Kline and Freyhan and Lehmann who were important figures but never made it academically in this country. But Kety did make it and Brady did too.

Michael Shepherd said he sat in on a few of the meetings with yourself, Kety, Gerard and Jon Cole, who all tried to organise what were the issues – how do you actually structure up this meeting, what should we be doing etc. There was a feeling that the whole thing was about trying to contain Kline.

Well, Kline got the money appropriated by Congress for the Psycho-pharmacology Service Center and he was very bitter because he had wanted the money to come to him to do a trial comparing reserpine and chlorpromazine. He had done this study on reserpine and with huge numbers showed a statistically but almost biologically insignificant difference between reserpine and placebo. Then he and this journalist from the Mid-west, Mike Gorman, and Mary Lasker, had an enormous impact on Congress because they were smart and articulate. The Psychopharmacology Service Center was started in large part because of Gorman and Kline's testimony.

Then there was a committee for doling out the money and, oh the early applications were pitiful in quality! I remember asking the Head of the NIMH at one point – Bob Felix – what do we do if we don't have anybody that we want to give the money to? And he said the money will be spent. Under no circumstances was money to go back to Congress. So in those days, in contrast to today when terrific researchers have a hell of a time getting funded, it was almost too easy to get money.

But there was this desire on the part of people like Kety and Gerard, who were sort of super-academics, to have a discipline and rigour and to avoid both the hucksterish folks, in which category they would put Kline or people who just did it the old-fashioned way like Frank Ayd, people who treated patients and reported anecdotally that they all got better. They had a scornful attitude towards these Johnny-come-latelies, who professed to be scientists but who in the minds of the super-academics were not. Some of the criticism was deserved but some of it was unfair.

On that point reading through the volume that came out of the meeting, there was a point where Kline at one point on the issue of rating scales and endpoints and things like that said the risk was that really all they would do would be to put the rabbit into the hat and then think they had done something wonderful when they pulled it out again. That what we should be doing is looking at endpoints like discharge from hospital or moving from the backward to one of the open wards. Anything else is a con job. No one actually took the message on board – they went ahead and they created all sorts of rating scales but in many ways this surrogate endpoint is a tricky thing, isn't it?

I remember when Cade came up with lithium, what was persuasive was that the first patient had been on the back ward for so many years and everybody had given up hope. It's what I call the Lazarus phenomenon. It isn't quite bringing the dead back to life like Jesus did with that leper but it's analogous to it and its damned impressive when it happens. Unfortunately it doesn't happen all that often. Jesus only did it once, as I recall.

A lot of folks these days are very critical about things like the Hamilton scales. For example, they say well they are not all that great – just because we have got used to them we think they are wonderful. People who know more about them than I do go through a list of criticisms to show how you can get misled by it. It is probably a tribute to our willingness to keep doing things because they are acknowleged by the gurus to be what you should do instead of thinking how could we make it better, how do we measure meaningfulness?

I know when I started in the analgesic game there was a man in Britain, whose name I can't remember, who had a way of calculating analgesic performance where you got points for pain relief and you took points away for side-effects. I remember thinking that's dreadful because a patient could end up with zero score and it might mean no relief and no toxicity but it might mean significant benefit and significant toxicity, the two neutralising each other.

An early cost-utility approach?

Yes, but I changed my mind with the passage of time because now I think the most important question you can ask about a drug like an analgesic is, what did you think about that drug? Was it good, terrific, moderate, trivial, terrible? You should ask subjects about benefit and harm separately so you can analyse them properly but ultimately it's this weighing of the good and the bad by the patient which determines whether you would want to have it again. And this is an important question to ask. When I was doing hypnotic trials, for example, at first I was amazed that somebody who had got a dose of secobarbital fell asleep quickly and slept soundly all night through, but when asked how it was would say terrible. Why? 'Well, because I felt sort of raped by the drug. I was no longer in control of my brain. It's yielding to a chemical Svengali.' Well, that's an interesting reaction and it's a very important question because if you have a lot of people who feel that way you have either got the wrong dose or the wrong drug.

You appear to me to be entering into an area there that we have completely neglected for 30–40 years, which is the whole area of self-assessment of drugs. We don't let the patient make assessments. Have we made a mistake?

It's a terrible mistake. There is a wonderful article in a British journal by a man named Jachuk from Newcastle who did a study on hypertensive patients on medication and their relatives. He asked the doctors and the doctors all thought it was splendid because they were studying the manometer. He asked the patients and some of them were positive and some were negative. But the relatives, to a man and woman, thought that the medications were terrible. They had had no trouble with Dad before he was on this medication – he was behaving perfectly alright and what did they know about his hypertension – it wasn't affecting anything. Dad was not sick until he started taking these pills but now he's a hypochondriac. He's a pain to have around and he is muddled. Three quite different answers – each of them right and wrong in its own way. But if you don't ask them all, you get a bizarre version of the truth, or at least only a piece of the truth.

But the pharmaceutical industry are not into that, are they? And no one else has the resources to run the studies.

Now they are into a different ball game in this country and in Australia. Now you have got to do pharmacoeconomic studies to get a drug successfully on the market and that is because third party payers, whether they are HMOs or Health Insurance Plans with the Government or what have you, are asking of a new medication, in what way is this better than what I have been using? Why should I use your drug at all, let alone at the price you are asking for it? So the essence now is comparative performance against what is already available. The problem is that we are not very good at doing these studies yet and we are not as sophisticated as we need to be in trying to evaluate benefit or harm.

A colleague at MIT here in Boston says that outcomes research is like teenage sex – everybody talks about it, a few people are doing it but no one is doing it well. There is a certain truth in that because there is this great impetus to do something. At launch you must have these studies available and because you have done them prior to launch they have to go to the FDA as part of your new drug application and because of that you have the FDA wandering into the economics of reimbursement, which they are not supposed to do legislatively. But if your economic claims are based on science, the FDA is perfectly competent to evaluate that. If you want to claim that your drug is better in some way then you will have to show it to the FDA's satisfaction. So we are probably going to move more in this direction as people get more sophisticated and they realise what are the important questions to ask. Up until now we have not often been asking these questions.

Let me chase thalidomide – you were involved in trials for it, weren't you?

I only did one study with thalidomide as a hypnotic and concluded that it was an effective hypnotic and, thank God, said something like we don't know enough about safety. This was before 1962.

Did it actually send people to sleep?

Oh yes. It was an effective drug and you couldn't kill an animal with it unless you covered the animal with enough powder to keep it from breathing. It was clearly an effective hypnotic.

In Germany it was sold over the counter. Now before 1962 there was a certain pressure building up as I understand it to reverse the idea that these new drugs should be on prescription only which came in with the 51 Humphrey-Durham Amendments to the 1938 Act.

Prior to thalidomide there was a push to have over the counter anything that could be used safely by individuals if they paid attention to the labelling. So if the consumer could make a judgement about the indication and the treatment it should be available over the counter. But in fact I can't think of any drugs, at least in my lifetime, that have been approved for over-the-counter sales that weren't first prescription drugs.

No but if thalidomide hadn't happened ...

Would they have gone more in that direction? I don't know. Thalidomide was what made the 1962 amendments possible because those amendments were dead as a doornail until Dr Helen Taussig testified showing pictures of deformed babies. All of a sudden you had both houses of Congress unanimously passing this Bill. They hardly ever pass anything unanimously and it was peculiar in that the Bill had nothing to do with thalidomide babies. It had to do with all sorts of things like getting the FDA into the act earlier and what you needed to document benefit. Safety had been part of the earlier 1938 Act.

Of course some companies had been doing teratogenicity testing before thalidomide but it was not part of the mystique to do it, and prior to that time people interested in teratology were folks who used drugs in animals as methods of producing abnormalities and studying how the abnormalities were produced without worrying about clinical usage. But I am not sure that today we couldn't have another thalidomide. I am sure that the tests we do on animals are not perfect for predicting harm. You occasionally get a drug killed because of the animal findings without knowing whether it would be a problem in humans. By the way, thalidomide is likely to come back on the market because it works for leprosy and a number of other diseases – graft–host disease and so forth. I think the drug could be used safely with proper attention to avoiding its use in pregnant women.

We have a compound on the market in this country, Accutane, which is supposed to be used only for severe acne but I am sure it is used for less than severe acne at times and it is clearly a teratogen. To get it a physician has to go through an extensive informed consent procedure having people sign off and so forth. I mention it because acne strikes me as a less bad disease than some of the things thalidomide is now acknowledged to be useful for. So if you say, well it can't be on the market because it is capable of being a teratogen then what about Accutane? If we are rational we will allow it on the market with all sorts of warnings. If you are a male it is hard to say that you should not have thalidomide if you have got diseases that would benefit. If you are a postmenopausal woman, likewise. And for pregnant women or women with the potential for pregnancy it is going to be a warning problem. By the way, it is bizarre to me that we are now hearing we *must* study new drugs in women of childbearing potential because it's their civil right to be studied because otherwise you won't know how to label the drug for them.

This is tremendously risky.

Well, I think it is. The Institute of Medicine has come out for this; the FDA has too and I keep wondering are they going to be co-litigants, when some woman who has a deformed baby – and we know that 1–3% of babies are born deformed in some way anyway – says post hoc ergo propter hoc, I want $10 million now. Who is going to foot the bill for that – not the FDA; they would say we are part of the Government, so you can't sue us. And then there is this question that you must study children, you must study blacks, you must study Hispanics, there is no end to it. I am not saying that one should not try to study these subpopulations at least pharmaco-epidemiologically after the drug is on the market. You can't study everything. We know in the UK 4% of approved drugs are withdrawn from the market for previously unsuspected toxicity. In the USA, cautious as the FDA is, slow as the FDA is allowing time for trouble to surface in other countries first, 3% of our drugs are withdrawn from the market for such toxicity. So we ought to be studying drugs in the real world after registration because that is the way you stumble on the pleasant surprises as well as the unpleasant surprises.

By the way, I should have mentioned something about Beecher. You know he is the father of the informed consent movement in the USA with an article he wrote in the 1960s? He sent me the manuscript to read before he submitted it. He had asked me for examples from the literature and I sent them to him not knowing what he wanted. I said, Harry, you know we never got consent when I was working with you. And he said, I didn't say I was without sin. Well, but you don't have anything in here about the fact that in your own laboratory you never got consent from subjects. And I said, you know it also hasn't been traditional to mention these things in scientific publications. It is conceivable to me, not likely perhaps but conceivable, that some of these investigators got consent but didn't put it in the paper. He said no, if they got consent and didn't put it in the paper it's as bad as if they did not get consent at all. Now I cite this one as an example of Harry not wanting fact to interfere with drama. I think most people would have said that if they got consent the fact that they didn't put it in the paper wasn't an indictment against them.

Now if you ask why weren't we getting consent, it wasn't that we were Nazis saying well, if we ask for consent we are going to lose some subjects and it is going to be harder for us to do our research. We were so ethically insensitive that it never occurred to us that we should get consent. If you had asked us how these people were benefiting, we could have said truthfully that the patients we studied were interviewed by a technician every hour and if they were not doing well they could get something else, which is more than you could say for people not in our study who might be lying in bed for hours having received no benefit from the first dose of morphine and having to wait four hours for the next dose.

When I had a haemorrhoidectomy at Hopkins I came roaring out of anaesthesia with the worst pain I ever had in my life. They gave me a shot of pethidine but it didn't work so I said I need another shot, but they said no, you've got to wait 3–4 hours. I said, go and get one of your bosses and tell him that I know about analgesics and if I haven't got pain relief by now I am not going to get it in the next 3 hours and so they acceded to my request but ordinarily you would have to live with it. So there were some benefits from being in our studies but also we trampled on the rights of people who didn't know they were in a study. We never asked whether they were willing to participate or not. That is another thing that makes Harry Beecher controversial to me.

When you said he was the father of the informed consent movement... what did you mean?

He wrote an article pointing out that people were not getting it and that this was not right. Now later on it's interesting – having started this revolution in a sense by this article – he then went on to say that the principal, the true safeguard for an experimental subject was an ethical investigator. Consent forms notwithstanding, if you had an unethical investigator that was bad. But he did start the revolution and deserves great credit for it.

It seems to me that we just have not paid enough attention to how well or bad we are doing this and the bioethicists are right in a way when they say it is imperfect, but what the hell is perfect in this world? Those ethicists who say that informed consent is a sham should be ashamed of themselves because I feel much better about research that is being done today than I did before. Yes, it is imperfect but at least our patients or our healthy volunteers who are approached are being told that this is a research project, laying out the risks and benefits, which often are minimal, so in a sense people are sort of sacrificing themselves for the benefit of science or other people. They are told they don't have to participate and if they do participate they are told how they will be compensated. There is at least an attempt to level with people and I find that so much better than what we did back in the 1950s. What's the alternative – not to do any research at all?

When Hopkins set up its first institutional review board, we met with the lawyers to the hospital who said it's very easy, we just won't do any human research. We said no, that is not an option. So they retreated and we set up these safeguards. We don't approve everything. We usually re-write the consent form. We sometimes will be attacked by angry investigators who say they are part of a multi-clinic study and everybody else has approved already and yet the review board wants to change it and we say well, that's too bad if other people have approved it, it's not good enough for us. There was one investigator whom we approved a few years ago but because we did not trust him to get consent honestly we insisted that the consent must always be obtained with another person present. So we do try our best to do it more ethically than has been the case in the past.

You mentioned the issue of the pain you had after an operation and being in a sense able to prescribe for yourself, which brings me back to the 1962 amendments which copper-fastened in place the idea that these drugs were going to be by prescription only. One of...

The prescription only came about in the 1940s. The FDA was responsible for that really because they had a problem getting the information out to patients. They felt that if there was a learned intermediary then we wouldn't have to worry about putting all sorts of things on the label because there would be this learned intermediary that would intervene between the patient and the medication.

But of course it means that the average patient has not got the advantages that you had when you are there in the bed in pain and you can say look, to hell with this, if I actually

have to prescribe this myself I will do it. There was a case that was in the news lately –
Mahlon Johnson, a physician who has AIDS who claimed to have cured himself because
he tried all sorts of combinations of cocktails, which of course he was able to do because he
was able to get access to these things which the average person can't do.

I chaired a committee that got to be known as the Lasagna committee because
people could not remember its long name and we were addressing the issue of
how to speed the approval of drugs for cancer and AIDS and possibly other life-
threatening illnesses. The AIDS advocates were the most effective advocates I
have ever seen in my life – articulate, impassioned, well informed, willing to
be obnoxious if necessary. When we were having the hearings their general
attitude was, we want access to anything that surfaces anywhere on the globe
that is possibly beneficial.

An AIDS activist named Martin Delaney said being an AIDS patient is like
being on an aeroplane, the engines have knocked out, you are plummeting to
earth, there is a parachute on the seat next to you, you put it on and somebody
from the Government taps you on the shoulder and says, by the way, that has
not been fully tested yet or approved – the response is well, I'm going to take
my chances because I am facing death. Our interviews with AIDS and cancer
patients show that most patients with lethal diseases know that they have got a
bad disease and are willing to take risks. But what we were hearing at the hearings was more or less let's have access to everything. Now we've got surrogates
– you get a drug approved on the basis of a good effect on CD4 lymphocyte
counts without any proof that that makes a clinical difference and now at least
some AIDS patients are beginning to say gee, I think we were wrong. We
should have some evidence of clinical benefit and some knowledge about safety and toxicity or otherwise we may not be doing ourselves a favour. That fits
in with my own philosophy as well.

When I chaired this committee we had a member named Thomas
Merigan, an infectious disease expert from Stanford, and he and I sat down
one evening and asked 'What if we were God or we were commisioner of the
FDA, which is more important than being God, what would we demand of
an anti-AIDS drug?' And we concluded that we would like a good impact on
a surrogate like CD4 lymphocytes or circulating antigen *plus* something clinically beneficial – like feeling better, requiring fewer transfusions or having
fewer infectious diseases. Something which might or might not be a surrogate for survival but which would be a good end in itself. I still think that is
the way to do it because if you approve a compound on the basis of surrogate
endpoint only and it turns out to be not beneficial and, even worse not beneficial and toxic, you embarrass the agency, you embarrass the manufacturer
and you get a hell of a lot of patients who are angry with you. There has been
a turn in sentiment there.

With anticancer drugs there is a move towards what the oncologists have
been recommending for a long time, namely use of a surrogate endpoint such
as tumour burden, because in general compounds that diminish tumour size
do turn out to have potential for benefit. It's a tricky business, this use of sur-

rogates, but clearly if there are short cuts to approval then we ought to be using them provided we are doing the right thing.

You were obviously one of the people who pushed hard for the 1962 amendments taking the shape that they did. Peter Temin in his book put you down as one of the people who changed their view as to whether the 1962 amendments were a good thing or not. Your view in the early 1960s was that the whole field of medicine had got so complicated that the average doctor can't really know what to do and has to be told by the expert.

Its not really reneging on my conviction about controlled trials, its just that I think we have gone overboard with believing that it is the only way to come up with any useful information. My feeling is that Bradford Hill was right about that and that we should not be ignoring other ways of getting useful information. I am just asking for a sort of broadening of the evidence required to get a drug on the market. I also think that the process has gotten enormously complicated because the FDA is now in the act all the way through from the request to go into humans to the very end. This has to do not just with clinical trials but with preclinical toxicology and so forth. It is now taking 10–15 years from discovery to marketing and costs hundreds of millions of dollars – the number keeps going up every year.

Our figure in 1987 dollars was $231 million. Half of that was out-of-pocket expenses, the other half was what they call the cost of money – what you could have got if you had invested the money and it was paying a reasonable return. We have gotten to the point where a company might well say, what the hell are we in this business for? These days a me-too drug is not going to sell at all – in the old days we could make a little bit of money at least by having a compound that was no worse than those already on the market – but those days are gone. The generic industry is out there bigger every year. How can we justify to our stockholders looking for cures for Alzheimer's disease and all the other things that are badly treated?

By the way, everybody says you only need two trials to get a drug on the market. In fact the average number now completed before filing an application is 60 or more. Some of that is looking at children and what have you and some of it is pharmaco-economics, but I can't believe that all of those trials are necessary. What I have been saying now for about 3 years is, why can't we have early and continuing collegial relations between the FDA and the sponsors, plus an appeal mechanism in case there is disagreement where the sponsor would have a chance of winning were he or she in the right, so that when you get to the new drug application it is self-reviewing because you have asked and answered all the appropriate questions and not asked and answered inappropriate questions. Because I am sure that some of what is being done now and contributing to the cost and the time are either unreasonable demands by the Agency or mistaken perceptions by the sponsor of what the agency will ultimately require. We shouldn't put up with that. I am not talking about cutting corners, I am talking about asking, is this trip necessary every time we are considering doing something? I think that would serve the public well, would serve the industry well and serve the FDA well too because their mission is to protect the public health, which means worrying about frauds and crooks and poor-quality drugs but also promoting the public health – that's another dimension and that has to do with getting drugs on the market.

I guess the current climate in the public is that you don't actually promote health by getting drugs on the market...

It depends who you talk to – if you talk to cancer and AIDS patients – they are dying for new drugs to get on the market. The public doesn't want the agency to shirk on protecting the public – they want to be protected from frauds. In fact one of the first things the present commissioner did when he took over was to try and get over the shame of the generic drug scandals where some of these generic companies were paying off with trivial amounts of money FDA employees to give their compounds preferential treatment in the process and filing fraudulent data. The agency lost some of its reputation because of this bad publicity.

When was that?

That was 6 or 7 years ago. There were a few instances of shameful behaviour by generic companies. There was one company who took a SmithKline & French compound and instead of comparing it with their generic version compared it with the SKF compound in another capsule. I am not sure if there is any evidence that the public was ever harmed by this but it made it look as if the agency had people that could be bought. And the first thing the commissioner did was to apply a cops and robbers approach with massive crackdowns, having inspectors going to visit plants with pistols – a little bit hammy but it worked and the FDA now is back in good odour.

I don't want to diminish that and I don't want the agency to stop looking for crooks and frauds but up until AIDS, by and large the agency was only accused by the Congress of poor performance if they approved a drug that later on caused trouble that nobody predicted. Until AIDS they weren't besieged by pressures from Congress – why aren't you getting drugs on the market sooner? And the agency to this day I am afraid still think that type 1 errors are worse than type 2 errors and that the worst that they can do is to allow a drug on the market that doesn't deserve to be on the market – refusing a drug access to the market that deserves to be on the market or slowing it down is less important.

That's always the bureaucrat's response really, isn't it?

There was a former Assistant Secretary in the Department of Health Education and Welfare, as the department was called in those days, who said that if you're a bureaucrat you find that you're like the whale – if you don't surface you don't get harpooned. So stay below the surface of the water. This is true for university bureaucrats too. It isn't just the regulatory agencies.

The 1962 amendments said that drugs would remain prescription only and they said that we want to evaluate the drugs in the way that the experts say they should be evaluated, which was the randomised controlled trials, but they also said we don't want drugs that are non-specific – we want drugs for indications that experts say we should have drugs for. In other words for a disease entity. We want to do away with drugs for halitosis and ton- ics and things like that. Was that a mistake, because you could arguably re-classify all of the antidepressants as tonics but called tonics they might have been a lot more acceptable to people than antidepressants – a disease indication can be problematic with the public.

I don't think it has actually been a problem. It's true that you are in bad shape if you go to the agency with trials where you say well, we had multiple end- points. They want you to pick a primary endpoint that you have settled on in advance of doing the trial. They look at other endpoints as a way of compen- sating for failure by coming up with something totally different.

But there are an awful lot of people out there – 10–15% of the population who have a generalised anxiety depression type of thing – they've fatigue and nervousness and it was OK during the 1960s to take a drug to the FDA which was going to be an anxiolytic. You can't do that now because of the benzodiazepines. So these people have all of a sud- den become depressed and we are doing trials with antidepressants which involves a cer- tain fraudulence ...

There is a problem because, as you were just saying, in real life these things don't exist in pure form and you ought to face up to the fact that they don't exist in pure form.

But the 1962 amendments at least for psychiatry don't do that.

I think you're right. I had not thought of it that way but I think that's right. And it's again part of this desire to keep things as clean as possible, which is not a stupid experimental approach when you do experiments in the laboratory. You want to have the variables under your control – if you use rats of different strains and dogs of different strains you just make it a bit more difficult and so I can see why you would want to study – if you could – pure anxiety or pure depression. On the other hand, if you do studies of those patients it seems to me the very least you have got to worry about is, will these findings also apply to impure anxiety and impure depression?

It seems to me that the clinical trial process for neuroleptics would be so much easier if the FDA were prepared to accept tranquillisation as an indication. In actual fact it's quite clear that the drugs we use for schizophrenia are relatively non-specific to schizophrenia. They will treat any psychosis, they will even treat people who are depressed or anxious. What these cases all have in common is some form of tranquillisation which we have not looked closely enough at because of the fact that we have been focused at the disease endpoint the whole time.

At one point there were ads run by I forget which company for a major tran- quilliser which had elderly patients kicking chairs – obstreperous, cantanker- ous you know. And that got into bad odour because if you have elderly patients come in and you ask what's bothering you, they don't say I'm cantankerous. I know myself, having worked in hospitals, that if you have a patient, especially if he is across the hall from the nurse's station who every 15 seconds is bellowing, after a while there is a desire to write a tranquillisation order. Who is being treated in that case – is it the nurse being treated or the other patients? It's a real life problem but if you demand evidence that that tranquillisation benefits the patient then that's a lot harder than is it benefiting the nurses for example or the other patients on the ward who finally have a chance to sleep at night. That has been part of the problem.

Sure, but the way the amendments have gone again at least in psychiatry has been to say well, we want drugs for schizophrenia. This is the indication the experts say we should be trying to develop drugs for. And we end up with the idea that these drugs are anti-schizophrenic in some sense whereas in actual fact what we have at best is a therapeutic principle that may be useful in schizophrenia. Have the amendments forced us too far down the road of an illusory therapeutic specificity?

Yes, it is probably what Alfred North Whitehead, the philosopher, called misplaced concreteness. Probably the psychiatric profession are accomplices of this by their use of scales and what have you.

We want to be part of real medicine. Can I hop to another theme? You took up the first Chair in pharmacology in Johns Hopkins.

The first division of clinical pharmacology in the USA anyway. A group of people devoted entirely to the study of drugs in humans, sometimes going to animals, but always with a focus on humans. That was 1954.

Were there any other clinical pharmacologists in the country then?

There were, here and there, and shortly thereafter other groups formed. There were some leaders – a man named Leon Goldberg who used to be at Emory and moved to the University of Chicago. A man named John Oates who ultimately became head of the Department of Medicine in Vanderbildt. A man named Daniel Azarnoff who was the group leader in Kansas City. So there were a few of us early in the game who were charismatic leaders who got training programmes started. We got training funds from the National Heart Institute, because a man named Bob Grant there thought that clinical pharmacology was a good thing even if it wasn't entirely cardiovascular.

So we got off to a good start but I have been disappointed in the evolution of clinical pharmacology. I think the Swedes and the Brits have done it better. You have Chairs in Great Britain. The Swedes have Chairs and infrastructural support for a unit in every one of the Swedish Medical Schools. In this country we haven't achieved that. My guess is that in Britain and Sweden if one of the leaders of one of these units or the occupants of a Chair died or retired they wouldn't hesitate for a moment to replace that person. In this country not infrequently what has happened is if the charismatic leader leaves – had he been a haematologist or a cardiologist the academic leadership would say well, we have got to have a haematologist, we have got to have a cardiologist, but they don't say that about clinical pharmacology. Partly I think it is because clinical pharmacology is a generalist speciality or can be unless you focus on just one kind of drug and the other specialities say, who are these guys who know everything about everything? They must be dilettantes at best.

It has been disappointing to me especially because I would have thought that in the year 1996 every hospital of any size would want a staff clinical pharmacologist, who might, on the one hand, be a therapeutic conscience for the institution and on the other hand help to make cost–benefit judgements. It is true we do have doctors of pharmacy in this country – PharmDs – I don't know whether you have them in Britain or not – and they sometimes play that role in hospitals. I am not decrying their use but it seems to me that having a medical degree ought to augment the ability to do that, provided you don't lack the proper training in pharmacology. So I can't say I feel happy about what has happened to clinical pharmacology in this country. I am sometimes called the Father of Clinical Pharmacology but I don't feel as if I've spawned a discipline that is properly appreciated.

In this country a clinical pharmacologist has more of a future in government – the FDA – or in industry, neither of which would dream of trying to function without clinical pharmacological expertise. Now it is true that if you are an MD or PhD or a PharmD or anything you are poorly prepared for a career in drug development and drug regulation. You have to do things that you have not learned in the process of getting those degrees. But once you have learned them you will be very useful in the FDA and in a drug company, whereas in academia there are plenty of institutions who say, we can get along without a clinical pharmacologist. To me that's a pity.

One of the awfully curious things at times when you go along to ACNP or BAP meetings which are supposedly for pharmacologists is that you find anything from 300 to 1000 clinical psychiatrists or behavioural biologists and you can probably count the number of actual proper card-carrying pharmacologists on the fingers of two hands.

I think you're right. A lot of the sessions are rather esoteric for many of the people who go to the meetings – and lots of people don't go. The ACNP prides itself on having good scientists, be they biologists or epidemiologists or clinicians or what have you. But in fact over the years it is fair to say that some of the folks who got in early in the game wouldn't get in today – they would be seen as 'just clinicians'. Frank Ayd, who was president of ACNP at one point, would probably not get in today.

Is it a problem that groups like ACNP are becoming almost neuroscience societies?

You are right. I don't go to the neurosciences meetings but my guess is that you can overlap them with ACNP without any trouble at all. Part of the trouble is that – Einstein used to worry about this – as science gets more and more complicated it's hard for the human brain to cover a lot of territory. If you get a research grant in this country from the NIH, God forbid that you should strike out in a whole new direction that isn't well circumscribed. That is part of the problem – how to you avoid the specialist versus generalist tension. And there is no doubt in my mind that for certain kinds of molecular biology you damned well better not be a dilettante. Do it well or don't do it at all. We have always had this need for something that over-arches and brings people together but how we achieve that linkage I don't know.

One hears a lot of talk these days about cytobiology and molecular biology and receptorology and computer-assisted design and whatever, as if ultimately you didn't need whole animal research and whole human research in order to see how things work out. No matter what the 3D configuration looks like, if the molecule doesn't get into the brain it is not going to have any effect. Sooner or later you have got to move away from cells and molecules to the big picture.

I heard that put awfully well by Silvio Garattini, who said you have all these people arguing that we should not be doing work with animals because it is so far away from man, but he said the same people then say that we should be doing work with cells, which is even further away.

Well, that's right. Would to God we had good models for the Merck man that I mentioned earlier. He would love it if somebody had an animal or a cellular model that worked. That to me has always been the definition of a useful model. I have a slide of this beast, that I call the Hound of the Baskervilles, straining on a leash and the next picture is of him tranquillised by amphetamine. I don't care whether this dog is the canine analogue of clinical hyperactivity and attention deficit disorder, if it predicts efficacy in attention deficit disorder it is a good model regardless. I am not going to go around looking for schizophrenic mice because I don't know that I can find them even if they exist. So I am left with models that are usually chosen on the basis of something that has been stumbled upon serendipitously in the past. Then the question is whether this model is only going to allow you to predict more things like what led to this model, whereas what you may want is something quite different.

In the field of analgesia my nalorphine experiment wasn't predictable in animals and to this day wouldn't be. There are no good animal models for the agonist–antagonist analgesics or for the non-steroidals. I remember one time going to Upjohn and they'd had for years a screening programme going to come up with a substitute for aspirin. They said, one problem is we can't pick up aspirin in this screen. So I said well, what are you using it for then? And they said, the girls are terribly good at running these assays.

One is left with a desperate 'Where the hell are we'? We can't just pick compounds off the shelf. You have got to pick them for some clinical trial somehow. We do the best we can and the trouble is we are not terribly good at it. Some things we are better at than others but in the field of oncology, which I have been forced to get into for a variety of reasons, for the traditional cytotoxic drugs we have models that are not so bad but if you come up with new things – anti-angiogenesis factors or whatever – things that don't affect a tumour but affect the spread, those are different models that will have to be tested empirically. It's a constant challenge – how the hell do we use theory or serendipity or common sense to allow us to pick candidates, knowing that thousands of chemicals are synthesised for every one that goes into humans and of the ones that go into humans only 20% or 25% ever make it to market? So it is a risky inefficient business but what else can we do? I wish I knew.

Can you account for the explosion in health care that has happened post-World War II and perhaps in this country more than any other country in the world, there has been an exponentially rising number of general physicians, surgeons as well as psychiatrists?

Well, medicine has always been a good profession to go into even today, when people say we ought to close every fifth medical school and cut the class sizes and so forth. Yet there are more applicants this year than we have ever had. I think it is because they say well, compared to what is medicine bad? We have had the greying of the population which means more people needing medical care. We have had explosions of transplants, new hips, new knees, new CAT scanners, new MRI machines, new drugs, new surgical procedures. Science has come up with a lot of things that could be delivered to the public if society is willing to pay enough for them. So our health care expenses are up to 14% of our gross national product at the moment, which is pretty high. A lot of people are saying 'That's enough.'

Now my prediction is as follows: we will go through a period, which we have already entered, where there will be strong attempts to cut the fat out of the system. Knock out the prescribing of unnecessary drugs, unnecessary surgery, unnecessary CAT scans, MRIs and what have you. This is a finite move pitted against the infinite ability of science, unless we stop supporting research, to come up with all sorts of ways of spending money. Now some of those ways will actually save money – for example, now that we know that peptic ulcers are caused by *Helicobacter pylori*, we can cure it and I am sure that the ledgers will look good. But for many things you are not going to save money. You are going to make people feel better. If you have got a painful hip and you get a new one, you feel a lot better and you are more mobile but economically it may not mean all that much. So what does that mean? I think it means rationing but a different kind of rationing from what we have always had.

First of all there is the rationing in wartime on the battlefield or in floods, earthquake, typhoon, where you triage. If I take care of those two dreadfully sick people I can't save 20 less dreadfully sick people. And that engages us in a statistical morality. But today we are facing something quite different. We are now talking not about our ability to deliver but whether we can afford it. That to me means that we are probably going to keep the safety net where it is so that there are certain things that everybody is going to have access to and then other things that not everybody will. There are two determinants of access which I have seen in every country. One is geography. If you are an Eskimo on the shores of Hudson Bay you don't get the same kind of treatment as if you were living in Toronto. The other determinant is personal wealth. If you are wealthy enough, you don't have to wait in line to have your cataract operated on. You go to another city, another hospital or another country. Now is that anti-egalitarian? You're goddamned right it is.

But lots of things in this world aren't egalitarian. We don't all live in the same size houses or drive the same cars or have the same boats or what have you. You might say that health is different from having a car. Yes it is and no it isn't. So I see an increasingly painful scenario at least for the older docs who grew up in the days when you did what was best for the patient. Early in my career I worked in hospitals where we undercharged the poor or charged them nothing and overcharged the rich – if you want you can call it the Robin Hood School of Medical Economics. At the end of the year if the hospital had a deficit you passed the hat in the community and raised the difference. It worked pretty well actually but that isn't the situation any more.

Now we have managed care which some people have said is really managed cost, not managed care, where we have outrageous guidelines such as you are entitled to two days of hospitalisation, if you come in with pyogenic meningitis. That's ridiculous, after two days to go home with a serious illness like that. That should never have been allowed. Now they do say 'Use your judgement, if a patient needs more than two days' but then you may not get reimbursed for the extra stay. It is a gloomy scenario that I see ahead of us. But if our society insists on capping the percentage of GNP spent on health I don't see any alternatives.

In Oregon 5 years or so ago Medicaid had just so much money to pay for the health of the indigent – most of whom were women and children – and they decided that they wouldn't do any liver transplants on chronic alcoholics because they're expensive and the money for one liver transplant could vaccinate a thousand children, a socially more justifiable use of the money. Now that is reasonable enough unless you are the alcoholic needing a liver transplant. It is very tricky. But the one good thing that is happening is that people are beginning to talk about it as rationing. For quite a while nobody talked about rationing. The R word was a bad word because it connoted wartime, petrol, etc.

You have been looking at the psychiatric business from right at the start – the 1956 conference – where you were able to look at this bunch of people trying to work out their problems. Who has impressed you in US or world psychiatry as a real player, people who have actually contributed anything substantial – or has there been anything substantial? We've got the trappings of being part of medicine now but has there really been anything...

I would give credit to people like Delay and Deniker, Lehmann and Freyhan, and Nathan Kline and Frank Ayd and Cade and Schou – the people who opened up the field. I would give Jonathan Cole a lot of credit too because the psychopharmacology service centre he set up, while it existed, did stimulate excellent research. I would credit Max Hamilton for his scales, imperfect though they are. I had a colleague who, borrowing from Max Beerbohm who used to be referred to as the incomparable Max, used to refer to Max Hamilton as the comparable Max. Hamilton was a curmudgeonly man but he worked hard and he did contribute some techniques for quantification. Michael Shepherd was important in getting the concept of trials going and Joel Elkes also had an impact there. In this country, Elkes started the ACNP and he deserves credit for that. Maybe part of the problem today is that there are not a lot of giants around who can go out there and grab our Society and shake it and say, come on let's do something about our problems.

Is there a change within the industry? 40 or 50 years ago you would have had people who were possibly medically qualified to span the whole range of drug development and now you've got the MBAs running the show and looking at the bottom line money-wise.

Well, on the other hand I would say that during my lifetime I have seen the quality of the physicians in both the FDA and the industry improve considerably. They were often dreadful in the old days. Many were people who could not make a go of it anywhere else. That was responsible in part for the fact that even good people in the industry were often shunned by their academic colleagues. There was a time, believe it or not, in this country, in the 1940s or 1950s, where if you were a member of our pharmacology society and you went into industry you were thrown out of the society. It showed how pejoratively the industrial side of things was seen. I remember one man who went to Eli Lilly saying to me that he was accused by his former boss of selling his soul for a mess of potage.

Things are better in part because life in practice is not as attractive as it used to be. If you are in research you may say today in industry somebody else is going to come up with the money so I don't have to get a research grant from the NIH or the MRC. So it has gotten better but I can't say that we have a plethora of giants. Maybe it is that our society does not have many giants in general. I was at a meeting recently where they were talking about the history of pharmacology and it was pointed out that May & Baker's sulphonamide was given credit for winning World War II because Winston Churchill's pneumonia was successfully treated with it. It's hard to imagine the outcome of World War II being the same had Winston Churchill not been around. When I look at the people running governments these days it's hard to say the same, although Margaret Thatcher, for all her faults and ego problems, was a super woman of sorts.

One of the unfortunate things that has happened in my view is the *p* value madness. It was just an arbitrary decision that resulted in 0.05 being the magical barrier. As far as I can see there is nothing magical about it. It is encouraging that a few journals like the *British Medical Journal* and some others have begun saying look, don't talk about things being statistically significant or not just give us the *p* values and confidence intervals and let people judge for themselves because in this world we do a lot of things with less certainty than 95% of the time. It seems to me that the more rigorous you are about that the more likely you are to make type 2 errors.

If you look in the psychological literature and the statistical literature you will find a lot of folks who are opposed to the magic 0.05. Editors by and large are religiously devoted to it and most clinical scientists are. The FDA is as well and it just seems silly to me – a bit like intention-to-treat analysis. You ought to be able to live with something a little more giving than that.

On the other hand, the literature used to be full of underpowered studies that could clearly miss clinically important findings, but a good thing that is happening these days is that the pharmaceutical industry is unlikely to start a trial these days without some sort of power analysis. They ask themselves what would we be unhappy missing 80% of the time. That is all to the good if one thinks back to our failure to do that in the past and the fact that most people, if they came up with a 0.10 value, act as if there is nothing suggesting activity.

Did the analysis of variance idea mislead us to some extent? It gave us false confidence that we can pick up differences that are statistically significant but maybe not clinically.

Yes, that's the other bad part. If you have a trivial difference and you study enough patients, you come up with biologically insignificant but statistically significant figures, which again is obviously another reason for putting more reliance on confidence intervals, where you say well, it might be as little as this or it might be as much as that. That to me as a clinician is more helpful than knowing that some trivial effect achieves this magical level of statistical significance.

The bad thing that is happening these days is I've noticed that the editor of the *Lancet* recently talked about how he might turn down a paper if it did not have women in it, for example. He is following this tendency to study everyone – women, the young, the old and so forth. When I read it I thought, I hope the paper isn't a study of prostate cancer. It would be a pity if the *Lancet* got to that kind of Gulliverian craziness. I remember one time going with Beecher to a meeting of biological editors. They had decided that if something had been learned through an unethical experiment it should not be published. And I asked the question what if somebody came up with a cure for lung cancer that had been discovered in an unethical way? Would you really feel good about hiding that from the public or would you not prefer to publish it with an accompanying editorial denouncing how they had done it but thanking god that a breakthrough had come?

Select bibliography

Beecher HK, Keats AS, Mosteller F, Lasagna L (1953). The effectiveness of oral analgesics (morphine, codeine, acetylsalicylic acid) and the problem of placebo 'reactors' and 'non-reactors'. *Journal of Pharmacology and Experimental Therapeutics*, **109**, 393–400.

Hill AB (1966). Reflections on the controlled trial. *Annals of Rheumatic Disease*, **25**, 107–113.

Lasagna L (1954). A comparison of hypnotic agents. *Journal of Pharmacology and Experimental Therapeutics*, **111**, 9–20.

Lasagna L, Beecher HK (1954). The analgesic effectiveness of nalorphine and nalorphine–morphine combinations in man. *Journal of Pharmacology and Experimental Therapeutics*, **112**, 356–363.

Lasagna L, Mosteller F, Felsinger J von, Beecher HK (1954). A study of the placebo response. *American Journal of Medicine*, June, 770–779.

Lasagna L (1960). The clinical measurement of pain. *Annals of the New York Academy of Sciences*, **86**, 28–37.

Lasagna L (1960). Thalidomide – a new nonbarbiturate sleep-inducing drug. *Journal of Chronic Diseases*, **11**, 627–631.

Lasagna L (1962). Controlled trials: nuisance or necessity. *Methods of Information in Medicine*, **1**, 79–82.

Lasagna L (1989). Congress, the FDA, and new drug development: before and after 1962. *Perspectives in Biology and Medicine*, **32**, 322–343.

8 Linford Rees

The place of clinical trials in the development of psychopharmacology

Can we start with why you were interested in medicine and what then led you to do psychiatry?

I came from a family of teachers. My father was a teacher, my grandfather a headmaster, my uncles and aunts either teachers or directors of education. They were all teachers. When I was at Llanelli Grammar School, I found that almost everyone in my class intended to become teachers. Wales exports teachers in fact! In view of the competition, I decided to think of something else. I therefore wrote to the Welsh National School of Medicine for a prospectus and was very attracted by the curriculum. I applied for entry and went through the medical training there. I was fortunate in the course of my training to win a variety of prizes in anatomy, physiology, medicine, and months as a resident student clinical assistant at Whitchurch, which gave me my first real contact with psychiatry. I enjoyed it tremendously. Of course, the irony is that I entered medicine to avoid becoming a teacher but ended up becoming one just the same.

What year was this?

This was 1937/1938. We were given a variety of types of work. For example, if the social worker was away on holiday, we would carry out the detailed social histories of outpatients as well as inpatients. Similarly when the pharmacist was away we did all the dispensing. It was very good experience. I used to do two rounds each day, accompanied by the senior nursing staff, who treated us with great respect and made us feel very important.

We also attended the outpatient clinics at the Cardiff Royal Infirmary and were given patients to treat. There is nothing like being given clinical responsibility to stimulate the interest of a medical student. I enjoyed the work and this gave me my interest in psychiatry.

After I qualified and after a period of house jobs and general practice I went to Worcester County Mental Hospital in Powick, where my first post was to look after the annexe containing 800 chronic patients. I examined all these and found a number of cases of general paresis which hadn't been diagnosed. During that time, there was a great interest in Birmingham and in the

Midlands in the role of focal sepsis in the production of mental disorder. This was treated by surgical procedures including tonsillectomy and washouts of sinuses and the removal of any other focal sepsis. I had to give the anaesthetics. One or two patients seemed to get better, but it was probably the non-specific effects or the stress of the operation which helped.

What other treatments were in use at that time?

I was the first to introduce convulsive therapy at Powick, using intravenous Cardiazol. The first patient I treated by this method was a chronic schizophrenic, who surprisingly showed considerable improvement. At that time, it was given for schizophrenia because of the belief that there was a biological antagonism between schizophrenia and epilepsy. Other treatments included producing pyrexia by TAP injections or by the intramuscular injection of a colloidal solution of sulphur in oil, which was called Colsul, which would also produce a temperature. These obviously were very empirical non-specific methods of treatment.

Were they used for general paresis only or would they be used for anything else?

Anything, really. In the case of general paresis, there was malaria therapy of course. But some people improved with Colsul. I think it may have mobilised the acute immunological system in some way. Anyway they weren't very scientific treatments but they were the only ones available. ECT hadn't come in at that point. Intravenous Cardiazol was used to produce convulsions but it was frightening for the patient, much more frightening than ECT.

When did you move to London?

I came up to London to the Maudsley, to do a Diploma in Psychological Medicine in 1940. I was appointed to the Maudsley Hospital, which was at Mill Hill in 1940. At that time, there were a lot of famous people there – Aubrey Lewis was the Clinical Director, Walter Maclay was the Medical Superintendent and Aldwyn Stokes his deputy. Other distinguished people included William Gillespie, Russell Frazer, Maxwell Jones and others. Maxwell Jones started his Therapeutic Community there.

I found Mill Hill very stimulating. During the war, we took about 500 service people suffering from neurosis from the army, the navy and the airforce and from the women's auxiliary armed services. There were also some civilian casualties. One interesting thing was that although London was being bombarded at that time, I, a young psychiatrist, looked after nearly all the outpatient clinics for the whole of London. What that shows of course is that there wasn't a tremendous demand for outpatient treatment. I had clinics at St Mary's Highgate, Mile End, St Charles and one or two other places.

It was during this time that the future Institute of Psychiatry was planned. We had meetings on a Monday evening to discuss what was required for the future psychiatric services at the Maudsley Hospital and the needs of postgraduate psychiatric training. Aubrey Lewis brought these plans to fruition after the war and the new Institute subsequently led to a tremendous expansion of research, with new Chairs, new Departments and a great expansion of postgraduate training.

You did some early work with Eysenck?

I was the principal psychiatrist who worked with Eysenck. We did a great deal of work on the effects of narcosis produced by nitrous oxide and other agents on suggestibility. That was our first collaboration. Subsequently, I did a lot of work with him on physique using anthroprometric measurements on various groups of psychiatric patients, people with effort syndrome and various normal control groups. I did most of the work and he helped with the statistical application of factorial analysis. We devised various indices of body build including the Rees–Eysenck Index for men and there's another for women called the Rees Index. These studies were all based on measurements of patients at Mill Hill.

What were the findings?

I think the work provided precise methods of assessment and therefore helped to standardise the assessment of physique. We showed that there were two main factors accounting for variations in physiques; the first factor was a general one of body size which affected all measurements, and there was a second bipolar factor which governed the shape of the person's body – whether it was narrow or broad. The broad type correlated with manic-depressive disorder, whereas schizophrenia was associated with a variety of types of physique. There was also a correlation between hysteria and anxiety states with totally different kinds of physique. Our findings only supported Kretschmer's views in part. There was, as I have said, some correlation between manic-depressive disorder and a broad physique but this was partly due to age – a lot of the manic-depressives were older and one tends to put on weight as you get older.

I also studied physical constitution in effort syndrome. I worked with Paul Wood on that – he was a cardiologist, whose recommendations that the syndrome be called Da Costa's syndrome were widely adopted. It was also called neurocirculatory asthenia. What I found was that the narrower the physique the greater was the constitutional predisposition to effort intolerance, autonomic instability and so on, whereas the broader types of physique were correlated with external stress such as bombardment and other forms of battle stress or sometimes precipitated by infection.

Is effort syndrome the same thing as ME?

No, quite different. Although in some of the Da Costa's syndrome patients, infections played a precipitating role, most of them were in ongoing military service and the clinical picture was quite different. The ME syndrome is characterised by intense fatigue and muscular pains, whereas Da Costa's syndrome is characterised by intolerance, autonomic dysfunction and various neurotic symptoms and is quite different from ME.

I worked very closely with Aubrey Lewis, who took a great interest in my research on physique. He used to come with me to the Mill Hill barracks. I would carry out the measurements on various groups of soldiers and he'd record them. We also worked closely in studying involuntary movements in post-encephalitic Parkinson's disease. This interest was stimulated by a patient who presented as suffering from what seemed to be an obsessive-compulsive symptom – tongue protrusion. This involuntary tongue protrusion had developed after eating Ryvita bread with ants on it.

Ants?

The insect – yes! The ants stung his tongue and the referring military psychiatrist thought that being stung on the tongue by ants was the triggering or precipitative mechanism for his obsessive-compulsive symptoms. I noticed that this man's pupils reacted to light but didn't react on accommodation which gave me the clue that this was a post-encephalitic type of neurological disorder.

Aubrey Lewis then arranged for us to visit Winchmore Hill Hospital, which was a centre for post-encephalitic parkinsonian patients. We examined a number of these patients and found in addition to general features such as rigidity and tremors, a number did suffer from involuntary movements such as tongue protrusion. We filmed a number of these patients and it was interesting that occasionally we detected oculogyric crises, which had not been observed clinically. It should be remembered that this was before the introduction of the phenothiazines and other neuroleptic agents and this was a rare phenomenon. Now of course, it's commonplace to see tongue protrusion. It was very interesting.

In addition to looking after the soldiers, I also looked after units of women, who were members of the auxiliary armed forces from ATS, WAAF, and Wrens. I was told I was given this particular assignment as I was married and they thought it was safe to have me in charge of these beautiful young service women from the forces. I had to do a round everyday, inspecting these lovely girls. It was very pleasant.

Another of my units was devoted entirely to conversion hysteria. This was very interesting. There was a whole range of conversion symptoms affecting special senses and various other functions. Physicians who had no experience of these severe hysterical conversion symptoms had tended to discount hysteria as a diagnosis and referred to it as illness behaviour. All these patients were thoroughly investigated neurologically as well as physically and I found no evidence to support the view of Elliot Slater, who considered that hysteria did not merit consideration as a separate nosological entity and that in his experience it tended to occur on the basis of somebody having a pre-existing neurological condition. But that's because he worked in the National Hospital, Queen's Square. If he'd worked in Mill Hill he'd have seen clear-cut cases of all types of hysteria – paralysis, blindness, and all the classic symptoms, without any underlying neurological disorder. The underlying disorder sometimes was a depression or occasionally schizophrenia but very frequently anxiety states with no evidence of neurological disorders. In addition to having all varieties of conversion symptoms we also had dissociative states, including fugues, amnesias and hysterical fits.

When Mill Hill closed down, I then went to the Southern Hospital, Dartmouth, with Maxwell Jones, where we were in charge of units of re-patri-ated prisoners from Japan, the Far East or from Europe, suffering from a variety of psychiatric disorders. This was interesting work, but the service was only needed for a limited time until the patients were sufficiently improved to be dis-charged. I was still on the staff at the Maudsley Hospital, and was asked by Aubrey Lewis to undertake continuing postgraduate training full-time of a group of 50 ex-service psychiatrists at St Ebba's Hospital, Epsom.. This was one of the most exciting and stimulating posts I have ever held. Teaching consisted of indi-vidually supervised clinical investigation and treatment of patients, the presenta-tion of patients at case conferences and daily seminars covering the whole field of psychiatry. The group greatly enjoyed the course, were highly motivated, worked very hard and were extremely diligent. It was a great success and I am still in touch with many members of that group, some of whom achieved high eminence and leading posts in the health service and academic institutions.

The next step in my 'career' was to go as deputy medical superintendent to Whitchurch Hospital. I enjoyed teaching undergraduate and postgraduate stu-dents and at the same time began research on schizophrenia and on the evalu-ation of treatments for it, including deep insulin therapy, electronarcosis, which was a new thing then, and electroconvulsive therapy.

Electronarcosis?

Yes. It was introduced at that time as a new method of treating schizophrenia and it consisted of bilateral application of the electrodes, which gave a contin-ual stimulation of the brain over a period of seven minutes. It was a bit fright-ening for the patient and for the rest of us, with lots of funny noises, stertorous breathing.

Did they actually have a fit?

Oh yes, but it was an inhibited fit. It came on right at the end. They were kept in a state of tonic contractions during most of the seven-minute period and then the clonic movements came at the end. It was not a very effective treat-ment for schizophrenia – no more effective than ECT. At that time deep insulin therapy seemed much better and I know the reason now. Research in this field needs a prospective, random allocation of patients by controlled methods. But at that time, the advocates of deep insulin therapy recommend-ed that patients should have a good previous personality, a shorter illness and acute-onset florid symtomatology, and these in fact were features indicative of a good prognosis anyway. Therefore, it was bound to be better than the results for other treatments. I published results controlling all these various factors in schizophrenia and matched groups by these means, and insulin achieved bet-ter results than ECT or electronarcosis, but the main reason for this still lay in the initial criteria for the use of insulin treatment.

What about Harold Bournes' article that questioned what was actually going on?

Yes. I had many discussions with him, and arguments. His views were empirically derived. Later at the Maudsley they did a prospective study, which threw doubt on the value of deep insulin therapy for schizophrenia. So insulin went out of favour.

How big a role do you think randomised controlled clinical trials has played in the development of the treatments we now use?

A major role really. I'll develop this in the context of talking about the early days in psychopharmacology. The beginning of the era was in 1952 when chlorpromazine was used in a French hospital called Valdegras. As you know, chlorpromazine was different from the previously available drugs treating psychiatric disorders. Anyway, from Valdegras its use spread throughout France and in 1955 Pichot, Jean Delay and Deniker held an international congress in Paris to discuss chlorpromazine and other neuroleptic medications. This was the first conference on chlorpromazine and other neuroleptic medications. This was the first conference on chlorpromazine and I had the honour of presenting three papers on it detailing three studies in which strict double-blind control methods had been used. Pichot showed a great interest in this methodology development, partly, it must be said, because he was interested in this British 'preoccupation' with double-blind clinical trials. It may be a little unfair but the French favoured a more 'impressionist' approach.

I had carried out a double-blind controlled trial in anxiety states in the first place because when I read about chlorpromazine and its actions it appeared that on pharmacological grounds it might be useful in treating anxiety states. I was working in south Wales at the time and I was running a number of outpatient clinics. It didn't take me long to get a hundred anxiety states. Colleagues in London were flabbergasted but it was different there because I had an unlimited supply of patients. So I carried out this double-blind control trial, and although it helped anxiety to some extent, its value was strictly limited because of the anticholinergic and hypotensive side-effects and also because people with executive or responsible positions had their anxiety relieved but it also eroded their enthusiasm and motivation.

Then I tried it out on asthmatic patients who had severe anxiety. These were patients that I collected from St David's Hospital. I was working there with DA Williams, a distinguished expert in allergies. I found that it helped the anxiety but it didn't help the asthmas very much and the dryness of the bronchi was a disadvantage. That was a double-blind randomised controlled trial. The third paper was a study on autonomic functions as a prognostic aid in the treatment of patients with chlorpromazine.

Not many people realised that this first international conference on chlorpromazine was in fact the beginning of the science of psychopharmacology. I think there were about 150 papers submitted. Mine were the only double-blind control studies. The next step was at the World Congress for Psychiatry in Zurich in 1957, where Nathan Kline organised one session in collaboration with Denber and others. This was the first time that the World Congress of Psychiatry had sessions devoted specifically to drug treatments. That then stimulated people to form an International College of Neuropsychopharmacology and its first meeting was held in Rome in 1958, where I presented a paper on a fully controlled trial of iproniazid in the treatment of depression. Since then the CINP has met every two years in different places.

I think my contribution to psychopharmacology is in the field of scientific controlled trials. I wrote a chapter in a book edited by Nathan Kline entitled *Factors in Depression* and there was an article in *Nature* in 1960, which gives you all the methods used in controlled trials at the time. The iproniazid trial, for instance, was a crossover trial.

How did that work, you'd cross people over from iproniazid to placebo?

That's right, yes, by random allocation of active drug and placebo and crossover.

It must have been pretty well the first trial on antidepressants in the UK?

It was, yes. Then I did the very first trial of phenelzine (Nardil) in the world with Brian Davies. Although these were severely depressed inpatients, the results were very good. But the dose we used was comparatively high. It was 90 mg a day, which was also the dose that both helped depression but suppressed REM sleep. In the Medical Research Council controlled trials on depression, unfortunately a dose of 45 mg was used.

I also did a trial on imipramine – not the first but an early one. Then it so happened that Brian Davies and I did the first trial of haloperidol in this country on mania and schizophrenia. It wasn't a fully controlled trial but it was the first trial. We also did the first trial on amitriptyline but the results were very disappointing which, I think, had to do with the severity of the depression we studied. A certain proportion improved but quite a lot of them didn't improve. I will come back to this point later. We later did a double-blind control trial with nortriptyline and that showed better results than placebo but not very dramatic. I did the first double-blind controlled trial of dothiepin with Maurice Lipsedge and a statistician and we then compared dothiepin to amitriptyline, which was a very interesting trial. Dothiepin came out better. Less side-effects than amitriptyline. Then I did another trial comparing the full daily dose of dothiepin at night compared with a divided dose during the day. Giving the full dose at night was as good as divided doses.

As a result of all these double-blind trials on tricyclics and monoamine oxidase inhibitors, we had an immense number of probands and a big number of first-degree relatives, so Michael Pare, Peter Sainsbury and I carried out a pharmacogenetic study. Taking the patients who had participated in double-blind trials as the index cases, we studied the development of depressive illness in the first-degree relatives and the outcome of their treatment. The results were very interesting. There was a high correlation between the results in this group and the first-degree relatives in the following ways. If the index case responded to monoamine oxidase inhibitors, the first-degree relative did so also. There was a similar response correlation with tricyclics. If they responded to both or neither, the same correlation held. This was a very clear-cut result. Jules Angst in Zurich and other people have carried out similar pharmacogenetic studies. So it seems there may be a genetic basis for responding to a particular group of antidepressants.

Another study was to carry out a sequential design trial on diazepam compared to amylobarbitone. The sequential method of studying became available only at that time. This gave a potentially quicker method of detecting differences between treatments. We also studied diazepam by a new method of assessing anticonvulsant therapy in relationship to convulsant therapy – with EEGs and a range of other measurements.

After that we were involved with the beta-blockers. In my department at St Bartholomew's Hospital the first trial of propranolol in anxiety states was carried out by Granville-Grossman, who worked with me, and Paul Turner. It was a double-blind controlled trial and this was the first trial to demonstrate that beta-blockers had a role to play in anxiety states. John Bonn did a similar trial with other beta-blockers, some of which have now been withdrawn because of the adverse side-effects.

Then we did another study comparing oxypertine with a placebo. That showed that oxypertine was an interesting drug. It's an indole derivative produced by scientists at Winthrop for the treatment of schizophrenia but it never became popular – there were so many other agents available. We used it in a trial for anxiety states and it was found to be better than diazepam. But when they promoted it for anxiety generally, the response was not favourable because people had been on diazepam. They were taken off diazepam and put on this and of course some of them then were suffering from withdrawal symptoms of various sorts.

Where did you get your interest in double-blind placebo-controlled trials from?

Well, looking back, Ralph Picken, the Professor of Preventive Medicine in Cardiff, taught us the pitfalls of uncontrolled trials. He was talking about controlled trials in hygiene and in treatment, when I was a student, and I think that's where the seed was sown. Before I did any work with chlorpromazine, when I came back to Cardiff after the war I did a number of controlled trials in schizophrenia, a lot of them with Dr King in Caerleon – evaluating treatments which the Americans had recommended such as cortisone in the treatment of schizophrenia. It was ineffective but somebody had to prove this. Desoxycorticosterone acetate was another one, as was hydrocortisone. So they required a double-blind trial. I think the very first one I did was a study on the substance betasymine in the treatment of anxiety. There were theoretical reasons why this could be helpful in depression or anxiety. So I organised a double-blind study but the results were totally negative. I think I should have published that, but people were reluctant to submit negative results. It's important to publish negative things but a lot of people don't want to waste time. That was one of the earliest trials.

That was when?

That was about 1950.

So these were pretty well the first placebo-controlled double-blind trials of any sort in psychiatry?

I think probably that's right. Yes, in psychiatry. Then the drugs came later. The comparisons of insulin, ECT and electronarcosis were not fully controlled studies but they were partly controlled because I managed to match groups for all prognostic and clinical features. What was missing was the initial randomisation of treatments. Anyway, it at least showed that electronarcosis was not effective. This paper was presented at a meeting of the RMPA, at which Spencer Patterson enthusiastically advocated electronarcosis. I gave my studies which contradicted these claims. The response to my paper was one of great interest. Most people there hadn't heard a paper given like this before in which all the prognostic factors were controlled and evaluated. I don't call that a properly controlled study but it had quite a big impact.

Did the industry help at all in terms of organising such studies?

The industry came on board for the phenelzine study. I told them how it should be done. I was ahead of them I think then. I don't think they were at all au fait with the principles involved. Later in some trials they helped by funding the salary of a research assistant.

Obviously when the first compounds were introduced, this didn't happen through double-blind methods. When do you think the industry got the message that they should be doing them?

Oh I think after the initial trials of chlorpromazine, iproniazid and so on. They realised that in order to get through the Committee for the Safety of Drugs and later the Safety of Medicines Committee – I was on both committees – results of double blind control trials became obligatory.

Let me put this to you – Roland Kuhn would say that the industry now spends billions of pounds on all these controlled trials, but they don't discover anything new; that, taking the impressionistic approach that he took, he was the one that discovered antidepressants and most other psychotropic drugs.

Well, that's all right. I think that the drugs are discovered by basic research, animal experiments and then from the profile that emerges – there is a feel for whether this drug is useful for depression, anxiety or schizophrenia. So, that's got to be true, but the only way you can prove it then is by proper controlled trials. Controlled trials only prove whether a compound is efficacious or not for a particular condition – they don't discover the compound. But even if new agents are discovered by other means they still have to be tested. There are different varieties of controlled trials but you cannot dispense with randomised double-blind trials.

Now, I think one fault with these double-blind controlled trials is the heterogeneity of clinical conditions. You see, they're all heterogeneous – schizophrenia, depression and anxiety – so that's why you allocate at random. What you're doing is expecting that unknown factors are equally distributed in the two groups. But you don't know. That's the best you can do really.

I have advocated many times, that what we still need is to be able to identify subgroups of depression, subgroups of schizophrenia, which are specifically susceptible to different treatments. I mentioned this to Aubrey Lewis in 1955. He agreed, but it still has not really been resolved. Once we are able to identify subgroups with specific susceptibility to particular treatments, much better results will be achieved. The same thing applies with neuroleptic drugs in treating schizophrenia.

Can I take you back to 1955? What was the mood as regards new drugs? What did people make of chlorpromazine?

Oh, I think people got quite excited. Because here was a drug which seemed to alleviate psychiatric symptoms without making patients fall asleep and from the basic sciences viewpoint it was interesting in that it had a wide range of novel pharmacological actions. Chlorpromazine enabled people to be discharged from hospital earlier and more frequently.

Now I don't think it was entirely due to chlorpromazine. I think there was a change in the composition of the patients going on at the time. A lot would have probably been discharged anyway. The therapeutic enthusiasm of the staff also undoubtedly contributed and chlorpromazine must take some credit for that.

Michael Shepherd's study published in 1956 seems to suggest that it was as much a question of changing patient–staff ratios as anything else?

Oh yes, but you see even then reserpine was available.

Yes, on that point, there's a paper by Davies and Shepherd, a prospective trial using reserpine to treat people who were anxious and depressed – showing that it was quite good.

Yes, this trial was carried out.

Which is all very odd given its reputation for causing people to get depressed.

Ah yes, but reserpine was really not suitable for a number of reasons – you do get a tranquil phase, due to the release of the biogenic amines, I suppose, but then there is a reactivation phase in which all the symptoms get exacerbated. It was very interesting. It occurs about a week or two after starting reserpine – if you're treating schizophrenia, all the symptoms can get worse before you get a resolution, but the other danger of course is severe depression – very severe, sometimes needing ECT. So I think there was a great deal of enthusiasm. And really the enthusiasm was something new and useful even though it was really not based on proper controlled trials.

Who were the key players in 1955?

Well, before that we shouldn't forget the work of Cade in 1948, who introduced lithium. But that really didn't shake the world at the time. It only became much more important when Mogens Schou found it to be of value in preventing recurrences of affective disorder. Anyway, to some extent it contributed, but only in retrospect. The other drug was lysergic acid (LSD), which was the most powerful drug available. It was active in minute doses, producing profound changes in perception, thinking, feeling and so on. Bradley in Birmingham did very important work on this. And then later Sanderson and a few people utilised lysergic acid to facilitate psychotherapy. So I think the three drugs which stimulated my main interests were lithium, chlorpromazine and lysergic acid, all in different ways. But the main boost to the start of the whole science of psychopharmacology was the use of chlorpromazine in France.

Did people at the 1955 meeting know that they were at the start of a new era?

I think so, yes. There was no doubt about the efficacy of chlorpromazine or about its wide range of pharmacological and clinical action – that's why they called it Largactil. So then attempts were made to find new phenothiazines with equal efficacy but greater safety in terms of side-effects and adverse reactions. A large number were then produced and I wrote an article for the *BMJ* on phenothiazines. Most of us just tried the whole lot of them in an ad hoc manner.

I was also asked to write an article for *Nature* on the use of drugs in the treatment of depression. That was a new idea at the time. For *Nature* to invite this article showed they were very perceptive. They could see in the treatment of depression the shape of a new era emerging.

This was when?

1960. The new antidepressants created a lot of enthusiasm because there were no useful drugs before the discovery of imipramine and iproniazid for depression.

It takes a particular kind of personality usually to get a field going – one thinks of a person like Nate Kline – he was obviously an enthusiast. Who were the other people in the field that you felt were the ones who were actually responsible for contributing a certain dynamism to what was happening?

I think Nathan Kline especially. He discovered or at least popularised reserpine and later discovered the antidepressant iproniazid. Heinz Lehman of Montreal was another one. Bradley certainly in his own specialised field, and of course Paul Jannsen, introduced lots of new drugs early on – haloperidol, droperidol, pimozide, and many others and he is still producing. But you're really talking about clinicians who contributed to the excitement.

What about Axelrod?

Well, Axelrod was a pioneer in basic research on monoamines. Kety was also important in the area of basic research and genetics. Biff Bunney was another – he was partly clinician, partly basic researcher. Then there was Derek Richter and his team who carried out important research on many fundamental areas relevant to psychiatry. More recently there have been people like Jules Angst and Julian Mendlewicz, who have both been very prominent in the areas of clinical, epidemiological and genetic research. Alec Coppen worked mainly on the electrolytes early on and later on antidepressants, and someone whom I mustn't forget is David Shaw.

Mogens Schou and his team were very important and they did very good research, but they more or less restricted themselves to lithium and its prophylactic actions. Another name I should mention is Stuart Montgomery. He's carried out a great deal of work in the field. Hans Hippius from Munich was also a leading figure. There was an Anglo-German symposium in London in 1956 and Hippius and I gave papers on psychotropic drugs, and that is where I met him for the first time. He is one of the people who discovered the efficacy of clozapine, now marketed as clozaril. He's been using it for years and he found it to be effective in schizophrenia and relatively free from extrapyramidal side-effects. I was on the Committee for the Safety of Medicines when we considered it and were put off by these reports from Finland – although this may have been a selected group of people who were genetically susceptible to agranulocytosis. One still has to pay attention to these things but under the special monitoring scheme they seem to be controlling it.

What weight would you put on the contribution of clinical people, basic scientists and the pharmaceutical industry to the way things have gone?

I think the pharmaceutical industry must take credit for the introduction of new compounds because they increasingly have to steer new drugs through complex and long and rigorous procedures – animal toxicity, human pharmacology and trials – before submission to the Committee for the Safety of Medicines or the FDA. Sometimes, 10 or 15 years of intensive work and expenditure go into development of a drug by the pharmaceutical industry. Now I think in the application of drugs, clinicians have played a much bigger role than the scientists, the biochemists, the pharmacologists, because they can do clinical trials and these provide essential information on efficacy, clinical applications, side-effects etc. On the other hand, scientists like Arvid Carlsson have been outstanding in actually discovering new types of compounds – zimelidine was a very good antidepressant; it was a pity it had to be withdrawn – but he was exceptional. He developed a lot of new things and he had also done a lot of relevant research on receptors and biogenic amines, so I think his contribution has been very important. Another person to mention in this regard is Paul Janssen. But apart from those two I would have to give most credit to the clinicians.

The operations of the CSM and the FDA now mean that drug companies have to come up with vast amounts of money in order to bring a drug to the market and because of that they are less inclined to look for unusual uses of a drug – they only want drugs for the larger conditions like schizophrenia and depression where they are guaranteed to get their money back. Do you think we've come to a point where perhaps because of the CSM and the FDA we're inhibiting the development of the field?

I think that drug development takes far too long, really. I think we could speed up the whole process. You see, once they've done the basic tests and trials I think then the Committee of Safety of Medicines should accelerate things and try to allow a new compound to go to a limited trial rather than hold it back until everything has been cleared. For instance, the new reversible monoamine oxidase inhibitor, moclobemide, was waiting for a terribly long time to be released. But having said that, there has got to be a regulatory machinery, otherwise all kinds of drugs would be brought to the market. It must be there for public safety.

It seems to me that for 10 or 20 years after the introduction of the first new drugs, there was great hope of progress and there was co-operation generally between all concerned in the enterprise. Things though have gone a bit sour of late partly perhaps because there aren't any truly new drugs, partly because the public has become more concerned with the risks of treatment. Have you any thoughts on whether the whole thing has gone sour, and if so why?

No, I do not consider that the situation has gone sour. Valuable and exciting new drugs are still being produced. The 5HT reuptake inhibitors were one such; risperidone is another, as is the resurrection of clozapine. But there is a public aspect to it. Nowadays when the public are given a drug they want to know is it safe, has it got any drawbacks or dangers? ... and of course they are entitled to know this. But they are tending to prefer alternative medicine, which they feel is much safer without knowing anything about its efficacy and safety.

Why do you suppose they prefer the alternative treatments? This is quite a mystery in a sense.

Yes, but I think many people are reluctant to take drugs. There's resistance even to take an aspirin and therefore when they read about adverse effects or the risks arising from drugs, they tend to go for herbal medicine or homeopathy, which is relatively speaking even safer than herbal medicines. Then of course, the teratogenic effects produced by thalidomide were disastrous. Because of that the Safety of Drugs Committee was formed.

When the Prince of Wales was made President of the BMA, he mentioned in his Presidential address that we as doctors don't own patients but yet we give them drugs without necessarily knowing how they work and we haven't given sufficient attention to the alternative methods of treatment. The BMA took this seriously and formed a working party on alternative therapy. I was a member of the working party, which met for four years. We interviewed representatives of all alternative methods of therapy, including acupuncturists, psychotherapists, hypnotherapists, reflexologists, all kinds of therapists. Anyway, we concluded that the attraction of alternative methods of treatment was the relationship between the therapist and the patient. They would listen to the patient – spend time with them – they'd touch them and they were sympathetic and they provided some symbol of treatment which the patient was willing to accept, but on analysing the evidence we concluded that there were only three methods of treatment which had any scientific basis of true value. One was osteopathy – of certain specific skeletal abnormalities; acupuncture because of its role in producing endorphins, and hypnotherapy, which is effective but which isn't really alternative medicine. The other therapies we felt were based on other factors, mainly to do with the interpersonal relationship – because the therapist was a nice person.

I think the other thing is that apart from the 5HT reuptake inhibitors, which have had an interesting development, freedom from the anticholinergic side-effect, no cardiotoxic effect and are effective, there have been as you say no other truly new compounds. Although there again, you see, with fluoxetine you get scares from America that people who take this commit suicide. I think what the American psychiatrists forgot about was people with severe depression are at suicidal risk and the greatest risk for putting this into action is when they start feeling better. And then there's another example recently. Somebody took a huge dose of fluoxetine and murdered someone. I think all of these reports can put people off.

Then of course were the embryonic effects produced by thalidomide – that was a frightener. Because of that the Safety of Medicines Committee was formed. But, I think the real reason is that we haven't really discovered entirely new effective and safe drugs. All current drugs have got certain disadvantages – side-effects and adverse reactions. I gave a lecture the other day on Executive Stress and Alcoholism. One physician got up and said what we need instead of alcohol is a drug which relieves our anxiety and stress, stimulates our brain and enables us to work better. I said, 'Yes, it'd be lovely if a drug could do all of those things' but will there ever be such a drug?

In Barts, between yourself, Michael Pare and your links with people like Merton Sandler, you were a very strong group of people.

I should have mentioned Merton earlier as a research person who has done an immense amount of work in the clinical field as well as in the lab. Then, of course, there was also Trevor Silverstone whom I should have mentioned; he also contributed a great deal, so much so that he was given the title of Professor of Human Psychopharmacology.

Was there any reason why the department you had there was so strong in this area? It was probably the strongest department in the country.

Well, my interest in psychotropic drucgs started in Wales before I came back to the Maudsley first of all in 1954. I joined Barts in 1958. I did a lot of the early trials in the Maudsley and the Bethlehem. So, I had a strong interest in all this and I suppose was fortunately joined by Michael Pare, Trevor Silverstone, John Bonn and Paul Turner later, all of whom had similar interests. I suppose the fact that Pare and I had been enthusiastic and keen on research into these drugs probably stimulated more general interest.

My links with Merton Sandler were first through Michael Pare and then later as a member of a research group called the Denghausen Group. This was founded by an American family that suffered from recurrent depression. Nathan Kline knew them and he suggested that they ought to finance a group of leading people doing research on depression to meet once a year to discuss their researches and to discuss the implications for practice and treatment. So the first meeting occurred in New York about 1958.

How large a group?

It was a small group then. It consisted of Nathan Kline, Heinz Lehman, Biff Bunney, Per Vestergard who worked in Nathan Kline's laboratory, Jose Delgardo who worked on animal experiments and myself – we were the first. The first meeting in New York was devoted to factors which determined cyclical activity and Curt Richter, who worked a lot on rhythms, attended the meeting.

After that we usually met in one of the Caribbean islands and later on Alec Coppen and Merton joined on my recommendation. Mogens Schou, Jules Angst and L Gjessing were also members. We used to meet at 8 o'clock in the morning in our bathing costumes with a blackboard underneath the coconut palms and then each one would present his work and results from the previous year. It was all informal, but we worked continuously from 8 in the morning to 1 o'clock and then had the rest of the day off. It was an ideal way of running a scientific meeting.

Talking about the BAP, is there any particular reason why you haven't been very involved with it?

I did join it. I was a member from the beginning and I think I was asked at one time whether I'd be prepared to stand for President, but at that time I was so busy with other commitments that I had to decline. Max Hamilton became the first President, which was an excellent choice.

These days it's all a question of time. The meetings are always held in July and in Cambridge and I'm always on holiday then. That's nothing against the Association; as a society I think the BAP is very good – it's purely in terms of the timing that I have problems. It's funny, when I was working before I retired I managed to find plenty of time to do research and teaching and go to conferences. But once I retired I found I didn't have time. It's very strange that, isn't it? But when you work at the university, you've got a big team, Nathan Kline, who was often away, was once asked who did his work when he was away and he said the same people who did it when he was there. There's a lot of truth in that.

What role do you think the BAP has had in this country?

Oh, I think it's had a very important role in fostering and encouraging proper scientific studies and presenting them in an acceptable and scientific way.

Where do you see it fitting in with the Royal College of Psychiatrists? Is there room for the two groups?

I think there is because there isn't really a proper biological psychiatry forum within the Royal College. There's a group for addiction and alcoholism and so on, but there isn't one specifically for psychopharmacology. So I think the BAP serves this purpose. Special interest groups are encouraged to develop by the college and if such groups grow and become well established they can be converted into sections of the college. There is, in my opinion, room for psychopharmacology to develop on these lines.

Before we finish, I'd like to bring you back to something you mentioned before we started the tape: your article that's buried in New York.

Yes, I was approached about one of my articles by the Academy of Sciences in New York as to whether I would be happy to have it included in a time capsule. This was buried in New York in 1965 and is to be opened five thousand years from then. As English is unlikely to be in use in 5000 years, they have converted the contents of the capsule into mathematical symbols. They have also copied the contents to various parts of the world, including the tops of mountains, in order to keep them safe from nuclear explosion, for instance. The capsule contains the work of Einstein, Churchill and others as well as a contraceptive pill, a polythene bag, a Beatles record and of course my article.

Select bibliography
Linford W, Healy D (1997). *History of Psychiatry*, **8**, 1–20.

9 Joel Elkes

Towards footings in a new science: psychopharmacology, receptors and the pharmacy within

Where were you born?

I was born on 12 November 1913, in Koenigsberg, East Prussia, Germany, just across the border from Lithuania, the country in which I grew up until I left it for England in 1931. My father, a native of Lithuania, had studied medicine in Koenigsberg and rose to become a leading physician in the, then, Lithuanian capital of Kovno, later known as Kaunas. My mother's family lived in Koenigsberg, hence my birth there. I should add that during the Holocaust my father was elected leader of his ghetto Kovno community, becoming a legend in his own time. He died in Dachau. Most members of my family, with the exception of my mother who survived the camps, my sister who was with me in London, and a few uncles and cousins who had escaped, were killed.

Perhaps I should say something about my early education and interests. I received a superb high school education in a new school, the Gymnassion Ivry, Kovno, founded by a group of young, dedicated, and exceptionally gifted teachers. All subjects, from Trigonometry to Voltaire, were taught in modern Hebrew. I was sent for a 'finishing' year across the border to a German school, which by that time, 1930, was becoming palpably Nazi. Then came another semester in Lausanne, Switzerland, where I gave full rein to my first love, atomic physics. Professor Perrier's lectures were an intellectual feast. I still recall the strange fascination exerted on me by cloud chamber photographs of particles colliding and separating on their mysterious ways. Perhaps it was then that I began to delve into particles – atoms, molecules, and the like. Having had only an elementary mathematical training proved to be decisive in my not following physics. I could only imagine and visually present to myself the subatomic and molecular dance. Most of it was sheer fantasy, yet this inclination to visualise has stayed with me all my life. To this day I see tiny channels opening and closing, molecules folding and unfolding, 'active groups' seeking out their niche. To put it another way, the good Lord appeared to be a Great Folder; an Origami Artist of sorts – all this being part of the economy of nature. Perhaps this inclination also accounts for my pursuing physical chemistry and immunology in my medical student days, and my drift into pharmacology later.

My father and I discussed my future. While not pressing, he asked me to think about medicine. There was a double pull there: the art of healing and the science – a Biology of Man in Health and Disease. For Healing, I had a fine role model at home; but for Science I had to look to physiology and an emerging biochemistry – a world that was still new in the early 1930s. We decided on England as a venue for my studies. One dark October evening in 1931 I arrived in London. The culture shock was enormous. I was accepted at St Mary's Hospital Medical School, supporting myself from my allowance and from tutoring. Later, I had to support my sister as well. Because of this, my training took much longer than the usual time. Things became particularly hard towards the end. I still recall the day when I had to pawn my precious microscope. But at St Mary's Hospital I had magnificent teachers. Alexander Fleming (penicillin) taught me bacteriology; and Sir Almroth Wright – pioneer of the typhus vaccine – taught me immunology. There were also clinicians in the great tradition represented in this country by William Osler. I recall particularly Charles Wilson, who served as Dean of the Medical School and later became Churchill's personal physician, better known as Lord Moran; and Aleck Bourne, senior gynaecologist, a brilliant teacher of the subject, and a seer of the shape of things to come in the transformation of health care services. He later became my father-in-law.

While a medical student I was apprenticed to my mentor, tutor, and dear friend Alastair Frazer, Reader in Physiology. He was later invited to found the Department of Pharmacology in Birmingham and I went with him to Birmingham, as a pharmacologist in 1942.

I had brought with me from my student days a deep interest in membrane structure, macromolecular interaction and stereochemical fit. I was interestingly enough much more attracted to immunology than to psychiatry. Psychiatry had a deep appeal but immunology seemed more precise. With my bent for visualising, I saw molecules interacting ...

The antibody–antigen locking fit?

Yes, precisely. I had started reading avidly Marrack's monograph and Paul Ehrlich's early papers. I had no training in physical chemistry – medicine, is a very poor preparation for chemistry – but I was fortunate enough to be apprenticed for one glorious summer in Cambridge to the Department of Colloid Science, where Eric Rideal was the Director. There I studied lipid–protein interactions, and was spreading monomolecular films on a Langmuir trough, and measuring zeta potentials.

I got recruited into research by Alastair Frazer. He was the nephew of the great anatomist Ernest Frazer, who taught Anatomy in St Mary's. He was a very fine physiologist. His field was fat absorption and he had a theory about the way in which the fat in the gut was emulsified and then absorbed in particulate form, to form the chylomicrons which appear, in great numbers, in the blood after a fatty meal. How does a particle like this survive in the blood? He asked me to begin a study on the surface coating of these particles, which had to be a lipoprotein. I invented a small micro-electrophoretic cell, on which we published while I was still a medical student. It had two gold leaf plates and you watched the migration of the particle under a dark-ground illumination. When we changed the pH, you could show quite clearly that the migration was charge-dependent. Then began an enquiry of what this coating consisted of, so we began to study the interaction between lipids and proteins and the formation of a lipoprotein coating, or membrane, and to develop models of its more precise structure.

So that's what sent me to Cambridge to study the whole idea of lipoprotein layers. In a Langmuir trough, you spread a polar lipid, a long-chain detergent, and inject a protein underneath. As the protein crowds into the membrane, you get a measurable shift in the lateral pressure exerted and a change in the zeta potential. I had no training in all this, but I had an avid interest. Sir Eric Rideal was a wonderful Director and left one very much alone. With him there was also a great physical chemist, Jack Shulman, who became very prominent in this field. We published a paper in the *Proceedings for the Royal Society* – two papers, as a medical student.

When did you become aware of the work of Francis Schmitt, who was also working on membrance structure?

I should back up before I answer this question. I came to Birmingham in the spring of 1942 to help Alastair Frazer to establish a department of pharmacology. My preoccupations from medical school followed. I was pulled equally to cell biology, particularly membrane physiology, as I was to psychiatry and scanned the horizon for some linkage between the two. But in those days, there were few bridges leading from cell biology to psychiatry; and it was not easy to convince university authorities that the subject – 'mental disease research' as it was known – was a worthwhile enterprise. With very few exceptions, the leading laboratories were small, not very well equipped, and usually functioned outside universities, being mostly supported by local hospital boards. Yet, in retrospect, I was most fortunate in Birmingham. Birmingham in those days was a vital, teeming university, very much engaged in the war effort. There was Randall, who pioneered radar. Rudolph Peierls one of the great figures of subatomic physics who later left for Los Alamos, only to return after the bomb had been detonated. Solly Zuckerman, later Lord Zuckerman, professor of anatomy – zoologist, planner, confidant of Lindemann, Churchill's principal science advisor and a power in the war establishment. There was Peter Medawar, zoologist – later to win the Nobel Prize for his work on the genetics of graft acceptance and rejection; Howarth, Nobel laureate in chemistry; and Lancelot Hogben, mathematician and essayist. In short, the company in the university refectory was always worthwhile, although the food was, at times, quite miserable. The other thing about the place was a magnificent comprehensiveness of the campus. Within 5–10 minutes, you could walk from the medical school at Queen Elizabeth Hospital to the Department of Physics, or Chemistry, or the Department of English, or the Barber Institute of Fine Arts.

In that university, Alastair Frazer and I were trying to establish a Department of Pharmacology. The department had four people when I began, and 40 when I left. I was teaching courses, including a course in hypnotics, analgesics, and anticonvulsants. My interests in psychiatry and chemistry of the brain were never far away. There were, though, only a few reference points in brain chemistry at the time – Page, Quastel, and Richter provided guide-posts. As for drugs used in mental illness, chloral hydrate, paraldehyde, bromine, barbiturates, and later the anticonvulsants reigned supreme. I still remember the pungent smell of paraldahyde as one walked through the wards. There was also, of course, insulin coma, and ECT. Dark days.

The great thing about Alastair Frazer was that he let me stray. I had worked on lipoproteins and their role in membrane structure, and suddenly realised that the nervous system was full of lipoprotein. It's name was myelin, so I strayed into the structure of myelin. It was at this time that I became aware of the work of Francis Schmitt. He was in St Louis at the time and sent me a beautiful set of reprints describing X-ray diffraction studies of dried myelin. The papers gave the exact dimensions of this ordered, lamellar structure. The question I posed to myself and my colleagues was whether X-ray diffraction of *living* myelin was possible. And there, I had one extraordinary stroke of luck. Bryan Finean walked into our lab as my first PhD student. The chemistry peo-ple told us that 'You can't do X-ray diffraction studies on a living structure.' Typically, though, Bryan said simply 'Let's give it a try.'

He developed his cell, which involved irrigating a tiny segment (about 3 mm) of frog sciatic nerve and shooting an X-ray beam through while altering the environment, through warming, through drying, through alcohol, ether and so on and seeing whether the X-ray diffraction picture had changed. This was, as far as I know, the first X-ray diffraction diagram of a living nerve . It showed up quite clearly the paracrystalline aspect of myelin structure which was very ordered and fell apart at certain stages of drying, when the water hold-ing the polar groups in place was removed.

I remember Finean and I, with our hearts in our mouth, going to see the great physicist JD Bernal. Bernal looked at these films and said, 'That's very interesting. Go on, just go on; this is worth doing.' Rideal by that time had become the Director of the Royal Institution so we had at our disposal the great X-ray tubes which Sir Lawrence Bragg had used for his famous crystallography studies. We had to cool the tube because we had a long exposure. I remember standing on a ladder putting ice around the tube to cool it sufficiently for the 15 minutes which we would need for exposure without the thing blowing. We got very good photographs, which we took to Alan Hodgkin. Hodgkin had not yet published his three great papers on nerve conduction. I remember him sit-ting there in the lab with a thermos and a sandwich looking at these pictures and saying, 'That's interesting. You should go on.'

That was all we needed – just a little encouragement. We were totally alien corn. We were neither in medicine, neurophysiology, nor physical chemistry, we just didn't belong anywhere. That was when I became really interested in the chemistry of the nervous system and started reading avidly what I could find about the action of CNS drugs. Dilantin had just come out.

Now why was that important? You refer to it often but don't really say why it was important.

Because from our studies, which I will come to in a moment, on catatonic schizophrenic stupor, which Charmian, my late wife had carried out, we had begun to regard schizophrenic stupor, and perhaps schizophrenia, as a state of hyperarousal. Hill and Pond had already begun to study the effects of the relationship between epilepsy and aggressive behaviour and we wondered whether an anticonvulsant could possibly reduce the state of arousal without impairing consciousness. But then we had a visit from Dr Thrower and we got Thorazine and began to work with it, rather than the anticonvulsants.

But let me just backtrack on the chemistry. The war had just begun. I was an alien, with a white card, curfew, the whole bit, and one day two men came to see Alastair Frazer, clearly on official business. They sequestered themselves for an hour with him. I was anxious. I was alone, I had to support a sister. The only protector I had was Alastair Frazer. He called me in and said these gentlemen had come to do a security clearance on me. They'd like us to work on cholinesterases, anticholinesterases, and antidotes against nerve gases, atropine and the like. So I began to attend meetings at Porton Down, the Chemical Defence Experimental Establishment, as one of a team. Later we had the good fortune of Archibald Todrick, formerly of the CDEE, joining us to take charge of these studies.

At this stage Quastel had gone to Canada, hadn't he?

Yes. Derek Richter succeeded him, I think. There was Weil-Malherbe at Runwell Hospital whom I invited later to join me at the Clinical Neuropharmacology Research Center in Washington. That was a very critical step not only for him but for the field because the conversations between Julie Axelrod and Hans Weil-Malherbe in our laboratory and at the NIH proved very productive for both.

Who was Hans Weil-Malherbe?

A Jewish refugee from Germany. He worked in a very modest laboratory at Runwell Mental Hospital. Hans was a very fine neurochemist. He worked particularly on amine, glucose and glutamine metabolism. An extraordinarily gifted but extraordinarily shy, retiring, self-effacing man, with the gentlest of smiles. Not appreciated at all; but mighty in his writings. We celebrated a 'Salut to Hans Weil-Malherbe' in Washington after I had moved to Hopkins. Julius Axelrod gave the celebratory address.

Perhaps I should digress at this stage and recall a crucial event in my early career – reading a sentence in a monograph by Henry Maudsley (1882). It read, 'It is interesting to notice that different nervous centres manifest elective affinities for particular poisons ... that medicinal substances do display these elective affinities is proof at any rate that there are important intimate differences in the constitution or composition of different nervous centres, notwithstanding that we are unable to detect the nature of these ... we may have, in the effect of poisons, a promise of a useful means of investigation into the constitution of the latter.'

I still recall the shock of recognition at this particular reading. For it spoke of pharmacology leading us to the source, to physiology. It shadowed out the regional differences which one suspected, even then, to be the chemical foot-prints of the brain's long, chemical evolution. The sentence gave one courage. Drugs could be tools, possibly connecting some ill-defined areas of the fledg-ling neuropsychiatry of the day. I remember looking at my hand. Five fingers, Five areas. *First* functional neuroanatomy, leading to the *second*, neurochem-istry, leading *third* into neurophysiology, leading *fourth* into animal behaviour, and animal behaviour bridging into *fifth*, the clinical experiment and a clinical trial. For the next few years in Birmingham, these overlapping, interacting areas assumed a life of their own in our little world, in the department of phar-macology. Slowly they became footings which guided us into an emerging new science in which we appeared to be engaged without quite knowing it. Let me give you a few glimpses of what it was like.

Take neurochemistry. No Beckman, no fraction collector, no radio-immunoassay in those days. So, you get the chilled brain, sit down patiently and dissect it into 13 regional samples, blowing on your freezing fingers as you go along. You grind up each sample with a substrate and incubate it in the Warburg machine. Then test the resulting eluate for neurotransmitter yield, usually acetylcholine, against the guinea-pig ilium. Slowly, slowly, you build up a regional map of a particular area. 'Elkes,' a senior colleague tells me, 'don't be a fool. Work on the heart, work on the gut, but get out of the brain. The brain is a sticky mess, and you'll come to a sticky end.' Indeed, David, these were precarious times. But area one soon led into area two. For, by an act of extreme good fortune, Philip Bradley walked into our lab and became my sec-ond PhD student.

Philip had been trained in zoology and had carried out micro-electrode studies in insects. He seemed interested in the problem and a salary was avail-able. By 1949, Philip was working alongside, developing his pioneering tech-nique for recording the electrical activity of the brain in the conscious animal; a procedure that in those days – the days of sulphonamide, not penicillin – was quite a trick. Using this technique, we started mapping the effects of drugs on the electrical activity of the brain – which, I say this without any undue humil-ity – proved classic studies of their kind. Results tumbled out day by day and night by night. Atropine, physostigmine, amphetamine, and later, LSD-25 all suggested powerful regional effects. About the same time, Morruzzi and Magoun published their ideas on the reticular activating system. They were beginning to talk about the waking brain and we about waking amines and families of neuroregulatory compounds, grouped around acetylcholine, nor-epinephrine, and serotonin, and later the synaptically active amino acids, particularly GABA. We began to talk of uneven regional distribution of families – and the operation of chemical fields in relation to consciousness and mood.

Allow me to quote from a paper in 1957: 'Perhaps rather than thinking in unitary terms, it may at this stage, be advisable to think in terms of the possible selection by chemical evolution of small families of closely related compounds, which by mutual interplay would govern the phenomena of excitation and inhibition in the central nervous system. Acetylcholine, noradrenaline and 5-hydroxytryptamine may be parent molecules of this kind; but one has only to compare the effects of acetylcholine with succinylcholine, or noradrenaline with its methylated congener to realise how profound the effects of even slight changes of molecular configuration can be. The astonishing use which chemical evolution has made of the steroids is but another example of the same economy. It is likely that neurones possessing slight but definite differences in enzyme constitution may be differentially susceptible to neurohumoral agents. Such neurones may be unevenly distributed in topographically close, or widely separated areas in the central nervous system; these differences probably extending to the finest level of histological organisation. Phylogenetically older parts, and perhaps, more particularly, the mid-line regions and the periventricular nuclei may, in terms of cell population and chemical constitution be significantly different from parts characteristic of late development. ... It would perhaps be permissible to speak of the operation of chemical fields in these regions, which would depend on the rate of liberation, diffusion and destruction of locally-produced neurohumoral agents. The agents in question may be either identical with or, more likely, derived from neuro-effector substances familiar to us at the periphery. Their number is probably small, but their influence upon integrative action of higher nervous activity may be profound. The basic states of consciousness may well be determined by variations in the local concentration of these agents.'

While these things were going on, we were directly propelled into the third area of animal behaviour. There we had the good fortune of meeting Michael Chance, who as an ethologist/pharmacologist was studying the effects of amphetamines in relation to the social field. He showed conclusively that the toxicity of amphetamines was related to crowding and introduced the strange new term – social pharmacology – into our vocabulary. We carried the goods into the Pharmacological Society. We got most peculiar looks.

But the best was yet to come. For, in a modest little clinical base in the local mental hospital, Winson Green Hospital, my late, beloved, former wife Charmian studied the effects of sodium amytal, amphetamine and mephenesin, in catatonic, schizophrenic stupor. I should add that we owed our entrée to Winson Green Hospital to a splendid, and most co-operative superintendent, Dr JJ O'Reilly, who really opened the door to us in a way which we never expected. At the time, catatonic schizophrenia was not uncommon in our hospitals. We were struck by the combination of mask-like rigidity, cyanosis of the limbs, and withdrawal. The syndrome then involved voluntary musculature, the autonomic system, facial expression, speech, attention and states of consciousness. Charmian suggested that we plan a study. When we proposed this to Dr JJ O'Reilly, he quickly agreed and remained a firm supporter and friend in the years to come. Dr O'Reilly put a small research room at our disposal and allowed us to choose patients, using criteria which we carefully worked out. He also gave us nursing help. Our aim was to study mental functioning in relation to muscle tone and autonomic function. Muscle tone was measured by a home-made gadget, a sling attached to a patient's wrist, going around a bicycle hub and leading to a pan into which weights were put. It took about three kilograms or so, as I recall, to change patients with extreme rigidity from full flexion to semi-extension. Temperature was measured by thermocouple and photographs of skin colour were also taken at the time. We gave the patients an opportunity to draw for ten minutes without prompting, under the influence of drugs, putting in front of them a drawing tablet and some coloured pencils. Also in the room was the steriliser and glass syringes – no butterfly cannulae in those days!

The effects of drugs were really striking. Sodium amytal administered in full hypnotic doses, which would send you and me to sleep, led to a paradoxical awakening of patients from catatonic stupor and a relaxation of muscle tone and a rise in foot temperature. The phenomenon was not unlike the awakening phenomenon in Oliver Sacks' film. The effect of amphetamine was equally paradoxical. It led to a deepening of the stupor, increased muscle rigidity, and deepening cyanosis. We also tried mephenesin, which had been shown by Frank Berger to be a powerful spinal internuncial, neuron blocking agent. When tested in catatonic stupor, mephenesin produced marked muscle relaxation. There was, however, little effect on psychomotor response, or overall temperature. The ability of patients to draw proved particularly interesting. Amytal in doses which would send you or me to sleep, markedly increased this ability while amphetamine inhibited it. The experiments thus suggested *selectivity* in the action of drugs on catatonic stupor and raised the question of the relation of hyperarousal to catatonic withdrawal and thus possibly to schizophrenia.

At that stage, the university became interested in the programme and asked us to name it. We called it a programme on 'Drugs and the Mind'. But, among ourselves, another term began to steal into our conversation. We began to talk of Experimental Psychiatry to remind us of the importance of the experiment in psychiatry and the continuity between the Lab and the Clinic. In 1950, while on a SmithKline Fellowship, and a Fulbright Grant, at Norwich State Hospital, Connecticut, I received a telegram informing me that I had been appointed Director of a newly created Department of Experimental Psychiatry in the University of Birmingham. As far as I knew, this was the first department to be so recognised. I owe this development entirely to three people – Alastair Frazer, my beloved mentor and friend; the Dean emeritus Sir Leonard Parsons; and Professor AP Thomson, then Dean of Medical Faculty. The new department was to comprise laboratories in Neurochemistry, Electrophysiology, Animal Behaviour, and though this happened later, a 44-bed Clinic set in the gorgeous grounds of the Cadbury chocolate family mansion – the Uffculme Clinic. For the first time, the university had given us, and the field, recognition. This department, devoted to what we would nowadays term psychopharmacology, was founded in 1951, some years before the discovery of the role of Thorazine in the treatment of mental illness.

So why did the university take the step? Was it that the authorities were particularly enlightened or were you particularly persuasive, or was it some combination of both?

Yes, as you say, a bit of both. I attribute it clearly to the people I mentioned. It is also fair to say, I suppose, that I had an instinct. I thought that the drugs we were working with, and the drugs still to come, could be tools of great precision and power depending on whether one was lucky to find one or two overriding properties. It is this precision pharmacology in the central nervous system that made me hope for and take up my stance in the face of many raised eyebrows which I encountered, not only in the Physiological Society, but in psychiatric circles where I was regarded as a maverick, newcomer, and curiosity. More important was the idea that families of neuroregulatory compounds had arisen in the brain in the course of chemical evolution that were chemically related to the powerful neurohumoral agents familiar to us at the periphery. At that time there were only three or four parent molecules, the cholinesters, the catecholamines, and the indoles. Implicit in this concept of families of compounds was the concept of small local, regional, chemical fields and above all, the *inter*action and *inter*dependence between molecules governing, modulating, gating storage and flow in self-exciting nerve loops. I had read Sherrington at the time and had absorbed many of his key concepts. He regarded reciprocal inhibition as an agent of structure in the nervous system. I had modified these ideas somewhat in various papers. The concept of families of compounds derived and evolved from a respective common chemical root governing the physiology of the brain and by implication the chemistry of awareness, perception, and affect now was a steady part of my thinking as we worked away in Birmingham. To the best of my knowledge, this represents an early formulation of these ideas. It gives me special satisfaction to reflect on Philip Bradley's illustrious career and the influence he's exerted on the course of neuropsychopharmacology in Europe and the world.

At one point you looked like you were going to say that while you earned your spurs in science, your role has been to come up with ideas ...

Yes, I suppose, this is a fair assessment. However, I can honestly say my passion in this field has been to try and develop talent as well as giving some ideas to work in. I tried to be a good gardener – create environments in which people flourished. Sometimes this required greenhouses. In those days, the glass was fragile.

Let me ask you about that because that's clear from some of your contributions to meetings that were put together by Derek Richter and others in the 1950s. In the UK at the time you were mixing with people like Dale and Feldberg and Marthe Vogt. Now as late as

1960, Arvid Carlsson was saying that he came to a meeting in the Ciba Foundation in London, while they had all the evidence on the drugs and he was able to show depletions of neurotransmitters etc., Dale and Gaddum and all of the other big names did not accept what was happening.

Let me refer you to another Ciba Symposium Foundation which I attended in 1957. The title of my paper was 'Drug effects in relation to receptor specificity in the brain: some evidence and provisional formulation'. It speaks of families of neuroregulatory compounds and the uneven distribution of receptors in the brain. I got approval from some, including Wilder Penfield and Geoffrey Harris, but there were quite a few raised eyebrows, too.

Why should this have been the case? Was it because the power of the neurophysiological paradigm was so dominant?

I suppose the partial answer lay in the enormous success of neurophysiology. But, neurophysiology had not yet confronted behaviour. The only exception was the great Wilhelm Feldberg whom I admired from the time I first met him. With Sherwood he developed an intraventricular cannula and was studying the effects on cat behaviour of direct injection of acetylcholine and allied substances into the ventricle. It was he who with Marthe Vogt in a classical paper in 1948 showed that there were areas in the brain which were relatively low in the enzyme concerned with the synthesis and destruction of acetylcholine. This paper had a profound impact on me because I had already begun to think of families of neuroregulatory compounds and implicated norepinephrine and, later, serotonin. Marthe Vogt in a later paper demonstrated the regional distribution of norepinephrine which coincided very well with the distribution of the Magoun and Morruzzi reticular activating systems and with Philip Bradley's and my own ideas on the neuropharmacology of arousal and the effects of amphetamine. Extraordinary exciting times!

Can I put it to you that perhaps the reason you were able to see this was because along with people like Brodie and Axelrod you weren't a neurophysiologist? Because you hadn't been trained in that discipline, it became feasible to see what the physiologists couldn't see.

This is possible. I was an outsider. Some of the theories and some of the assumptions, especially the more rigid assumptions, made no sense at all to me. Possibly, I was clumsily and crudely intruding into a cherished terrain. However, fairly early I defined the criteria for the presence of a naturally occurring, neurohumoral transmitter in the brain. These were presence of the agents, presence of enzyme systems for synthesis and destruction, the demonstrable effects of specific inhibition and the physiological effects on behaviour of a hypothetical agent. I felt from the beginning that drugs acted by interaction between naturally occurring substances binding selectively to receptors or displacing in some way naturally occurring substances. Hence, the title of my paper in the Ciba Symposium of 1957 and a paper at a Macy Symposium in the same year. Drugs interacted with naturally occurring substances and thus affected behaviour.

How did this relate to chlorpromazine?

Thank you for an important question. I suppose the dates are quite significant here. Our programme on 'Drugs and the Mind' was established in the late 1940s and the new Department of Experimental Psychiatry, devoted totally to the study of the effects of drugs on mental function and behaviour was established in the summer of 1951. This was some years before the discovery of effects of the first major chemical tranquiliser.

I should, perhaps, now backtrack a little. At about this time, another pivotal event took place. A small unit, 'Mental Disease Research', loosely administered from the dean's office, became available and fell under the aegis of the Department of Pharmacology through the retirement of it's director, Dr AP Pickford. I was put in charge of two rooms in the medical school. There were also some seed monies. An enormous step in my life had been taken, and I knew that I was in biological psychiatry for good. I began to prepare myself avidly, reading, attending psychiatric meetings in London, and seeing patients at a local mental hospital, Winson Green, to familiarise myself with the drug treatments then available and with the syndromes. I had some excellent role models in the dedicated staff at the hospital. I confess, despite administering ECT and the trinity of drugs that we used, troubling questions beckoned everywhere. I felt like a naturalist advancing into a strange continent. I was deeply moved by the patients' histories, as I interviewed them and by what I saw and heard in the ward, and over lunch. I found myself discussing my bewilderment with Charmian, who was in general practice at the time. We talked into the night, pulled by the same curiosity, and concern. One day, after a meeting in London, I believe it was the first Anglo-French post-war meeting which Jean Delay attended, catatonic stupor was discussed, which at that time, we saw all around us and as I've mentioned we were intrigued by.

Now I must bring us back to our encounter with chlorpromazine. I remember the critical meeting very well. Sometime in late 1952, or early 1953, I honestly do not remember which, there walked into my office Dr WR Thrower, Medical Director of Messrs May & Baker. He carefully unlocked his briefcase and presented me with the early reports by Delay and Deniker of the effect of a new drug, chlorpromazine. He told me that May & Baker had acquired the British rights from Rhône-Poulenc. They had a supply in their safe and could make up the necessary placebo, and active tablets. Would we care to perform a blind, controlled trial? Being very impressed by Delay and Deniker's path-breaking studies, I said, 'Yes, we certainly would,' and suggested that we do so at Winson Green Hospital. Again, I asked Charmian whether she would be interested. Quiet pioneer that she was, she said she would, and assumed full responsibility for the management of what has proved to be, I think, a rather important lesson to us all in clinical psychopharmacology. For, as I think back on it, all the difficulties, all the opportunities, all the unpredictable qualities of conducting a trial in a mental hospital were to show up clearly and to be dealt with clearly in that early trial. This included the selection of patients – we decided to err on the heavy side and chose some

194 The Psychopharmacologists II

grossly overactive and disturbed patients – the preparation of the ward, the training of personnel, the gullibility of us all, the so-called halo effect, the importance of the careful use of words and terms, of training attendants, patients themselves and relatives as informants, the use of simple rating scales and calibration of such scales. All these elements came into their own once Charmian, and to a much lesser extent, I, were faced with the realities of working in a chronic mental hospital ward, a reality we had already been exposed to through our catatonia study.

I still remember the morning when we all trooped into the boardroom of the hospital, spread the data on a large oak table, and broke the code after the ratings of effects and the side-effects had been tabulated. The trial involved 27 patients chosen for gross agitation, overactivity, and psychotic behaviour. Eleven were affective disorders, 13 were schizophrenic and three senile. The design was blind and self-controlled; a drug and placebo being alternated three times at six week intervals. The dose was relatively low – 250–300 mg a day. We kept the criteria of improvement conservative, which was reflected in our discussion. Yet, there was no doubt of the results, after the code had been broken and the results tabulated. Seven patients showed marked improvement, 11, slight improvement, and there was no effect on nine patients. The side-effects of chlorpromazine in those early days were significant and astutely observed by Charmian. We published a short paper, which conclusively proved the value of chlorpromazine in overactive states. It was a blind and self-controlled trial but to us it was also a statement of the opportunities offered by mental work of this kind.

Please allow me to quote again. 'Perhaps we may be allowed to draw attention to one last point – namely, the lessons we feel we have learned from the trial itself. The research instrument in a trial of this sort being a group of people, and its conduct being inseparable from the individual use of words, we were impressed by the necessity for a 'blind' and self-controlled design and independent multiple documentation. Furthermore, we were equally impressed by the false picture apt to be conveyed if undue reliance was placed on interview alone, as conducted in the clinic room. The patient's behavior in the ward was apt to be very different. For that reason the day and night nursing staff became indispensable and valued members of the observers' team. We were warmed and encouraged by the energy and care with which they did what was requested of them, provided this was clearly and simply set out at the beginning. A chronic 'back' ward thus became a rather interesting place to work in. There may well be a case for training senior nursing staff in elementary research method and in medical documentation. This would make for increased interest, increased attention to, and respect for detail, and the availability of a fund of information, all too often lost because it has not been asked for.'

I recently had occasion to attend a meeting in my old haunts in Birmingham, and I sat in the room at the same oak table. It was a poignant moment.

Were you aware of any of the other trials that were happening at the same time? Schou did something very similar. Double-blind placebo control with a crossover design with lithium, which started in 1952 and published in 1954, and Linford Rees had done some trials with cortisone in 1951/52 but they hadn't shown that it worked. He did a chlorpromazine trial in 1954 which was published in 1955 and Michael Shepherd had begun a trial on reserpine in 1953 that was published in 1955.

No, I was not aware of those trials.

It seems that a few people came to the idea of this control design around the same time. It's curious how these things happen.

Yes, synchronicity and coincidence. But as far as we know, we acted independently.

Were there any other influences? The idea of a placebo had been around with Harry Gold and the double-blind idea was also there, but putting it all together, what influenced you? Had you been influenced by the 1948 streptomycin trial?

No, I was not aware of the streptomycin trial. It simply seemed an obvious way to go. The only person I spoke to when we were well into the trial was Lance Hogben, who, with Myre Sim, was engaged in a theoretical thinkpiece on the subject. After our paper came out, Aubrey Lewis was very encouraging. I was examining at the time for the DPM at Maudsley and remember attending a lecture by Michael Shepherd, before he had become the shining light in psychosomatics. But people were busy with their own things.

I should backtrack a little because there were many other stirrings in the woods at the same time. I started to commute to the States pretty regularly, visiting colleagues, companies, and comparing notes as things were shaping. One such visit had great consequences. I believe it took place in 1952 or early 1953. Seymour Kety, by that time Director of the Intramural Program for the National Institute of Mental Health, Heinrich Waelsch, Professor of Neurochemistry at Columbia, Jordi Folch, Director of the McLean Hospital Laboratories at Harvard, Lou Flexner, Chairman of Anatomy at the University of Pennsylvania, and I met to discuss the need for and the possibility of an International Symposium on Neurochemistry. In England, I got in touch with Derek Richter and Geoffrey Harris, who later was to emerge as a father of modern neuroendocrinology. The joint hope of our committee was to organise an International Neurochemical Symposium, the first of its kind. As the theme of the symposium, we chose 'The Biochemistry of the Developing Nervous System'. As a place to hold it, we chose Magdalen College, Oxford. I was charged with being the organising secretary but could not have done so without the help of my British colleagues. The symposium took place in the summer of 1954. 69 colleagues from nine countries participated. It was a fine symposium, and it may very well be, though I am not sure of this, that at this symposium the term 'Neurochemistry' was used officially for the first time. Heinrich Waelsch and I wrote the foreword to the *Proceedings*.

A second symposium on 'The Metabolism of the Nervous System' was held in Aarhus, Denmark, in 1956. The *Proceedings* were edited by D. Richter. A third, on the 'Chemical Pathology of the Nervous System,' followed in Strasbourg, France, in 1958. The proceedings were edited by Jordi Folch. The fourth international symposium, where Seymour Kety and I introduced the term Regional Neurochemistry, as a formal title for the first time, was held in Varenna, Italy, in 1960. It is hard to convey the excitement and productivity that attended these meetings. Functional cellular neuroanatomy was leading into neurochemistry and neurochemistry was being related to electrophysiology and electrophysiology to animal behaviour, particularly in relation to arousal and the reward system of Jim Olds. Joe Brady and Peter Dews brought an application of behavioural analysis to the study of drug effects and drug metabolism was being related to behaviour. There was a steady refinement of the clinical trial. In a word, things began to connect. This was also borne out by the WHO study group in 1957, which I convened and of which I wrote the report. The report carried the first classification of psychoactive drugs by Eric Jacobsen.

Actually I should backtrack again and say a little more about the new department. As I mentioned, it was founded in 1951 – the Uffculme Clinic came a little later. I invited William Mayer-Gross, co-author with Martin Roth of the leading textbook of psychiatry in Britain, to serve as Director of Clinical Services; and John Harrington of the Maudsley to head up the Uffculme Clinic. It was a marvellous setting. There was a small Ethology Laboratory in the coach houses in the gardens, where Michael Chance did his work on 'social pharmacology'. A little later, we had a small space built for the department by the Queen Elizabeth Hospital and some labs in the medical school, so that in a way the department extended from the laboratory to the clinic. All in embryonic form, but somehow the shape of it all seemed right. It was a Department of Psychiatry where we tried to maintain context and continuity between the laboratory and the clinic. It was, I suppose, this sense of continuity which later on attracted the Rockefeller Foundation, who gave us a very considerable grant, and the NIMH who invited me to come to Washington to establish a similar unit on a larger scale at St Elizabeth's Hospital.

Can I ask you about that, because what you've elaborated is a different vision to Francis Schmitt's vision. Schmitt is often credited these days as being the founder of the idea of neuroscience and it seems to me that he had a key role but in a non-clinical neuroscience. You began in very much the same area but seem to have moved in a very different direction.

Francis Schmitt was a giant and saw much further than what he wrote. His ultimate hope was that neuroscience would serve people and ever since his students have been carrying that banner. But, yes, I was more interested in function, illness and well-being . I was deeply influenced by Sherrington and his seminal volumes on reciprocal inhibition in the nervous system. Also I am very much a people's person. I always felt that if we are to help people, we must work in context. We must provide an environment where there is continuous conversation, and that is how the idea of the Department of

Experimental Psychiatry arose. Experimental psychiatry is clinical or it is nothing.

Why did SmithKline & French give you a fellowship, because this was before they got involved with chlorpromazine or anything to do with psychiatry?

They visited me in 1949/50. I still remember Dr Ted Wallace's kindly face. They thought, I suppose, there was a future in the field. Don't forget, SmithKline & French made money on Dexamyl, Amytal and Dexedrine, for which Ed Fellows was responsible. So they had moved around in this area before chlorpromazine. They gave me a Fellowship and when I got a Fullbright Grant I went to Bellevue first, where I met Sam Wortis, then to the New England Center, Boston, where I worked with John Nemiah and later to Norwich State Hospital because I wanted to see an American State hospital from within. They found that they couldn't employ me because I was an alien; so they gave me the lowest assignation, an intern. So on the roster by the Superintendent's officer there was this list of 20 staff and right at the bottom, 'Intern, J Elkes'. Then, one day, I got a telegram from the University of Birmingham, which I mentioned. I went to the Superintendent and I said, 'Look, Dr Kettle' – showing him this telegram. He slapped his knees and said, 'My God, that's the fastest promotion I've ever known.'

I suppose it was the principle of maintaining continuity between the laboratory and the clinic which moved me to accept the invitation of Seymour Kety and Robert Cohen in 1955 to join the NIMH. Robert Cohen was Clinical Director and Seymour Kety was Director of Intramural Research. They invited me to come over in the spring of 1955. From Birmingham and our little office in Winson Green Hospital, I suddenly found myself in Building 10 of the NIH campus, the proposed site of what at that time was termed the Laboratory of Clinical Science. In the laboratory there was Julius Axelrod, Ed Evarts, and many other young people who have since become famous. I remember listening with fascination to Robert Butler, then quite a young man, speaking of the need of the elderly. He is now, I suppose, the senior gerontologist in the United States and his book on the subject won a Pulitzer Prize. David Shakow, the great psychologist, spoke of set and vigilance in schizophrenia. He was right next door. A few doors away, later on, was Paul McLean, father of the limbic system. I was totally overwhelmed by the talent and by the opportunity; but I had a difficulty. By that time, the Medical Research Council in Great Britain had been very good to our unit and the Rockefeller Foundation had made us a large grant, one of the largest grants in Europe. Dr Maier of the Rockefeller Foundation came over and told me he would like to support our unit because 'we think it could be another centre like Penfield's Center in Montreal – we're investing in him and we're investing in you.' I felt that I could not really leave at this time. A terrible conflict was churning inside. I lay awake at night, wondering whether I was foregoing a tremendous opportunity. I felt, however, that England had been very good to me and so I said 'No.'

A year later, Seymour called me up and said, 'Joel, we've offered you the best job we have at the NIMH. In fact, it's so good that I'm resigning from my Directorship of Intramural Research to become the Chief of the Laboratory of Clinical Science, which we offered you.' Their laboratory was where Kety and Sokoloff expanded their famous work on cerebral circulation and Julie Axelrod began his pathbreaking studies. Seymour Kety then invited me back again, but this time we thought about things and decided to do it differently. Let us put the labs where the patients are, rather than bringing the patients into the labs for special studies. In fact, I remember, thinking how good it would be to have laboratories in a mental hospital environment where every worker – no matter how esoteric their field – was exposed to the realities of psychiatry and the needs of psychiatry in a mental hospital setting. So we started to develop what was later to become the Clinical Neuropharmacology Center, now the Center for NeuroScience.

Dr Winfred Overholser, Superintendent, proved extraordinarily co-operative and offered us a huge building, the William A White Building, as a site for our centre. I remember one day – it must have been in the spring of 1957 – standing in front of that vast edifice, awed by the sheer size of the building and wondering how best to accommodate neurochemistry, electrophysiology, animal behaviour, and clinical studies into the building. The logistics were fairly simple. The labs below, human studies above, and patients between and all around us. Seymour Kety sent me the catalogues to Birmingham, because they had to be included in the same year's budget. So there I was designing labs in Washington while I was still in my job in Birmingham. However, the key was not space, or equipment, or even number of positions, but people and communication. How, we asked ourselves, could people, colleagues, best live the interdisciplinary nature of our field? We were used to working in teams. How could we train a new kind of psychiatrist who was superb in the lab and who would also listen? How could we put a team into a single head? I don't quite know how it happened, but happen it did, both in the Intramural Program in Bethesda under Bob Cohen and Seymour Kety's leadership and in our satellite centre at St Elizabeth Hospital, and for that matter, later at Hopkins.

One of the first people to arrive to run the experimental Lab was Nino Salmoiraghi from Montreal, who had worked on the physiology of respiratory neurons and who later, soon after his arrival, recruited Floyd Bloom. Both later succeeded me, and Floyd Bloom is now Editor-in-Chief of Science, one of the most influential posts in science in the world. Hans Weil-Malherbe accompanied me from England and set up his neurochemistry lab. Conversations, and, later work, began both with Julius Axelrod and Steve Brodie. Steve Szara joined me from Hungary; and as the years flew by, in a flurry of activity, colleagues came from all over the place to work with us. It was a wonderful time. Before long Fritz Freyhan joined us from Delaware to assume a post as Director of Clinical Studies. Paul Wender came, Posner and Shepherd Kellam, now Head of Mental Hygiene, at the Hopkins School of Public Health. Max Hamilton wrote some introductory lectures on research and psychiatry and gave them to a very attentive small group. Others came, too numerous to mention. I still remember clearly Nino Salmoiraghi and Floyd Bloom showing me the pulling of the new five-barrel micropipette with which they mapped the chemical susceptibility of the neurons in the hippocampus, proving again the extraordinary, uneven distribution of certain types of neurons in special regions. I remember, for that matter, Fritz Freyhan sharing with me the early issues of his 'Comprehensive Psychiatry' and I clearly remember Max Hamilton pounding RIGOUR and research methodology into frightened residents.

There were weekly seminars for which people prepared and rehearsed like for a big public event – wonderful discussions and enormous productivity. I was particularly moved when I saw developing cooperation between Steve Szara, a neurochemist working on psychoactive indoles, and Herb Posner, who had been trained in Skinnerian reinforcement techniques. There was also Herb Weiner, who ran a fine lab and developed some studies on operant conditioning in man, and there was a star colleague, Richard Chase, who developed a really outstanding lab on what he termed Neurocommunication – an area which he then carried forward after he accompanied me to Johns Hopkins.

The invitation from Johns Hopkins came, after a visit by a Search Committee for the chair vacated by Seymour Kety who had been there for a year and was returning to NIH. I went through quite familiar pangs. I had just settled down in Washington at the centre and was very reluctant to move. Charmian had established herself in private practice and we both loved Washington. One element which I missed, however, were students. I loved to teach and get young minds involved in our subject. I was also thrown into conflict because I was being considered for a Fellowship at the Salk Institute at La Jolla. When I got back from La Jolla, I found a letter from the President of Johns Hopkins, Dr Milton Eisenhower, formally inviting me to Hopkins. With a heavy heart, I called up Jonas Salk and told him I would go to Hopkins next spring. He was very gracious about it. We have been very good friends ever since. He asked me a little later to suggest names and organise the first Symposium on the Neurosciences at the Salk Institute, which was still held in the temporary buildings in, I believe, 1964. It was a good meeting and I felt that I had played a little part in bringing neurosciences to the Salk.

At Hopkins I moved, again, into an older building. The famous Phipps Clinic founded by Adolf Meyer in 1913 had seen many illustrious men and women pass through it. I felt on hallowed ground when I moved into Adolf Meyer's, later John Whitehorn's and Seymour Kety's old office. Next to it was Adolf Meyer's old library, where I spent many happy hours. In the building, too, there were, on the third floor, Dr Curt Richter's laboratories where he did his classical work on biological clocks. I found it fascinating that the labs were across the hallway from the wards. Curt was meticulous in the hygiene of his animals – they were in some ways looked after as well as very special patients. Also, in the basement, there was Horsley Gantt, the only American pupil of Pavlov, who ran a Pavlovian laboratory in the very same institute. Both had been recruited by

Adolf Meyer, who was a living legend. He coined the term psychobiology, which was the subject of his Salmon lectures, published posthumously. Another valuable colleague was Jerome Frank, author of the classic *Persuasion and Healing* anticipating, by decades, literature which appeared later. There was John Money, a national figure in research on sexual function and dysfunction, a New Zealander with a sharp wit and an extraordinary grasp of his subject, ranging from genetics to neuroendocrinology. Quite a group.

The best part, however, was the student body, and the residents. We changed the name of the department to 'Psychiatry and Behavioral Science'. We introduced a course on Behavioral Science in Relation to Psychiatry. The course was significant because, along with myself, the chiefs of Obstetrics and Gynecology, Pediatrics and senior members of the Department of Medicine and Surgery participated in it, bringing out the significance of psychiatry, not only as a speciality, but as a very important component in the practice of medicine. When the chiefs of their respective departments were involved, the students listened. And then came some labs in a new building, and I had the great good fortune of an extraordinary array of colleagues joining us. I still can't quite grasp the good fortune when I think back. Dr Ross Baldessarini, Joseph Brady, Lino Covi, Joe Coyle, Len Derogatis, Richard Hall, Nelson Hendler, Dennis Murphy, Candace Pert, Elliott Richelson, Solomon Snyder, Nathan Spinner, Joe Stephens, Daniel Von Kammen, Bill Webb, 'Uhli' Uhlenluth, Herbert Weingartner, and many others. Sol Snyder is now Distinguished Service Professor and Head of the Laboratories of Neuroscience at Johns Hopkins. Joe Coyle is Chairman at Harvard. Ross Baldessarini, Director of the Mailman laboratories at McLean, Elliot Richelson, Director of a major enterprise at the Mayo clinic. We celebrated the 25th anniversary of the ACNP under the presidency of 'Uhli' Uhlenhuth.

I could say the three major developments began to take shape in my time at Johns Hopkins. Sol Snyder established his group in Neuropharmacology from a laboratory initially jointly supported by our department and the Department of Pharmacology under Dr Paul Talalay, Chairman of Pharmacology and a true friend, who showed a real understanding of the emerging new field of psychopharmacology. I might say this was quite unusual at the time among departments of pharmacology. It is a matter of deep joy and satisfaction to have watched Sol Snyder's group grow to the world leadership it now occupies. Joe Brady, who joined us from Walter Reed, brought us another important component. As a clinical psychologist with a Skinnerian background, he developed behaviour analysis and operant conditioning as a major research approach to the study of the effects of drugs on behaviour. Bringing his great originality and boldness of approach into the clinical area, he rapidly created at Johns Hopkins the Division of Behavioral Biology and Behavioral Medicine, foreseeing clearly the shape of things to come. At the same time, 'Uhli' Uhlenhuth and later Len Derogatis established much of the technology for quantitative clinical trials in an outpatient setting. We also revived an old interest in the use of anticonvulsants, particularly Dilantin, in anxiety and depression. We maintained close contact with Al Kurland and Stan Grof's group in the Maryland State Psychiatric Institute. Stan Grof was, what Roland Fisher later called, a 'cartographer of inner space'. I felt that equal insights could be gained by studying states of sensory deprivation, and allied states of extreme relaxation. As you know, he has written nearly a dozen books and has produced some experimental evidence of Jungian concepts. His concentration on holotropic breathing came much later after he'd gone to California.

At Hopkins, we tried, as I said earlier, to breed a new kind of experimental psychiatrist who was also a sensitive clinician. We tried to be trans-disciplinary rather than multi-disciplinary, breed a fine experimentalist who would also listen. I tried to set the tone. I was always there on grand grounds, and summarized the discussion. I looked around to see who was there; they knew if they were not around, they would be asked why. Slowly a conversation developed. I outlined these concepts in a memorandum for the Search Committee before I accepted the job. The message was well received and understood by the administration.

You've touched on a huge range of things, but can I take you back to Jean Delay? What was he like?

He was a very cultured man. A savant in the French sense, an author. He wrote impeccable French and was a great friend of Andre Gide. When he spoke one had the sense of deep culture. Deniker was magnificent in his fiery, practical activism – in a sense a complementary counterpart. I was on several committees with Deniker and Pichot in the WHO study group etc.

On the thorny issue of who actually started the CINP, Philip Bradley suggests that Ernst Rothlin came to Birmingham before the CINP started and that even at that stage he had the idea for a CINP. This is interesting because others had the impression that Rothlin at the start was against the idea of the CINP.

Yes, I can attest to that. In the Spring of 1955, or 1956, I cannot remember which, Ernst Rothlin and Mrs Rothlin paid us a leisurely three day visit in Birmingham. Rothlin delivered a fine seminar at the Uffculme Clinic and I confess, I was heartened by his comments on our trans-disciplinary enterprise. I was quite impressed by his scholarship. The conversation ranged from his compatriot, Carl Gustav Jung to Goethe and Pavlov. It was a fine time to take stock and to attempt to look into the future. During these conversations, in which Charmian, Philip Bradley, Willi Mayer-Gross and I participated, two broad ideas kept surfacing. One was the need for an International Forum to discuss and serve the advances in our emerging field. The other was the need for an international journal. I do not rightly recall whether the Latin name of Collegium was used in our discussion, but the need for an organization certainly kept on recurring. As for the journal, preliminary work had already been done. Willi Mayer-Gross had been in touch with Richard Jung of Munich and Springer, the publishers, had been approached and appeared interested. Further discussions involved Jean Delay, Pierre Deniker and Pichot in Paris and most importantly Abe Wikler. It took quite a number of telephone calls and letters to persuade Abe to assume the co-editorship of this new journal. I served on the Editorial Board, and still recall the excitement when the first slim, yellow issue of *Psychopharmacologia* landed on my desk.

Can I pick up on Fritz Freyhan?

He was Director of Research at Delaware State Hospital and I invited him to join us about two years after I had arrived at the NIMH St Elizabeth Center. He was slight in stature, always immaculately dressed, cultured, given to a lovely dry sense of humour and benign and gentle irony. A pleasure to be with. He had a view of psychiatry very much akin to my own which was reflected in the title of his journal, *Comprehensive Psychiatry*. He was deeply surprised, when I invited him out of the blue to come to Washington. I confess, I was a little concerned, because I did not know how he would get used to the ways and politics of Washington. He was methodical, clear, and became a most articulate advocate of psycho-social factors in relation to drug effects and of the need for social rehabilitation as part of pharmacotherapy. He wrote on that extensively. The American informal ways did not come easy to him; but inside, he was a warm and deeply caring person. We had at the same time, at least partially overlapping, with him, Drs Horden and Lofft, so clinical care for our patients was in good hands.

Fritz played a significant part in early CINP meetings. He was clearly one of the people who was thinking about the field and the implications of drug treatment for theories of psychopathology. But he died early – what from?

Yes, that is so. He died of a heart attack. I do not remember his age. He was in his second marriage, which was a very good one. Charmian and I saw a lot of them in Washington. I cannot really tell you much about him except the pleasure I had of drawing on his philosophical streak. He was very well read, particularly German literature, and often quoted Jaspers to me. He was very encouraging to me personally in another respect. When I came to write a paper on 'Schizophrenia in relation to levels of neural organisation and information processing in the brain', I could have no better oracle than to test it against Fritz. He wrote me an extraordinarily warm and encouraging letter after he'd read it. In that paper, I elaborated on the role of regionally organized chemical control mechanisms in relation to information processing in the brain. I mention the possible role of dopamine, norepinephrine and serotonin and the role of the thalamus, corpus striatum and hippocampus in the organisation of information-in-time whether it be applied to perception, ordered movement, or thought. It was a good synthesis and I liked having his OK on these rather, at the time, far-fetched theories.

What about Willy Mayer-Gross?

Willy Mayer-Gross was a wonderful man. He had been Director of Research at Crichton Royal Hospital, Dumfries, and was on the point of retiring. We spoke at the same symposium, and we got quite chatty. I asked him, 'Would you care to consider having a quiet corner in Brimingham?' 'Yes, I might think about it,' he said. A few days later, I called him up and said, 'Dr Mayer Gross, I have the money together, will you come?' 'Yes, I will' he said. And so, Willy Mayer-Gross and his dear wife Carola, who was non-Jewish, arrived in Birmingham. It was a tremendous difference to have him around. Compact in stature, muscular, vigorous, with a strong walk and strong gestures, he radiated 'joie de vivre'. His face was quite remarkable. It was dominated by a massive forehead, a large Hebraic nose and wonderful eyes, always with a twinkle, peering at you through large gold spectacles. The conversation was always lively. He was a tremendous phenomenologist. He was also a very sensitive man, insightful into the nuances of interpersonal relationships and very much a supporter of psychotherapy. His book with Martin Roth was at that time the standard textbook of psychiatry in Great Britain. Willy was a tremendous support to me, a young head of a very young department, feeling his way into the unknown. I remember particularly, when after a disappointing committee meeting, I would retire to my room, dejected, wondering what to do next. There would be a knock, the door would open slowly, and there peering through would be an enourmous nose mounted by gold-rimmed spectacles and eyes twinkling with good humour. 'Ach' he would say, 'Don't take it serious!' – 'Ach – nimm es nicht ernst.' I wrote at his behest a major chapter for Jung's *International Handbook of Psychiatry* where in nearly one hundred pages and 500 references I summarised my view of the status and future of psychopharmacology. It contained a good many of my views, but did not get wide circulation because it was sequestered in a volume mainly familiar on the continent. I regard that paper as one of the hardest papers I've ever written, and also one of the most comprehensive. It covers, I think, a fairly good view of psychopharmacology as seen at that time. It was in part modelled on the WHO study group report, which I had also written some years before. I passed both these papers to Willie for his approval. It meant a great deal to me.

Willy stayed there after you left?

He stayed behind and died in Birmingham. As I said, he was a refugee and his wife was Catholic. They were going back to Heidelberg, where he had a house and his wife's whole family were still living. He was packing to go when he had a massive heart attack. He is buried in Birmingham. When I was there some three years ago, I spent an hour looking for his grave in the Jewish cemetery, but could not find it. He really was a very special person, one as we say in Hebrew 'of blessed memory'.

Another person early on was Abe Wikler, who seems to have been very important in the early years but who has been written out of the history. What was his role?

Thank you for bringing up the great Abe Wikler. I pay a tribute to him in all the invited lectures that I give. To my mind, he was a central figure. 'Written out of history' is a very good term, for he belongs right squarely in the middle of the beginnings of psychopharmacology. When he spoke of the relations between pharmacology and psychiatry, he had a sense, a prescient vision of psychopharmacology. I still remember a letter he wrote to me, after a chapter in which I wrote on the 'Study of regional processes' in the brain and of 'synaptically active amino acids'. His work on addiction and dependence was a model of rigour and clarity, seen from the vantage point of someone working at the bench and in the clinic. He saw ahead, long before most of us. Maybe I am attributing something to him because I liked him so much, but the 'Relation of pharmacology to psychiatry' was a landmark. He had great vision and definitely belongs in the early history of our field.

What about the 1956 Conference on the Evaluation of Psychotropic Drugs?

Let me back up a little before I answer this question. In 1953 Hudson Hoagland organised an important interdisciplinary symposium at the Battelle Institute in Ohio, at which we began to talk of, among other things, social setting in relation to drug effects – socio-pharmacology and other new conepts. Both academia and industry were represented at that meeting. In 1954, a Symposium of Neuropharmacology initiated by Harold Abramson brought a number of us together and at that symposium I talked of some of Bradley's and my own work and also reported Charmian's work on catatonic schizophrenia stupor and touched upon the work with LSD. The Macy Symposia in Neuropharmacology were tremendous meetings of the time, building the footings of a new science. Then came the meeting in 1956 under the joint chairmanship of Jonathan Cole and Ralph Gerard, which proved to be, in my mind, a milestone conference in psychopharmacology. It was held under the aegis of the National Research Council, the National Academy of Science, and the American Psychiatric Association, and I believe was instrumental in bringing together the most active people in the field in the United States at the time. It was soon thereafter that the Psychopharmacology Service Center was created – a step of enormous consequence in the future development of our field. I looked recently at the *Proceedings*. I remember it was a very big meeting. I was there even though I had not yet moved to the States at the time. I regard it as a crucial meeting because for the first time tools of evaluation were emerging. What was a dimly lit landscape gradually acquired topology.

One of the odd things about the meeting is that none of the key organisers – Kety, Brady, Gerard, Lasagna – were psychiatrists, which seems extraordinary.

Yes, I suppose it seems odd, but in a sense quite natural. Seymour Kety and Ralph Gerard were physiologists. Brady was a pupil of Skinner, a behavioural scientist and a senior pharmacologist; so was Lasagna. All, however, had a common interest in the brain and were approaching psychiatry from the scientific base of their own discipline, including myself. Psychiatry had not yet begun to train the kind of person who was to lead the field later on. Some psychiatrists were eager to know more, and enthusiastic about developments – I mean psychiatrists like Heinz Lehman, Nate Kline, and others. Please recall that the predominant model in American psychiatry was the psychoanalytic model. Some enlightened psychoanalysts, among whom I could count Karl Menninger, who later came to see me, were deeply interested, eager to learn. Others were stand-offish. The new wave was led by newcomers outside the field.

Also internationally, official bodies began to stir. Late in 1956, the Mental Health Section of WHO, of which Dr Kvapf was Head, invited me to think about a study group on ataractic hallucinogenic agents in psychiatry. I compiled a list by phoning around and taking advice including input from WHO, which was indeed comprehensive in its representation. There was Ludwig von Bertalanffy who represented systems theory, Bovet, later a Nobel Laureate to represent pharmacology, Erik Jacobsen from Denmark, also a pharmacologist, Morton Kramer, who represented epidemiology and statistics, TA Lambo from Nigeria, later to become Deputy Director of WHO and a student of mine in pharmacology in Birmingham, who represented transcultural psychiatry, Erik Lindemann of Harvard who represented psychiatry, Pierre Pichot who represented quantitative psychopathology working with Jean Delay, David Rioch who represented neurosciences, RA Sandison, England, who we thought we should include because of his work on the possible therapeutic effects of LSD, PB Schneider from Switzerland, a clinical pharmacologist, and myself as rapporteur. I wrote the 1958 report, which incidentally carried Erik Jacobsen's pioneer classification of the main drugs according to their pharmacological properties. In the meantime, the scientific commands of the US Air Force through a Colonel James Henry had catalysed important work in the neurosciences in several European laboratories. Through these meetings the importance of brain research became steadily more apparent. And another thing I may recall here, after preliminary meetings, 1958–1960, a number of us met at UNESCO House in Paris to draft the statutes and by-laws of the International Brain Research organization (IBRO). The disciplines of neuroanatomy, neurochemistry, neuroendocrinology, neuropharmacology, neurophysiology, behavioural science, neurocommunication and biophysics were represented. Daniel Bovet and I represented neuropharmacology on the first central council of IBRO. In short there was quite a context of events between 1954 and 1960. The meetings fed into each other, and, of course, laid the foundations for what happened in the CINP and ACNP.

I recall a very moving letter I received after I wrote the first working paper for the WHO report. It came from Dr Wolff, head of the section of Addiction at the time. It simply said that 'your paper (and I'm paraphrasing) sent my heart beating faster which was not very good for me'. Six months later, I was in Geneva to chair the meeting. I wanted to thank him personally, but he was quite ill. I insisted and was taken to his flat where he was drifting in and out of coma with an oxygen mask on his face – a memory which will never leave me.

Can I take you to the foundation of ACNP?

For more detailed history, I refer you to the accounts available through the ACNP but it was sometime in 1960 when some of us, convened by our beloved and gentle Ted Rothman, began to discuss the idea in earnest. Ted Rothman is really the originator of the idea and it is very important that credit be given to him. On 12–13 November 1960, a conference for the advancement of neuropsychopharmacology was held at the Barbizon Plaza Hotel in New York City, organised by the convening secretary, Dr Ted Rothman, under the chairmanship of Paul Hoch. The main purpose of the conference was to stimulate critical discussion and to suggest proposals for the advancement of neuropsychopharmacology. There were about 20 participants present – amongst them I recall, Ted Rothman, Paul Hoch, Heinz Lehmann, Paul Feldman, Jonathan Cole, Bernard Brodie, Abe Hoffer, Eugene Chaffey, Joe Tobin, Arnold Scheibal, James Ferguson and myself. The most important outgrowth of this was a recommendation for a committee to organise an American College of Psychopharmacology. Ted Rothman was elected chairman of that committee, with a key role being played by Frank Ayd, Bernard Brodie, Jonathan Cole, Paul Feldman and Paul Hoch. The committee met on numerous occasions.

Plans were laid for an organisational meeting of interested individuals for the creation of the college. The draft constitution and by-laws were formulated and steps taken to form a non-profit, scientific, research corporation in the state of Maryland to be known as the American College of Neuropsychopharmacology. These preparations led ultimately to the first organisational meeting of the college which was held in Washington DC at the Woodner Hotel on 7 and 8 October 1961. Ninety participating members at the meeting recommended that the multi-disciplinary group of 123 be accorded temporary Charter Fellowship. A credentials committee was set up to approve the final membership and report to the members at the next meeting. During this meeting I moderated a symposium on the contribution of basic science to neuropsychopharmacology, Fritz Freyhan moderated a symposium on the contributions of the clinician to the science of neuropsychopharmacology and Jonathan Cole spoke on the current programme of the Psychopharmacology Center in NIMH. The participating members represented 22 States and two Canadian provinces. They approved the constitution and by-laws of the college. All disciplines immediately concerned with neuropsychopharmacology including pharmacology, psychiatry, psychology, neurophysiology, and biochemistry were represented at that meeting. It was during this meeting that the Assembly elected as President elect Paul Hoch, Claus Unna as Vice-President, Ted Rothman as Secretary/Treasurer and Milton Greenblatt as Assistant Secretary/Treasurer. They did me the immense honour of electing me their first President. Council members elected were Frank Ayd, Bernard Brodie, Jonathan Cole, Heinz Lehmann, James Toman, and Joseph Zubin.

In keeping with its mandate from its first organisational meeting, Council proceeded to structure the college by way of various committees. We also, during my tenure, created the Study Groups. Some of the early topics chosen were on 'Individual variation in the metabolism of psychoactive drugs', 'The analysis of the effect of drugs on the electrical activity of the brain', 'Individual animal differences in drug responses: determining factors, social factors and individual expectation in relation to drug responses in man', 'Advantages and limitations of the controlled clinical trial in psychopharmacological investigations', 'The effects of drugs on communication processes in man, with special reference to problems of verbal behaviour', 'The pharmacology of memory and of learning' and 'The toxicity of psychoactive drugs'.

Why did they pick you?

You must ask them. I suppose it was in part because I had negotiated some of the initial difficulties in establishing psychopharmacology as a discipline in my own life. Also because I was heading up a rather large centre that was becoming internationally known, which comprised within its walls the footings of our new science: neuroanatomy, neurochemistry, neurophysiology, animal behaviour and the clinical trial. I had advocated this comprehensive approach to psychopharmacology and again and again had spoken of context and training a new kind of psychiatrist. I said we must train people who listen as they do and doers who listen. But, you must ask the people who elected me why they elected me. All I can say is that it is the deepest honour I've had in my life. When the Joel Elkes International Awards were created by ACNP and laboratories were named after me at Hopkins, this was, so-to-speak, the frosting on the cake.

There was a fork in the road around the late 1950s or early 1960s. LSD or that kind of compound were much more experimental psychiatric compounds, whereas chlorpromazine was for therapeutics. We've gone down the therapeutic road it seems to me to the neglect of an experimental approach. Would you agree?

Yes, I would agree up to a point, though I confess that experimental psychiatry means to me more than the study of a chemically induced experience in the laboratory. The mode of action of chlorpromazine and reserpine were slowly elucidated by studying their interaction with dopamine and norepinephrine. No, there should be a continuum between the lab and the clinic. The term 'experimental' here simply suggests for me an attitude to psychiatry, a sort of robust scepticism which would account for the usual and the unusual effects which one sees in the clinic. The experimental study of long-term after-effects of the phenothiazines is a case in point. Much of it emerged from the clinic, but also from long-term experiments in the laboratory. We now understand tardive dyskinesia much better because of the supporting experimental evidence.

But I might perhaps digress a little, into a field which has become very close to my heart – the whole area of the behaviourally silent, deeply subjective experiment and experience. I have been preoccupied with these from my youth, thinking as I did at the time of the origins of the poetic imagination. I read a good deal of Goethe, and various authors of the late 19th century who were preoccupied with this area. I was bowled over by reading Williams James' *The Nature of Religious Experience*. I mention this because it bears on a lecture which I gave, I believe in 1961 – a Harvey lecture, which I regard as quite an important piece of mine. The origins of this lecture were as follows. One day I had a visit from the chairman of the Harvey Lecture selection committee, Dr Richards, a Nobel Laureate. This lecture was held in the New York Academy of Science. He invited me to give a lecture for the following year and asked me to speak, of course, on psychopharmacology. I sat down, starting to write this lecture, and was about to churn out the usual stuff about our work; but suddenly the idea of complexity of the non-verbal, deeply subjective experience hit me and also the difficulty of expressing or conveying or actively sharing this profound non-verbal experience. I suppose this harks back to my interest as a medical student in meditation and intensive states of concentration. I switched the subject and talked about 'Subjective and objective observation in psychiatry', examining among others the function of language in science, especially in physics, and the need for new languages for accurate description of the biology and the metamorphoses of the inner life. The lecture was a very formal affair. Somebody had forgotten to tell me that you were to come attired in a dinner jacket. I arrived in the august halls of the New York Academy of Science to be met by the reception clerk, who told me that 'There's a room in which you can change, sir.' I asked him what he meant. 'Well, sir, I suppose you have your dinner jacket.' 'No, I do not.' So there I was, in a business suit, sitting among the august society delivering my lecture. My audience was comprised of some of the crowned heads of psychiatry and neurology. My closing argument was that it 'seemed advisable to give early thought to the development of an adequate symbolic system for the exploration of these very rapid subjective processes and to relate these whenever possible to existing instruments in psychological sciences'. I also said that the creation of such new systems would require long-term planning within small groups; it would require highly trained observers and highly trained subjects capable of self-observation, to whom unfamiliar phenomena become familiar through practice as maps are to seasoned travellers, and who are capable of developing operational definitions of states experienced and observed. Such an endeavour, which I called at the time, Inner Space Laboratories, could be engaged in the training of a species of 'intronaut'. They would require close co-operation between psychiatrists, psychologists, linguists, mathematicians and communication engineers. It may require training in more than one discipline to ensure a more direct personal contact with a phenomenon. It would require, I said, much debate and much crude trial and error and it would require money, which I thought at the time that Congress could regard as a wise investment. The history of science suggests that, once a beginning is made, progress can be quite rapid.

I mention this because this interest in subjective phenomena harks back to my youth, to my medical student days, and is very much with me now. My introductory lectures in the behavioural sciences course were always on these subjective phenomena and centred on the writings of Jung and William James. They performed a useful counterpart to the empiricism of the course which followed. I've always felt that students had a laboratory 'within' and that the day could be an experiment. Training in awareness was very much needed. It took some 30 years before an attempt to develop this approach could be pursued in Louisville. I mention it, simply to round out the picture. One had to go through personal analysis to gain full respect for these phenomena. But the average student can acquire a great deal of personal knowledge by some quite simple exercises practised every day which incorporate awareness into daily life. This is not psychopharmacology but it really leads me to a subject which preoccupies me greatly: 'the pharmacy within'.

I believe that the drugs which we have and the generations of drugs that will follow them will give us much deeper insights into how the body manages its own health and healing without the chemical prostheses which we are using at present. For all drugs, as we know now, interact with naturally occurring neuroregulatory substances. The neuroregulatory families of old have grown from three to about 60 or 70 members. They play an enormous role in the regularities of mental life – thought, behaviour, mood and subjective experience. We know a good many of them already. The danger is that we may again, in a typical way, overdo it, 'attack' from without, ignoring the enormous healing powers which reside in the body – what Norman Cousins and I and the late Brendan O'Reagan used to call the 'inner mechanisms of healing'. About those we know very little. But the enormous advances in neuropharmacology, neuroimmunology and neuroendocrinology suggest an astonishing economy in the way nature uses certain ancient key families of neuroregulatory compounds which have emerged in evolution again and again and about which we will hear much more in the next decade. It would be very surprising if the agents promoting wound healing and tissue repair in the body were not very similar to the agents which turn up in the brain and help us in the healing of the mind. I still remember the excitement I experienced when I read the draft manuscript of Candace Pert's and Sol Snyder's first paper on endorphins. Also, I would say, that in the events we are studying now, which revolve around a chemical and electrophsyiological model, we're missing something quite important. I believe that what we regard as fast events are a very slow readout of much faster events which take place in the central nervous system at a quantum level. Quantum biology and modern genetics will have their day in psychopharmacology; and it is then that it will become a much more comprehensive and precise science than it has been hitherto.

Well, this comes back to the point I was making, which is that psychiatry has seemed to become reduced to therapeutics only which, while it is of crucial importance, can't sustain the whole enterprise.

Yes, psychiatry is still looking over its shoulder, anxious to be counted as a medical science. In fact it is in a position to lead rather than to follow. In terms of its clinical use it is a speciality but in terms of theory it is a generality. Where in medicine do you find an area as broad, as deep, as rich as ours? Modern psychiatry ranges from molecular, and I believe submolecular, biology to the subtleties of subjective experience, thought and behaviour, into psycholingusitics, social psychology and anthropology. A very cultured human being can go on learning psychiatry to the end of their days and still remain ignorant of the vastness of our enterprise. It is the quintessential science of man and it belongs in the very heart of medicine and should be taught as such. It is this comprehending comprehensiveness which is psychopharmaology's great gift to contemporary medicine. Medicine still does not know quite what to do with this gift, but gradually it will dawn on medicine what it has in psychopharmacology. Our humanity will follow us to the deepest recesses of our molecular search. That is the beauty of our field and that is why I feel so lucky to be in it.

When I retired from Hopkins, in 1972–73, I went to my little house in Sarasota, Florida, sat for awhile and got bored. I then got an invitation to come for a few months as McLaughlin Visiting Professor to McMaster University Medical School, of which I'd heard a great deal, and where a former Chief Resident of mine, Nahum Spinner, was a member of the staff. I came and gave a talk and liked the atmosphere very much – I thought I'd get them interested in behavioural medicine. I might add that McMaster is one of the most inventive medical schools in the world. Lately copied by Harvard, it advocated self-directed learning and a mixing-in of clinical exposure with the earliest days in medical school. I loved it. I functioned as a tutor – all the education is done in small groups. I drew the attention of the head of the department, Dr Nate Epstein and later the late Dr Jock Cleghorn – a wonderful and supportive friend – to the prospects of behavioural medicine in psychiatry. It was well received, and having come for only six months, I found myself staying for five years and am now an Emeritus from that university.

At McMaster, I also followed another interest. You will recall my interest in immunology in my school days. Psychoimmunology was being pioneered from George Solomon's laboratory at Stanford and Bob Ader's work in nearby Rochester. I gave a seminar on the emerging area of psychoimmunology. I confess it was received with some scepticism. But I am glad to say these things are changing now. I mentioned earlier my preoccupation with the healing powers and biology of the states of relaxation: those profound anabolic events about the chemistry of which we know so little. We created a small and rather secret society of about seven of us, residents and a few members of the staff, particularly Tony Bellissimo, who has since written a very good book on behavioural medicine. We met privately to teach each other meditation. We called our secret little group the 'Inlookers'. I was reading avidly on the physiology of the relaxation response, which was about that time. When I spoke to people with similar interests I got warm responses but from my own brethren I got a familiar, glazed look.

I then left Canada to return to Sarasota, but somewhere along the way I got an invitation to give a lecture in Louisville. I gave my lecture looking forward to a nice respite in the evening; but I found that the President of the university James Greer Miller, and the Chair of the department, John Schwab, had other plans. In my lecture, I had thrown out the idea of a small, preliminary course – a sort of self-inoculation for students in processes of personal awareness and self-care. The President asked me whether I would care to carry it out in Louisville. Again, I said I'd stay for six months. I was there for 11 years and with an exceptional dean of students, Dr Leah Dickstein, began our now very well-known programme on health awareness for medical students. The programme is voluntary and lasts for a week before student registration. Year after year, 92% of the students or more attend this exercise, which teaches subjects like psychobiology of stress, relaxation, nutrition, exercise, listening skills, spouse troubles and the value of the arts as a very effective tool in self-repair and enhancing self-awareness. It partly didactic but largely experiential, very much like the course I tried to introduce at Hopkins in 1963. So again, there is a return, and the message about the 'inner pharmacy' which belongs in the practice of the good life – one day at a time.

More recently I had the great privilege of being invited as Senior Scholar-in-Residence to the Fetzer Institute. This is a remarkable institute in Kalamazoo, Michigan, conceived by a visionary electrical engineer, John Fetzer, who, among other things, was senior communications officer for the US Army in World War II. He established an industrial empire of radio and TV stations in Michigan. He had deep insights concerning the function of electromagnetic fields in the organisation of life processes. He inspired the themes of the institute, now directed by Robert Lehman. The themes lie in the areas of health, education and self-care, the place of electromagnetic fields in living processes and the study of states of consciousness. All these activities are permeated by a deep spirituality. I feel privileged with other guests to share Mr Fetzer's old house. So here again there is a sort of closing of a cycle – a return. The pharmacology without leading to the 'pharmacy within'. As new generations of drugs of immense precision and power emerge our ethical dilemma will be as deep as any we have encountered. Are we ready for it? I do not know whether we are.

Joel, you very strikingly call people to meet in a place that most of them are only dimly aware of and challenge them in ways they don't associate with psychopharmacology. You have been doing this for a long time. Your address at the foundation of ACNP in 1963, which I would like to end with, is a marvellous statement of this vision.

'In looking back over its short history from that early meeting at the Barbizon-Plaza to the present day, it is hard not to be encouraged by the vigor and variety of programs developing within our small association. It is not uncommon for any one of us to be told that Psychopharmacology is not a science, and that it would do well to emulate the precision of older and more established disciplines. Such statements betray a lack of understanding for the special demands made by Psychopharmacology upon the fields which compound it. For my own part, I draw comfort and firm conviction from the history of our subject, and the history of our group. For I know of no other branch of science which, like a good plough on a spring day, has tilled as many areas of Neurobiology. To have, in a mere decade, questioned the concepts of synaptic transmission in the central nervous system; to have emphasized compartmentalization and regionalization of chemical process in the unit cell, and in the brain; to have focused on the interaction of hormone and chemical process within the brain; to have given us tools for the study of the chemical basis of learning and temporary connection formation; to have emphasized the dependence of pharmacological response on its situational and social setting; to have compelled a hard look at the semantics of psychiatric diagnosis, description and communication; to have resuscitated that oldest of old remedies, the placebo response, for careful scrutiny; to have provided potential methods for the study of language in relation to the functional state of the brain; and to have encouraged the Biochemist, Physiologist, Psychologist, Clinician, and the Mathematician and Communication Engineer to join forces at bench level, is no mean achievement for a young science. That a chemical text should carry the imprint of experience, and partake in its growth, in no way invalidates study of the symbols, and the rules among symbols, which keep us going, changing, evolving, and human. Thus, though moving cautiously, Psychopharmacology is still protesting; yet, in so doing, it is, for the first time, compelling the physical and chemical sciences to look behavior in the face, and thus enriching both these sciences and behavior. If there be discomfiture in this encounter, it is hardly surprising; for it is in this discomfiture that there may well lie the germ of a new science.'

Select bibliography

Bradley PB (1953). A technique for recording electrical activity of the brain in the conscious animal. *Electroencephalography and Clinical Neurophysiology*, **5**, 451.

Bradley PB, Elkes J (1957). The effects of some drugs on the electrical activity of the brain. *Brain*, **80**, 77–117.

Elkes J, Finean JB (1953). X-ray diffraction studies on the effect of temperature on the structure of myelin in the sciatic nerve of the frog. *Experimental Cell Research*, **4**, 69.

Elkes J, Elkes C (1954). Effects of chlorpromazine on the behavior of chronically overactive psychotic patients. *British Medical Journal*, **ii**, 560.

Elkes J (1957). Some effects of psychotomimetic drugs. In *Neuropharmacology*, Transactions of the Third Conference of Josiah Macy Jr Foundation, New York, pp. 205–294.

Elkes J (1958). Drug effects in relation to receptor specificity within the brain: Some evidence and provisional formulation. In *Ciba Foundation Symposium on the Neurological Basis of Behaviour* (G Wolstenholme, ed). Churchill, London, pp 303–332.

Elkes J (rapporteur) (1958). *Ataractic and Hallucinogenic Drugs in Psychiatry*. WHO Tech Rep Series 152, World Health Organization, Geneva.

Elkes J (1961). Schizophrenic disorder in relation to levels of neural organisation. In *Chemical Pathology of the Nervous System* (J Folch-Pi, ed). Pergamon Press, Oxford, pp 648–665.

Elkes J (1962). *Subjective and Objective Observations in Psychiatry*. The Harvey Lectures, Academic Press, New York, pp 63–92.

Elkes J (1967). Behavioral pharmacology in relation to psychiatry. In *Psychiatrie der Gegenwart* (HW Gruhle, R Jung, W Mayer-Gross, M Muller, eds). Springer, Berlin, pp 931–1038.

Elkes J (1995). Psychopharmacology: Finding one's way. *Neuropsychopharmacology*, **12**, 93–111.

Elkes J (1970). On beginning in a new science. In *Discoveries in Biological Psychiatry* (FJ Ayd, B Blackwell, eds). Lippincott, Philadelphia.

Feldberg W, Vogt M (1948). Acetylcholine synthesis in different regions of the central nervous system. *Journal of Physiology*, **107**, 372.

Maudsley H (1882). *The Physiology and Pathology of the Mind* 3rd edn, New York, p 195

Waelsch H (ed) (1955). *Biochemistry of the Developing Nervous System*. Academic Press, New York.

Elkes J (1963). The American College of Neuropsychopharmacology: A note on its history and hopes for the future. *ACNP Bulletin*, **1**, 2–3.

10 Leo Hollister

From hypertension to psychopharmacology – a serendipitous career

Why did you go into medicine?

During the 1930s an American journalist, Paul de Kruif, wrote a series of books such as *Men Against Death*, and *The Microbe Hunters*, largely about the advances in medicine such as the development of the concept of bacterial diseases and nutritional deficiency diseases. I thought it was tremendously inspirational to see how research could make a difference in the lives of many people. So that was one of the influences. I had had a tendency to think in terms of law because my stepfather was a judge. I will never forget sitting in the judge's chair when I was about 9 or 10 looking over the majesty of the court room thinking 'God, what a powerful thing the concept of Government by laws is!' But I later came to the conclusion that lawyers tended to try to distort the truth whereas scientists tried to find it. I found the latter much more appealing.

So despite considerable obstacles, because I didn't have a whole lot of financial backing and had to work through both my pre-medical and medical career as well as go to school, I decided to go into medicine. It was curious that the work I did then had a later influence on my career. During the pre-medical years I worked in a pharmacy and learned a lot about drugs. And then during my medical school I worked in a neuropathology laboratory, where we had quite a number of interesting people who would come by for seminars, including Albert Sabin of the Sabin vaccine. This was exciting – it indicated the complexities of the brain. So those two things, drugs and the brain, tended to gel and ultimately more or less by accident influenced my career. It is strange what influences can occur that you are not even aware of but later on play a role in your choice of career.

In the recent History of the CINP, you reviewed the 1955 Paris Colloquium on Chlorpromazine that was organised by Jean Delay – essentially the first meeting of the new era; were you at it?

No. I had occasion to review that meeting for a book *Toward the CINP* written by Tom Ban and Oakley Ray but I was not at the meeting. My beginnings in psychopharmacology were quite fortuitous. I was working as an internist in a Veterans' Administration Hospital largely devoted to psychiatric patients. A detail man, one of the salesmen who come around to tell you about drugs, from Ciba Pharmaceuticals came by my office one day and said, 'We have a new drug that we think is going to be very useful for treating hypertension' and I said, 'Gee, I know every hypertensive in the hospital and I've had a long interest in hypertension. Why don't you give me some and let me try it?' So he merely walked out to his automobile, pulled out some reserpine tablets from the trunk and gave them to me. About two days later the first patient was being treated with reserpine. So much simpler to do clinical research than it is today.

Somewhat to my surprise the drug worked. It was a very effective treatment. I had already tried many other drugs to treat hypertension and saw nothing like this before. About 3 months later he came by and said, 'We have some reports that this drug may also be useful for psychiatric patients.'

This was when?

This was in 1953. I don't precisely remember the month. So I said, 'Well, psychiatric patients are not my cup of tea but let me see what I can do.' I went to the chief of psychiatry and told him the story. He somewhat patronisingly said, 'Leo, you know, in psychiatry we have had these drugs come and go and nothing ever has come of them, I wouldn't waste my time.' So obviously he wasn't interested. Then I asked him if it would be all right if I asked some of the psychiatric staff, most of whom were golfing buddies, if they would mind trying the drug under my direction. He said, 'No, not at all, go right ahead.' What I proposed to the psychiatric staff was that they would send me their schizophrenics to my medical ward and I would keep them there as long as we needed to get them started on their treatment, then send them back with a supply of oral medication. It was their duty to tell me whether the patients were improved or not. I didn't feel confident to make that judgement. What I did then was to treat some of the patients with the active drug and some with placebo. I believe that these were the first parallel-group double-blind studies that were ever done with antipsychotics.

Curiously enough, I had already done two placebo-controlled double-blind trials in patients with what I then called 'psychoses associated with old age'. The first was with oral pentylenetetrazole (Metrazol) and the other was with combined hydrogenated alkaloids of ergot, known better as Hydergine. Metrazol was not very effective. Neither was Hydergine, with the exception of two patients who had what was then called 'hypertensive brain disease'. So I wasn't exactly a novice, although I felt more competent to judge progress in patients with senile psychoses than in those with schizophrenia.

Where did you get that idea from? Because that was very early to be...

The idea of doing double-blind studies originated in the 1940s, largely propelled by Harry Gold, a pharmacologist at Cornell University. It was widely used in the postwar period to evaluate the new drugs for tuberculosis. So I was familiar with these developments and I thought this was one occasion when it would be very informative to try. Needless to say we did not have to make too many passes. Some of the staff were coming back to me and saying, 'I don't know what you're doing over there but some of the patients you sent back are vastly changed.' I said, 'Well, that is good news.' We kept that up until we had accumulated a reasonable number – 30 or 40 – patients treated that way.

Why was there no difficulty with the other psychiatrists whose patients you gave reserpine to?

It is curious but despite the pessimism of the chief of psychiatry, the other staff were fairly amenable to joining me in this. As I said, most of them were people with whom I played golf, so we were on friendly terms. They were willing to go along with me although I don't know what they expected. It didn't take too many turnarounds after they sent their patients to my ward and I sent them back before they knew something was going on. And quite correctly they said only some of them got better but not all of them. So in a way I was lucky. I guess if they had turned me down I would never have pursued the idea. But it turned out that I was fortunate. So many things happen in your life that you can't predict.

By this time it was 1954 and I had heard rumours of another drug, called chlorpromazine, which might be equally effective in such patients. In those days it was ridiculously simple. I just contacted SmithKline & French and in no time at all I had chlorpromazine and placebo. We could then do the same thing with that drug as we did with reserpine.

By the end of 1954, a meeting of the American Association for the Advancement of Science (AAAS) was to be held in Berkeley, California. I had been invited to tell of our work with these two drugs. At that meeting I gave a rather brief paper describing what we had done but pointing out that this seemed to be a revolution in the treatment of mentally ill patients and that undoubtedly there would be a lot more work done with these drugs. One can't be entirely sure but this might have been the first meeting sponsored by a major scientific group that dealt with the new antipsychotics. Others whom I recall being at that meeting were Nate Kline, John Kinross-Wright, who later became a drinking buddy, and Murray Jarvik.

How did you get asked to that meeting? How had people heard about your work?

I suppose the organisers, Jonathan Cole and Ralph Gerard, must have found out through the drug company because up till that point I had never published anything on the work. I was extraordinarily naive in those days. I thought that having given the paper at an AAAS meeting and knowing eventually the proceedings would be published that there was no need to publish any further. The proceedings came out in 1957 in a small book which probably only 15 people ever read, so my pioneering work remained widely unknown.

If you had published them as early as you could have done, would you have published before Nate Kline?

No. Nate had used reserpine before we did. He had used a very small dose, doses that were usually appropriate for treating hypertension. In his initial study he had not seen a whole lot change. But by that time Ciba had come to the conclusion that you needed much higher doses. By that time Ciba had a research physician, Dick Roberts, who came to the West Coast and was charged with setting up studies of the drug on the West Coast. He was invaluable in telling us what the proper doses should be. The dosage schedule that we used started with a 5 mg loading dose intramuscularly given for several days, followed by subsequent oral doses of the same magnitude. This increased dosage schedule was much more effective than the smaller dose that Nate had used. Of course, Nate got the same word so by the time we were using that dose he was also using it. A third chap, Robert Noce, working at one of the California State hospitals, had also started using reserpine in his patients.

By the middle of the 1950s the New York Academy of Sciences, prompted by Ciba, held a meeting in New York to get together the people who had studied reserpine. I was invited to that meeting where I reported work we had previously done plus the work we did subsequently. This report was the only one at that meeting that involved a controlled study. This approach attracted a great deal of interest on the part of the press so the study was widely reported throughout the country via the wire services. There were articles in almost every newspaper in the country about reserpine and schizophrenia.

This was a sobering experience because subsequently I received literally piles of correspondence from various people throughout the country saying that they had a husband, son, daughter or whatever who had schizophrenia and they were looking for something to do for them. I made it a point to answer personally all these letters, telling them that essentially there was no need to send people to California to get the treatment because there were very few secrets in medicine and the drug would be widely available throughout the country. It was a rather sobering experience to see what tremendous effect the press had on stirring up hopes for a cure among people who suffer dire diseases.

Again I hadn't published any of this work in regular journals. The New York Academy of Sciences usually produced *Annals* that published the papers of their meetings. In 1957, a couple of years after the meeting, the *Annals* appeared and my paper was in there. So in a nutshell this was the strange beginning of my career in psychopharmacology. I always liken it to the saying attributed to some well-known writer who said, 'When I started writing I really didn't think I had much talent but after I sold a few books and was making a pretty good living out of it, I decided to keep it up.' In that sense I was hooked on psychopharmacology and proceeded after that to study many drugs in the field. We studied prochlorperazine, Compazine, which was the next SmithKline & French entity, which was an effective antipsychotic drug. But what is a company going to do with two drugs competing with each other for the same indication? So SKF promoted it as an antiemetic drug. It was highly effective for that indication, as most antipsychotic drugs at the time were.

Later Sandoz had a drug, thioridazine – Mellaril. We studied that one and it proved to be as effective as chlorpromazine. Mellaril may very well have been the first so-called atypical antipsychotic. Like the current group it was a weak dopamine receptor-blocking drug. In fact, many basic pharmacologists at the time doubted that it would be an effective antipsychotic. But it was. The weak effect on D2 receptors also made the drug unlikely to produce extrapyramidal motor reactions, though most of us at the time believed that this difference was due to its strong anticholinergic effect.

Didn't Sandoz very early on market it almost as much for mood disorders as for schizophrenia? It had an antidepressant flavour to it.

I think that came later. I may have contributed to that notion. Because it was a phenothiazine, and generally speaking drugs within a chemical group have somewhat similar actions, it was tried as an antipsychotic. The remarkable thing about thioridazine was that it rarely produced the extrapyramidal reactions associated with other drugs. By this time, of course, reserpine, which was not under a patent because of being a natural substance, fell into disuse because the phenothiazines seemed to do as well or perhaps even better than reserpine with fewer disagreeable side-effects. Reserpine produced a kind of flu-like syndrome! Diarrhoea, aching, feeling rather unpleasant, including a somewhat depressed mood. So by that time the pendulum was swinging towards the phenothiazines.

We studied another SKF drug, trifluoperazine – Stelazine – and again it looked to be like an effective antipsychotic. With this drug, we used a variant on the double-blind technique. Patients were all started on trifluoperazine and then, after having responded, were continued on treatment under blind controls with either the same drug or an active placebo – a small dose of phenobarbital. This technique was somewhat different from what Joel Elkes had done early in the game with chlorpromazine in which patients were simply crossed over to placebos.

The impetus for Mellaril being tried as an antidepressant came from clinical experience in Europe. People were using it for that purpose. We did a controlled study under what might be called triple-blind conditions – because the participating physicians didn't really know what drugs were being used – Mellaril versus imipramine both in schizophrenics and depressed patients. In the schizophrenic patients Mellaril was clearly superior but in depressed patients the two drugs looked somewhat similar. This result gave a considerable boost to the idea that Mellaril could be used for treating depression. I'm not sure whether that was a correct conclusion – there were probably many reasons why we couldn't show a difference.

When was that, because it sounds something similar to what Don Klein and Max Fink did in Hillside where they randomised everyone regardless of diagnosis to imipramine or chlorpromazine?[1]

Yes. That would have been probably around 1958. I remember both Max and Don approaching me and saying, 'Why don't we do our studies together?' I said that mine was already under way and I was happy with the design, so why didn't we do them independently, which would probably give more force any-

[1]Klein DF (1996). Reaction patterns to psychotropic drugs and the discovery of panic disorder. *The Psychopharmacologists*, Vol I.

way to whatever consistent conclusions emerged. But you're correct that it was about the same time.

There was then the large Veterans study of chlorpromazine that you were involved with.

Yes, by 1959 the Veterans Administration had decided that, because they were the biggest operator of psychiatric beds in the country – they had more psychiatric patients than perhaps all the institutions put together – they should look into these new drugs in a systematic way. I was approached to join the planning group which included a multidisciplinary group of statisticians, psychiatrists, psychologists, neuroscientists and so on. We then planned a series of co-operative studies among a group of many hospitals. The first study was a comparison between chlorpromazine and another phenothiazine, mepazine – Pacatal, that had been reputed to be an antipsychotic. At my insistence we used phenobarbital as a kind of active placebo. Much to our gratification, this study showed that chlorpromazine was effective, that Pacatal was almost ineffective, and that placebo was totally ineffective. So we had a technique that was sensitive enough to distinguish between phenothiazines with different levels of antipsychotic action, which was really encouraging. From then on a series of studies over the next several years extended the first one and we started the study of antidepressants. So the VA co-operative studies group was a highly productive group in defining the uses of these drugs.

There were also a number of studies done by some of the larger State hospitals in New York and California, modelled on the VA studies, which came to virtually the same conclusion. Then the National Institute of Mental Health (NIMH), under a subunit called the Psychopharmacology Service Center, had planned to do a study in acutely admitted schizophrenics – people who were presumably having their first break – and I was invited to consult with that group as well. That study got more publicity and more references in the literature than any of the VA studies, which many of us found somewhat offensive. But because the Psychopharmacology Service Center had the purse strings for grants, obviously people wanted to cite their studies. Their study was somewhat similar in the sense that they studied two phenothiazines, both of which were effective compared with placebo.[2]

The NIMH study indicated a high number of these patients, perhaps 20%, spontaneously remitted. This result led to the erroneous conclusion that there is a high placebo effect in schizophrenics. The fact of the matter is that in those days it was not easy to make a diagnosis. I am quite sure that a lot of those so called acute schizophrenics were really manics who probably went into spontaneous remission. Besides for everyone who got better an equal number got worse. The net effect of placebo on these so called schizophrenics was essentially a stand-off. The study has been misinterpreted in respect of placebo effects.

---

[2]Cole JO (1996). The evaluation of psychotropic drugs. In *The Psychopharmacologists*, Vol I.

When the Psychopharmacology Service Center began they held a large meeting in Washington in September of 1956 which was convened by Ralph Gerard and Seymour Kety; were you at that?

Yes. When I mentioned the multidisciplinary group that had been associated with the VA studies, Ralph Gerard was a consultant to the VA group before he became a consultant to the NIMH group. When I used the word neuroscientist among the disciplines represented I was thinking of Ralph, who of course was well known for his wonderful aphorism that behind every twisted thought is a twisted molecule. In a way that was the essence of biochemical psychopharmacology in those days. He consulted with the VA group in 1956 and the NIMH group in 1959. I don't recall Kety's participation in either group.

The 1956 meeting I was referring to was organised when the funding came through from Congress and it was out of that meeting that the psychopharmacology centre came.

I may be wrong. I was commuting back and forth to Washington to both the VA and the Psychopharmacology Service Center groups. The latter was then honchoed by Jonathan Cole, who had been one of Ralph Gerard's protégés. The Psychopharmacology Service Center aided immeasurably in elucidating the mechanism of action of these drugs because of their grant funding. Their first grant programme was for the study of acutely newly ill schizophrenics. They recruited about 10 or 11 hospitals and gave them a considerable amount of money to participate. From that point on they had a more open grant system where investigators could apply. I don't know when I first actually got a grant but it was probably not until around 1961 or thereabouts. That grant went over 27 years. I remember that in my last reapplication I said, 'I am not trying to get the largest numerical suffix on my grant but if you give me two more years I promise never to come back.'

Those were exciting days. You might wonder why all these different agencies, the VA, the NIMH, the State systems and numerous independent investigators worked so hard, using controlled studies to prove these drugs were effective. All you had to do was look at your patients and improvement was obvious. People who were mute began talking. People who were attacking ward personnel were no long hitting people. Even now when I hear about the older drugs not being effective for negative symptoms, I don't believe it. I remember quite well very early in the game I asked one of the psychiatrists participating in my study, 'Would you like to have some more of your patients treated with chlorpromazine?' And he said, 'Leo, I have so many patients talking to me now who never talked to me before that it's all I can handle to keep up with them.' Now if that is not improving a negative symptom I don't know what is.

Some years back I pointed out to John Overall, my long-time colleague, that we had abundant data showing that negative symptoms as well as positive symptoms were amenable to improvement although they did not improve as much as the positive symptoms. I wanted to resurrect some of our old data and write a paper about it but John was even more lukewarm about publishing than I was, so we never did that.

Can I ask you about John, since you have introduced him?

John and I first met in 1960 at one of the annual VA meetings on chemotherapy in psychiatry. These meetings described the progress of the co-operative studies as well as other studies being done within the system. I had never known him before, but we hit it off very well. We both liked to drink a bit and over a few drinks we managed to generate all kinds of possible ideas. So that began a collaboration that exists up to the present time. I recently joined the University of Texas in Houston Medical Faculty where John is also a member, so we are now together. He was the main reason I came from Stanford to Houston. It was an excellent collaboration because he knew everything I didn't about rating patients. Of course, his Brief Psychiatric Rating Scale has become the most widely used rating scale ...

Where did that come from?

It was a derivative of a scale called the In-patient Multi-dimensional Psychotherapy Scale (IMPS) that Morrie Lorr had brought out a few years before. In this scale the domains of psychopathology were rated in a more particulate way and what John and Don Gorhim, his colleague, did was simply to take the same domains and make rating them more global. That made it a much more useful scale but it was somewhat derivative from the IMPS. Subsequently John and Don made some other refinements by putting in two or three other domains. John knew about psychometrics as well as being a superb statistician. I knew something about drugs, medicine and experimental design, so we meshed very well. Once when we were having some conversation and I pointed out something about the statistics of the situation and he was pointing out about something about the drugs, we seemed to have learnt much from each other. I refer to John as one of our national treasures as they do in Japan, because he is an outstanding researcher. I feel very fortunate to have had a chance to work with him over the years. Most of the time, not having the credentials of psychiatry, I have felt that I have needed psychiatrists or psychologists to evaluate patients.

Did you not ever go back and get a psychiatric training or did you just stay straight medical?

No, I never felt the need to. I'm a great believer in self teaching – you can learn on your own a lot of things. Sometimes I point out to students, trying to give them an idea that learning is a never-ending process, that I am probably the only person who has been a Professor of Psychiatry and Pharmacology at two different medical schools who has had absolutely no formal training in either discipline. These days you simply have to keep learning all the time and be willing to cross disciplines. After some years I began to feel confident that I could make diagnoses and make appraisals of patients. In fact, having come from internal medicine, where we are more precise about our diagnoses, I was more conscious for the need of accurate diagnosis than most of my psychiatric colleagues. At the New York Academy of Science meeting on reserpine, people were talking about '150 psychiatric patients' – no diagnoses at all. Psychiatric diagnosis is terribly imprecise and, despite setting up various diagnostic criteria it is still so. Further it has become increasingly evident that diagnoses don't exist in pure culture. You see a patient and you can make three or four diagnoses on him – personality disorder, psychosis and affective disorder. So there is a tremendous amount of overlap due to comorbidity, which is still rather vexing. One of my colleagues at the University of Texas, whom I think is a very able clinician, said, 'When I see patients I don't know what to call them.' There is such a mixture. So there are many remaining problems in regard to diagnosis.

Let me take you back to the late 1950s. What was the impact of Nate Kline at the time?

Well, Nate was a very opportunistic fellow who wanted to make a big name for himself, which he did. He also had a great deal of showmanship – I wouldn't say charisma because he was not universally liked. But he was able to project himself in the public eye – like going to Haiti to start a psychiatric system where of course most people didn't have enough food, clothing or shelter. But he did a lot to put psychiatry in the public eye in a somewhat favourable way. He didn't stay too long in academic psychiatry or at least investigative psychiatry. He had been director of research at the Rockland State Hospital in New York and had done very well. But by the early 1960s, the mental hospital system was beginning to shift to an outpatient mode, so Nate started a private practice in New York.

My first encounter with Nate was rather unusual. The physician from Ciba, Dick Roberts, had also helped Nate. At the AAAS meeting Dick and I were sitting together when just before the meeting was to begin Nate came in. Dick stood up, which he did with some difficulty because he had a residual of polio in one of his lower extremities, and I did too, to greet Nate. Dick introduced me to him. Nate was very high handed – he acted like we were peasants gathering crumbs from the master. As he departed to go up toward the podium, I turned to Dick and said, 'Who the hell does that guy think he is? Does he think he is going to get the Nobel Prize simply because he used your drug?' Well, it turns out that might not have been too fanciful an idea. A couple of years later Nate got one of the first Lasker awards for using reserpine.

And why not you?

Because Nate knew how to cultivate people. He got to know Mary Lasker very well and she was interested in psychiatric illnesses so I am sure that contributed to the selections. In those days the Lasker was not nearly as prestigious as it became later on. Mary alone could name the awardees. Heinz Lehmann was another of the awardees at that time as well as Bob Noce, whom no one has heard of since.

Anyway, Nate was always somewhat controversial. After my rather rocky beginning with him, it remained rocky throughout the course of my acquaintance with him – sometimes it was pleasant, sometimes not. He was that way with many people. He always seemed to have a provocative approach. If there was a chance to get into an argument, he would do so rather than try to resolve differences. Despite these character faults, he certainly had a big impact on psychiatry and hastened the acceptance of biological psychiatry into the mainstream. At that time psychoanalytic theory dominated the area and virtually every chairman of a department of psychiatry in the US was either a psychoanalyst or psychodynamically oriented. Now of course the pendulum has swung completely in the opposite direction. One current chairman, Joe Coyle at Harvard, has also been president of the Society for Neuroscience.

As far as the Collegium, the CINP, is concerned I missed the first two or three meetings. Finally my family was getting old enough to enjoy a trip abroad so I took my wife and three of the children to Birmingham, England, for the 1964 meeting. After that I have attended most meetings. When you are president you have a big say as to who comes next. I lobbied for Arvid Carlsson to be my successor and next for Paul Janssen, two indisputable choices. Later, I was influential in having Ole Rafaelsen, one of the brightest people I have ever met in medicine, named as president. My last influence was to support Paul Kielholz. We have had some excellent people as president and I feel very fortunate to count myself among them.

What role do you think the CINP has played? There are certain strains at the moment but I guess there always have been various strains.

There are all kinds of neuropsychopharmacology groups formed around nations or regions. The first of these was the American College of Neuropsychopharmacology. One of the prime movers in getting that organisation started called me up and asked me if I would like to join. I said, 'Oh God, we have so many organisations now, who needs another? But if you insist put me down as a member.'

Who actually called you?

Ted Rothman. Ted was a very nice man who suffered from rheumatoid spondylitis but that did not impair his sense of humour a bit. At one ACNP meeting we shared digs. He was one of the prime movers in getting ACNP started. I missed the first two meetings, which according to the by-laws should cause you to lose your membership. But I went to the third meeting in Washington. As we were signing out of the hotel, Ted was nearby and I walked over to him and said, 'Ted, I was dead wrong, I am so happy you persisted in getting me as a member of this organisation because I think it's great and it will become even greater.' Since 1962 I have not missed a meeting. The next such society was the German-speaking one. The Canadians had their own society and I just learned at this meeting that there is one in Latin America, in which one of my former foreign students is now the president. The CINP serves the purpose of integrating all of these groups by bringing everyone to share a wider viewpoint.

I used to give a lot of papers and I have done as much travelling as anybody giving lectures to medical schools, societies and various other groups. Now I rarely give a paper. One of the problems with a meeting like this is that only so much is new. Most has already been published somewhere and is old hat. But maybe it isn't old hat to everybody and even repetition may serve some purpose.

In the US ACNP and psychopharmacology have seemed to be more an East Coast than a West Coast thing.

It may have started off that way but I don't think it's that way now. In fact there have only been four people from the US who have been president of both the ACNP and CINP. The first was Paul Hoch from New York but the next three were me, Biff Bunney and the current ex-president, Lew Judd. I was pointing out to Biff yesterday that the only three living people who have been president of both societies are all from California. So things have shifted a bit from the East Coast. This may be just part of the general demographical redistribution over the last 30 years – with an enormous shift towards the West Coast.

You were one of the first people to describe a benzodiazepine withdrawal phenomenon. Can you tell me how that came about?

That was a fortuitous situation. In 1960, just before the introduction of chlordiazepoxide, Roche had a closed meeting in Princeton, New Jersey, where the people who had been studying this drug reported on it. I had been invited to the meeting, not because I had studied the drug, but as an outside impartial observer. All the reports were quite favourable. As I listened to them I kept thinking, if this drug is as good as these people say it's going to be abused. So I thought, how can we study this possible problem? One of the studies not yet done was to use it in large doses for schizophrenia. Thus we could justify larger doses not only to test this indication but also to study any withdrawal syndrome. We pushed doses up to 300 mg and 600 mg a day, at which time most people were ataxic. Then under very carefully supervised conditions we would switch them to a placebo while taking blood for measurements of plasma concentrations, EEGs and a number of clinical observations. We only tested 11 patients but 10 or the 11 showed a very clear-cut withdrawal reaction comparable qualitatively to that which had been discovered a few years earlier for alcohol and barbiturates. The big difference was it was attenuated in time. For the first couple of days after withdrawal not much happened and then about the third day patients began to develop clinical symptoms which generally peaked at about the fifth day. We had two patients with seizures on the eighth day. This timing was quite different from short-acting barbiturates or alcohol, where seizures usually occur within the first 48 hours.

We had drawn blood for measurements of plasma concentrations, which in those days were rather primitive compared to current measurements. The data were not complete because I had no idea we should follow plasma concentrations for eight or nine days. However, we deduced that the half-life of this drug after discontinuation was approximately 48 hours. Consequently the delayed onset of withdrawal and the late occurrence of seizures were attributable to the long half-life of the drug. Incidentally, although chlordiazepoxide alleviated some of the behavioural symptoms of schizophrenia, it was not truly an antipsychotic.

These results were published in *Psychopharmacologia*, in 1961. I was fully confident that nature would imitate art and that a lot of spontaneous withdrawal reactions would be subsequently reported. One of the reasons for the paucity of reports was doubtless the attenuated time course. Many patients resumed taking the drug and managed to abort the full withdrawal reaction. Or some of them probably went through without knowing what was happening, as the withdrawal reaction was relatively mild. Much later in the 1970s and 1980s it became a much bigger issue but by that time my original report was somewhat forgotten.

Possibly of much more clinical significance was the concept of therapeutic dose dependence – that even smaller doses multiplied by a long period of exposure could lead to some sort of modified but definite withdrawal reaction. This recognition came during the 1980s.

Had you thought right from the start that these drugs would cause a withdrawal reaction?

Oh yes, that was the hypothesis. If they were going to be abused they would cause a reaction. The surprising thing was the time course. Earlier we had studied withdrawal reactions from meprobamate. These were much more like the classical ones, with early onset. We figured the half-life to be in the order of 11 hours, which is comparable to the short-acting barbiturates. Later when the meprobamate congener, tybamate, came out we tried to produce withdrawal reactions but we couldn't because tybamate has a half-life of 2–3 hours. There was no way short of keeping patients awake during the whole 24 hours of the day to sustain a high level of the drug. This experience led to a formulation which I think has held up pretty well; that is, that the onset and severity of withdrawal reactions are a function of the half-life of a drug. Those with a shorter half-life will have a more abrupt onset and a more severe reaction and those with a longer half-life have a delayed onset and are less severe. There had, for instance, been a lot of clinical use for phenobarbitone before the newer sedatives came along, but withdrawal reactions were never a problem. Phenobarbitone had such a long half-life, in the order of 96 hours, that it had a built in tapering-off action. That formulation has generally held over the years.

What response did you get from Roche when you showed this potentially significant drawback to their treatment?

They were not particularly happy about it. I just told them that I wasn't trying to kill their drug but that it was worth knowing about the possible withdrawal reaction before the drug was marketed so that people could be aware that following long-term use of the drug they might taper it as they stopped it. A couple of years later, in one of my small collaborative groups, we also studied diazepam in schizophrenics, again with large doses. Unbeknownst to me one of the hospitals decided they would run all patients up to the maximum dose with 120 mg a day and then abruptly stop the drug. It turned out that diazepam produced exactly the same withdrawal reaction – with a somewhat delayed onset and late-developing seizures. We reported that in a little paragraph on adverse effects in the original paper but never as a separate publication. But that too was known before diazepam was put on the market.

There was another observation of withdrawal reactions which I neglected to publicise. I can't imagine how naive I was in those days. Sidney Raffel, a professor of microbiology at Stanford, had done some *in vitro* experiments where he showed that chlorpromazine in concentrations of about 5 μg/ml could kill *Mycobacterium tuberculosis*. Now in the 1950s, we didn't have too many drugs for tuberculosis, so we decided to add chlorpromazine to the existing regimen of isoniazid and other drugs that tuberculous patients were being treated with. We did that for six months with two three month evaluations and saw absolutely no change in the progress of the tuberculosis. Our doses were 300 mg a day of chlorpromazine. We then said OK, let's quit. It was a placebo-controlled study. None of the placebo-treated patients had a bit of trouble stopping but 5 of 17 chlorpromazine patients had a clear-cut withdrawal reaction which was mitigated by either restarting chlorpromazine or starting another sedative drug. I reported those findings in a very brief paragraph in a paper reporting the whole study – again not publishing it separately. In retrospect it was an unusual situation. First, it was the only placebo-controlled withdrawal study. Second, it was the first study in which a withdrawal reaction occurred with therapeutic doses of the drug. And third, it was the first study in which a withdrawal reaction occurred in the absence of any abuse potential, because nobody in their right mind would ever abuse chlorpromazine. I missed the boat.

What do you think the withdrawal syndrome with chlorpromazine is?

Well, I suspect that at any time you disturb the chemical equilibrium in the brain, some compensatory mechanism will try to overcome it. Then when the drug is stopped the over-developed compensatory mechanism produces the opposite effect. That's been shown for tricyclic antidepressants and I am sure it would be the case for many drugs that affect the brain. The manifestations in the case of chlorpromazine were somewhat the opposite to the therapeutic effects – nausea and vomiting as well as restlessness and sleeplessness. So I suspect that this is a generalisable phenomenon. It goes back to a number of theories about tolerance and withdrawal that were adduced in the late 1940s from a number of groups.

Talking about withdrawal brings Abe Wikler to mind. You reviewed his book Pharmacology and Psychiatry, which came out in 1955 for the recent History of CINP and called one of the key early texts in the field.

I didn't know Abe at the time because he worked at Lexington and I never had any experience there but his book on the relationship between psychiatry and pharmacology was a monumental effort and it certainly opened my eyes. Having come into this thing with no training in either pharmacology or psychiatry his book not only helped bring the two together but summarised the state of the art as it existed in 1955. I always felt that it was rather strange that Abe, whose primary interest was in substance abuse, would come up with such a complete volume covering all of psychopharmacology but he was an avid student and he had many interests. Even today his theory of conditioned abstinence is very useful in treating substance abuse and explaining it. Later on I got to know him but at the time I read his book I had no idea who this chap was who was doing such a comprehensive job. The paperback version is still on my bookshelf.

In fact the work of the group at Lexington provided the model for most of the studies we did. They did some studies in the early 1950s on alcohol which proved that alcohol withdrawal was exactly that and not some mysterious ailment caused by some toxin or whatever. They also did studies on the withdrawal to barbiturates, mostly the short-acting ones, so when I started my study on meprobamate the essential model was what they had done at Lexington with the barbiturates. It was a great group at Lexington. Harris Isbell was there. He was a remarkably quiet and unassuming man who had a wealth of knowledge.

In a book called Storming Heaven, *which is about the LSD phenomenon in the US in the 1950s and 1960s, there is a minor mention that Ken Kesey of One Flew Over the Cuckoo's Nest fame was an orderly on one of your wards at one point and got some of his ideas from your work on LSD.*

Around 1960 I had a look at the literature on LSD. At that time there was a lot of talk about LSD producing a model psychosis and that it was a way to understand schizophrenia. I wasn't very happy with the work I saw published and I thought maybe I could do a little better. So over the next 5 or 6 years, up to 1966, we did a series of studies on various types of so-called hallucinogens or psychotomimetics. We studied not only LSD but also mescaline and psilocybin, which in a series of clinical and biochemical comparisons were essentially identical, give or take a few orders of magnitude difference in the dose, so we presumed they must have rather similar modes of action. We studied LSD as a therapeutic agent in alcoholics – we compared it with dexamphetamine – and found that while there were minimal benefits after 3 months this was gone after 6 months. The idea of curing alcoholism with LSD perhaps now sounds naive but we demonstrated that there wasn't much clinical benefit there.

Ken Kesey approached me early in our studies, saying he was writing a book and needed to know what it might be like to have schizophrenia. He thought the psychotomimetic drugs would provide such an experience. I told him I wasn't so sure but that if he wanted to try some, I'd enlist him as a volunteer subject. I was very interested at the time in delineating clearly the clinical syndromes produced by such drugs. We would leave a tape recorder in the testing room and periodically I would venture in after giving a time cue to ask about what was being experienced. Later, in a labour-intensive fashion, it was possible to reconstruct the sequence of the clinical phenomena. Most subjects needed such promptings but not Kesey. He was at the recorder constantly, dictating what later turned out when listened to to be the most beautifully written and imaginative descriptions. There was no doubt that he was a master of words. He later took a job as an orderly at the hospital to gain more first-hand experience. His subsequent novel, *One Flew Over the Cuckoo's Nest*, became one of the most magnificent and successful first novels in history. Alas, he became hooked on the drug culture and despite his enormous talent never produced anything of note thereafter. In retrospect, I consider him to represent the worst result of our studies with psychotomimetics.

What was the idea behind using LSD – was it that it allowed you to cut into the depths of an individual's fantasy life and this might allow you to undo the complexes that were leading to alcoholism?

There were probably various rationales at the time. What prompted me to do the study was there was an off-beat group headed by an engineer, who was not medically trained, who was going round the country giving 600 μg doses of LSD to alcoholics and charging them $1500 or some astronomical amount for this treatment. This sounded rather phoney to me and that's why we subjected it to a controlled clinical trial. Curiously enough, at the same time there were two other groups also working on the problem and independently we all came to the same conclusion, which I think stands up pretty well. One group was Arnold Ludwig and Jerry Levine. We all came to a meeting in 1964 and presented our papers independently. All came to the same conclusion, even though we used vastly different techniques to test the hypothesis.

You alluded to the possibility that LSD or similar drugs might be useful for facilitating psychotherapy – we tried our hand at that too. We gave people who were already in psychotherapy a series of trials where they were randomly assigned to either LSD, mescaline, psilocybin, placebo or no treatment and we taped their interviews and had them rated independently and blindly by experts in psychotherapy as to what they thought the productivity of the interview was. There again we could find very little evidence that these drugs increased insight or brought about a confronting of problems or any of the other things you try to achieve in psychotherapy.

Another of our experiments was to test the model psychosis hypothesis – did the LSD state have any resemblance to schizophrenia? What we did there was to record interviews with schizophrenics as well as interviews with people who were under the influence of these drugs and edited out any reference to drug action in either group. We then had them audited by psychiatrists who were experts in diagnosis and the batting average was almost 100% in terms of distinguishing between who were schizophrenics and who were not. We went to psychologists and they did just as well. We went to social workers and they did as well, as did the nurses. It seemed that almost anyone could tell the difference between the line of thinking of a schizophrenic and the line of thinking people had under the influence of these drugs. To my mind that scotched the model psychosis hypothesis. Danny Freedman and I used to quibble about that because he was in favour of the model psychoses. He thought it might be more applicable in first-break or newer schizophrenics than it might be in the older ones that we were studying but this hasn't been followed up very much.

Just about the time we were ready to sign off on our studies of hallucinogens it became possible to get synthetic delta-9-tetrahydrocannibol (THC). To illustrate how things can happen by accident and how casual things were in those days, I was in Washington for a meeting and I ran into a chap named Milton Joffe who was with the Food and Drug Administration. He said, 'We have a big problem with something called STP out in San Francisco – we really don't know what it's all about. I have some in my desk drawer.' I said, 'Give me your supply of STP and we'll study it', which he did. It turned out to be one of the amphetamine homologues. Sol Snyder also started studying it but he had a grant for it. I had a protocol set up for LSD so we simply switched to studying STP instead. Within a few weeks we had shown that it was a hallucinogen very similar to mescaline and LSD and that group, secondly that tolerance could develop very quickly to it and that it was not amenable to treatment with chlorpromazine or any of the antipsychotics. Because Sol had also done some work, he and I decided to publish jointly and a first account came out in *Science*. Subsequently we each gave more detailed separate accounts.

My last excursion into hallucinogens was when synthetic delta-9-THC came along. Again it was very simple, I just had to go to Washington and ask them for it. I remembered that there was a compound called synhexyl, which was a THC-like structure that had been studied very extensively in the 1940s on the assumption that it was equivalent to marijuana. Nobody ever had a chance to compare it directly with THC. I was working then with a pharmacologist friend who had retired from Abbott Laboratories and he said, 'We had some of that in the refrigerator for a long while.' He was able to put his hands on some 25-year-old synhexyl which looked like a bit of tar. We reconstituted it in aqueous alcoholic solution and gave it to subjects in a blind comparison with THC and what we found essentially was that they were the same even though structural differences existed between the two compounds. Synhexyl was somewhat weaker than THC and had a lag-time in its onset of action but qualitatively it was quite similar.

Marijuana is more of a political issue these days than a scientific issue. Ten years ago I published a review in *Pharmacological Reviews* on health aspects of cannabis, looking at the possible adverse effects but also the possible medicinal uses of it. At that time I was roundly criticised by Gabriel Nahas, who is on the ultra-conservative wing of the substance abuse question. I and the editors of *Pharmacological Reviews* pointed out to him that I had tried my best to be impartial and fair but that didn't satisfy him. I have become acquainted with the philosophy of trying to turn an enemy into a friend and over the years we have started to collaborate. One project is a re-review some 11 years later covering the literature that has appeared in the interlude. This may be very timely now that there is a big push in the US to liberalise its use in the medical field and possible first steps in a campaign to legalise the drug. I anticipate there is still some interest in what the health aspects of cannabis really are.

I have belonged to several organisations but I think the one I was most effective in was the Committee on Problems of Drug Dependence, which was the oldest scientific organisation set up for drugs of dependence in the US. I was invited to join it by Nathan Eddy after my study on STP came out. Within a few years I became chairman of the committee while it was still under the National Academy of Sciences. Owing to some political shenanigans within the Academy they decided to drop some committees including that one and it was my job to shepherd it along through another channel, which has now evolved into the College on Problems of Drug Dependence, which is continuing the tradition of good science in this field.

How much have the behavioural pharmacologists contributed to the field of drug dependence?

I am not terribly impressed with this. One of the thrusts of the Committee on Problems of Drug Dependence was to make sure we didn't market any opioid analgesic that might be abused. God knows how many were turned down because monkeys would self-administer them. I often wonder whether we didn't keep a lot of potentially useful drugs off the market. When you look at it, it isn't the medical use of opioids that causes the addiction, its the social use. It has little if anything to do with medical use. You could count the number of medically addicted people on your fingers and toes so I wonder if the thrust of that committee wasn't misplaced.

Furthermore it seems to me that a lot of behavioural studies have shown that drugs that will be abused by man will be self-administered by animals, which is no surprise. It's usually been that way around rather than the other way. They have contributed something to the clarification of the tendency to abuse a drug by tests such as determining how hard an animal will work to get a reinforcement but I see that more as cleaning up the situation after it's already known. Maybe I have a biased view on that.

Did you meet up with Jim Olds at any point?

No, he died shortly after his work on the reward centres in the brain. That was one of the seminal discoveries in the whole of neuroscience. Had he lived I'm sure he would have been a candidate for a Nobel Prize. Here I am contradicting myself because that was behavioural pharmacology. But I'm sure it was completely unexpected. Insofar as one can get it from the history they were just feeling around in the brain, putting in these probes to see how animals responded without any idea that there would be this systematic division between reinforcement and punishment. That's the way so many discoveries are made.

I didn't think I would pursue a career in psychopharmacology. I would have bet that it would have been in hypertension. Sometimes I wonder which would have been better. By and large we can treat hypertension somewhat better than we can mental disorders as well as having a better idea of the pathogenesis. But it's not all that different. I think the interesting thing about being in psychopharmacology has been the multidisciplinary nature of the field and the fact that we are dealing with an extraordinarily complicated mechanism compared to what causes your blood pressure to elevate. What causes the brain to go awry is much more complex. So I don't think we need to hang our heads.

A book published in 1954 called *American Medical Research At Mid-Century* reviewed progress in 10 major public health problems, including schizophrenia. After comparing progress in schizophrenia to progress in other areas my conclusion is that schizophrenia isn't all that far behind. It has been an exciting 50 years but I expect in another 50 years people will consider our current approach primitive. But that is the nature of science.

Let me float this past you. In the case of hypertension, there was a study from Newcastle about 14 years ago which showed that from the point of view of the physician treating hypertension treatments worked awfully well – blood pressure fell – but the patients were not so happy because they were not clearly aware of any subjective improvement in how they were feeling and quite a few felt worse. But from the point of view of the relatives treatment was a disaster because the patient had been converted into a hypochondriac and they had symptoms that they never had before. Does that apply to psychopharmacology?

No, I don't think so. The paradox about hypertension is that it has no symptoms. You can have fairly severe hypertension, which puts you at risk for a myocardial infarction or stroke, and never know it. Furthermore hypertension is absurdly simple to diagnose. Unfortunately many of these drugs that we use to treat hypertension produce side-effects, so a patient who is feeling pretty good starts on these drugs and they develop new symptoms that they don't particularly relish. Nevertheless the complications of hypertension have been enormously reduced over the years due to the fact that we do have effective treatment. It is hard to think these days that there is any kind of hypertension that could not be managed by drugs. When I was younger we used to have people with malignant hypertension whose life expectancy was measured in months. But you hardly ever see those patients any more. We don't have any less hypertension than before, nor do we have any less schizophrenia, but we can treat both of them better.

What role did Gerald Klerman have in the field?

I first ran into Gerry when he was a Fellow at Jonathan Cole's Psychopharmacology Service Center while they were planning the first NIMH collaborative study on schizophrenia. Gerry was very sharp, very much with it on the development of the study. He probably had more influence than any other single individual on the form that it ultimately took. Gerry had an amazing good humour about him – he could always tell some joke or find something to laugh about. He also had a facility for a good phrase – such as 'Pharmaceutical Calvinism'. We were in Geneva a few years ago at a panic disorder meeting and somebody mentioned that term without giving it an attribution. I told Gerry that this place might be the most appropriate to use that term, but I objected that he was not given the credit for the statement.

I was sorry to see him get so disabled in the latter years of his life. His diabetes caused a lot of complications so that in the last two or three years of his life he had to get around in a wheelchair. Despite that he travelled all over the world. His second wife, Myrna Weissman, was an angel so far as he was concerned. When he died I wrote Myrna and told her how much I admired what she had done for him, because without her I don't think he would have been anywhere near as productive as he was. The other gratifying experience in this field is that over the years you meet so many bright nice people – people you admire, people you value as personal friends and sometimes who have an influence on broadening your own perspective. Gerry is just one of many that I can think of.

Anyone else you want to include there as the people who have influenced you?

I have always had a tremendous amount of respect for Arvid Carlsson. We were at a reception a couple of nights ago and I told Arvid that a few years ago I had a chance to nominate somebody for the Japan prize and I nominated him. He said, 'Gee, that is maybe why I got it.' I thought he was kidding. The next day Brian Leonard introduced him for a Guest Lecture and said that he had won it. I was dumbfounded because I would have congratulated him the night before if I'd taken his statement seriously. Arvid has been an enormously fertile thinker. I have always said his genius was that he knows just how far beyond his data he can extrapolate to come up with novel ideas. Another genius is Paul Janssen. Janssen has been a genius in business as well as in science. I had a chance to nominate some people for the Nobel Prize for several years running. One of my nominations was a trio of Black, George Hitchings and Paul Janssen for developing drugs, each one with a different approach. Hitchings used them as antimetabolites, Black used homologues for receptors, and Janssen exploited structure–activity relationships. Well, those two won it and Paul didn't. Paul is one of the richest men in Belgium, which probably turned the Nobel committee off, because the theory behind the Nobel Prize is that it is to help people who need help. Paul certainly didn't need help financially. He is a very modest man, very congenial and very bright. I could go on and on but those are two of the giants in the field.

I got to know Julius Axelrod tangentially. I never worked in his lab but I knew a lot of people who had. I knew Bernard Brodie, whose heart must have been broken when Julius got the prize and he didn't. I remember a pharmacologist friend of mine came up one morning and said, 'Guess who won the Nobel Prize?' I said, 'von Euler, Sutherland and Brodie.' He said, 'You're close: von Euler, Katz and Axelrod.' I said, 'Oh my God, Brodie must be shaken to his core.' But they were virtually equal. Very pioneering in their work. Brodie was the founder of biochemical pharmacology. But these were the top dogs in the field. There are many many others who aren't that prestigious but who also had very good ideas and were quite influential.

Anyone else who stands out for you?

Frank Ayd is one. He and I became acquainted early in the game and have long been friends. My favourite story about Frank concerns the Christmas cards he sent while he was resident at the Vatican. One Christmas, my secretary after sorting out the mail said, 'You have a card from the Vatican.' I replied, 'No doubt that's from Frank Ayd and if it isn't a signed photograph of the Pope I'll be disappointed.' It turned out not to be – merely an appropriate Christmas card. The following summer in 1964, while attending the CINP meeting in Birmingham, I lunched with Frank and told him the story. He remained rather non-committal. The following Christmas another card arrived, somewhat different from the previous one. It was a photograph of Frank, his wife and 12 of their 14 children with Pope Paul. Talk about one-upmanship. I think my second son still has the photograph.

I have on occasion co-authored papers with persons who, though great in their own fields, were not close colleagues. These came about because of my belief that one paper on a subject is better than two. For instance, in the early 1960s, there was flurry of excitement about a 'pink spot' in the urine of schizophrenics. As it turned out to be a compound closely related chemically to mescaline, the thought was that this represented the residue of some endogenous psychotogen. Arnie Friedhoff had been investigating it in animals but I decided to see what it would do in humans. I was the first human to take it. It did nothing to me or subsequent volunteers, it turned out, given in progressively higher doses. Arnie found that it was immediately metabolised, accounting for its inactivity. Arnie and I published jointly two papers: one on the clinical activity of the compound and the other on the reasons for it. Nearly at the same time, there were implications that alpha-methyltyrosine, a specific blocker of tyrosine hydroxylase, might be useful in treating schizophrenia. We found it not to be so and so did Sam Gershon, who was working with it at the same time. Our studies were halted prematurely because dogs formed renal stones when given the drug – they have highly alkaline urine. So Sam and I decided to combine our two incomplete studies and publish together. I commented elsewhere on the impromptu collaboration with Sol Snyder. One would think that these collaborations would be encouraged, especially in this day of universal and rapid communications.

One of my greatest regrets is that I did not leave a greater legacy of students. Only two have become major successes. Ken Davis returned to his Alma Mater, Mt Sinai, and turned it from a backwater into a major department of psychiatry in the US. John Csernansky was offered an endowed Chair at Washington University. I have no doubt that both would have succeeded without me. Perhaps the most a mentor can do is to provide encouragement and support early in the careers of rising students.

How does the field look after 35 years?

I must confess it is frustrating because the rate of progress has been so rapid with the neurosciences in the last 15–20 years. We have a totally new vocabulary spawned by molecular pharmacology and molecular biology – it's almost impossible for any individual to keep up with it. Much of the programme at an ACNP or CINP meeting these days, perhaps 80%, would be as appropriate at the Society for Neuroscience. The promises of this new knowledge are so important in allowing us to have a fundamental understanding of mental disorders and the rationale for using drugs that nobody can short-change the possibility that we will soon have very selective drugs for these disorders, in contrast to the non-selective and accidentally discovered drugs we had in the past.

But on that score the evidence of the last 35 years is somewhat discouraging. The difference between not having chlorpromazine and having it was enormous. The difference between having chlorpromazine and risperidone, clozapine or olanzapine is not that great. There is a lot of hype now about the new drugs for depression and schizophrenia. But if you look at them from a historical point of view they don't represent a benchmark advance. I have only been present in three medical miracles – in my internship I had a patient with bacterial endocarditis who was one of the first treated with adequate doses of penicillin. She survived an otherwise totally fatal illness. The second one was having a patient wheelchair-bound from rheumatoid arthritis being able within a week to walk around the ward after getting corticosteroids. Though corticosteroids are not now the treatment of choice, they certainly had a tremendous impact. The third was the marked changes seen in schizophrenic patients with the antipsychotic drugs.

I don't think we have reached another point that is as sharp as not having chlorpromazine and reserpine and having them. Risperidone may have less side-effects but there is a very very narrow margin between the therapeutic dose and the dose that will produce extrapyramidal reactions. Clozapine perhaps over the long pull has some effect on re-socialisation and of course it works for many patients who don't respond to traditional drugs but that's always been the case – every time you get a new drug you find people who respond that did not respond to something before. And as far as the atypicality of the profiles I am not quite sure what all this means. Nobody has ever been able to claim that a D1 receptor antagonism has anything to do with schizophrenia and the purest $5HT_2$ antagonist, ritanserin, has been of little use in schizophrenia. So it is pretty hard to believe that D1 or serotonin receptors are all that important in the action of atypical antipsychotics.

You're saying the neuroscience has advanced but the therapy hasn't?

No, I don't think the therapy has and in that sense that's perhaps why the balance of the programme for these societies has moved more in the direction of neuroscience than clinical science because there is nothing so terribly new coming along clinically. Thirty-five years ago before anybody was sure how to study these drugs John Overall and I were trying controlled trials and objective measurements of change and so on. He provided many novel statistical analyses. You had some feeling of contributing something but these days that's all old hat. Every drug company has its staff that will produce an excellent protocol that will fly through the regulatory agencies. They have the statistical help in-house to process the data. They farm it out to some professional writing house to write up the manuscript. So these days the clinical investigator is relegated to data gathering, which is a dull enterprise, if you ask me. We really ought to be more experimental in trying to break out of the traditional parallel group double-blind design which 35 years ago was news but is news no longer and find ways that may be more expeditious and cheaper to screen these drugs and get them on the market.

Select bibliography
Hollister LE, Krieger GE, Kringel A, Roberts RH (1955). Treatment of schizophrenic reactions with reserpine. *Annals of the New York Academy of Science*, **61**, 92–100.

Hollister LE, Traub L, Beckman WG (1956). Psychiatric use of reserpine and chlorpromazine: results of double-blind studies. In *Psychopharmacology*, (N Kline ed). American Association for the Advancement of Science, Washington, DC, pp 66–75.

Hollister LE, Motzenbecker FP, Degan RO (1961). Withdrawal reactions from chlordiazepoxide (librium). *Psychopharmacologia*, **2**, 63–68.

Hollister LE, Degan RO, Schultz SD (1962). An experimental approach to facilitation of psychotherapy by psychotomimetic drugs. *Journal of Mental Science*, **108**, 99–100.

Hollister LE (1986). Health aspects of cannabis. *Pharmacological Reviews*, 38–220.

11 Michael Shepherd

Psychopharmacology: specific and non-specific

You were in the US in 1956, just after your reserpine trial was published, just when things were beginning to roll psychopharmacologically speaking. How did the field look to you then? Were you at the Conference on the Evaluation of Psychotropic Drugs in 1956?

Well, I can tell you what happened. I was working at the time at Johns Hopkins. I was on a postgraduate fellowship in the School of Public Health. Because of my other interests I had made contact with a lot of people in the States and one was of them was Louis Lasagna, who was really the driving force behind clinical pharmacology. He was familiar with some of the work that I had been doing and was still doing. He was the editor, at the time, of *Journal of Chronic Diseases* and he was also a very nice man. Clinical pharmacology is a very curious subject. You are squeezed between the God-like figures of medicine who believe they know all about treatment and the pure pharmacologists who are only interested in receptors and so on. You need to have a certain element of determination and he had it.

He and I got on very well and it was he, I think, who first told me about this conference. There was set up, in Washington, a Steering Committee of quite important people – Seymour Kety was one and Ralph Gerard, Joe Brady, the experimental psychologist, and Lasagna. The Secretary was Jonathan Cole, who at that time was a public health employee of the US Public Health Service. He proved to be very efficient as a manager. I was invited to sit in on the planning discussions. I used to go to Washington every month and these rather high-powered people would come together and they actually planned the structure of the conference. By virtue of the fact that I was there, I participated. From time to time they would ask me about somebody or some point of view. So I had a ringside seat at that conference, which was the first major national conference in the area.

It also set the seal of academic respectability on this subject. You see in the States at that time there were a number of mavericks. People like the late Nathan Kline. They were pressing for the mass introduction of psychotropic drugs everywhere. It was about that time that the Brill and Paton paper was published from New York State, in effect initiating the era of de-institutionalisation but attributing it to the mass introduction of drugs, which of course was meat and drink to the pharmaceutical industry. I think that these hard-headed scientifically inclined people, who came from several disciplines – they weren't by any means only psychiatrists – had become aware of the need to begin to take a hard look. That was the first overall attempt to look at the issues within the United States. I suppose I played a minuscule part by just knowing the people and being able to discuss some of the matters. Of course, in the process I did form contacts with many of them which were very helpful later on.

You'd run the reserpine trial before that? Was that the first properly run randomised double-blind study in psychiatry or was Mogen Schou's lithium study which reported in 1954 or Joel Elkes' study the first?

The truth of the matter is Charmian Elkes should have had the credit for that study. She actually did the planning. I was involved with two studies. One was the reserpine study, that you mention ...

How did that come about? The subsequent history of reserpine is, of course, that people become depressed immediately on it and throw themselves out of windows but ... the results of your study were entirely the opposite. How did that actually come about and how do you account for the fact that it has vanished without trace?

Those are two separate questions. I'll try to answer the first because I was involved. The answer to the second question raises the question of why some studies last and others don't when there's no essential difference between them. I don't think it has anything to do with the quality of the study, it has to do with the receptivity of the scientific and medical community at a point in time.

As far as the first question goes, what had happened was that I was a senior registrar at the Maudsley Hospital, on the Professorial Unit. The drug industry was just becoming alert to the possibilities of something quite new in psychiatry. They were bombarding, on a very small scale compared with what we now have, people in the teaching hospitals to peddle their wares. They sent material to Aubrey Lewis. I don't think they realised quite who he was. I think we had a patient who in some way had either taken reserpine or was taking reserpine and, talking to him at the time I raised the question how difficult it would be to know, whether if we did give this patient reserpine, there would be any difference. And he said, 'Well, have you seen all this stuff?' which had come through the mail, which I hadn't.

When we talked about it it was clear that the whole question of the clinical evaluation of treatment was appallingly low in psychiatry. It was one of those areas that it's difficult now to realise how primitive it was. To give you an idea of how appalling it was, people took William Sargant seriously. In discussing this with Aubrey Lewis, who was very closely involved with the MRC, we naturally got on to the whole business of the clinical trial – Bradford Hill and so on. During the discussion I remember saying, well, intrinsically there is no reason why we shouldn't try and do this and he produced some material from, I think, the New York Academy of Sciences, which was written by a well-known bio-statistician, I think Mainland or some such name, and out of that came the idea of trying to see how far you could, at a very simple level, apply these principles to a psychiatric issue. I now realise I couldn't possibly have chosen a more difficult group ... the idea of taking anxious depressed outpatients makes one shudder because one now knows how difficult it is to construct criteria and refine them and measure them, which are essential.

At the same time I did another controlled trial in chronic schizophrenia with David Watt. Now that was much easier in many respects because you were dealing with a relatively homogeneous population of inpatients. And although I wouldn't compare them with tuberculosis or rheumatoid arthritis, in terms of the measurements, the principles were much more easily applied. I think the value of these things in retrospect was simply to show that you could do it. This was doing it with no money. We had no money from the industry, we did it ourselves. That meant the co-operation of the nurses, a lot of hard work in collecting the questionnaires and doing the statistics. I certainly learnt an enormous amount about the problems that arise, which stood me in very good stead later on and I suppose historically they certainly do have some value, simply because they were so early. There's nothing especially original about that in itself but it did draw the attention of people who were more academically inclined to the need for this and it stimulated the pharmaceutical industry. I had a lot to do with the industry at that time and they were very aware of the importance of this sort of thing for the large programmes that they were preparing then for new drugs in the future. So I would have thought that it made a modest contribution to the subject at the time.

In terms of trying to parcel out which came first – were you aware of any other trials being run before that within psychiatry? Linford Rees was doing some controlled trials on desoxycortisone and things like that. Did he influence you at all?

No, not at all no. I didn't regard them as meeting the criteria that I felt had been laid down by the people who were responsible for the model clinical trials which had been applied in somatic medicine. You bring back these distant memories. When I started working with reserpine, I had to familiarise myself of course with what was going on. A lot of it was in the field of hypertension. The psychiatric side was very subsidiary. There had been a meeting at the New York Academy of Sciences in which Nate Kline, as always, played a prominent part and I went to him and he sent me everything. I think it was Ciba who was producing reserpine and he had access to the unpublished material. There wasn't anything. I was looking for some sort of predecessor on which I could base our own study and there was nothing that was available.

You actually used placebo, didn't you, which the original Bradford Hill trial hadn't? So the idea of using a placebo was new.

I think placebos had just come in later on after the early MRC studies.

Harry Gold hadn't been doing an RCT but he had been using placebo. Was there anyone else?

Well, I wrote a little thing about the placebo recently. That was a very interesting experience itself. When I read that paper, which was about 3 years ago, the

Chairman of the session was Louis Lasagna, now the distinguished Dean of Tuft's University and of course one of the original collaborators with Harry Beecher on the work that really put the placebo on the scientific map, although it's had to battle to stay there. It was very interesting because I read this paper to a virtually all-American audience and as you may know the Americans are not modest at question time – there are no polite this, that and the other. When I finished he, as the Chairman, said, 'This paper is now open for questions.' Nothing happened. Half a minute elapsed, a minute elapsed and nobody said anything at all. Lasagna then said in his characteristic way that in the circumstances we would have to move on to the next paper but he couldn't refrain from commenting on this unnatural silence. 'There are three possible explanations' he said. 'First you were all asleep and therefore you heard nothing. Secondly it was so bad that since this speaker has come 3000 miles you didn't want to embarrass him. Third it is genuinely so original and new that you don't quite know what sense to make of it. I'll leave you to decide which it was.' Afterwards we had dinner together. He confirmed, because he's a man who knew all about it, that this whole area of the placebo is totally neglected. Did you know about Beecher?

No.

Oh, I can tell you about Beecher because that's highly relevant. He was Professor of Anesthetics at Harvard. He was a footballer. I think he played American football for Harvard. Now that puts you in the first division as far as American life is concerned. He was a powerfully built solid character, very much in the mainstream of medicine. During the war he was in charge of a base hospital when the Americans were fighting the Japanese in one of the Pacific islands. There was a terrible battle going on and the casualties were coming in and emergency surgery was going on 24 hours a day and they ran out of morphia. Well this, of course, is a disaster because they were in shock and pain and you couldn't operate. The story, as I recall it, was that accidentally one of the nurses gave an injection of still water and the patient came out of shock and lost his pain. And Beecher, who was an extremely observant clinical scientist, was struck forcibly by this observation which was repeated. I think for a time they had to use distilled water because the supplies were not coming in.

This was a sort of Pauline conversion as far as he was concerned because he was very much a bread and butter physical doctor and when he came out of the services he decided to study the placebo. Lasagna was one of the group that worked with him in his laboratory. He had psychologists, physiologists, pharmacologists, clinicians and so on. Because of his reputation they all had good positions. He wrote a paper which was very influential in *JAMA*, called the Powerful Placebo in the mid-1950s. There was then the beginnings of a serious interest in the placebo, not as the bit that gets left behind, but as something you really must take in its own right.

The moment he retired the group broke up. I knew several of them. Some of them worked at Hopkins. I remember talking to them one evening and what they said was, 'Well, it was all right as long as Harry was there because he looked after us. But if you want a career in American medicine it's better not to study the placebo, its not really a topic that is popular with anybody.' They all drifted into different areas, in the process neglecting the basic work that had been done. And if you look at Goodman and Gillman, 2500 pages, you find four or five paragraphs on the placebo. It's chalk that you give because irritatingly about 30% of people do get better on it in clinical trials but they pay no regard to the fact that underlying the whole issue of the placebo is the crucial issue which I tried to bring out in my paper on specificity in medicine, specificity of action. The idea that the disease is due to a specific agent which can be counteracted by a specific substance which eliminates the toxic features.

On that basis which is really Claude Bernard's basis for experimental medicine, the whole of the natural science approach to medicine is constructed and it's quite wrong, not in itself but because it's so limited. It cuts out the non-specific factors which are in fact at least 50% and probably more in the aetiology of disease and of treatment and among them is the placebo and the nocebo, both of which are extremely powerful.

When you come to psychiatry, where the bacterial model, which is really what underlies this, is largely inapplicable, you find that the non-specific component of both causation and treatment gets bigger and bigger. This is where all the rubbish about psychotherapy, social treatment and alternative medicine comes in – this is all non-specific blah, some of which may be empirically valuable but you can't tease it out if you begin with the assumption that your only aim is to look at specificity. It all gets obfuscated. So you have psychiatry virtually shattered by pointless discussions – are you a psychotherapist or are you a physical doctor and all this nonsense that goes on. If you shift the ground of the argument to say we are actually talking about degrees of specificity and non-specificity which have to be given operational meaning and then evaluated, in just the same way that you would penicillin or anything of that sort, then things become scientific. We don't have many answers but at least you can approach it.

My personal view has always been that there should be a Chair of Placebology which I think would save the National Health Service huge sums of money. It would improve medical education and it would take all these factors into account and give them their correct weighting. Whereas, as you know, so much in medical schools and medical practice is hopelessly weighted in favour of this quest for specificity.

Do you not think though that the introduction of drug treatments as we've had them has worked heavily against that model? With DSM-III and DSM-IV we're heading towards a psychiatry that's dominated by a categorical model of disorders and the industry invites us to line up and provide magic bullets to hit particular targets.

We are now moving into a much broader area because it concerns treatment, and treatment is what doctors are supposed to be concerned with. As far as psychiatry goes my own feeling is equivocal on this. I gave a talk about Kraepelin recently, who is really the representative of all this in psychiatry. This is where psychiatry went down the wrong road completely. There was a misapplication of natural science. Not that there's anything wrong with using natural science, of course, that is one of the most important areas of conceptual thinking. But the assumption that natural science is it, ignores all philosophy. It ignores subjectivity. You can't put subjectivity into the natural science model – you dismiss it. Psychology is Wundt and Wundt is animals and twitching and what is psychopharmacology – it's updated Wundt's pharmacopsychology, which is where Kraepelin cut his teeth. And what did they do, they measured work curves, tapping and so on. This would now be regarded as physiological psychology and it's fine. There's absolutely nothing wrong with it. But when you say that this is a model that you use for studying bereavement or anxiety states or something of that sort, there's a gap which is only bridged if you assume that you can extend the natural science model to encorporate everything else.

Kraepelin is responsible for this. I don't mean Kraepelin personally, he was merely the representative. And Kraepelin was a fascist – the whole subsequent development of the genocidal racial hygiene policies in Germany stem from this. His successor was a member of the SS. So one could actually see if you look at the facts, which have been very carefully obfuscated, that psychiatry took the wrong road and is still taking the wrong road. It's got a much wider aura, this question, than just what drugs you give for what patients. It underlines a whole attitude to the subject and it's been woefully misrepresented, which I think is a pity.

Talking about Kraepelin naturally brings Adolf Meyer to mind. Was he still at Johns Hopkins when you were there?

No, he wasn't. Mrs Meyer was there. He had died. I was doing some work on a completely different subject, a clinical subject, and I went to the library at Hopkins where I was confronted with large numbers of dusty volumes. The librarian told me that these were some of Dr Meyer's volumes but they were only a small number and if I got in touch with Mrs Meyer, who lived in Baltimore, I would get more. So I got to know her. I used to go out and spend long periods in his library. I learnt about Adolf Meyer through his library, just as years later, when I brought Willy Mayer-Gross' library here, I spent 2 days in his house in Birmingham looking at his library. You get to know a person when they've got 5000 books and you see them.

Meyer's trouble was that he was stranded between the English and German languages. He could not express himself. If you read his papers, they're extremely difficult to follow but he was a vastly erudite man. When Kraepelin first produced the fifth edition of his textbook, Meyer invited him to Baltimore and wrote a review in glowing terms saying, 'This is an advance. This is a man who has actually given some order to the chaos of clinical psychiatry.' But 15 years later Meyer wrote a review of Kraepelin's contribution which is really very interesting. It gives him all credit for what he did and then points out how hopelessly inadequate it was. But because Meyer wasn't a polemicist who would rush around and make a fuss, I think his views were accepted as those of a distinguished person but when he retired he was swept away by other forces.

His understanding of the situation actually was best represented by people like Aubrey Lewis who took over this broad psychobiological standpoint and tried to put it into practice. Meyer himself, I think, was so hopelessly handicapped by his inadequate mastery of the English language that he didn't really make these points clearly enough but he appreciated what was going on.

Let me take you back to one of the other trials in this period which used something of a randomised design and also placebo – Mogen Schou's first study with lithium. You obviously weren't aware of that while it was happening but it appeared in 1954. I'm trying to chase where the idea of the randomised trial came into psychiatry from. As I say, there's probably about four people we need to look at. There was yourself, Linford Rees, Joel Elkes and Mogens Schou.

I was aware of Schou's study. I was aware of most things going on at the time. Yes, I suppose they were for quite different reasons all moving in the same direction. If you take the general view that after all what determines what goes on is events and the climate of opinion rather than some shattering individual that sees through it all, this sort of thing was probably in the air and it was a question of who and how it would be introduced. If you take just those four people, I don't know if there are any more, but if you just take Schou, he went through the motions and then in effect said, 'You don't need this, it's evident, I know.' Rees never really focused on just one thing.

I think I became more and more convinced that this was a fundamental axiom in the way you look at the theory and practice of psychiatry. How you applied it was another matter. I was reinforced in that view when the MRC Clinical Trials Committee was set up because then I spent nearly 20 years in close collaboration with Bradford Hill, which was an unforgettable experience. He was a most remarkable man.

Why do you say that?

Well, I'll tell you a little story. When the Clinical Trials Sub-Committee was set up – this itself caused a little flutter in Park Crescent – the MRC, what were they doing with all this strange stuff? But George Pickering, who was very influential, was Regius Professor of Medicine at Oxford and he gave the blessing. He had worked a little bit with Bradford Hill and Doll, of course. So they set up this Committee with Bradford Hill as the Chairman and I was the Secretary. Bradford Hill was not medically qualified but he had been born and bred into medicine, he thought like a doctor and knew a great deal about the medical profession. I had only met him two or three times. He was a very charming man.

It was suggested that if we were going to mount a trial we had to soften up opinion. This is the way the Council thinks. One of the things that was decided was that it would be a useful thing to have a group of eminent senior psychiatrists, professors and mental hospital superintendents come along to the Council for a morning, have coffee and biscuits and be asked what they thought of clinical trials and the possibility of evaluating this. I was merely the Secretary, so Bradford Hill did all the talking. The assembly arrived and there were about 10 of them. You could imagine who – they were the people at the time. They were all asked their opinion and they virtually all said the same thing which is that, of course in theory, clinical trials must be supported, after all it's science, but this doesn't replace real clinical knowledge. I mean the bed-side manner, the understanding, the experience – in my unit I always teach that, etc., etc. Well, one after the other said this and Bradford Hill was polite-ness itself. He just nodded and so on. I suppose they were there for about 2 hours and as the door closed on the last of them he and I were left alone. There was a sort of silence and I remember, we were sitting at opposite sides of the table, and he suddenly looked at me and said, 'We're going to have trouble with this bunch' and I realised that he was spot on. He knew exactly who he was dealing with.

He always said he didn't understand sums. He had difficulty in multiplying things and so on. He wasn't a high-powered statistician. But he had a feel for what was going on. He and I spent a long time talking about the design of the 1965 multi-centred trial. I was very impressed by the speed with which he picked up the issues. He knew nothing about psychiatry. He had been asked by the Council to come in because you couldn't trust … psychiatrists … so you had a Professor of Medicine and a Professor of Biostatistics and a young nobody, myself, there for the ride just to keep the show on the road. But he understood, in a way that Pickering never did, what the problems were.

He was fascinated by the issue of how you measured subjective phenome-na. If a chap says 'I'm depressed' you can't break that down to some physio-logical correlate and assume that this is the core of the disease. For him this posed a real problem and I was very impressed with the speed with which he grasped the situation, the way in which he helped to design a realistic study and then in the analysis of the data and the discussion of its implications how he brought to bear his vast experience in other fields of medicine to make sense of what we'd done. I've never come across anybody who has been able to do it quite as efficiently as that. Right up to the end of his life, he was as sharp as a needle, and he was courteous and helpful and in every way a pleasure to work with, and you can't say that about everybody.

One of the offshoots of the RCT has been the current craze for evidence-based medicine, which stems from the Archie Cochrane book I guess – the idea that if only we were to restrict ourselves to procedures which were demonstrably effective then we wouldn't be wasting all the money in the health services that we are wasting and we wouldn't be doing some of the awful things to patients that we are doing.

We would also, of course, never make any advances because all advances depend on guesses which we call hypotheses – most of which are wrong but some of which are right. In terms of the logic of the scientific process the evi-dence comes after the hypothesis. You must begin with a hypothesis and that is a guess. I knew Cochrane but this again is pushing the thing to, I think, an absurb extreme. Of course, it's true that the whole discipline is cluttered up with procedures for which the evidence is meagre at best and there is a case for trying to make quite certain that that is minimised. If that's what is meant by it – certainly – but it eventually stiffles everything else.

I was talking to somebody about this just the other day. If you take what I suppose is the biggest issue in medicine at the moment, which is the AIDS pandemic, there's an enormous amount known about AIDS. There's an enormous amount of stuff which calls for tidying up, not least the psychiatric aspects of AIDS, but the biological advances in AIDS don't have any evidence yet. You've got to pursue the matter with guesses and experiments and research and so on. Sticking to the available evidence at the moment simply leaves us in a static situation and I think that's true of most forms of mental disease as well. The value of this evidence-based medicine is as a method of thinking. If you could really get into medical schools this notion it would help considerably to improve the intellectual calibre of practising doctors. I think there's a strong case for every medical student to be very familiar with one well-conducted clinical trial, or even participate in one if possible. If that's evidence-based medicine I agree, but its role is limited.

One of the concerns that I would have with it is I think most of the evidence today is generated by the pharmaceutical industry so this becomes means for the industry to take over larger chunks of the health care. But on that score, the MRC study in 1965 was fairly independent. I think by virtue of its independence and the eminence of the people involved, it had a huge impact, but did you get the dose of phenelzine wrong?

You have to choose a dose and the dose was chosen on the best evidence that was available at the time. This, of course, is an issue with every clinical trial. If you ask questions at that level I think everybody concerned would say, well, of course we should have done another study with another dose. And when we get evidence-based medicine widely accepted no doubt that sort of thing will be feasible. But you have to put these things in their social context – you have to realise what an extraordinary event it was to have done that trial at all and in that climate of opinion.

Imagine this for the moment: I told you roughly what happened with the 10 dignitaries. We then had the 40 or 50 people who were going to fill in forms and they were summoned I think, rather than invited, to the MRC headquarters from mental hospitals all over the country and they were herded into one of the rooms. George Pickering came in and made a speech. What he actually said to them was, 'I want you to understand that you are privileged to participate in an MRC study. It's going to be a lot of work for you and you're not going to be paid and we expect a high standard but do remember that this is an honour.' And they took it. I remember sitting and thinking surely somebody is going to have the guts to get up and say, 'Who do you think you're talking to?', which is what would happen now. Because all these people now would be paid by the industry to do trials for money. It didn't exist at the time. You couldn't repeat that trial. Because what has really happened is, as you said, the industry is taking over the profession. Money is drying up from every other source. It's being done subtly, it's being done sometimes even benefically but in the long run it's disastrous because it's being done for the shareholders in the industry – it has to be. And therefore a study like that one which was absolutely independent simply couldn't be done now.

It's odd because one thinks of this country as having a socialised medical system and the US system has been market driven but the NIMH really has done some fairly independent studies to its credit.

But I can tell you – we used to have Steering Committees for this multi-centre trial and Jonathan Cole, who I mentioned earlier, had recruited an assistant, Gerry Klerman, which is how his career began, and he wrote and came over from Washington to sit in on our discussions on how this was going. Many of the NIMH-funded studies were actually modelled on the original MRC study. Then their system of course made it in some cases easier and some cases more difficult to introduce studies on a large scale.

The MRC study reported in 1965 but you must, presumably, have been actually planning it from ...

From 1960. It was a huge undertaking. We recruited the first patients, I should think, in 1962. I am speaking from memory.

What about Klerman?

When I gave this lecture on the placebo that I mentioned, which was in New York, it was at the invitation of, I think, the American Psychosomatic Society. I had made arrangements to go just for 3 days or so to give this talk and see one or two people. I got a telephone call from Klerman a couple of weeks before saying that he'd heard that I was going to be in New York and he would very much like, because I hadn't seen him for some time, to meet as he had one or two suggestions, if I could stay on for a couple days. So I agreed.

When I got there, I went to Cornell to have lunch with him and I was absolutely horrified. I hadn't seen him for 3 years. He was in a wheelchair, he was dying. He looked absolutely appalling. I didn't know anything about his illnesses and so on. But his attitude was unchanged. He had just been to Japan and he was planning a trip to Europe and wherever he went there were ambulances and dialysis machines and goodness knows what. He was a highly intelligent and what the Americans call an abrasive character but he learnt from his mistakes. Ever since I have known him, which was when he was Jonathan Cole's assistant, I think it was perfectly clear that I represented something quite different from him, which in one sense annoyed him but on the other hand made him want to try and grasp it. What he suggested at this meeting was two days later for me to go out to the Westchester division of Cornell and not give a lecture but for he and I just to sit together in front of an audience and argue. I think he really wanted to learn more about some of the issues that troubled him, by rubbing off against somebody whom I think he repected in spite of himself.

I agreed to this but 24 hours later he was dead. He collapsed and was admitted to hospital. I remember I was flying back on the Sunday evening and his wife, Myrna Weissman, who I also knew well, phoned me and said that his funeral was going to be on the Sunday morning and she asked me to attend if I could. Well, I had a plane to catch and I had, in fact, to go directly from the funeral parlour straight to the airport but I felt that was the least I could do. It was very instructive because they had rustled up half a dozen people, quite apart from all his colleagues. The Director of the NIMH, Danny Friedman, flew out from Los Angeles. David Hamburg was there. Leon Eisenberg came from Harvard and they all gave these speeches. They don't do that here and it was really quite touching. There was a sort of rugged honesty about him and he admitted when he was wrong, which is not all that common.

There's no doubt that he played a very considerable part in the NIMH studies as the Director of ADAMHA. He had administrative skills and he was a shrewd operator. He got involved, as you may know, in the last year of his life with this business of the case of psychotherapy in which he really went ...

The Osheroff case.

Yes, He didn't pull his punches. On the sad occasion that we met for the last time he was just beginning to tell me some of the background and how disillusioned he was as to how many of his colleagues, when it came to the point, did not back him up. He wasn't afraid of sticking his neck out and you have to respect people like that. There aren't all that many in his position who would have done that sort of thing. So I had a soft spot for him.

Do you think he was right to stick his neck out on the Osheroff case the way he did?

Yes. I think somebody had to, just to sharpen the issues. A lot of people in his position would have muttered and said, 'Well, these things go on' but he was uninhibited when it came to that sort of thing and I respected him for it. So he undoubtedly played a considerable part. On the other hand he swallowed that whole business about panic disorders and alprazolam.

Yes, but do you think the agenda there really was he wasn't so much interested in perhaps panic disorder or alprazolam per se as in how much the DSM-III formulations could be internationalised?

Well, that was one factor. But you see this comes back to another fundamental divergence of opinion. The DSM system, whatever you think about it, and I don't think personally very highly of it, which has the impertinence to call itself atheoretical, is essentially an attempt to standardise Kraepelinian categories. Klerman called himself, as you know, a neo-Kraepelinian, and wrote about the neo-Kraepelinian movement. About a year ago, in the *American Journal of Psychiatry* you know, they have a thing called Images in Psychiatry and Nancy Andreasen, whom I also know well and who is now the editor, herself, wrote the piece about Kraepelin. I was in correspondence with her about something altogether different and this thing arrived, so more or less as a postscript I said I was very sad to see that you've turned this man into an icon. He was a monster who has done a great deal of harm. You're the editor of the journal, you're writing this for 50,000 people – you've wasted a generation or more knocking down Sigmund Freud and now you're just sticking Emil Kraepelin in his place. In the long run you're doing a disservice to the profession.

I got back a long letter saying: why do you say this, don't you realise this is science and after all the whole of the APA DSM system is based on neo-Kraepelinism. Of course this is true – you are dealing with a movement. Now Gerry Klerman was one of the key players. I think that if he and I had been together as you and I are now, and this issue had cropped up and I had said to him what I have just said to you, this would have generated an outburst of annoyance and a few personal comments and so on but he would have thought about it and maybe 6 months later he would have said, 'Well, you know I do see a little bit about.' You see he could do that.

But because he suffered from the disease of being American – we've all got our diseases, the Irish have their diseases, the English have their disease – the American disease is that you've got to be in the mode. You've got to be seen up there as being representative. And he was driven to be there, so he had his psycho-analytical phase and his psychopharmacological phase and then his Kraepelinian phase and so on, which broadly corresponded to what was going on in the States at that time. It's very difficult to buck the system because you then get frozen out. You don't fit in to any recognisable group and above all you don't get grants, which is what matters. So in a way he illustrates I think a general process but actually I liked him just as person.

There are extremely few people I think in the US of the period who were as broadly based as he was. He had a foot in all the camps really.

Yes. He had immense influence in the last 10 years of his life. He never stopped working and he was learning all the time, which again is unusual. Most people stop when they get to about 20. He didn't. He was extremely bright. One of the people who spoke at his funeral, apart from all these dignatories, was his longest extant friend who was in school with him. I found his address very interesting. He was well recognised as top of the class in everything and there's no doubt that he was a man of superior intelligence but something of a rough diamond as well. So that was really what I felt about him.

I'm sure you've been asked ad nauseam about the lithium controversy. Do you want to say anything about it?

I've told you a little bit about the way in which it seemed to me that clinical evaluation was a basic component of my idea of clinical practice. I had known Schou for years because we were members of the CINP and I was the vice-president or something glorious for a time and we used to meet at different places. On these occasions at CINP meetings there were always the big plenary sessions and so on and there was a little group of people who always talked at a symposium of their own, talking about the use of lithium and the treatment of mania. They were really no more than a dozen and nobody ever went to these symposia because they were largely dominated by biochemical measurement and mania was not regarded as a major issue. Schou was prominent among them because of his laboratory contributions to the work.

He was a genial man. He could be in the members' stand at Lords; he wears a blazer; he speaks perfect English; he has considerable charm, he's got this Danish humour and you know we had always got on very pleasantly but he always disappeared to these symposia on the treatment of mania and I never understood quite what was going on. Then what happened was that I was invited to Gottingen to a little meeting organised by the Chairman of the Department, who I knew quite well, and this was to the German psychiatric Group or whatever. There weren't many people and when I arrived there was Schou with his wife. We chatted away and we went into this room and I was asked to give a talk on something like the principles of clinical evaluation, some general topic, and all I did was to try to indicate really what the structure of a clinical trial was, what it could do, what it couldn't do, how little it had been applied to the study of mental disorder etc.

Then Schou got up and he was billed to talk about lithium in affective disorders. I expected to hear about mania and whatnot. But what I got for the first time was this view that lithium was everything, that it prevented the disease, that it treated the disease etc. I remember it very well because I was sitting at the back of the hall and one of the Germans wrote me a little note and he said, 'This man is contradicting everything you've just been saying.' As I listened I could see that this was absolutely true. I remember also thinking, 'I hope to heaven that I'm not asked to participate in the discussion.' I tried to make myself as inconspicuous as ... but of course I was asked as a guest. I tried as gently as I possibly could to indicate that this was not good enough on the evidence which had been presented. It might or might not be true, but it wasn't good enough.

This would be 1961, 1962, 1963?

It would be about 1962. I tried to be as tactful as I could and said, 'No doubt the figures will show etc.' Afterwards Mrs Schou took me aside and said, 'You know, you were very severe and you've upset Mogens very much.' I said, 'Well, what have I done?' and she said, 'You've implied that what he was saying was doubtful and that more evidence was needed' and I said, 'Well, surely that is the case', still not fully realising. Then he came and joined us and I can remember it very clearly. I realised that I was in the presence of a believer – somebody who knew. There were a lot of them about in most fields. I hadn't realised this because I didn't go to the symposia on mania and lithium. He told me that a relative had been ill and that he was taking it and that really there ought to be a national policy in which everybody could get lithium. Because he has this jovial manner I wasn't altogether certain that he was serious but then I realised he was.

In order to try and mollify him I said, 'Well, obviously you've done this study, if I can help in any way send me the manuscript and I'll make what comments I can.' So he did send me the manuscript. I took a bit of trouble and made a number of suggestions. What then happened was the paper was published encorporating my suggestions but twisting them. It gave the impression that he had taken account of all these factors and after due deliberation had decided on scientific grounds that this was so. This I found unacceptable. At that time I cared about these things perhaps too much. I thought, this is an appalling thing to happen, which is why Barry Blackwell and I wrote a piece really as a warning. We made the mistake of trying to depersonalise it but of course you can't do that when this is a faith for some people. Quite inadvertently we sparked off a nightmare which went on for years. From my point of view it was completely unnecessary. I had to restrain Blackwell otherwise there would have been further trouble. But it didn't make any difference because Schou simply went on and on about this and then, well, we had other factors. We had the people who joined in like Coppen ...

And Kline and ...

That's right, because they saw a killing here and of course the industry. The industry had ignored lithium because it's an element, it's cheap and suddenly they saw money. You combine lithium with any other antidepressant and you sell it as both therapeutic and prophylactic. We got involved as a sort of scapegoat in all this because we'd had the affrontery to raise the questions. Well, at least it did force them to do a more scientific study. I didn't think that the evidence from the trial justified the conclusions that certainly some of these people took from it, but it was never an important matter to me, whereas it was a very important matter to Schou because it challenged an article of faith and of course his reputation was built on this. Baestrup was an honest, straightforward clinician and he apologised. Schou has never apologised. Baastrup got involved because he was the co-author of the original paper and he's a very modest, retiring chap who I suspect supplied the patients and was probably rather horrified at the lengths to which all this was going. I don't regret having done this in any way but I am sorry that it should have generated the emotion that it did. It completely distorted its significance but the underlying principle is the right one.

Can I push you on that a bit because one of the big arguments from the opposite camp was that we cannot randomise to prophylactic trials because people will die. There will be suicides. Now the prophylactic trials have since been done, including the MRC one. There have been some suicides haven't there?

I don't know. To be quite frank I forget all this. I did publish a piece devoted entirely to the ethics of this issue. I don't believe that's insuperable. I mean, this is one of the issues that arises from clinical trials.

Can we switch to primary care depression, which you more than anyone else really first raised the profile of? Do you ever think that all you did to some extent was make a mar-

ket for the industry – enlarge the size of the antidepressant market? Is there any way to avoid making markets for the industry?

Well, you're really asking a question which again has to be put in a broader context. What you say is absolutely true. The background in brief was that I had become interested in what is now called the epidemiology of mental disorder, which was not a word that was used then. In fact, I was reprimanded for using the word epidemiology by a professor of bacteriology who said you can't have an epidemiology of a non-infectious disease, which shows you how rapidly things have changed. It became clear to me, in brief, that if you study psychiatric institutions you learn nothing because most mental disorder doesn't come to them. I learnt a lot of this when I was in America because there was a small group of people in the States completely outside the ordinary run who were interested in surveys and counting and measuring and I knew them all – they were mostly in the public health field and many of them were not psychiatrists. They were just interested in the burden of morbidity on populations – this is what epidemiology is all about.

I thought that the direction was right but it hadn't a chance of succeeding. You can't do that sort of thing in the States because everything is chaotic. Everybody is moving. They won't answer questions. You haven't got a centralised statistical service and the more I thought about it, the more it seemed to me that the National Health Service provided the perfect sampling frame in general practice because GPs had to fill in the forms in order to get their capitation fees and they covered 98% of the population. So why not apply the standardised survey methods to general practice? – and this is what I did. When I started I was told by everybody I spoke to that I was wasting my time. What very quickly emerged was that far from wasting my time I had, call it what you like, stumbled on a horrifying fact which was that psychiatrists knew very little about mental disorder because they never saw more than a tiny segment of the thing.

This resulted in all sorts of difficulties, I can tell you. When we started to publish, which was in the early 1960s, I think I might just as well have published it in Serbo-Croat for all the impact it had. It was extremely relevant to public health people, to bio-statisticians and to people who are interested in policy. What they didn't understand was that my personal interest was entirely in collecting information on the nature and distribution of mental disorder but as I reluctantly pointed out in the monograph that we wrote, it had vast implications. I didn't care about them. That was not my job. What I then did was to thank the Lord that we were so side-tracked because it meant that nobody took it seriously. I had quite enough money from the Department of Health, which in those days you got by going up and having a cup of tea with a senior civil servant and somebody saying, 'How much do you want for the next 5 years?' There were no site visits, nothing. They were interested because it helped their statistics. They didn't think it mattered very much but it wasn't doing any harm.

We were given about 15 years' grace in which to really work on our own. We were cold-shouldered by the psychiatrists, who were horrified at the implications. We were ignored by the GPs, who were dominated by Michael Balint on the one hand and the pharmaceutical industry on the other. We just got on with it and in this time I was able to build up a unit and publish 400 odd papers and so on as though we were in a vacuum. Then in the 1980s the bubble burst when it became clear that the whole of the psychiatric service policies was falling to pieces – that terrible errors had been made about mental hospitals. As is always the case with governments and administrations, they look round and here was a cache of nearly 20 years work which was solidly based, impersonal, simply giving the size of the problem, the nature of it and among other things the extent of depression. This resulted in a flood of publicity and the work was then ripped out of its original setting and used and misused galore.

Over the weekend, Rachel Jenkins, who used to work with me and is now the Senior Medical Officer in the Mental Health Division and the Advisor to the Minister, has been going over with me the agenda for a conference, next month, organised by the Department, WHO, the college, and some other body with about 50 speakers from all over the world on 'Prevention in Primary Care'. It's totally unrecognisable in terms of the sort of things that we were doing but it's inevitable because primary care psychiatry is now a large grow- ing body all over the world – even more outside than inside the UK.

Somebody asked me about this the other day and asked me what I felt about it. I feel like the magician from the *Sorcerer's Apprentice*, who went out of the shop and comes back and finds chaos. It's everywhere. If you say, well you know you're responsible for this, this is not necessarily a compliment but I have to say it's not mea culpa – I'm not responsible for this at all. What we did was to outline the whole area. We developed the methods, we did a number of studies, we had them replicated and we trained a generation of people, not only here but all over the world who have confirmed this.

Who were the key people you trained?

David Goldberg, who is Professor here. Brian Cooper, about 20 Chairs, most of them psychiatrists. Robin Eastwood in Canada and Henry Dinsdale. Paul Williams, who's now with Glaxo. Tony Clare, Neil Kessel, Greg Wilkinson, three Chairs of Biostatistics, two of Psychology. There has been Michaele Tansella in Italy, Gia Marie in Sao Paulo, Andrew Cheng in Taiwan and a num- ber of attached workers who picked all this stuff up and through WHO and other fellowships have spread it all over the world. So the indirect influence has been vast actually. Over the years we must have had I should think 30–40 people who went on to senior academic positions of one sort or the other. The entire policy of the mental health section of the Department of Health in this country is now geared towards primary care. Rachel Jenkins is honest enough to say she's been dining out on this for the last 5 years.

There would be other people you would know about. For example, you will never have heard of Debbie Sharp, who is now Professor of General Practice in Bristol who did her doctorate with us. The way we functioned was to get these people to do supervised doctorates either abroad or here and then go off and spread the word. I think that this is very difficult to measure actually, but the influence is vast and if you look at textbooks and so on, it has brought an awareness that psychiatry is more than schizophrenia and manic-depressive psychosis. Unfortunately, it doesn't give you a clear enough picture of just what is involved and this is particularly true of the non-psychotic disorders, which of course is meat and drink for the pharmaceutical industry. They have quickly latched onto this, distorted it out of all recognition but that's what they are there for. So you can say, yes, in one sense I was unwittingly responsible for this but I take no blame for it. It's what was done to our studies that I think you're seeing now. Sooner or later it will settle down and the wheat will be separated from the chaff.

Talking about wheat and chaff is the right note for introducing the next question, which is this – Ronald Knox, looking at the history of some of the Protestant churches in a book called Enthusiasm, said that the greatest danger of all is enthusiasm but of course the most important thing of all is also enthusiasm. Now enthusiasm connects to the Oedipus effect, to which you have ascribed an important role in the history of the period. Do you want to pick this one up?

I would say that if you want to sum it up that what you need is controlled enthusiasm. Without enthusiasm nothing happens. Unrestrained, Auschwitz happens. The inquisition happens. The atomic bomb happens. So you're caught. You have to accept that this is part of the motivation, the actual mechanism of human activity which keeps people moving, but God help them if they don't ask where is it going – on the assumption that you can control it. You see, if you take the general practice story as an example, I had absolutely no way of controlling the way that this happened. As it got better and better known, we were approached by more and more people. We were offered more and more money but at a cost, which is that we produced results and now you have another issue which crops up, which is that many of the people who latch on to this sort of thing, which has got public health and policy implications, are paid to produce the right results.

The advantage of the work that we did in primary care was that it didn't matter at all. It was a piece of academic research, a series of studies which were designed to add to knowledge. Now it so happened that they had implications which is, after all, true of high-speed physics – the atomic bomb came out of it. Not that I'm comparing what we did to that but the same process is there. It's curiosity really which is a form of enthusiasm. You become wrapped up in 'my goodness that's interesting, I never realised there was so much psychiatric morbidity in general practice'. That's interesting because it leads on to other things which have got nothing to do with how many antidepressants do you give or what would be your profit ratio if you doubled the antidepresant dose to anxious people, say.

I think what is true about this particular thing is that it is very unusual to have a series of studies which were published and lay fallow for nearly 20 years with nobody realising just what was implied by them if you took them seriously. This comes back to your earlier question – why didn't the reserpine paper have an effect? The reason was that people were not thinking like that. It looked very strange, that you're writing a paper about treatment in the *Lancet* and what's the paper, it's half a dozen tables, statistics and chi squares and so on. It wasn't what people expected in the clinical field and certainly not in the psychiatric field at that time.

There's also the other bit there, which is that in order to make the catecholamine hypothesis the idea that reserpine made you depressed was quite crucial, so contradictory evidence wasn't going to be particularly welcomed. And it's a curious irony in that the preceding piece to your paper is one of these anecdotes about people becoming depressed on reserpine.

That's right. But you are interested in my work only insofar as it opened up the awareness that there was this issue?

Well yes, but one of the things that happened when Kuhn introduced imipramine first of all was that it took 2 years before Geigy decided to actually market it. The reason seems to have been that people thought that there were only very depressed people out there, people who could be treated with ECT and the drug wasn't going to be as good as ECT, so where was the market? It took a person like Kline with his flamboyance to some extent to force the companies down this route.

He did, and not only that. I once went with him to hear him talk to a congressional committee in Washington in 1955. Henry Brill and Frank Ayd were also there but he was the driving force. He was full of what the Americans call pazazz, which is an untranslatable word. He made these congressional characters feel that if they didn't take this on board they were doing the gravest disservice to the American nation since King George III with the British Army. It was a wonderful performance. He undoubtedly played this enormous role. I knew him quite well. There were his counterparts in this country, people like Sargant, but Sargant was restrained by the system. I remember thinking at the time that if you had behaved in that flamboyant manner with television appearances, the girlie magazines, the whole business, ... at that time you'd have been drummed out of the profession. The GMC would have said this is unprofessional behaviour.

His private practice was like something out of a Holywood movie. It was hardly describable but this is what you paid for. His sales pitch to all these rich suckers who would go to see him was that they were going to get the latest drug which nobody else had access to. But of course what they didn't know was that these were drugs that were still on trial and he was using them as guinea-pigs. And he got away with it. He became famous and a rich man and so on in a way that is inconceiveable here. He was a public figure in the national press. I once went with him to a television studio to listen to him give a talk and it was like listening to an advertising agent. But in a funny way, he too, was sincere. This was the American way of doing things. And of course it raises the even bigger issue, if he really believed this, as to how far was this self-deception to chime in with his own well-being and the system and how far was it actually related to reality, bearing in mind that he was a doctor and he wasn't selling toothpaste? There have been a lot of others who have clambered on to the bandwagon since but Kline made the bandwagon. He was rather a different phenomenon.

Heinz Lehmann puts it in terms of liking the way Kline didn't stand for any kind of pretension – that he was a little bit of a joker to some extent.

Well, there are many funny things about Kline. First of all he was an unexpectedly intelligent and educated man. He had a degree in philosophy and he had a taste in people. For example, he had the highest regard for Aubrey Lewis, which is extraordinary, when you think you couldn't possibly have two more dissimilar figures ... They are hardly of the same species but he was a bit like Klerman. He would respect something that was however different if it felt right. And this is what made him more than just another salesman. There was that side to him but he was a much more interesting and complicated person.

One of the impressions that comes through the literature is that the scientifically minded approach that you had seemed to people like Kline and others as though you and people from the Maudsley were negative as regards drugs. This sort of insistence on scientific ...

Well, it is now generally accepted that the core of the scientific method turns on the concept of refutation. If you want to call that negative, then all of science is negative. If you can't refute a contention you are not talking about something scientifically. If I say schizophrenia is due to rhubarb, which it may be for all I know, you have to test it in some way and you can't test a positive. This is now widely accepted ... if you call that negative you're playing with words and ...

But what comes through in the actual correspondence between Blackwell and Kline, for instance on lithium, where Kline says, 'I've heard this tone before. It was used when we introduced the drugs in the first place and we didn't have RCTs to introduce them. But of course, Dr Blackwell, in addition to thinking that lithium doesn't work, perhaps thinks that none of the other drugs work either.'

But that's a standard rhetorical game – you hear it in the parliaments of the world. Its chop logic. The real issue is that these topics have a scientific core and if you look at the scientific side of them there is only one way to proceed and that is to attempt to put forward the hypothesis and refute it, and if you fail you've got something positive which you can then build on etc. That's true in every branch of science. But these topics have spin off's – like money, reputation, fraud and publicity and 101 other things, which you can take out of the issue and make your own without ever actually getting involved in the scientific issues concerned. That is I think where the conflict takes place and it can't be resolved. It's got nothing to do with whether drug X affects condition Y. It's a question of whether Mr A or Dr A or Professor A wants to get something which is non-scientific out of an issue which has a scientific basis. That's true in every business. Think of Cyril Burt. This sort of thing goes on and on and it's part of the process. You must recognise that it exists, that is always has existed and that it always will exist and if you don't separate from that the fundamental scientific issues, you just get lost and the whole thing gets degraded. That's happened, sadly.

Where do you think things will go from here? We may be at the end of an era. Perhaps we will have time to stop and take stock.

It's anybody's guess obviously and mine is no better or worse than anyone else's but I would have thought that if what you say is true, that this penny in the slot approach has paid good dividends and it's no longer working, I would have thought there would be two barrels to fire. One would be to approach the whole issue from the biological side in a different way. I would be personally inclined to follow the molecular genetic line to see if any of these suggestions should materialise what their pharmacological implications would be. Pharmacogenetics would be a potentially productive line. The other would be to take the opportunity of the pause in the propaganda and so on and start looking at the non-specific factors sensibly. Begining with the placebo and then the environment and interpersonal issues – not in the haphazard way that they have been done.

To do that, would we have to have an independent psychiatric profession? Do we have one still?

I'm talking about the issues in theoretical terms. If you're asking who was going to do it? ... well, it will only happen if there's a need for it. I could see for example an enlightened pharmaceutical industry saying, 'Well look, we'll call it a day for 20 years and go back to the laboratory, we'll buy up the best people and we'll tell them to get on with it.' Which is what the MRC used to do. The MRC is finished as a serious element in this. But the industry could if they were far sighted enough because they could pay the best people the requisite salaries and not put pressure on them. The other thing is looking at the issues, as they are now, calls for a body of clinically informed scientists, who are able to appreciate what the issues are and put them to the test. I don't think they exist in the psychiatric profession. I don't think the standard is good enough. So either you do something radical to lift the whole thing up or you admit defeat – look at the fate of mental subnormality – it's ceased to be part of psychiatry.

I think the psychiatrists have now got to show what they're made of. I think it's anyone's guess as to how it will materialise – fortunately I am not going to be responsible. We have to raise the right questions – you don't have to give your own answers but the questions are important. We must first define what there is to be done.

Is there any hope that Meyer's kind of thinking will come back? That the wheel will turn yet again?

The real problem, if you're asking about this, is that if you are to influence people within the profession, you've got to stand up and be counted. You've got to be seen to do more than talk about it. I can remember, for example, week after week in this building here, at 12 o'clock, on a Monday morning,

Aubrey Lewis took the clinical conference. The first two rows of the conference room were occupied by every consultant in the hospital. The registrars were at the back and the discussion was between the professor of psychiatry and his senior staff. There they all were, hand picked, so that you would get the Jungian view, the biological view, the eclectic view, this, that and the other view and the registrars would be transfixed listening to this and realising that nobody knew anything. These were all people expressing personal views. The actual substance of the material was extremely tenuous. But it was an educative experience and this is psychobiology in action. To be able to do this you've got to be respected enough and to have sufficient authority to get away with it. If you don't, it's a farce.

It just so happens that last week I happened to see the weekly programme here. There's still something called the clinical conference on Monday at 12 o'clock but it isn't taken by the Professor of Psychiatry. It's taken by a mixture of people and the thing that really struck me was the words '12 o'clock clinical conference, presided over by so and so, 12.30 p.m. lunch by whoever' and that is what's happened. I'm sure people go there for the sandwiches and once this happens, you're lost. The only way that anything carries any force is by example. After all, as anybody who has been to a medical school knows, we all remember our professor of neurology, or a paediatrician and so on, who impressed us by their bearing, by their authority, by their this, that and the other, in addition to their clinical knowledge, because medicine is an apprenticeship. You have a model which is in a medical school. That's where you pick it up. Not from reading and certainly not from libraries or anything of that sort. You've got to see the way the boss actually behaves on the ward with the patients, because that's the only argument that's going to carry any force. The psychobiological example is very difficult to define and to carry off – not as a theoretical matter but in practice. When it works it's unforgettable.

Select bibliography

Beecher HK (1955). The powerful placebo. *Journal of the American Medical Association*, **159**, 1602–1605.

Davies DL, Shepherd M (1955). Reserpine in the treatment of anxious and depressed patients. *Lancet*, **ii**, 117–120.

Shepherd M, Watt DC (1956). A controlled trial of chlorpromazine and reserpine in chronic schizophrenia. *Journal of Neurology, Neurosurgery and Psychiatry*, **19**, 232–235.

Shepherd M *et al* (1965). Clinical trial of the treatment of depressive illness. *British Medical Journal*, **i,** 881–886.

Shepherd M (1981). Reserpine as a tranquilizer. In *Psychotropic Drugs in Psychiatry*. Jason Aronson New York, pp. 55–66.

Shepherd M (1981). A multicentred clinical trial. In *Psychotropic Drugs in Psychiatry*. Jason Aronson, New York, pp 143–151.

Shepherd M (1993). The placebo: from specificity to the non-specific and back. *Psychological Medicine*, **23**, 569–578.

Shepherd M (1996). The two faces of Emil Kraepelin. *British Journal of Psychiatry*, **169**,

12 Mogens Schou

Lithium

When and why did you begin to do medicine?

I started medicine in 1937 at Copenhagen University after having finished school, and I graduated in 1944. My goal was to go into psychiatry because my father, Hans Jacob Schou, was a psychiatrist, and I had 'caught' it from him. My father was medical superintendent at a provincial mental hospital, which had psychiatric and epileptic patients, and he himself built in addition a so-called 'Nervesanatorium', a clinic ostensibly for neurotic patients. In fact most of the patients suffered from light psychoses and mild depressions. The patients were treated with rest cures, baths, supportive psychotherapy – but not psychoanalysis – etc. There were no effective somatic treatments at the time, and I remember clearly those depressive women and men wandering in the surrounding park with their drooping attitudes and disconsolate faces. Then in 1938-39 my father told me about the advent of ECT, which had a marked therapeutic effect on both manias and depressions and in addition on acute delirium. He was delighted because not only did we now have an effective treatment. He also felt that when we could treat the illnesses, we would soon find out what caused them. That was about 60 years ago, and look at us now, really not much further in understanding disease causes.

Delirium isn't usually thought of as an indication for ECT these days. I guess because we use haloperidol.

Right. Acute delirium was not widespread but it was not infrequent before the neuroleptics. It could arise in any psychosis that progressed strongly enough. The patients became very agitated and developed fever, and eventually they died of exhaustion. The mortality of acute delirium was very high, especially among the young.

After my graduation from medical school I took 3–4 years of clinical psychiatry in, among other places, St Hans Hospital in Roskilde and Dikemark Hospital in Norway with Rolv Gjessing. But at that time there was so little one could do therapeutically for the patients that I became frustrated and decided to specialise. I could either go into psychotherapy or into biological psychiatry, and I chose the latter. Although primarily a clinician my father had founded a

260 The Psychopharmacologists II

research laboratory, where he and his associates did biochemical work with patients.

Did Gjessing's work on the periodic psychoses influence you?

My father and my medical superintendent at St Hans Hospital, JC Smith, both knew Gjessing, and at one time I changed job, salary and house with a colleague at Dikemark for three months. I admired Gjessing for his exactitude and painstaking work with the periodic catatonics. One weakness with him was his reluctance to share his experiences with his colleagues in an understandable way. He did publish a lot of data and curves and a text written in heavy German. Fortunately his son Leiv Gjessing, together with Alec Jenner in England, later translated some of his work into English and made it more palatable.

When I had finished my years of training in clinical psychiatry, I trained in experimental biology with Herman Kalckar in Copenhagen and with Heinrich Waelsch in New York.

Who was Herman Kalckar?

He was a student friend of Erik Strömgren's, who had worked for a number of years in the United States and made quite a name for himself there, especially for work on energy-rich phosphate bonds. Now he had returned to Copenhagen and set up a laboratory there, and he gave me an opportunity to work with him for almost a year. I studied xanthopterin, a compound found in butterfly wings with some interesting chemical properties.

How did you come to go to New York and work with Heinrich Waelsch?

Here again Strömgren was of great help. When I approached him, he had recently been in New York and visited Heinrich Waelsch at the New York State Institute, Columbia University, and he helped me to obtain a US postdoctorate fellowship for a year. Waelsch was, together with Derek Richter in England, among the pioneers of neurochemistry, and together they founded the *Journal of Neurochemistry*. What I worked on there had nothing to do with psychiatry. Waelsch at the time studied the synthesis of proteins. He was particularly interested in glutamine and glutamic acid. He was energetic and made clever studies, and he was a forceful personality who did me a lot of good.

Joel Elkes, was he ...

Elkes and Kety were pupils and admirers of Waelsch, so I knew them from that time.

Given your role in clinical trial development, when you were in New York did you have any contact with people like Harry Gold?

No, but Waelsch took me to lectures and symposia in New York, and I met interesting people there.

Among my professional mentors I count my father, Rolv Gjessing, Herman Kalckar, Heinrich Waelsch and, last but not least, Erik Strömgren. Strömgren made a position for me as a research associate in biological psychiatry at the

Psychiatric Hospital in Risskov near Aarhus, where I built up a research laboratory. I later became its director.

You have had a research appointment pretty well from the start, which seems extraordinary in a relatively small city like Aarhus.

In addition to establishing, slowly and gradually, the research laboratory I took over the leadership of the hospital's clinical chemistry laboratory. The former was my main interest, the latter I took as a duty.

When did you get your Chair at the university?

For a number of years I functioned as Reader in Psychopharmacology at Aarhus University. In 1971 I got the first Chair of Biological Psychiatry in Scandinavia. Ole Rafaelsen got the second in Copenhagen about six months later.

Strömgren, who was behind that as behind so much else, was a remarkable man, respected in international as well as Danish psychiatry. Rather than take a more prestigious Chair in Copenhagen that was offered him, he chose to build the hospital in Risskov as a comprehensive institute with units for clinical psychiatry, psychiatric demography and genetics, psychotherapy, social psychiatry, child psychiatry, geriatric psychiatry, brain pathology, and biological psychiatry with psychopharmacology. The diversity of activities gave the individual researchers, me among them, freedom to be one-sided without having a bad conscience. Strömgren was at all times very supportive. I, and many others, owe him a huge debt of gratitude.

You came back from the US and started work at Risskov. What brought you to lithium?

In 1951 Strömgren drew my attention to the Australian publications about this drug. In fact I first read the paper by Noack and Trautner and then within a short time got hold of Cade's paper.

How could someone working in Aarhus at the time have been aware of papers published in the Australian Medical Journal? Wouldn't there have been a feeling that new psychiatric treatments were unlikely to be discovered in an out-of-the-way place like Melbourne – prophets from Galillee and all that?

Well, here in Risskov we were not exactly in the so-called centre of things – wherever that may be. I mean, discoveries can be made anywhere if there are original minds. And you must remember the situation around 1950. Apart from ECT we had no active treatments for manic-depressive illness. Barbiturates were used for mania and opium drops for depression, none of them ever proven effective. So understandably we welcomed this chance of something that seemed better, and that is why we did a trial here. Strömgren and two other clinicians selected the patients and observed them during the trial. I didn't see the patients but planned the trial procedure.

Before we come to the trial, though, to some extent the way the history has been written, it has all been about Cade and you. Noack and Trautner have not made an appearance in the historical reports.

I do not know much about Trautner, who was the leading author of the joint paper, but Samuel Gershon has repeatedly stressed his importance. He was a

German physiologist who took an interest in psychiatry. I met Cade but never Noack and Trautner, although I corresponded with the latter. Cade came and visited us here in 1972. A few years later my wife and I visited the Cades in Melbourne, and thereafter he and I met in various places, including New York, where we shared the Kittay prize.

But while Cade made the breakthrough, he didn't ever do anything else really, whereas Trautner recruited other people to lithium – Sam Gershon, for instance.

John Cade recruited me. But it is true that he himself left the field. Cade was a very special person, who had multiple interests and an insatiable curiosity. For example, when he came here in 1972 we asked him to give a lecture and of course expected him to talk about lithium. Instead he talked about the psychiatric effects of strontium, because, as he said, there might be another fish in that lake. Nothing, however, came of it.

John Cade was a keen naturalist. His wife told me that she and John once walked through the woods around Melbourne and there found an animal dropping. 'There has been an elephant here', Cade exclaimed. 'But John, have you gone mad. We are in Australia', she protested. Half an hour later they came to a circus. She asked him how he had been able to recognise the dropping. 'I have been to the zoo and looked and photographed.'

Another story. When he and Jean Cade visited us here, we wanted to show them a bit of our country. Danish nature is pretty but not spectacular, so we chose to show them something that was old and took them to a stone age burial place, a mound, in the countryside. John became interested and started sighting along the stones and asking where North was. He wanted to find out whether this monument had been functioning as an observatory like the 2000 years younger Stonehenge. I am afraid that Jean, my wife and I pulled him away before he had reached any conclusions.

Then we went to look at the two medieval churches in Aarhus: the cathedral and the church of Our Lady. The latter has an interesting feature, namely a crypt beneath the main church. This is infrequent but not unknown in larger Danish churches, but this case was special because the crypt had been filled up and forgotten for many years, the small curved windows along the ground having been covered with ivy. The crypt was discovered accidentally when the ivy was cleared away, and it turned out to be the oldest existing church in Denmark, dating from about AD 900. This of course interested John very much, and when we came up from the crypt into the main church, he went around stamping on the slabs of the floor to find out whether perhaps another crypt was hidden underneath. These two experiences told me something about John Cade as a man and a scientist – the wide-ranging curiosity, the inventiveness, the eagerness to find something new, the willingness to risk making a fool of himself. This is the stuff innovators are made of, and of course fools. John Cade's contribution was not foolish. In a way he and I supplemented each other admirably. He was the curious innovator with bold ideas, whereas I was less daring but perhaps more systematic.

But if Noack and Trautner hadn't written their paper, would lithium have vanished again?

I don't think so. Cade's paper would soon have become known, and it unavoidably struck the clinical reader by its vivid descriptions of the patients and their response to the treatment. Incidentally, Sam Gershon worked for a time with Cade and observed how he became so frightened by cases of lithium poisoning that he stopped the treatment altogether. Sam Gershon was the one who brought lithium to the attention of American psychiatrists by publishing a paper about it in 1960, and he has been an important figure there.

The French began to pick lithium up at about the same time as yourself.

Some of them in fact before I entered the field. There were some fairly brief clinical reports confirming Cade's finding of an antimanic action, but no systematic trials. I became aware of the studies after we published our 1954 paper, but they are all mentioned in my review of 1957.

You did what was perhaps the first placebo-controlled study in psychopharmacology.

Since lithium was the first psychotropic drug, as we understand the term now, that was wasn't so strange.

But someone like Linford Rees had been doing controlled trials on deoxycortisone and things like that. They weren't things that worked, but they were agents for which claims had been made. Now that was around the same time as your trial. What I am trying to push at here is where did your idea to do this kind of trial come from?

From general medicine; there was nothing original in it. The procedure was new only to psychiatry. I also thought of Gjessing's work which was not a controlled trial but which studied the effects of long-term treatment with thyroxine in patients with periodic catatonia. Our paper in 1954 was in fact a mixture of, on the one hand, controlled treatment with double-blind shifts between lithium and placebo in patients with more prolonged manias, and, on the other, more or less continuous treatment in patients with shorter and more frequent episodes. We felt that this procedure would provide a maximum of information about manias with different courses. So in a way the study had elements of both a therapeutic and a prophylactic trial. We didn't look at it that way at the time, because we took it for granted that if a therapeutically active drug were given continuously, it must also prevent further recurrences. It was only later, when we found lithium not very effective therapeutically in depression and yet prophylactically effective against not only manic but also depressive recurrences, we felt we must distinguish between therapeutic actions and prophylactic actions. The antidepressant drugs began to appear in the latter half of the 1950s, and they clearly had a therapeutic action. Prophylactic trials with continuation treatment came later, possibly under the influence of the experiences with lithium.

A number of other placebo-controlled trials were published in the following years. There were the Elkes and the Linford Rees studies on chlorpromazine and the work by Michael

264 The Psychopharmacologists II

Shepherd using reserpine which was published in 1955. Were you aware of any of these other trials happening at the time?

It was natural that I was interested in other agents that acted antimanically but without the sedative effect of the barbiturates. I was particularly impressed by the later multi-centre MRC study on antidepressants organised by Shepherd.

But that was much later. I am just trying to get some feel as to why you employed this kind of trial design. You say it was happening elsewhere in medicine, but was there any particular area of medicine you had in mind? Was it the streptomycin trial?

It wasn't any study in particular. The controlled trial was just a technique that was around which attracted me

How did your clinical colleagues cope with the idea of this kind of trial?

Some of them were against it. But Professor Strömgren together with two other senior psychiatrists, Juel-Nielsen and Voldby, supported it. Of course there was uneasiness about the possible toxicity of lithium. We knew about the experiences from the United States with patients on a low-salt diet, who were given lithium as a taste substitute. Several of the patients became intoxicated and some died. So the scare was around.

But were there any problems with the idea of the special kind of trial you were proposing?

The psychiatrists had no objections, but I wouldn't say the nurses were entirely happy with the knowledge that some of their violent manic patients might be given placebo. Some of them even broke the tablets and tasted them. However, we had foreseen that and by adding various constituents to the placebo tablets made them similar to the lithium tablets in taste, colour and consistency. So we fooled the nurses.

Did people like Strömgren wonder why you took this approach?

Strömgren knew the literature and had read about controlled trials, and he applauded and supported the study. As I mentioned, he himself participated as one of the clinicians. However, the design was entirely my own, and I did not see or assess the patients. I sat in the laboratory and flipped a coin to decide who were to receive lithium and who placebo.

We started treating the first patient in 1952 and submitted our manuscript in 1954. It had an odd fate. We first sent it to Eliot Slater, but he did not think much of this report about an unknown drug and suggested that we send the manuscript to a more out-of-the way journal, the *Journal of Neurology, Neurosurgery and Psychiatry*. It was accepted there and published later in 1954, but few psychiatrists read this journal, and it would be less than the truth to say that the treatment became a hit.

Can you recall matching the code to the clinical findings and seeing what the results looked like? Can you recall the moment when you became aware that lithium was actually working?

This came gradually. Looking at the diagrams of the patients' disease courses I soon realized that in most of the patients the course was altered radically.

At that point you must have been operating without blood levels. When did the idea of a target lithium level begin to play a part in practice?

In the 1949 reports about lithium intoxications some of the authors determined serum lithium concentrations at the height of the intoxication and found values of 2–4 mmol/l. Cade didn't monitor his treatment with serum determinations. He increased the dosage gradually until improvement of the mania occurred or side-effects developed and then gradually reduced the dosage. Noack and Trautner determined serum lithium levels with the purpose of finding concentrations indicative of impending intoxication but failed to establish such values. The concentrations were too variable. In Risskov we determined serum lithium levels during treatment of mania from the beginning and found effective doses to produce concentrations between 0.5 and 2 mmol/l. Higher concentrations sometimes led to signs of toxicity, sometimes not. Later my associate Amdi Amdisen suggested a fixed time interval of 12 hours between the last lithium dose and the drawing of blood. At the present time we recommend serum lithium concentrations between 0.6 and 0.8 mmol/l in most patients given prophylactic treatment.

In the 1954 paper you wrote that lithium treatment is symptomatic. The idea that it might be prophylactic did not occur to you at that time?

Symptomatic is the converse of curative and prophylactic the converse of therapeutic. We must retain these distinctions. Yes, we considered the antimanic lithium treatment symptomatic and not curative, because when we stopped lithium the manic symptoms reappeared.

When did the idea of prophylaxis appear to you?

Among our patients in 1954 there was one with rapidly recurring manias and depressions, a bipolar with an almost circular course and very few and short neutral intervals. When we gave him continuous lithium treatment to keep away the highs, we saw that also the lows disappeared or were considerably attenuated. However, at the time we did not pay much attention to this observation.

Then in 1959 I was approached by GP Hartigan from Canterbury and PC Baastrup from Vordingborg in Denmark. Simultaneously and independently of each other they wrote to ask whether long-term lithium treatment might perhaps keep away also depressive recurrences, because this was what they had seen in a dozen patients. I visited each of them and saw their patients. Having our own above-mentioned patient in mind I felt that we might be on to something new and important, and I urged Hartigan and Baastrup to publish. Not exactly as a proof of anything but as an observation that might spark further work. They were, however, both reluctant. Not having published before they were afraid of what the academic centres would say to this. Eventually, and after I had been at them several times, they published two short papers in 1963 and 1964. At the same time I wrote a note drawing attention to the articles and pointing out their possible significance. None of our reports seemed to attract attention.

Hartigan sadly died a few years later. In Neil Johnson's book about the history of lithium treatment there is an interview with his widow, and in it she gives a vivid picture of this original person.

Baastrup then started giving lithium to patients with recurrent manic-depressive illness, both bipolar and unipolar cases. He followed them without lithium treatment for about two years and thereafter started long-term administration of lithium. Although living in different parts of the country Baastrup and I joined forces. He treated and observed the patients while I did the data analysis and eventually wrote our joint paper. The majority of the patients had a distinct drop in the frequency of recurrences, both manic and depressive. In fact the prophylactic effect was equally pronounced in bipolar and unipolar cases. About 10–20% of the patients did not respond to the treatment. Many of these were schizo-affective cases, but it was striking that even among these atypical manic-depressives a considerable number responded excellently.

Since most of the patients given lithium had had a large number of recurrences before lithium, on the average six to seven and at least two episodes within one year, and since the lowering in frequency or the complete absence of recurrences was maintained on lithium for up to four years, we found it justified to claim that lithium was the first agent for which a prophylactic, i.e. a recurrence-preventive, action had been established.

At this point the antidepressants were beginning to come on stream. Could Baastrup not have used an antidepressant for the unipolar patients?

The antidepressants were not widely used at the time of our trial, and no one seemed to have thought of subjecting them to a prophylactic trial. The study lasted 6½ years and included 88 patients. It was published in 1967 in *Archives of General Psychiatry* and made quite an impression. Psychiatrists from Scandinavia and continental Europe took up the treatment and came to the same results. In England and the United States psychiatrists were more reluctant, which may have had to do with different diagnostic traditions. In the Nordic countries we had inherited from Kraepelin the notion of manic-depressive illness as an endogenous psychosis with a course that is largely independent of external events. In Great Britain psychological factors were given more weight.

Let me take you back to Cade for a moment. When he outlined his rationale for using lithium in the first place he talks about it having a seemingly non-specific sedative effect on the guinea-pigs he gave it to, which led to its use in humans, but on the other hand after he had given it to people with mania he talks about it having a specific effect almost to the point where he gives the impression that mania must be a lithium-deficient disorder. There is a huge contrast here ...

I shall try to answer two points separately. To begin with his guinea-pig experiments which led him to try lithium on patients: I think he interpreted his animal experiments wrongly. We have tried to give lithium in high doses to rats and guinea-pigs but only found sedation or lethargy, when we gave high, probably very toxic doses. But never mind this question of the interpretation of animal studies, he did the crucial thing which was to try it on patients. This brings us to the second point. The effect he saw then in manic patients was clearly different from that of the barbiturates. The patients lost their excitability and talkativeness but they were not sedated or sleepy. It was this that led him to talk about a specific effect of lithium.

Did you ever hear anything more about the patients he treated with lithium? He gives a memorable description of the very first.

The first patient, WB, eventually died of lithium poisoning. This came out when Neil Johnson looked into the case notes while working on the history of lithium treatment. That death was not mentioned by Cade. Neil's book gives a very balanced assessment of the arguments for and against this policy. I was not aware of the event at the time.

Concerning the controversies about lithium prophylaxis. Michael Shepherd describes a meeting in Göttingen where he talked about the principles of clinical trials and you gave a talk about the prophylactic effects of lithium. He says it was pointed out to him that what he said and what you said were in contrast, and that he himself tried to point out politely the need for further research. The controversy seems to have started there because he got the impression that you wanted to skirt a randomised trial.

There was clearly a fundamental difference between Shepherd's and my approaches and interpretations of data, and I shall describe them separately. The design of Baastrup's and my trial was not ideal, i.e. double-blind and placebo-controlled, for it had started more or less on an exploratory basis and then grown gradually. We felt, however, that data collected in an open prophylactic study of mirror design need not be disregarded. In your interview with Jules Angst in 1994 he expressed the same opinion. The marked and long-lasting change in disease course coincided with the start of lithium treatment and was unlikely to have been fortuitous. Most of the patients were discharged, and it was accordingly the general practitioners, ignorant of the ongoing trial and therefore not biased, who decided when a recurrence had taken place.

Baastrup's and my observations did not provide final proof of a prophylactic action of lithium, but the evidence was at least sufficiently weighty to give hope about a new and effective means of treating patients suffering from a dangerous and devastating illness. When I told the colleagues in Göttingen about our findings, I expected them to welcome this development.

Michael Shepherd took an entirely different view. He was convinced that valid evidence could be obtained exclusively through placebo-controlled double-blind trials and that any other evidence must be rejected. He clearly felt that when I showed gratification with our findings I must necessarily be a 'believer', an enthusiast, naive and not to be trusted.

The crucial point seems to have been reached when I told how the disease course of my brother, who for 25 years had had depressions every spring, changed drastically on lithium. To Shepherd this was apparently the final testimony of my folly and more or less proved that lithium was ineffective. He did not seem to understand that my personal involvement made me extra motivated to put the efficacy of the treatment on the firmest possible ground and to study closely its side-effects and risks.

Things got very acrimonious. Can you explain why?

When Shepherd and I later that year met in Barcelona, he told me that he was working on a comment to our study, but he did not reveal its contents and did not send me a manuscript copy before its publication. That was the Blackwell and Shepherd paper which appeared in the *Lancet* in 1968. Baastrup and I wrote a rebuttal in which we countered Blackwell and Shepherd's arguments and pointed out how they had misread our paper. They counted, for example, the end of our observation period, 1 July 1966, as a time when all the patients relapsed. This of course gave statistics that were entirely different from those Baastrup and I had presented.

Critical debate is what science thrives on and should at all times be welcomed. But one does not appreciate having one's data, conclusions and ethics rejected totally and unfairly. Moreover, Blackwell and Shepherd continually made hints about Baastrup's and my motives for drawing the conclusions we drew. Conjectures about other scientists' motives are irrelevant in and should be kept out of scientific discussions.

What was the development after the encounter in Göttingen and the exchange of opinions in the Lancet?

Baastrup and I speculated about organising a double-blind study but were held back by ethical considerations. Could we, who found the evidence of a prophylactic action of lithium strong, expose patients who seemed to benefit from it, as for example my brother, to a 50% possibility of being given placebo, with risk of recurrences, possibly suicide? Blackwell and Shepherd, on the other hand, saw no ethical problems, but they did not themselves carry out a controlled trial.

Baastrup and I finally decided to subject the question under debate to further and more stringent testing through a double-blind placebo-controlled discontinuation trial, which we had designed so that the risk of recurrences was minimised. We used sequential analysis to end the trial. Statistical significance ($p < 0.01$) was reached within six months. At that time half of the patients switched to placebo had relapsed, while none of their lithium-treated partners had. That paper was published in the *Lancet* in 1970.

Shepherd and I met again at a meeting in Yugoslavia in 1973, and since the proceedings of that meeting were published in a little-known volume, it may be appropriate to present part of the discussion here.

Shepherd said: 'On the basis of such experience I would regard Professor Schou's question as reasonably straightforward. His original paper with Dr Baastrup was an example of an elaborate but uncontrolled piece of work, corresponding to a phase II investigation and clamantly calling for further elaboration by phase III studies. Had the manuscript been submitted to *Psychological*

Medicine it might well have been accepted as a preliminary communication in a suitably modified form. The problem created by Professor Schou was of his own making. He appears to have believed so firmly in his own judgement as to have concluded that independent assessment was unnecessary. The evidence which he presented was certainly incomplete, as we pointed out at the time, and the history of physical treatment in psychiatry has unfortunately demonstrated too often the folly of relying on uncontrolled studies only, however eminent and enthusiastic the clinical observers. Mention need only be made of deep insulin coma therapy and prefrontal leucotomy in this connection. For this reason I am very glad that Professor Schou eventually felt able to overcome his scruples and to accept the widely accepted ethos of the scientific community. The wisdom of his choice has been amply supported by the interesting studies, several reported in this symposium, which indicate that lithium should be regarded as a substance with exciting possibilities for scientific enquiry rather than as a novel form of panacea.

'While disagreeing profoundly with the argument developed by Professor Schou I am very grateful to him for having raised so important an issue for public discussion. Few investigators will disagree with the conclusion stated in the abstract of his paper that "ethical responsibilities must in the final analysis rest with the investigators". At the same time most workers agree that there are broad rules of conduct governing the way in which these responsibilities should be undertaken. The many codes of ethics which have been drawn up converge on the general principle: "First a warm and loving heart and secondly truth in an earnest spirit". Such lofty sentiments are clearly irrefutable but all too often very difficult to apply. In practical terms, therefore, it seems to me that there are advantages attaching to a consideration of the more specific everyday problems faced by the editors of scientific journals who constitute, after all, the final common path for the distribution of scientific information. What, in short, should they do when a manuscript is submitted which is scientifically respectable but ethically doubtful? In the case of my own journal, *Psychological Medicine*, the referees are routinely asked the following question about every paper: "Does the experimental work raise ethical problems? If 'yes', specify in your review". In this way it has been possible to build up a bank of experience ... on the ethical need to stabilise the climate of medical and lay opinion which has been so perturbed by the extravagance of the claims advanced by proponents of lithium as a "prophylactic" agent.'

My reply was as follows: 'I am in complete agreement with Professor Shepherd about our profound disagreement. We differ first and foremost as regards what was, and is, the central issue in the debate on lithium prophylaxis. According to Professor Shepherd's account the sequence of events appears to have been the following. In 1967 Baastrup and I presented an inconclusive piece of evidence. Its inadequacy and folly was pointed out by Professor Shepherd and his associates, but we believed stubbornly in our own judgement and even used ethical misgivings as an excuse for not carrying out the double-blind study that in his opinion was the one and only means of confirming or refuting our claim. When at last we did carry out such a study, this was because we yielded to the widely accepted ethos of the scientific community as pointed out by our Maudsley colleagues.

'In other words, Professor Shepherd ranks on the one side the double-blind trial, the wisdom, the objective truth, and the scientific ethos, and on the other side the non-blind trial, the folly, the uncritical enthusiastic belief, and the lack of scientific ethos.

'Alas, things are not that simple. The double-blind design is only one among other types of controlled trial. Its special virtue is to control for observer bias and the psychological effect of the treatment. If these sources of error are likely to be of significance for the outcome of the trial, its use is essential; if they are not, other types of controlled design may yield equally valid information. This is the whole point of the debate.

'We have repeatedly explained our reasons for considering it unlikely that observer bias and psychological factors could account for the results we obtained, reasons dealing with the particular type of patients studied, with the considerable length of the trial period, and with the operative definition of a relapse. The validity of our assumption is further supported by evidence provided by later studies; no data have been presented which would invalidate the assumption. Professor Shepherd chooses to disregard this altogether. He argues as if it was unknown to him, which of course it is not. Strange.

'At the present time double-blind studies on lithium prophylaxis have been carried out in Denmark, England, and the United States; they all support the conclusions drawn from the non-blind studies.

'Professor Shepherd chooses to disregard also this evidence, even though it is provided by studies carried out with the design he himself considers the appropriate one. Peculiar. Professor Shepherd refers even today to the "putative" lithium effect, an effect that is still "sub judice". To him lithium is not a useful drug, merely "a substance with exciting possibilities for scientific enquiry". Incidentally, we never claimed lithium to be a panacea. One wonders why Shepherd and his associates use so much energy fighting this entirely self-made dragon.'

Why did they spend so much energy trying to counter this self-made dragon?

I don't know. Of course you can more easily win a debate if you are able to present your opponent's claims as obviously ridiculous.

When was the last time you saw Michael Shepherd?

Presumably it was at the 1973 meeting. We haven't corresponded either. As Alec Coppen pointed out in your interview with him, Shepherd seemed unwilling to discuss lithium any further.

I wonder whether you and Shepherd were so different after all. You were both alert to the importance of clinical trials very early on, you both recognise pharmacogenetics as an important way forward and you even have the same initials! At least without him and the fuss that was created, would lithium have become as well known as it did? The discussion helped to create some of the publicity that did not come from the pharmaceutical industry, which had no interest in lithium.

Heinrich Waelsch used to say that you cannot become famous before you have had a fight, but I do not really agree with him. As regards lithium, Coppen and his group and Hullin and his collaborators had started prospective double-blind trials even before what you call 'the fuss', so lithium treatment would presumably have developed also without the controversy.

In an interview he did in 1991 with Greg Wilkinson, Michael Shepherd suggests that Baastrup apologised for overstating the case for lithium, whereas you never did. He quotes a piece Baastrup wrote to support his point.

Baastrup did not apologise. In support of the alleged apology Shepherd quoted a passage from a paper written by Baastrup. But he quoted only part of a paragraph. Read in its entirety and context the passage is clearly ironical, and the meaning of irony is reversed when the reader chooses not to treat it as irony. As for my own failure to apologise I find it difficult to see what I have to apologise for and to whom. To Michael Shepherd? To the psychiatric community? To the manic-depressive patients?

By 1973 the argument was no longer just between yourself and Michael Shepherd. There were a number of people on both sides. How important was it that for example people like Jules Angst and Nate Kline got involved?

In 1966 I met Jules Angst at a Denghausen meeting, and when I told him about our experiences with lithium, he said that he had observations about the spontaneous course of manic-depressive illness and statistics to deal with that kind of problem. So he, Paul Grof, Baastrup and I did a study together with pooled data from the clinics in Zürich, Praha and Risskov. Our paper won the Anna Monika first prize and was published in the *British Journal of Psychiatry*. The joint study showed that the assumptions Baastrup and I had made concerning the course of illness to be expected had lithium not worked were correct. The treatment results from the three centres were in agreement about equal prophylactic effects of lithium in bipolar and unipolar patients. There was also an effect in recurrent schizo-affective illness, but it was less pronounced.

You must have had a sense of déjà-vu when the British Journal of Psychiatry ran a critique of the prophylactic studies on lithium by Joanna Moncrieff last year.

So I had but her criticisms didn't make much of an impression on me. It was so glaringly one-sided. She obviously preferred the role of lawyer to that of scientist.

I happen to know that there are people within the Maudsley who explain your position by hinting that you yourself had manic-depression and are on lithium and that therefore you have a vested interest in seeing things one way. There also seem to be some people, mainly those working on schizophrenia research, who for various reasons feel that your work has interfered with their field of interest. Did you know that?

This is entirely new to me. Perhaps it explains why Shepherd always referred to me as an 'enthusiast', clearly meaning an uncritical person whose opinions couldn't be trusted. Well, I am not manic and never was in lithium treatment. But what difference would it make? Baastrup's and my data, arguments and conclusions are there for anyone to assess. Should data, arguments and conclusions presented by insane persons be disregarded rather than judged on their merits?

I do not know what you refer to when you talk about 'field of interest'. Do physicians in private practice blame a new and effective treatment for having deprived them of income? Psychiatrists working in schizophrenia research did in fact at one time blame me for having been responsible for the increased use of 'manic-depressive' disorder and the decreased use of 'schizophrenia' that took place in the 1970s. But that was of course said jokingly.

How is Baastrup nowadays, and what does he feel about the controversies?

Poul Christian Baastrup is a taciturn person, and he did not contribute directly to the debate. But we always agreed about the contents of our articles. Baastrup primarily took care of and observed the patients. I feel a lot of gratitude toward and admiration for him. As a clinical psychiatrist he was open to new ideas and to improved patient care. Our collaboration was a happy one, perhaps because our spheres of competence were so clearly divided. So in spite of close collaboration over many years under stressing conditions we have remained friends.

What is your position now on the ethics of placebo-controlled studies, especially as concerns prophylaxis?

One could not today do the kind of study we carried out in 1969–70. There would be the question of informed consent, and that would tend to make the patient group non-representative. Placebo studies would under most circumstances be considered unethical, because new and effective drugs are now available. I consider informed consent essential and necessary, but it cannot be denied that sometimes it impedes therapeutic progress.

In long-term prophylactic trials there is also the question – both an ethical one and a pragmatic one – of the patients who for one or another reason drop out of the study. Dropouts presumably do not occur randomly, so again we have a risk of being left with an unrepresentative sample. In the Pittsburgh studies, for example, when they extended the study period from 3 to 5 years there were so few patients left in some arms of the study that one has to question how representative that was.

There is a further ethical concern if during the trial it gradually becomes clear that one drug is distinctly better than placebo or the comparison drug. How long is it then ethical to continue the trial? That is why we chose a sequential analysis design which stops the trial as soon as statistical significance has been achieved. In our discontinuation study this happened in less than six months.

What about Nate Kline's involvement?

Kline was an ardent therapist and always after new treatments for his patients. Along with Jonathan Cole he put pressure on the FDA to acknowledge lithium. However, the FDA hesitated because there had been those bad intoxications back in the 1940s, and they had also burned their fingers on thalidomide. A decade later FDA did approve prophylactic lithium treatment of bipolar patients, but its use for unipolar patients has never come about.

What did you make of Nathan Kline?

One cannot but have many opinions about Kline. I'll start with his shortcomings. He could not resist money and publicity. But apart from that he was a marvellous and highly gifted person. One of your interviewees has already mentioned his memory for poetry; he could recite verse for a whole evening, all from memory. Kline was also a very generous person, and he had good connections personally and professionally. He could get to the legislators and to rich people. That was how he organized the Denghausen meetings.

Along with your and Shepherd's controversy, there was an exchange between Barry Blackwell and Kline.

I rather wish that hadn't taken place. Their dispute lowered the tone of scientific discussion, and I do not think it did either them or the lithium debate any good.

I understand you met Barry Blackwell in Frank Ayd's office once. Did you get to the bottom of what was going on?

No. It was only a brief meeting over a cup of coffee. Blackwell seemed to be a pleasant fellow, and Shepherd was clearly the leading spirit in their joint paper.

In 1963 you floated the idea of lithium and the antidepressants as being specific treatments for mood disorder.

I have ambivalent feelings about that paper. It was more speculative and less self-critical than most other things I have done, but some people, including Fred Goodwin, have told me that it struck them as original and interesting. The antimanic effects of lithium had been seen clearly. The therapeutic effect in depression was less clear even though the prophylactic action in recurrent depressions was fairly obvious. Akimoto in Japan had also observed antimanic effects of imipramine. This impressed me enough to suggest that lithium and the antidepressants might be acting on the manic-depressive illness as such. But the paper was a bit speculative and not in my usual style.

What do you make of recent suggestions that the SSRIs may be somewhat less effective than some of the older antidepressants when given for the current episode but perhaps better prophylactically against future episodes?

I am not sure I know what studies you are referring to. Excellent work about continuation treatment with antidepressants has emerged from Pittsburgh. My only misgiving about their publications is that they never mention lithium which, after all, was the first drug for which a prophylactic action on recurrent depressions had been demonstrated.

Is lithium more prophylactic than the standard antidepressants in this area? Michael Shepherd ironically later did a study (Glenn et al.) in which lithium and amitriptyline were compared and it seemed to be better than amitriptyline and there has also been recent work from Germany.

The German so-called MAP study involved a large number of centres and was co-ordinated by Waldemar Greil. This was a well-organised study, carried out with exactitude and involving a large number of patients. The study showed lithium to be significantly better than carbamazepine in recurrent bipolars. Lithium was also better than amitriptyline in the unipolar patients, but the dose of amitriptyline was only 100 mg daily, so perhaps this drug did not appear at its best. To my knowledge there has not been convincing evidence that these drugs are prophylactically superior to lithium.

You've also compared lithium and flupenthixol as prophylactic agents.

That was a multi-centre study where the numbers of patients provided by each centre varied widely. Many centres studied only one, two or three patients, and under such circumstances one cannot be sure that the patients used for the trial are representative. I suggest that in multi-centre studies the centres providing fewer than ten patients should be left out of the analysis. What came out of the study was that flupenthixol did not have a prophylactic action, but in some centres lithium did not either. That study was of dubious quality.

When Cade made his report in 1949 and also for a while thereafter, responses to lithium were quite high. In the first studies on prophylaxis the efficacy of lithium also seemed considerable, the response rate being in the order of 60–80%. In more recent studies the prophylactic response has been much lower, about 40–50%. How do you explain this?

Has the drug lithium changed its properties? Of course not. So what else can have happened? The early studies were mostly carried out in university units, where the staff had close relations with the patients. In all likelihood non-compliance plays a major role in the recent so-called 'naturalistic' studies. Moreover, if patients are not motivated and instructed very carefully they are apt to discontinue lithium, either because they feel that it does not work, or does not work as quickly and completely as they had expected, or because lithium works so well that there are no further episodes and the patients feel they no longer need the treatment. Before the start of lithium treatment patients must be told about the recurrent nature of the disease and the risk of dire consequences of not taking the drug.

One must also remember that when patients are referred to a psychiatric hospital this is often a secondary or tertiary centre, and the patients are likely to be atypical. Patients who respond well to lithium usually remain under the care of general practitioners or practising psychiatrists.

Another thing is that since lithium became 'popular' it is being used on wider and wider indications, especially after the diagnostic criteria have been changed. European psychiatrists working in the United States or Canada tell me that lithium often is used as a sort of antipsychotic in 'atypical' or schizo-affective cases, and this may be the reason why discontinuation of lithium is often and quickly followed by recurrence, mainly of the manic type.

This brings up the tricky question of rebound. In studies on rebound the discontinuation of lithium should always be physician-initiated and blind, i.e. a switch from lithium to placebo without the patients knowing about it. I have gone through the literature, and I found no methodologically acceptable studies providing evidence for rebound or the existence of a 'lithium withdrawal syndrome'.

But it is becoming widely believed that there is a rebound.

Sure. Impressive publications in the *Archives of General Psychiatry* with lots of patients seem to support such an idea. But the discontinuations were non-blind and largely patient-initiated.

That's a hard concept to explain to people outside the field.

Even to those inside the field.

What role did the Sheard study play in this? It seemed to broaden the indications for lithium when he said that it was an anti-aggressive agent.

This relates to the question of specificity. Lithium was claimed by Cade, and initially by myself, to be specific against mania insofar as its effects differed from those of barbiturates and neuroleptics. Later we found that it also worked against depression, prophylactically more clearly than therapeutically, which seemed to make it not only symptom-specific but also disease-specific. Further clinical effects of lithium turned up later, for example against cluster headache and then against aggressiveness. It has never become clear which component or components of manic-depressive illness lithium actually works on. One possibility is mood, another periodicity. Sheard claimed that the patients with outbursts of aggressiveness who responded to lithium were not manic-depressive. Apparently it was the aggressiveness as such that responded to lithium maintenance treatment, sometimes to the extent that the patients themselves would say, 'Now I can think before I hit him.' I found the data convincing, but replication is difficult because it is considered ethically dubious to do drug trials on incarcerated persons.

What component of the picture do you think lithium works on?

I don't know, and I have not speculated overmuch on it. I am not a theoretician. Lithium works in cluster headache but not in migraine. It does not protect against the most frequent psychiatric periodic disease, premenstrual dysphoria. There have been claims about such an action, but together with colleagues in Hong Kong I did a controlled trial and found no effect. Another interesting question is to what extent schizo-affective patients are treated with lithium. Hanns Hippius at one time said that whenever there was anything periodic they gave lithium and obtained excellent results. But the general impression is that lithium does not act on the core schizophrenic features.

There was work that came out of England in the early 1960s which looked like it was going to be relevant to the lithium story. This was the studies by Coppen and Shaw, which showed that there was a dramatic shift in electrolyte distribution during episodes of mania and depression. Did you think at that stage that the mode of action of lithium was close to being discovered?

They were interesting studies but they have not been replicated. There was also a problem about the interpretation of the findings. Alec Coppen suggested that the electrolyte changes reflected intracellular events, but they might as well have been extracellular, taking place in interstitial tissues which can bind a lot of ions. Anyway, they were intriguing studies that should be repeated. At one time we tried using muscle biopsies for this purpose, but that was too unpleasant for the patients and had to be given up.

It is curious how things can come into and go out of fashion, isn't it? These findings have never been refuted, they are just lying there. What about the Coppen studies on the pro-phylactic effects of lithium?

Coppen's were the first confirmatory study outside Denmark. To get priorities right, Coppen started his prospective prophylactic study before we did our discontinuation trial, but ours ended quicker and was published first. His results were of course spectacular, even better than ours. And he made it clear that one could use lower doses of lithium than we had used and get the same efficacy with fewer side-effects.

One of the other players in the prophylactic story was Pierre Lambert, who was the first to describe the prophylactic action of sodium valproate. Who was Lambert?

I don't know, I never met him. Interestingly his later studies on carbamazepine were based on observations made by a Danish neurologist, Mogens Dalby, who used carbamazepine for epileptic patients and noted a mood-elevating effect. That was in 1971.

When these reports began to come through about carbamazepine, what did you make of them?

I welcomed them, because we needed a prophylactic alternative to lithium. Then these anticonvulsants came and seemed to work in patients who didn't respond to lithium or patients who were troubled by lithium-induced weight gain or psoriasis. But according to the German MAP studies I mentioned, lithium still seems to be somewhat better in straightforward bipolar cases.

Neither carbamazepine nor lithium has been particularly promoted by the industry. What effect has the lack of industry support had on lithium therapy in your opinion?

The situation has been peculiar. The industry was never really interested in lithium because of the lack of opportunity to make money from it. So we have had to do a great deal of lithium work without support from the pharmaceutical industry. Carbamazepine and sodium valproate have had more support in terms of propaganda and economic help. I see nothing wrong in that, but it does make for selectiveness. As far as I understand from reports from the United States, students and young physicians there hear exclusively about the anticonvulsants and nothing about lithium, and that of course gives a bias.

Over the years I have speculated on whether it was good or bad that we were not supported by the drug companies. We lost many opportunities in terms of information distribution and drug company-supported symposia, but in other ways it has been good to be independent. What we wrote, positive or negative, was not censured or controlled by anyone. I believe I have published more about lithium toxicity and side-effects than anyone else. That might not have been permitted under drug company control. But I realise that drug company support and publicity have major effects, and these should be kept in mind.

At the moment valproate is being promoted very heavily in the USA, more than carbamazepine ever was, and this is having a significant effect on its market share, even though it is not any safer than lithium. Another point where it seems to me that an industry input might have made a difference was when the arguments about prophylaxis were raging. Studies involving many patients could have benefited by support from the industry.

That's true. We tried to get around that by combining resources and data from Denmark, Czechoslovakia and Switzerland. Of course with industry support we might have had thousands of patients, but then there could have been difficulties with diagnostic differences.

Because of the lack of company input another aspect of our work has been the collection and dissemination of information. I have here in Risskov a reprint library and a literature database with most of the lithium information. To increase the spread of information about lithium I have travelled and lectured a good deal, trying to inform and instruct general practitioners, practising psychiatrists, and hospital psychiatrists. I have also tried to reach the patients through their own associations, and I have written books in non-technical language for patients and relatives, books now available in nine languages. It is difficult to reach physicians directly. The good ones read journals and go to meetings, but the lazy ones do not, and for this reason it is important that the patients themselves are informed and when they come to the doctor can point out that 'Schou says ...'.

In terms of toxicity what was the first problem that arose during the use of lithium in psychiatry, apart from intoxication?

The first was the catastrophic effects in patients given low-salt diets. We later showed that the kidneys excrete lithium much less efficiently when there is a low salt intake. The next problem was the effect on the thyroid, which was observed simultaneously in Stockholm by Sedvall and in Risskov by us. This was a rather worrying problem until we found out that all adverse effects on the thyroid could be rectified by supplementing lithium with thyroxine. The goitres shrank and the thyroid variables normalised. So this isn't a problem once you have spotted the thyroid trouble. But hypothyroidism can to some extent mimic a depression, and treatment of myxoedema with amitriptyline is not very effective.

As regards the kidney problems, when did they begin to emerge?

Around 1969 a group here in Aarhus saw that some of the patients with lithium intoxication had morphological changes in the kidneys. This of course created a major stir, because many clinicians became concerned that long-term lithium treatment might destroy the patients' kidneys. We approached the matter quantitatively and studied the kidney function of many hundred patients, and the same was done in other places. What became clear from this was that water excretion and renal concentrating ability were significantly influenced by lithium – as we had known for many years, but in a manner that was in almost all cases reversible. The glomerular filtration rate was influenced only corresponding to the patients' advancing age. There is no convincing evidence that lithium has long-term effects of its own on the glomerular function. Only three cases have been reported of lowering of GFR in lithium-treated patients with subsequent haemodialysis, and how is it possible to know whether they were or were not caused by the treatment?

Ole Rafaelsen also worked on the effects of lithium on the kidneys. What did you make of him?

Rafaelsen and his associates followed a considerable number of patients over many years and had by and large the same results as we. One point on which they and we took issue was the dosage regimen. By tradition we gave lithium in two daily doses, morning and evening, whereas in Copenhagen they gave lithium only once a day. When they and we pooled data, it came out that their patients had less polyuria than ours. The Copenhagen people were convinced by this that once a day was best and even suggested that lithium every second day might be even better. We were less convinced, because theirs and our patients were not directly comparable. As regards the every-second-day regimen, there have been reports that this is less effective prophylactically. All in all, the magnitude of the daily dose seems to matter much more than how it is distributed over the day.

As regards the sustained release tablets we thought they offered advantages as regards side-effects when we introduced them, but it turns out that their effect is not significantly different from that of the conventional tablets. Of course the tablets with a controlled release of lithium interested the industry because they could be patented. But apparently neither the distribution of doses over the day nor the speed of release from the tablets is of importance.

Ole Rafaelsen, as everyone else, had plusses and minuses. The plusses were very evident. He was blond, tall, handsome, witty, and highly intelligent. He very easily became the centre of any group he was in. Rafaelsen was an excellent organiser, who wrote and talked easily, and he created a unit for biological psychiatry in Copenhagen with a special metabolic ward. However, I do not regard Rafaelsen as a particularly penetrating scientist. He was active and started many things, but in my opinion there was more promise than achievement in his own scientific work.

What about the stories of encephalopathy which were associated with the combined use of lithium and haloperidol?

In 1974 Cohen and Cohen published a paper about what appeared to be a catastrophic interaction between lithium and haloperidol. It scared many people. With this as with other reports about adverse effects of lithium we approached the matter quantitatively. Together with other clinics we studied the case records of many hundreds of patients having been given lithium and haloperidol concurrently, and we didn't find any signs of interaction unless the patients had been given very high doses of haloperidol. So if one wants to use the two drugs together, for example for the initial treatment of violent mania, one would be wise not to go higher than about 20 mg of haloperidol.

An advantage of having had a biological laboratory in a psychiatric hospital is that we have been able to do experimental work on animals and observe the patients at the same time. This has on several occasions been useful, because in animals you can have more stringent conditions and use larger doses of lithium and thereby gain experiences that may be applicable to patient treatment. And the observations made on patients during treatment may provide new ideas for studies on animals. The cross-fertilisation has been useful. For example, when we saw goitre in some of the patients, we could study thyroid function in rats. We also found in studies on animals that treatment with diuretics may lower the lithium clearance, and from clinical observations it appears that some intoxications arose because the lithium-treated patients were given diuretics. One of my associates, Klaus Thomsen, has extended the study of lithium clearance, and this has led to observations of importance for renal physiology. His lithium clearance method is now used all over the world.

In 1987 I got a Lasker Award. In my award lecture I emphasised that choice of study field may be determined more often by limitations and available facilities than by the bright ideas most acceptance speeches appeal to.

In contrast to Holland, Denmark seems to hold psychiatry in relatively high esteem, and there has been greater sympathy toward biological approaches to the management of mental illness. How do you explain this?

I can't explain but I may describe. Psychiatry in USA and apparently Holland and in Scandinavia seems to go in waves but out of phase. When I worked in New York in 1950 psychoanalysis was the thing, while the biological approach was looked down on. It was the other way here. In the 1980s the situation was reversed. Biological psychiatry grew in the United States, while in Scandinavia social psychiatry became a major issue. Psychoanalysis has never been widespread in Denmark.

Psychiatry as such has been fairly well accepted in Denmark and has retained some prestige. Of course there are some who disrespect it. As Professor Strömgren used to say, surgery and medicine are for specialists, but everybody has an opinion about psychiatry. We had some antipsychiatric activities after 1968 but not as fierce as elsewhere, and in addition there were patient and carer groups who were worried about the lack of funding for psychiatry.

Lithium augmentation became a recognised strategy in the 1980s following an article from Canada which suggested that some treatment-resistant patients responded instantly and almost miraculously to the addition of lithium to the antidepressants they had been on. The combination though was in use before that, wasn't it? When did you first become aware that lithium was being added in to regimens and what is your impression of the strategy – it is not of course a strategy that has ever been established by randomised double-blind methods.

There were a few early reports from Czechoslovakia and the United States suggesting that lithium might have an antidepressant action of its own but not strong enough to compete with the antidepressant drugs. There was furthermore a Scandinavian multi-centre study from 1974 with Lingjaerde as the coordinator, which indicated that the combined use of tricyclic antidepressants and lithium was therapeutically more effective against depression than the combined use of tricyclic antidepressants and placebo. The interest in what became known as lithium augmentation was, however, not really raised until de Montigny in 1981 reported that in eight depressed patients not responding to antidepressants alone the addition of lithium not only led to improvement in all eight but the improvement took place within 48 hours. Later replication studies confirmed the lithium augmentation but provided evidence that the improvement after addition of lithium might take several weeks. In 1990, I wrote a review pointing out that the evidence about augmentation was not yet good enough but later studies impressed me and by now I'm convinced of this effect. I believe that this is a useful strategy for those who are refractory to antidepressants alone.

I've always thought that de Montigny's claim had some of the characteristics of John Cade's original claim – it was striking. Now whether some people have a particular talent for making claims striking or whether there is a right time for certain things to be made a phenomenon, I am less certain. The irony here, I suppose, is that the claim that made a new field came some time after the evidence. Can I move on to something else though. Some people complain of lithium damping them down. What do you make of this?

I take these complaints seriously. There was a question once about how lithium affects creativity, which is one measure of vitality. I interviewed, by letter or personal contact, a number of manic-depressive artists who had responded to prophylactic lithium treatment, asking them what lithium had done to their creative ability. Out of 24 such artists six reported that they felt less creative on lithium, and four of them for this reason stopped lithium, two having to return to it later. Six artists saw no difference, and 12 reported that they now created more and better. They had less restlessness and more artistic discipline.

Obviously such a sample cannot be representative, but the interviews at least show us that different persons respond differently to lithium.

I also tried to dig into the question whether the experience of mania or depression might be of value for the process of creating. Being slightly manic appears useful, but if the mood becomes too high, the output is of little artistic merit. This is usually recognised by the artists themselves after the episode has ended, and they throw the products away. But what about the experience of going through the valley of the shadow of death? Well, for the artists I questioned depression was merely a barren period, but there are undoubtedly instances where the depression acts differently, at least in the beginning or toward the end of an episode. Kay Jamison has reported about such occurrences.

Coming back to the question of whether lithium acts on a disease process or on aspects of the constitution, in a volume by Antoinette Gattozzi, probably Nate Kline inspired, put together in the late 1960s, she talks about the fact that there are lots of people out there in the community who have episodes of hypomania which may be more destructive even than mania because they are not picked up, and all the while the person is spending money or having affairs or making irresponsible work decisions. Is it an American phenomenon to see lots of illness out there in the community? It seems to me they may be reproducing the same story these days with adult attention deficit disorder.

In the case of lithium treatment the patients themselves must see the need for it. I have observed situations where the patient yielded to pressure from relatives or physicians, and in almost all these cases the patient later stopped lithium or became non-compliant. I sometimes make the patients draw a chart of the episodes, and they are often very surprised to see how periodic their condition is.

You've mentioned Gjessing, Strömgren and others as being important in your development. Who else has been important in your subsequent scientific work?

In addition to Jules Angst and Poul Baastrup, already mentioned, I would like to point in particular to Paul Grof from Ottawa and Bruno Müller-Oerlinghausen from Berlin. They have been close friends for many years and at all times inspiring and supportive.

Ten years ago I started IGSLI, the international group for the study of lithium-treated patients. The group includes Grof and Müller-Oerlinghausen. Five or six centres in different countries with four to six researchers in each centre meet once a year, and we rotate the meeting places. There are no English or American participants, so we share the burden (or privilege) to communicate in a language that is different from our mother tongue. We also share a European tradition when making diagnoses, which is important for having reasonably homogeneous groups of patients when we pool our data.

One of the issues we have dealt with, suggested by Bruno Müller-Oerlinghausen, is mortality in lithium-treated patients. He and his group in Berlin were the first to report about a lowered mortality during prophylactic treatment with lithium. Coppen found the same in a large group of patients and so did the IGSLI group with still more patients. Whereas manic-depressive patients in general have a mortality that is two to three times higher than that in the general population, patients given long-term lithium treatment have a mortality that is not significantly higher or only slightly higher than that in the general population. After discontinuation of lithium one again finds a significantly increased mortality.

IGSLI is also doing a genetic study, which is headed by Paul Grof and Martin Alda in Ottawa. Most genetic researchers work with rather heterogeneous groups of patients with affective illness, but perhaps when limiting ourselves to so-called excellent lithium responders we may deal with something more homogeneous. This study is running at the moment, and I consider it very likely that it will lead to something interesting, even though the findings may have more to do with the genetics of responsiveness to lithium than directly with the genetics of manic-depressive illness. I'm sure that over the next few years a lot of the genes we pick up will relate to things such as treatment responsiveness.

I hadn't planned to go into the fascinating 'pre-history' of lithium with you until I read a startling little piece in Neil Johnson's book about the history of lithium treatment. It appears that Carl Lange, a Danish neurologist, had described the prophylactic use of lithium for depressive disorders in the latter half of the last century. This is interesting enough, but the twist lies in the fact that one of the people who later wrote a piece that seemed to 'debunk' this idea was your father HI Schou. What would he have made of you ending up in the 'enemy' camp?

Carl Georg Lang was born in 1834 and graduated from the medical faculty of Copenhagen University in 1859. He has been called 'Denmark's first neurologist'. He both practised and studied neurology. He described, for example, aphasia at the same time as, but independently of, Hughlings Jackson, and he was the first to establish the pathogenesis of tabes dorsalis. His observations concerning conditioned reflexes and learning by facilitation preceded Pavlov's studies by 20 years.

Among his main interests were physiology and psychology. In 1885, he published a book, *About Emotions: A Psycho-Physiological Study*, which was translated into German, French and English. It made him known internationally. The central hypothesis was the same as the one the American psychologist and philosopher William James had proposed the previous year – it has since become known as the 'James–Lange' theory of emotions. This was that our emotions exist only as a result of concomitant bodily changes. We are happy because we smile and sorry because we weep. This theory, which is no longer upheld, was epoch-making at the time because it introduced an objective physiological point of view that was radically different from the prevailing romantic belief in the superiority of the soul and the supreme value of introspection.

In 1886, Lange gave a lecture in the Danish Medical Society 'Concerning Periodical Depressions and their Pathogenesis'. It was published in Danish and later in German. Here he described the symptoms and course of what we now know as the unipolar form of manic-depressive illness or recurrent major depression and his descriptions are penetrating and comprehensive. He distinguished this disease from circular psychosis – today's bipolar illness – because he rarely encountered patients with manic episodes in his practice.

He hypothesised that the aetiology of the illness was a so-called 'uric acid diathesis', a metabolic disturbance which at that time was widely believed to underlie a number of diseases, chiefly gout. On this basis, he gave lithium to his periodically depressed patients. His younger brother Frederik Lange was the medical superintendent of a provincial mental hospital and had access to such patients and together they treated many hundreds of patients with doses large enough to lead to serum concentrations of the same order of magnitude as those used today. They claimed to see substantial improvements in their patients but in contrast to John Cade did not give detailed and convincing case histories. And of course the use of statistics and double-blind trials was not known at the time. The Lange brothers cannot be said to have presented conclusive evidence of a lithium-induced prevention of depressive recurrences. When the uric acid diathesis went out of favour, lithium treatment went with it.

When my father later made observations that supported Lange's notion of recurrent depressions as an independent disease, he did not treat the patients with lithium and in his paper from 1938 he did not mention it. On page 17 in Neil Johnson's book there is a passage quoted from correspondence he had with Amdi Amdisen which states that my father's 1938 paper dismissed and 'uncompromisingly denied' the success of prophylactic lithium treatment of recurrent depressions. Amdisen's idea is ludicrous. My father never even mentioned lithium. He could not know that Baastrup and I, 30 years later, long after his death, would provide evidence of a prophylactic lithium action in unipolar illness. It is a misconception that he and I should have held different or opposing views on lithium treatment.

[**Addendum.** After having interviewed me, David Healy let me read his interview with Michael Shepherd and asked what I made of it. The section about lithium is more or less what I had expected; the attitude, the tone, etc. speak for themselves. But some of the statements require correction. Shepherd claims that after the discussion in Göttingen in 1966 (not 1962) my wife came up to him and complained that he had upset her husband. That is pure invention. Shepherd further tells that he made a number of suggestions for my manuscript but that in my publication I twisted them. This again is misinformation. He never sent me any suggestions, so there was nothing I could have twisted. As he himself frequently said citing from Mark Twain – 'The older I get, the more vivid is my recollection of things that never happened.']

Select bibliography
Angst J, Weis P, Grof P, Baastrup PC, Schou M (1970). Lithium prophylaxis in recurrent affective disorders. *British Journal of Psychiatry*, **116**, 604–614.
Baastrup PC, Schou M (1967). Lithium as a prophylactic agent: its effect against recurrent depressions and manic-depressive psychosis. *Archives of General Psychiatry*, **16**, 162–172.

Baastrup PC, Schou M (1968). Prophylactic lithium. *Lancet*. **i**, 1419–1422; **ii**, 349–350.

Baastrup PC, Poulsen JC, Schou M, Thomsen K, Amdisen A (1970). Prophylactic lithium: double-blind discontinuation in manic-depressive and recurrent depressive disorders. *Lancet*, **ii**, 326–330.

Blackwell B, Shepherd M (1968). Prophylactic lithium: another therapeutic myth? An examination of the evidence to date. *Lancet*, **ii**, 968–970.

Grof P, Schou M, Angst J, Baastrup PC, Weiss P (1970). Methodological problems of prophylactic trials in recurrent affective disorders. *British Journal of Psychiatry*, **116**, 599–603.

Johnson FN (1984). *The History of Lithium Therapy*. Macmillan, London.

Schou M, Juel-Nielsen N, Stromgren E, Voldby H (1954). The treatment of manic psychoses by the administration of lithium salts. *Journal of Neurology, Neurosurgery and Psychiatry*, **17**, 250–260.

Schou M (1959). Lithium in psychiatric therapy: stock-taking after ten years. *Psychopharmacology*, **1**, 65–78.

Schou M, Baastrup PC, Grof P, Weiss P, Angst J (1970). Pharmacological and clinical problems of lithium prophylaxis. *British Journal of Psychiatry*, **116**, 615–619.

Schou M (1974). Ethical problems of therapeutic and prophylactic trials in manic-depressive disorder, In *Psihofarmakologija 3* (N Bohacek, M Mihovilovic, eds). Med Naklada, Zagreb, pp 323–334.

Schou M (1992) Phases in the development of lithium treatment in psychiatry. In *The Neurosciences: Paths of Discovery II* (F Samson, G Adelman, eds), Birkhauser, Boston, pp 148–166.

Schou M (1993). *Lithium Treatment of Manic-Depressive Illness, A Practical Guide*. 5th Revised Edition, Karger, Basel.

Schou M (1993). Is there a lithium withdrawal syndrome? An examination of the evidence. *British Journal of Psychiatry*, **163**, 514–518.

See also interviews with Jules Angst and Alec Coppen in Vol 1, *The Psychopharmacologists*.

13 George Simpson

Clinical psychopharmacology

Where and when did you train?

Well, I studied biochemistry in Glasgow and then I was directed to 'work of national importance' – that always sounds much better than it was. I went to work with Distillers, who, I think, made 33 Scotches and two antibiotics. I was lucky or unlucky enough to get the antibiotics. I worked in Liverpool for a couple of years and then went to Medical School in Liverpool. The Dean was Scottish and, when I went to apply, he let me know that I would be all right. That was important because I had a very poor record as a student in Glasgow. I would have to say that either he saw something that nobody else had or he was just being nationalistic. So, I did medicine in Liverpool and I interned there for a year and that was when I decided that I was going to go into Psychiatry. It is interesting how people decide a bit earlier, particularly in the States, you have to declare what you are going to do before you graduate, but I was still interested in paediatrics until my final year. When I decided on psychiatry it was a question of going to London because Liverpool was not very good.

Was Frank Fish there then?

No, Frank Fish hadn't arrived. We had Barton Hall, who was a very pleasant man, but a bit stiff. He was a Reader so there wasn't even a department. I always remember we got lectures in psychotherapy but I never had any clues what he meant by psychotherapy. I wouldn't have said he was a good lecturer either. London seemed more attractive. Then I think I was sitting at tea-time, while everybody else was looking at a test match, reading the *Lancet*, when I saw an ad from McGill about training there. I wrote a hand-written letter and I'm not sure whether I got a cable back or an airmail letter accepting me – from Ewan Cameron.

Which year was that?

That would have been 1956. When I went to McGill, my notion really was that I would spend a year in McGill and maybe a year or two in the States, end up in Mexico and come back to London with the notion of going to the Maudsley.

What did you make of Cameron?

Well, he was very unusual. He was a super-administrator. If he had gone into General Motors, the Japanese would never have penetrated the American market. His institute was his body image. If there was a crack in the stairs you always felt that more people would get ECT that day than if the institute had been whole. He had a lot of bright, stimulating ideas, except he was a terrible researcher. If he had seen himself as an administrator, I think he would have been top of the line. He did have a day hospital, which apart from the Marlborough Day Centre and centres in the Soviet Union was the first of its kind. He was very innovative and energetic but he just had wild ideas – naive and simplistic. You probably know about some of the wild things he did. Before I got there, I think he gave intrathecal hyaluronidase on the notion that depression might involve some abnormality in the blood–brain barrier and this would allow the flow back and forth of whatever it was to resume. You can imagine what his neurological colleagues thought of somebody just shoving hyaluronidase into CSF.

Do you know what the outcome of that was?

Well, I would guess it was positive, but there were never any controls and that was the worst part of it. For instance, another thing that he was giving intravenously was ribonucleic acid. I had a patient with Alzheimer's who had been in the hospital for three months and I don't know if she ever found her way back to her room. However, there was a psychologist who worked with Cameron who showed that her memory had significantly improved. Now some of these people had quite clear rigors probably from pyrogens in the RNA – I don't know where they got them from. There were wild leaps in the dark, I would have called them, that he did without much concern.

   Of course, he was more famous for his psychic driving which one or two people have written about. That was financed at least in part by the CIA, although whether Cameron knew about that or not history may or may not tell us. I was once approached by a foundation to let me know that they were interested in something I was doing. Now if I had pursued that I would never have investigated them to see from where they got their money. I would have taken the money and I think most people would. So, if the CIA were laundering money, it's conceivable that Cameron didn't know. But the research itself was just awful. It was uncontrolled. Some of it was bizarre. I remember a woman who should have worn a helmet with a radio receiver in the ear, transmitting 'I like people, people like me.' When I came in to see her one day, she was sitting on the bed, soaked in urine with her foot in the helmet, which was still going on making the pronouncements, literally in her case, 'I like people, people like me.' It was a male voice and she was responding, 'Well, of course he does and that is what has been the problem in our marriage.' So, part of this woman's problem was her husband who was successful in more ways than one and she felt the voice coming from the helmet was his voice repeating this about himself. There were other things like that. It was difficult because everybody felt it was strange but nobody did anything about it.

I was in my first year in psychiatry at the time and I would argue that the Allan was the most stimulating place in the English-speaking world at the moment even though the rest of the city spoke French. They were just a marvellous group of people around. You had Sloane, who became the Chair at Temple and then USC. Charlie Shagass did all his sedation threshold work there, which was well in advance of his time and probably is still more robust than a DST, but he did it at the wrong time. Cleghorn was there. The Department of Psychiatry had Murray Saffron, a steroid chemist, who actually had a doctoral candidate working within the Department of Psychiatry who I believe got a Nobel Prize later on. Ted Sourkes was there working on catecholamines.

Malmo was doing work on galvanic skin responses, which was interesting. We had to interview patients who were hooked up to this and so were we. I used to tell people in the United States that it was a great way to learn about transference. You would be asking some delicate question of the patient and you could see her GSR rising and you would look over and yours was rising in parallel. Kral was there. He wrote a very good paper on the amnestic syndrome at that time. Robin Hunter, Tom Boag and Jim Tyhurst who all became Chairs. Clifford Scott, who was president of the International Psychoanalytic Association was there and Miguel Prado, a pupil of Cajal's who came over to work with Penfield and got seduced by psychoanalysis. Eric Witkower and a whole bunch of other people were there – all of them in one department. It was a small building and everybody met, socialised and had tea together. You could talk about football or anything with them, which was very different from being a young doctor in England.

In the Maudsley ...

Well, I have never been to the Maudsley but even in Liverpool things were pretty formal. When I left England, I still had to meet the consultant on the steps even though it was pouring with rain. So it was a much more informal and stimulating atmosphere. You saw a lot of patients, worked very hard, and you did a lot of things. For instance, everybody gave amytal interviews; everybody gave amphetamine interviews; everybody gave LSD. All of these things were on the go at that time, so you had a lot of experience. When I came to the States, it was astonishing how little people knew about psychiatry. It was hard to believe. You almost felt grandiose. There was a trainee that I met taking a course that I went to for the Boards and at that time he had never heard of Bleuler. He felt that any book that had not been translated into English for all these years couldn't be up to much – he ended up working in a teaching hospital.

Tell me about Charlie Shagass and his work, because like you I think he has been under-estimated.

Well, Cameron, by administrative fiat, said that everybody who came into the hospital had to have a sleep EEG. You, as the resident, had to go and give the sodium amytal. That produced the data for Charlie's work. It turned out the sedation threshold was a good predictor of response to ECT. He continued working in electrophysiology until he died last year in his eighties. He left there and he went to Iowa. When Sloane, who had been at the Maudsley, took the Chair at Temple, he discussed with me at dinner in New York who he should bring in. He brought Charlie and he brought Joe Wolpe – I advised him against Joe because of the psychoanalytic sensitivity but to his great credit he ignored me and the two best-known people at Temple later were Joe Wolpe and Charlie Shagass. Charlie didn't go back to sedation threshold though he did study drug effects. He had a grant that ran for about 30 years and did a lot of interesting work and was the President of the World Biological Psychiatry meeting when we put on the 4th World Congress in Philadelphia.

Why did you come to the States?

Well, I made one or two goofs in evaluating things. I really would have liked to have gone to spend some time in France. I thought Montreal might combine the best of Britain and the best of France, but I think it probably combines the lesser part of both. But, at any rate, when I went there I got paid $85 a month and my rent was $80, so I ate in the hospital 7 days a week. I think I also had a bit of nostalgia, which would be called culture shock in the States, but it's not nearly as good a word, and I was a bit fed up with some of the things. Cameron came and offered me a Fellowship to stay on, which I felt he should have offered me beforehand. Though, retrospectively, it was up to me to have asked rather than him to have offered. So, one weekend, I just applied to every training programme in the United States that was approved for three years that took foreign medical graduates and paid $300 a month. I posted all the letters on the Monday and on the Friday Cleghorn came and told me that I had been naughty. I asked him what he meant and he said that he had just had a call from Nate Kline in New York.

On the Sunday morning I was wakened early – I remember being cheesed off – and there was Nate Kline on the phone, this very breezy person, talking to me about a Fellowship in research, because in my one-page hand-written CV I said I was interested in research. I went down to visit a couple of times and he just kept phoning so I didn't go anywhere else to be interviewed. I just went to Rockland. Not a well thought out plan – it was just easier.

What was Rockland like at the time?

Well, it was out in the country, pleasant grounds, a lot of space, horrible buildings. They were huge buildings; it was probably one of the last of the big hospitals where they felt that bigger was better. The wards were unbelievably crowded and in this place was a small group of people doing research.

You hear that the research labs were in their own building, which Nate had actually drawn the plans up for – there are all sorts of stories about him having marked out the floor-space.

No, what happened was this. Per Vestergard had come over to work with us from Denmark, where he had been very influenced by Gjessing of periodic catatonia fame. He was collecting and analysing steroids in urine. He seemed to think if he only had enough urine he could answer all the questions. So every time he got money he bought a new freezer and had a whole basement filled with frozen urine. Then came the great New York electrical 'brown out' and it all thawed. I don't know how Nate had finagled him into coming, but I think he expected he was going to have these marvellous labs and what he got was the toilets – it was a big room with 10 toilets with no seats and not even a curtain separating them. There was a picture of that in a Vestergard grant application, a picture of Per sitting on one of the toilets like 'The Thinker', then a picture of him with a hammer and then a picture of a smashed toilet. So Per built his labs in what would colloquially have been called the 'section' in New York. The actual ward was just a routine hospital ward – the only difference was that there were much less patients.

Later that ward was redesigned so that there would be much more observation. Somebody who was interested in space and territoriality came to work on that ward after me. They chalked up the ward into spaces so that they could have somebody continuously recording who was sitting in whose chair. They showed that people had their own territory and their own space. I had known that just by watching my grandfather – nobody ever sat in his chair.

The research building was a hospital building and they would break down parts of what had been wards and make labs out of them or a day room. Before that, some of the wards in the hospital had just beds and the beds were much closer. There were wards where you could not have walked on the floor since the beds were so close together. There was one ward in that hospital that should probably have held 30 odd beds in a way that would have passed today's standards but there were 100. I actually read *The Snake Pit* when I was there and experienced déjà vu and then I found out that yes, indeed, *The Snake Pit* was written in and about Rockland.

Tell me about the discovery of reserpine by the hospital glazier.

Right, this is something I really should have tried to document but I am inclined to believe it. Reserpine came from Jack Saunders, who was working with Ciba at that time. There had been other people who had done some work with it in the States, but I don't think they announced it as dramatically, or with as much flourish. Anyway we had the research ward where patients never got any drugs because they were being followed 'endocrinologically' and they were sort of almost untouchable. But on another of the very busy wards they had given patients reserpine. Now, no one noticed very much – they were not impressed. Then the glazier in the hospital told somebody, 'I don't know what they are doing on that ward but there has been less broken glass than in all the time I have been working here.' That was the rating scale that showed it.

It says something about how far we have or haven't advanced. At the time, I wrote a grant on the notion that thyroid status would be a predictor of outcome, particularly with drugs. So, we did a study where patients were actually given either reserpine or perphenazine or phenelzine to look at outcome and this involved a lot of rating. Many of the patients got better and I probably discharged half of that ward. I didn't like the 'Waiting for Godot' approach – just following

290 The Psychopharmacologists II

patients and not giving any interventions even though these patients had never been on drugs. But I also had another ward elsewhere because of another NIMH grant I was brought in to bolster up a bit. The psychiatrist who had been doing studies had a pocket diary and on one page of that diary was all of the material for each patient for the whole study – the patient's age, all the demographics and the outcome, and none of these pages were full. I thought that was awful. But before that, there was no documentation at all, so this psychiatrist had made a giant leap forward in terms of documentation of what had happened to patients. In practice, drugs were given to patients and then somebody said the patient had improved or hadn't improved and that was all the data.

Moreover, at least in some of the studies, patients were getting other drugs. Joe Barsa, who did some of the work with Nate Kline, ran a building with some 500 patients with another doctor. Now if you are responsible for 250 patients and have to give an annual physical and whatever else is required because you are responsible for the physical care of these people – there is no way you could do research. So, in point of fact, there were drugs that I know people got almost as a baseline treatment and then other drugs were added. That was the state of how things were at that time. It was only later that more sophisticated things were done. The studies that I did were predominantly open studies on patients whom one knew well and to whom you gave a new medication after they had been off medication for a month. Later we did some controlled studies as well. But all we were doing was saying a drug was active or was not active.

Can I ask you about Nate – who was he?

Well he was from Atlantic City originally. His family was made up of business people and he said that they were disappointed that he did not go into the business but went to medical school instead. I'm not sure if I really believe that. He did a Masters in Psychology before he went to medical school. Then, he went into the Navy and when he came out of that, he decided he was going to go into research. He applied for a job in research in Worcester, where they gave him the job of Director of Research – so he started at the top. He was there for a short while and then, somehow or other, he got this job at Rockland.

Actually, I'll tell you an interesting story that says something about Nate. I met George Nicklin at a cocktail party at the UN last night. George had been at NYU and he had a bee in his bonnet that there was a toxin that caused schizophrenia – a lot of people thought along these lines after LSD. His question was, what would happen if you got a hallucinating schizophrenic and transfused his blood into a normal subject and vice versa? George was a Quaker and he recruited another young Quaker who had volunteered for some public duties and he volunteered for the cross-transfusion study. So we did a controlled study in which tubes were coming in and out of the patient and the volunteer and they did indeed exchange half of their blood. I reported somewhere that the patient got slightly worse and the control got married but nothing else really happened. Now he had tried to do that study at NYU and was told that it couldn't be done. Eventually they told him that if you go to Nate Kline, he could probably do it. So that is why he came and did it at Rockland and that was Nate – he was open for that.

He was an enthusiast in many ways. Ewan Cameron didn't like him. I think Cameron felt he was too flamboyant and also made extravagant claims. I think Cameron was a more knowledgeable and a better clinician than Nate. Before reserpine, Nate had given a paper on 'normalcy', trying to define what was normal. I think Dick Wittenborn came and helped him with some rating scales at that time. This was in the early 1950s. Then reserpine came along and that catapulted him into the limelight. Now this has to be seen historically against a background where everything in America was psychoanalysis. When these drugs were discovered it was not easy to convince people that they worked. Clearly Nate did a good job of this.

Then, somehow or other the Laskers became interested in mental health, with Mike Gorman, and they endowed money and gave the Lasker award. They were very instrumental with one or two other people in pushing Washington to get money for mental health. So suddenly there was more money for research than anyone knew what to do with. Jonathan Cole was really running around looking for people to give money to. Nate had been involved in an early study of reserpine for which he got the Lasker award and there was a lot of hullabaloo, so it was natural research monies would go his way. He had a good relationship with the Director of the hospital so I think he could also get monies and positions from there and from the State and from other outside funding.

The grant that I wrote could very well have been the first NIMH grant that Rockland had. Jonathan Cole, when he came to site visit, told me that it was a good idea for us to expand and ask for more money, but that I was too junior to be the principal investigator – which was true. The only problem was that Nate became the principal investigator and he really saw it as a book. Some of the other very eccentric people who were working around the place just saw the grant as a way to advance their own work and so they did the work in passing rather than with any commitment. Eventually, that grant which must have added up to over a million dollars – a lot of money in those days – produced little or nothing at all.

You would have come there just after the iproniazid story had started rolling and presumably before Jack Saunders and Nate began to argue over who had really made the discovery. Did you get any impression over what had really happened? What was Jack like?

Well, Jack was a tall solemn gentleman who was apt to get bad tempered. I always found it was easier to deal with him face to face. He got more bad tempered on the phone than he did face to face. But, he was a bright guy and he had a lab and he did studies. Now Jack wasn't a psychiatrist, so in effect when I started doing the clinical work I took that away from Jack – even though I'm not quite sure how it came about that he was doing it in the first place. Thereafter, Nate was the senior and Jack the junior entrepreneur and the other people did the work. By the time I got a second grant, I was on my own and Nate never really interfered with what I did. Nate, at this time, was very busy going around the world, to Haiti and Tibet, giving lectures and he had a very busy private practice. Nate got into the limelight and Jack sort of stayed in the shadows.

Nate had a lot of the characteristics that would make him attractive company whereas Jack would have been a much more dull person socially. When iproniazid first came out, I remember Cameron talking about it. Nate had gone to some meeting where he was supposed to talk on one subject, but instead he made some pronouncement about iproniazid. Jack somewhere along the line got upset – I think it was when Nate got his second Lasker award. Somebody should check whether Nate was on the selection committee at that time. There always was a rumour that he had nominated himself. Jack gave a presentation at the New York Academy of Sciences, where he said it the way he felt it happened and that was that until Nate wrote an article for *JAMA*, when he got the Lasker, about how iproniazid had happened. That is where I think Saunders took exception.

Clearly also Harry Loomer had been the person who actually gave the patients the pills. These were inpatients, so some of them would have suffered from affective disorders and goodness knows what. I have no idea what the population was, but it was an open study on a busy admission ward. Nate had also used some of it on his private patients as well. Looking back at it, it was remarkable that they ever discovered anything. They nearly missed reserpine and, if you think about it, getting a new antidepressant when you have a busy ward or you have a busy private practice and you are given a drug openly could be very difficult.

So that was when Saunders got irate and in the *JAMA* article there were certainly things that, for me, were very dubious. In the article, Nate said that the next thing that happened was when Coppen in England and we here independently worked with tryptophan and 5-hydroxytryptophan and found it improved the rate of onset of recovery. Well, I had been in Bill Sack's office when he received a reprint from the *Lancet* by Alec Coppen about giving tryptophan to patients on monoamine oxidase inhibitors, showing that it had an added effect. Sack suggested using 5HT because he was doing biochemical studies with it. Nate started a study of 5HT after the *Lancet* article was published, gave it to quite a few patients very quickly and had his '24-hour cure for depression' published the same year as the Coppen study – but the idea was clearly Coppen's.

But he was quite happy to sell this as something he had come to independently?

Yes. It was cleverly written – independently; it certainly was not a collaborative study. I never particularly believed the finding. In a very naive way, I had gone in to cover Nate's private practice when he went to Europe for six weeks in the summer – he needed somebody in the office. The FDA had decided that if you treated patients they needed a case history to give them some information.

Nate had done a study for which he had no case histories. He might have had a page of longhand writing and that would be the admission history of a patient.

So the idea that you read in the obituaries that they got a very detailed work-up by him first ...

No. That came along later. At that time, essentially, I came in to reconstruct case histories. So we phoned and patients came in. I would ask them when they came here and that we were interested in getting information – which we were – and we asked them how they were feeling at that time and as best we could, we would get that information. And that was in many ways how I got involved. We did a study with desipramine ...

Well, I was about to ask you about that. That was you, Nate and Brodie. What did you make of Brodie and how did the two of them get on together?

I liked him. I only saw them together once in Paris. Brodie had shown that imipramine was demethylated to desipramine. He was a well-known scientist. Nate and I gave this drug openly to some 20-odd patients. I was a rather junior person who saw the patients and wrote it up but Nate added the conclusion which was that desipramine worked faster than imipramine and I was too junior and naive to argue about it.

This is the finding Brodie would have wanted.

Of course, but retrospectively, once one had got to know a bit more about depression it was silly. That is Brodie's only clinical paper, I think, which is quite amusing.

I went on working with Nate but I stopped after we did a controlled study in depression which I thought was foolproof. We had an independent diagnostician who saw the patient, did the initial interview and decided whether the patient would enter the study. Nate did the prescribing and then I saw them independently, and rated them. When I went to analyse the data, there were 39 patients and I think only 19 had no other drugs added to their regimens. I never wrote it up. That was when I decided that it was unlikely that we would ever do something controlled.

What was incredible also was the patients who came. I suspect that early on in his career, Nate had treated somebody in the Sephardim and so we had a lot of Sephardic Jews. Then we had patients referred by Albert Ellis and other, you could say almost fringe people, who were smart enough to know that a patient was not doing well and if there was an alternative treatment maybe that would be a good idea. Moreover, I think there were probably some other non-physician referrers. In all events we saw a lot of patients who did indeed make very dramatic responses. When you think of Listening to Prozac, you know we were Talking with Tofranil a bit earlier. We saw many patients because there weren't very many people doing that sort of work in the city. In that area, I'm sure that Nate had a very positive influence both in terms of treating patients and pushing pharmacotherapy against academic inertia as well as resentment by people who were not about to believe this.

He kept, at least through to about the mid-1960s, referring to the MAOIs as psychic energisers rather than antidepressants. Was this for legal reasons because of the Lasker court case or was it because a lot of people actually think that they were not the same kind of agent as the tricyclics.

Well, no. There was the paper from Mortimor Ostow and I think that concept probably was Ostow's. I would speculate that, to Ostow, the idea of a psychic energiser fitted in with a dynamic theory of depression. I don't see any legal angle in that.

But he had to use the concept later in court to sustain the case that he was the actual discoverer – he appealed to the paper that he had written with Ostow in 1956 so that he could point to the fact that even before he found the drug he had proposed that there could be this kind of a drug. Did you ever feel that he was trying to play that kind of game?

No I did not. In the 1958 paper, the presentation at the CINP in Rome, he talks about people resisting getting well and, to me, the concepts are very psychodynamic and very dubious. I think that there are indeed people who don't want to get well but they are not usually people with major depressions. No, I think that he was a person of his time. Did you know that Nate was psychoanalysed by Paul Schilder? I remember him saying that it never took. I think people didn't know how to describe these drugs at that time. Don't forget that in some of the original tuberculosis studies these drugs were called euphoriants and they were called stimulants and so on. It was some time before anything was called an antidepressant.

But oddly enough Max Lurie as early as the 1953 paper was talking about isoniazid as an antidepressant. He had been giving it to non-personality-disordered people and to people who were outpatient depressives and not to people on the backwards.

Well, this is fascinating because, if you read these early papers, neither Kline, Crane nor anyone else mentions that paper. Now I tried to follow up on this after I last spoke to you because the Lurie paper references Bill Turner. I spoke to Bill at the December meeting. He is high up in his eighties but he was there with a poster. He took down the details and promised to get in touch me but I haven't heard from him and I don't know his address. But anyway, Bill had used isoniazid as well and it is interesting that Lurie in Ohio knew of Turner's work and Turner was in Long Island and that is where Crane was working in the Tuberculosis Sanatorium when he picked this up. So it is strange that nobody mentioned these other papers.

Indeed, and the isoniazid story is quite believable because in Paris Jean Delay had used it as early as 1952 and had said it was an antidepressant. How do you explain the fact that Max Lurie is unheard of?

Well, I think there are two things. People don't read the French literature and vice versa. And Lurie published his work in a Mid-Western journal and not a national journal. Current contents or any of these things hadn't been invented. But you would have thought somehow or other that it must have caused some ground swell somewhere because there weren't all that many things that people were saying. The other thing that I liked about the Lurie paper is that he said that his patients seemed to take about 2 or 3 weeks to get better, which is much more impressive than these instant responses. But neither it nor Delay was mentioned and clearly that was in the literature and should have been available. It is fascinating to think about it given the fact that isoniazid is not a monoamine oxidase inhibitor. Wouldn't it be interesting if it had a totally different mechanism of action?

I worry about the fact that nobody knows very much about the kinetics of the MAOIs. There's very little work on that at all. It's conceivable that 85% MAO inhibition is going to be achieved by a dose of phenelzine that will give you enough phenelzine to do something elsewhere. With tranylcypromine you can get a tremendous amount of inhibition. In a study that I was a volunteer in I got over 80% inhibition after 10 mg, just one tablet. So that if we are really talking about getting 80% inhibition, one tablet a day would do most people and some people could do with one tablet once a week. This suggests to me that raising monoamine oxidase levels with tranylcypromine is not the mechanism of action and you have people like Jay Amsterdam who is treating treatment-resistant depression with 90, 120, 140 mg of tranylcypromine and certainly I feel that I have seen people who did not respond to 30 but did to 60. So I don't know what is going on there. It's an interesting area for somebody to look at.

Can I take you to one of the other things that began happening in Rockland, which was computers and Gene Laska? Can you fill me in on that development?

Well, essentially we had the RED grant, which was for the Research in Endocrinology and Drugs, which was the one I mentioned before – Nate abbreviated it to the Red Grant. Somebody, I think Ted Cranswick, said that you'll have to watch that Nate because you will have people investigating you. Ultimately, I had somebody from the FBI come to see me about one of my nurses. She had belonged to a poetry reading society out in the Bush in Australia and there had been some leftish person there, and then she came to London when the 'ban the bomb' marches were on. Anyway, she came to work with me and the FBI came and asked what the work was that I couldn't have had an American nurse do. I told them that she was working on what we called the RED project.

As it turned out, Sobell, who had been a spy, was in the same building. He was the guy who took off to Israel and was extradited from there to the US and then just before his plane landed in London he took an overdose of Nembutal and died in a London hospital. He was dying of leukaemia anyway. He had worked in the other half of the building and had an adjoining door – the phone was on our side. Sobell was a psychiatrist, who, when he had left Lithuania, had been pressured about his family. He had done some things donkeys years before and because of that the phone was tapped and I guess they checked up on everybody who came to work there, which is where the nurse story came in.

At any rate we were collecting masses of data because in effect patients had their thyroid status measured all the time. Their steroids and behavioural ratings were also done and by the time we had a year or so's worth of data, somebody said, 'Well, what are we going to do with it?' We didn't have a statistician. Then Gene Laska came from IBM to talk to us about the idea of having some computing skills there and eventually he came and joined us.

Why?

I think that it probably looked interesting. Of course very soon he had a huge grant for the multi-state information system – it was a 5 million dollar grant. They began computerising the hospital records and drug prescribing and all of that. Indeed, sometime in the early 1970s, I ran a hospital service, inpatient and outpatient, where everything was computerised so that nobody wrote anything. You just filled in a mental status or an anamnesis and your secretary put these forms into the computer. On the way home and in the morning you got a typed report with a differential diagnosis. I think Nate probably saw that computers would become important. But essentially Gene Laska's first task was to manage the RED data. Afterwards he built up this other thing on his own with Nate's support.

We published a computerised mental state in the 1970s which had a Hamilton and a Wing scale buried in it and then you had a narrative output – that was Scribe. It was a clever gimmick. I remember at a meeting in Madrid there was a NOSIE scale where you could get a narrative like a nurse's report from filling in this and you could get it in six different languages. You could fill it in in English and get the report in Russian or Spanish.

But there wasn't a big follow-through with it. The doctors didn't like the computerised records. When I left, that all disappeared. I think they felt that you were missing the human touch. Certainly there was no way that you could have done a Sherlock Holmes – if somebody did have a short leg or a cross eye you're not going to get that. But, they were all legible and they were there forever and it wasn't a bad idea. During it all through the WHO connection, places like Indonesia went from having no medical records to having them computerised. The bureaucrats loved it because their inventory control of drugs became efficient for the first time in history. When everything was done by hand how did you decide how much you would get in the way of drugs for your building's monthly order? If there were suggestions of rationing, people ordered more than they needed and stored, but in the first year when the computers were used thousands of dollars were saved just because nobody could order more than they needed, just in case. The computer told them, here's what you did last month and here's what you will need if your prescriptions are correct and that was that. So Gene came around that time and stayed. He has moved out of computers and into trial design and he has done a lot of work on carryover effects in analgesia etc.

When did you get involved with ACNP?

I got involved in the 1960s because of Nate, who said that this is a good organisation and I should join. In the days when I applied, nobody had to write gargantuan letters of recommendation and all of these things. They were always from the very beginning unique meetings. Unique because of the site in the first place – they were always in the winter in Puerto Rico in the week before high season. This was because it was cheaper and ACNP was essentially an East Coast outfit.

Why has psychopharmacology been an East Coast thing in the States?

I don't know. From the start, you had Heinz Lehman in Montreal, Fritz Freyhan in Delaware, Kinross-Wright in Texas and the others in the State Hospitals, Nate, Denber and Tony Sainz up in Syracuse. The drug companies also were here so it was easier to go to your own back door than go elsewhere. But the early people were all hospital based, which has always fascinated me. Psychopharmacology began in the State hospitals and the VA and had to almost hammer the doors of academia down. Everywhere else in the world, knowledge begins in academia and spreads outwards.

It isn't only in this country but it's throughout Europe.

Yes. It was because these were the people who were on the front line who had to do something and you are more likely to get the desperation treatments. I think people in the State hospitals had this approach so that when drugs came into the State hospitals they spread like wildfire. In order to control people at the time, you were using atropine, hyoscine and sodium amytal, as well as wet packs and ECT. When I came to Rockland, I couldn't believe that they gave ECT without anything. And, not only that, but the man who gave it wasn't very smart. When I talked to him about using muscle relaxants and so on he thought that was a bit silly. They simply had tongs and they went around just buzzing people. So there was a huge need for something to happen.

There had been a social revolution in Britain and other countries after the war, which drove mental health change. I think change in America came a bit later in mental health and it was driven here by psychopharmacology. It's hard to talk about British psychiatry without talking about the Maudsley, which certainly doesn't have the most therapeutic reputation. But you have to compare that with here, where in academic circles nobody was doing anything. The other thing that we do in psychiatry, which is strange, is that we send away the most difficult patients to the State hospitals. So, on the one hand, we look down on the State hospital doctors and think they're not very good but we send them the most difficult patients. This is a strange phenomenon. Usually you send the most difficult people to the Chair of the department.

Another thing that was good about the ACNP was the way it was kept small. In the beginning, it was small and then they realised that they had accidentally stumbled on a good idea. They had these siestas on the beach or at the pool and you could get anybody and have a long conversation with them. When you go to other meetings if you want a long conversation with somebody you end up having dinner with them. There are many people, however, that I would like to have a long conversation with that I might not want to have dinner with and you can only have dinner once a day but there you could have had this three hour thing and you could get two or three people together and get the information you wanted. And then there was a real interchange of information at the workshops and other sessions.

So, they deliberately kept the size down as it evolved. That has always been one of the tensions in the organisation because, on the one hand, it gets the name of being elitist and there are people out there who you know are clearly superior people that should be in any organisation but they are not in the ACNP. But I think it has worked out quite well.

You were the President of ACNP at much the same time as the American Society for Clinical Psychopharmacology was being formed?

I was President in 1992 and ASCP was formed, I believe, the year afterwards. The ASCP was really Gerry Klerman, Don Klein and Paul Wender who talked about it and invited some people to a meeting in Washington. I went along to hear what they had to say. It seemed to me that it was a good idea. The ACNP has an educational wing but it is a small organisation and by its very definition it has top-notch pharmacologists and psychiatrists, psychologists, statisticians, everything, but that's not a big deal for practitioners. So there was the question of the big gap between what we know and what is happening out there and who is going to try and narrow the gap. The idea was that the only way to do it was to have an organisation where people who are in the front line would have some say.

It was clear to me that there would be some tension as it would overlap with the ACNP. But they are two different constituencies. ACNP is a small organisation that is heterogeneous and they are never going to be able to do the educational job that it needed. It is conceivable that this organisation will be helpful because already they have twice as many members as ACNP. While most of the people who are on the board are people who have reasonably distinguished research and academic credentials, there is a hope that as the organisation progresses it will be less involved with name recognition and with democratic organisation, teaching and other problems as well as research. I think there is enormous room for doing this kind of thing because you have got dozens of people who have seen a lot of patients who could provide information if they agreed to do something jointly by electronic bulletin board or whatever. The organisation is still a fledgling organisation but I think it is pretty stable. Its not a breakaway from ACNP, but something in parallel.

Its probably many people's dream in medicine to go 'eponymous'. You've done this. How did the Simpson–Angus scale come about?

We first started measuring extrapyramidal symptoms in the early 1960s and already by 1964 had published a paper on this, which included a rudimentary rating scale. I finalised the scale thereafter and we used it from 1965 onwards but it was not until we combined a series of papers in 1970 that the scale was ever published. The reason for the delay was simply that we were a very busy unit. Scott Angus joined me at this time and he was a very pleasant fun person to work with. We did the writing up which then appeared as a monograph in *Acta Scandinavica*.

The reason for developing the scale was simple. In the early 1960s, little was known about the relative potency of antipsychotics. Given that they appeared safe, people were apt to give them until they saw some side-effects. To an extent everyone believed that if there were no extrapyramidal symptoms (EPS) you did not have an active agent. We evaluated new drugs continuously and it seemed to us, therefore, that if we could quantify extrapyramidal symptoms, this would be a better way to measure relative potency than the effect on psychotic symptoms.

I modified the scale further in the 1980s for two reasons. One was that originally all the work had been on inpatients and, therefore, we had items that required an examining table on which the patient could sit with their legs 'hanging down, swinging free' but I took this leg rigidity item out as it did not contribute very much. I also took out head dropping and substituted head rotation. The other major change was to include akathisia.

That leads nicely onto clozapine. As I understand it there was a point when shortly after clozapine was first banned in this country there were only about four people who were using it – you, Nate, Herb Meltzer and one or two others. What do you make of the clozapine phenomenon? I sense you are not as enchanted with it as some others.

Well, it clearly is a unique drug. The first time we gave it to patients, everybody in the ward knew very quickly that it was something different because we saw people getting better and we never saw any EPS. So I think it is more active than any drug that we possess. I think it is a drug of choice for people with akathisia or any tardive condition, particularly dystonias but also dyskinesias.

But can you criticise study 30 on the basis that half the patients were being poisoned with huge doses of comparators and, lo and behold, the other half who weren't been poisoned did slightly better.

That was certainly a critique here. You could make an argument, and I don't know that I absolutely believe it, but I think it is still up to somebody to disprove that the beneficial effects of clozapine are totally EPS-related. We have data from the 1960s where we just happened to have somebody rating EPS and somebody else rating psychopathology and we found that emotional withdrawal and EPS parallel each other beautifully. Other people have shown that too. But I'm not sure that anybody is clever enough to separate negative symptoms from the akinesia and parkinsonism. The question of how much more efficacious than other drugs it is is, I think, still up for grabs. We are getting figures in some places that a substantial number of people are going back to work. I haven't seen that. The dramatic cases I have seen have been affective disorders.

Oh, now that is interesting. Because it is a tricyclic of sorts ...

The people who took up the bed and walked have clearly been people with affective disorders or who were very sensitive to EPS from typical neuroleptics. I have a tape of a young woman who was very hebephrenic and would come in dishevelled and disorganised, talking gobbledegook. If you gave her any drug, she would turn into a beautiful, neat, tidy young girl but she couldn't stand any of them because of akathisia, so she was always coming back in. When we gave her clozapine she had no problem. We have done a study, which is unpublished still, a controlled double-blind crossover of 100, 300 or 600 mg of clozapine, where patients get 16 weeks of each dose, the idea being to find out which worked the best. The bottom line was that we got something like a 24% response – 12% of them during that study and the other 12% when we raised the dosage to 900 mg. Unfortunately the 900 mg was an open tail but I believe that after 48 weeks in a research ward you are not going to get much placebo response. We have blood level data and some of the people at 600 mg did not have adequate levels. This was an older and more chronic group of patients. I guess my bottom line would be yes, it is better than anything else we have got but perhaps not as good as some people are saying. In terms of clozapine and risperdal, John Davies in his met-analysis came up with about 30% extra benefit for clozapine and about 15% for risperdal.

Given that we are advancing on many fronts, I think that if you took a treatment-resistant population and did the original study over again you might get a lesser response because you have creamed off some of the patients and you are left with even more treatment-resistant patients. But this idea that they go on improving forever I think is just social learning – their symptoms are gone and they are beginning to do other things.

What about the question of akathisia and dysphoria with other neuroleptics?

Yes. Haloperidol produces a lot of akathisia, perhaps more than any other drug, though one would need to study this to say it more clearly. In our clozapine study we had 44% akathisia in a lead-in period with 10 mg of haloperidol and almost 0% with clozapine. One of the nice things about the new atypicals coming along is that they will finally teach us what the dose of haloperidol is. In the Sertindole studies, for instance, it is quite clear that 4 mg of haloperidol is active, not quite as good as 8 mg but the EPS at 8 mg are very substantial. We did a study comparing three doses of fluphenazine – 10, 20 and 30 mg – and we did not see any difference in outcome between the three dosages. When we looked at predictors apart from chronicity of illness the most important predictor of poor outcome was akathisia.

By akathisia you mean something other than just the actual movement of the feet – you mean something closer to dysphoria?

Well, perhaps. When you read the Barnes scale, you think that a lot of people have subjective distress. A lot of people do, but I think as you get more chronic patients, they don't complain at all. So our definition of akathisia was the one that was recorded by the staff, not by a scale.

Very often your average prescriber fails to appreciate the effects of this – having seen grown men cry on 4 mg of haloperidol, I'm sure that if you have that experience, even if you know there is an antidote for it, it is going to put you off taking the drug.

Oh yes. Well on the question of why patients do not take their medication, Ted Van Putten, who did not do controlled studies of these things, was I think absolutely right when he wrote that this was a big cause of people not taking medication. The young girl that I talked about would be a good example. People have difficulty describing it – we say people feel like jumping out of their skin. My explanation of akathisia to residents is that you feel like you have a constant infusion of adrenaline – just slightly more than you can tolerate. It is extremely dysphoric and indeed we wrote about that same little girl in one of our papers a long time ago when we discussed psychotic exacerbations caused by neuroleptics – iatrogenic psychosis you might call it. There she was crawling around on the floor until her knees bled and was importunate with the nurses. Illness or akathisia or both? Parkinsonism is easy to recognise compared to this. One of the problems with akathisia is you can get it on 1 mg of haloperidol – at a sub-therapeutic range. Phil May in terms of patient dysphoria and George Awad have done some nice things about this. But it may all go out of the window – it wouldn't happen with clozapine.

Let me take you back to your roots and ask you to comment as a Scot on either the Prozac or the Listening to Prozac phenomena and the whole ADDH thing. We don't have ADDH over in the UK. Perhaps we do but culturally at the moment we don't. Who is right?

You don't have Borderline Personalities either. I think the guy who wrote Listening to Prozac could have been Talking to Tofranil 20 years earlier if he had not been preoccupied with psychodynamics. There was no question that in the 1960s we were referred patients by good psychotherapists who knew they were stuck in treatment. The cases were mild endogenous depressions and you prescribed drugs and you got marvellous responses. Over my career, what I see is that what I once believed was not treatable, and then later might have said was personality merging into the tail-end of an illness, has come into the treatment range. Incidentally there was a poster yesterday claiming that fluoxetine was beneficial for some normals. Richard Belon was a co-author.

If people had asked me 20-odd years ago what sort of people responded to monoamine oxidase inhibitors, I might have glibly said, people that you think would do well on psychotherapy and who don't. I think Peter Kramer had a big investment in psychodynamics and that over time fluoxetine gave him a rationale to escape – it was something different so his old teacher wouldn't have been right and he wrong and so he used fluoxetine. The other thing about fluoxetine is that it didn't have the side-effects or dosing problems of tricyclics – one size fitted everyone. Now who are these people who respond? I think they are in the group I have just referred to.

I think of the Columbia people, Jean Endicott and Wilma Harrison, and the PMS studies. There was a certain subgroup of PMS people who were really chronic dysthymics, who really only become very symptomatic premenstrually, leading to their inclusion in PMS. Now these are the people you can treat with antidepressants. Clearly if you treat females with tricyclics, whatever else they get, they are going to gain weight, as with the the the MAOIs, so I think that Prozac got all of that market immediately. In the US non-psychiatrists were targetted by Lilly and the one-dose strategy carried the day with these people.

At all events physicians, including psyciatrists, who not have prescribed tricyclics began to prescribe fluoxetine. For some psychiatrists there had been a little bit of religiosity, a belief in the sanctity of the self which you invade when you give drugs, so that you have this notion that the real treatment is the talking. I think these people began to give drugs with fluoxetine. A good example recently was a case that a resident presented to me of a woman hospitalised for her diabetes. The intern, who had been a doctor for less than six months, realised she was depressed and gave her fluoxetine. She didn't respond. When the resident presented the history to me it was clear that she had been hospitalised a year or so before in our ward, had been treated with nortriptyline and did very well. So I said, well, you must promise me that you will phone that intern and say that we in psychiatry don't mind you treating depression but you must take a history. I doubt if that intern would even have treated a patient with a tricyclic.

When I was working in Philadelphia, I got referrals from some very good therapists. They would have somebody who did not meet all the criteria for major depression but had some of them. Now, if I had been seeing the patient for the first time, I probably would have waited a bit before I did anything. As they had done the wating, I would just give them an antidepressant, often with surprising and rapid results. So that is the area that people are getting into as part of the Prozac phenomenon. I'm also sure there are a lot of people who are getting Prozac for the wrong reasons.

ADHD is a different phenomenon. It has become a very respectable middle class illness. It offers the possibility that I didn't fail at school because of being stupid or I didn't fail this, that or the other because of my aptitude but because of course I had an attention deficit disorder and that makes it all respectable. I am being cynical but there is a lot of it going around with people self-diagnosing themselves but on the other hand it exists.

Yes, I would agree with you that it actually exists and it has always been there and should be recognised and there is the adult form too, but when did it begin to roll? How has it come to be such a huge thing now?

I don't know how much Paul Wender has to do with that. Paul Wender is a psychiatrist who was involved in the adoption studies in Denmark. He lives in Utah and came out with the Utah scale for attention deficit disorder and has done a lot of studies.

The areas that I would see that everybody should be aware of include having a history when they are young. And you do see cases who have difficulty concentrating and focusing who when you give them a stimulant do much better. I can think of one case I saw who I gave a stimulant to – the first thing he noticed was that he felt more relaxed. The second thing was that he could concentrate better. The third thing was that he could sleep better and the fourth thing was that he got a shift in his appetite so that he ate more. Everything it would have done to me, it did the reverse to him – it relaxed him, made him sleep more, had a contradictory effect on his appetite etc. He was a good case but it must be there when they were young, which it was in his case.

Clearly the diagnosis has been overlooked, but going back to the Prozac thing, how far do you guys here go over the top with these things? Enthusiasm seems to be a US thing. There is a ground swell from the critics of psychiatry that this is just one more instance of the pharmaceutical industry raping our children.

Well, I have heard people saying that but clearly you get lots of mothers who testify the other way round. When they showed that methylphenidate had an effect on growth, it was a big boost to the critics but then Rachel Klein showed that growth caught up over time. But clearly you would like not to use drugs if you can get away with it. When you ask Rachel Klein why the Germans or Swedes don't use these drugs, she would say they have more discipline in school. Now I would rather have kids getting discipline in school than getting amphetamines. But that is the choice and it is clear that the American people want it both ways.

It is just beginning to hit the UK now; the stories are beginning to appear in the media and the BAP are beginning to think that we should convene a round table to look at the question of paediatric psychopharmacology.

Well, you should do that anyway because there is a fair amount of research going on. Tom Cooper has been measuring methylphenidate levels and metabolites in these kids for some time. It would be good to draw attention to this and to conduct disorder, which is also a big problem and again, to me, something with huge environmental influences. A colleague of mine drew up entry criteria for a study of conduct disorder in terms of the aggressive acts and verbalisations but he had to reduce the entry criteria because few were meeting it and of those who did on admission, 50% didn't meet it after they were in the hospital for a week. Now in the new managed care setting they are all going to get drugs coming in the door and they are going to do very well because 50% at least would do very well anyway. The same is true of adolescent depressions. Willy-nilly you get the 50% response rate by changing the environment. But then, these kids with conduct disorder are sent back to the ghetto and behave the same way. What is the influence of drugs in all of these things?

What happened to Nate in the end? Something went badly wrong, didn't it?

Well, he got involved with the endorphin story and he was giving it to patients who were depressed – I think on a one-time shot – and that caused a bit of concern. Endorphin was very hard to get but CH Li, who discovered growth hormone, made endorphin and brought it over and gave it to Nate. Now I think a lot of people in the ACNP and elsewhere felt that it was a bit inappropriate to do this. The preparation had never been tested in any which way at all and it was precious stuff. But Nate finished the study on July the 3rd or 4th and it was read at the Royal College meeting on the 5th and published in *Archives* in September of the same year. I think he pulled in all his favours to get something published in *Archives* inside two months. Anyway the FDA looked into it and the upshot was, I believe, that Nate was not allowed to do any more clinical research.

How did you read the battles between Nate and the Maudsley over lithium with Michael Shepherd on one side and then Nate and Heinz Lehmann and others on the other side?

I think Nate would always be critical of anybody who questioned his clinical or therapeutic beliefs. When I teach residents about lithium I always give them the Blackwell and Shepherd paper to say that it doesn't matter that they were wrong because what they did was to provoke people into doing the right study and that is what we needed. There is no excuse for giving treatments that we can show are effective but haven't proven it. I think people felt that Michael Shepherd and Barry Blackwell were a bit highfaluting and anti-therapeutic.

It was extraordinarily bitter. I mean, there were some very nasty correspondence in one or two journals.

Yes, well, I think that Nate occasionally liked a good fight. I remember something that Linford Rees wrote about monoamine oxidase inhibitors and Nate didn't feel he got enough credit and he wrote to Aubrey Lewis to complain about Linford Rees. Now that just seemed a bit childish to me but there it was. But afterwards Nate invited Linford Rees to the Caribbean islands for a shindig to which some lady donated annually.

What did you make of the Haiti angle? Did running institutes there for the poor compensate for charging $500 an hour or whatever it was for his private practice?

Well, in Haiti, in the late 1950s, Nate somehow or other talked a group of pharmaceutical companies into building a hospital and he had a very good film maker do a documentary. I always remember when I saw it Ted Cranswick, an Australian who had been in New Guinea, sort of shuddered and said, 'That guy has got beri-beri.' The patients got perphenazine and multi-vitamins in Haiti. What you saw in the documentary was that before treatment they were living in a ruin and after they were living in a ward and they were washed and clothed and well fed and so on. That was the Haiti connection. People came back and forth. Nate, I think, got decorated but it sort of fizzled. I would just say it was an expedition that Nate went on and that he enjoyed it. I wouldn't have seen it as the most altruistic thing, even though there was altruism involved. You could say well, it doesn't matter what the motivation was, the outcome was important and it was good.

The $500 an hour was much later. I think he was co-opted into that by some of the staff that he was very friendly with. Even though he was a big name, for a long time he did not charge big fees until I think somebody told him that he was making a mistake. At least to begin with he carried a lot of people for years who were difficult patients and he did not raise their fees. Then they had a new broom in the office and raised the fee and there was an exodus of patients. Patients that I had not heard of for years phoned me.

Jack Saunders, by the way, is still alive. He just retired a year ago and I think he is living up near Nyack. He did a psychiatric residency later but he was never someone that people were very friendly with. Now Nate could be a lot of fun. With Nate you would have told jokes but I can't imagine telling a joke to Jack. There was almost a boyish awkwardness about him whereas Nate had all of the hypomanic characteristics and charisma.

Towards the end he used to go around with a poodle, is that right?

Yes, he had a dog and of course he grew a huge head of white hair and a huge beard. He looked like Hemingway at times, though he wasn't quite as robust. He was a bit eccentric with that. On the other hand, you always had a feeling that he did a lot of these things very consciously. He would usually dress quite conservatively before that, but somehow or other he got into leather pants or something in his 1960s.

So do you think you made the right move ending up over here as opposed to staying in the UK?

I think so. I intended to come back and I just kept postponing it. I did speak to Aubrey Lewis in New York about going to the Maudsley when I had some publications. He said that they were not taking anybody unless they had membership and then Max Hamilton would tell me that I should finish my DPM, do an MD and all of these things. I never did any of them and then when the Royal College was founded they made me a Fellow, so I told Max that he had been wrong, which was quite funny, since for once he could not argue.

14 Gerald Curzon

From neurochemistry to neuroscience

You've had a career that has spanned the development of neurochemistry in Britain.

Most of the important names of the first wave are now dead – people like Richter, Blaschko, Feldberg. I wouldn't remotely compare myself with any of them or indeed with some members of the second wave but I suppose I am part of this second wave. I have been fortunate in being in an area of research that has become particularly lively as I have got nearer to retirement. When I started working on 5HT, it was often seen as a poor relation of the catecholamines but over the years the balance has shifted, largely because of the realisation that there were so many different 5HT receptors, with so many potential roles.

How did you come into the field?

I wanted to do a degree in biochemistry but the biochemistry course at Leeds, where I lived, was four years and the chemistry course was only three, and a year at 17 seemed to be an awfully long time so I did a chemistry degree but remained interested in biochemistry and did my PhD in it. Going into the Biochemistry Department and having to do animal surgery was quite a culture shock. There was then no requirement or opportunity to do preliminary training. It was 'This is what you do, now get on with it.' My PhD was officially on the vasoconstrictor effects of protein breakdown products. It derived from an idea of my supervisor that the hypertension of blackwater fever was due to proteolytic degradation products of haemoglobin. It didn't get very far largely because the degradation products we were working on did not have a reliable vasoconstrictor effect. This was around the time that serotonin had been identified as a vasoconstrictor substance in serum and shown to be 5-hydroxyindole ethylamine.

This was when?

In 1948–9 by Rapport, Green and Page. Serotonin, being derived from an amino acid tryptophan, was, in a sense, a protein breakdown product, so there were a few lines on it in the introduction to my thesis. Subsequently, in 1953, I came to the Institute of Neurology, for an interview for a research fellowship with Dick Pratt, who was a psychiatrist. He showed me the chemical structure of lysergic acid diethylamide and said, 'This causes hallucinations, how do you think it works?' – I'd never heard of LSD. It was shortly before hallucinogens were publicised by Aldous Huxley's *The Doors of Perception* on mescaline and long before LSD became a street drug. I said, 'Its structure reminds of this new stuff in the blood called serotonin.' Dick said, 'Does serotonin exist in the brain?' and I replied, 'Not as far as I know.' I did not know that a few months before Twarog and Page had isolated it from brain. I also didn't know that a month or two later Gaddum et al. would report that LSD blocked the effect of serotonin on smooth muscle. So these things came together and started me off on my interest in serotonin.

Were you offered the job?

I was offered the job on the strength of guessing the link between LSD and 5-HT. At that stage, speculations on the neurochemistry of mental disease tended to be based on analogies with sharply defined inborn errors of metabolism such as phenylketonuria. The idea was that major psychoses were due to the absence of a specific enzyme and hence a gross accumulation of some harmful substance. So I was 'looking for the spot' in schizophrenia, the revolutionary technique then being paper chromatography. It was hoped that the substance would appear in chromatograms of schizophrenic urine. I found unusual spots but they turned out to be related to gut bacteria or a dietary peculiarity, like excessive tea drinking. Nevertheless, it was all quite exciting. Looking at the chromatograms fitted in with the romantic image of the scientist peering down the microscope and shouting, 'Eureka!' I guess I have always tended to get excited about the work I was involved in at any time. Then, because of the experience I gained of paper chromatography of indoles, I was given the opportunity of doing some of the early work on the elevated extracerebral 5-HT metabolism of carcinoid disease. I also became involved in work on amine metabolites in CSF of patients with neurological diseases such as Parkinson's disease and Huntington's chorea.

I was then working in the Department of Chemical Pathology under John Cumings, who eventually became the Professor of Chemical Pathology. One day he came into the lab and said, 'I have put you down for giving a lecture on the biochemistry of depression.' I replied, 'I can't do it, I don't know anything about it' and he said, 'Go away and find out.' So I spent the next few weeks reading everything I could find about the biochemistry of depression, which at that time was not very much. I came up with the idea that depression was not a sharply defined metabolic disorder like phenylketonuria, but was due to an interaction between individual metabolism and responses to environmental stimuli and that secondary metabolic effects of the illness could exacerbate or stabilise the depressed state once it was established. The main key was overactivity of the hypothalamo-pituitary–adrenal axis in response to stress. The specific idea was that stress activated the HPA axis, causing the induction of tryptophan oxygenase (then called tryptophan pyrrolase) so that tryptophan was diverted away from 5HT synthesis – hence depression. There already was some evidence from Ashcroft and Sharman that depressive CSF contained abnormally low concentrations of 5HIAA, the 5HT metabolite.

I thought this was very original when I published it in 1965. But there are very few really original concepts and around that time others were publishing rather similar thoughts. A few years later, Paul Bridges and I reported that a group of depressives showed abnormal diversion of a tryptophan load on the pyrrolase pathway. So we did get some evidence but a paper in the *American Journal of Psychiatry* disagreed. A problem in those days was that depression had not been as well defined as later and this increased the likelihood of disagreement in the literature.

What were the influences that led you to this? There had been early work by Harris on the hypothalamo-pituitary axis, the HPA, and by Quastel and Richter looking at glucose and things like that ...

There had already been a number of papers on overactivity of the HPA axis in depression, though some workers had discounted it as due to hospitalisation or secondary to the psychiatric symptoms and without causal significance.

But it's one of those curious issues that has not been solved even 40 years later. The dexamethasone suppression test seemed at one point to settle things but it was a false promise. It didn't in the end clarify things.

I wouldn't put it as strongly as that but I agree that what the primary HPA abnormality is remains unclear. Is there a single primary abnormality? There are many ways in which the HPA axis might be disturbed so that an abnormal sensitivity to stressful circumstances occurs. At that time, there were almost two separate communities in depression research – there were the HPA axis people and there were people like George Ashcroft in Edinburgh who suspected a defect in serotonin synthesis and that certainly made sense inasmuch as monoamine oxidase inhibitors, which were antidepressant, increased 5HT and reserpine, which had the opposite effect, decreased it. I was aware from the work of Knox and his colleagues that one effect of HPA overactivity was that tryptophan was metabolised more rapidly. This seemed to mesh together with the idea of a 5HT defect in depression.

Then Richard Green came to do a PhD with me and I set him to see whether stress would decrease rat brain 5HT synthesis. During this period we published a fluorometric method for determining 5HT and 5HIAA in rat brain regions. We felt somewhat diffident about submitting it as it merely combined things that were already known. In the event, the method became the most cited paper from my lab and was a standard method for about 20 years, though it has now largely been replaced by HPLC. Our experiments on stressed rats were not progressing so we tried to cut the Gordian knot by giving rats cortisol instead and looking at 5HT metabolism. Levels did decrease. But even with our new method we could only measure total regional 5HT and 5HIAA. The ability to repeatedly monitor the bit of 5HT that was out in the synaptic cleft was far in the future. Also, we didn't consider that increased HPA activity might have numerous effects as well as decreasing brain tryptophan and might hit 5HT function at many points. But in those days we knew nothing about 5HT receptors, for instance.

Looking back, it seems to me that most of the time almost all scientists follow the current fashion. I can remember various stages of the 5HT story. First of all it was exciting to be able to measure 5HIAA, the metabolite, and then 5HT itself, and for years hardly anybody gave much thought to the importance of the availability of tryptophan for brain 5HT synthesis. Even though it was known that tryptophan hydroxylase, the rate-limiting enzyme for it, was normally not saturated with tryptophan, the whole question of its availability for the enzyme was largely ignored except by Eccleston, Ashcroft and Crawford, who published on it in 1965, though we had in 1963 reported increased urinary 5HIAA in rhesus monkeys on chronic high tryptophan intake but made little of it. For a long time what happened at postsynaptic 5HT receptors evoked much less interest than the synthesis of the transmitter. Quastel visited the lab and said with great emphasis, 'The thing is Curzon, what's happening at the receptor? What's happening at the receptor?' I was simply unable to discuss this question.

He must have been quite old then. Did he do much after he left Cardiff and went to Canada?

He was old but mentally very lively. Quastel's major work was in the early stages at Cambridge and Cardiff, where he preceded Richter. He was diverted away from brain chemistry for some years during the war when he was recruited by the Ministry of Agriculture and was largely responsible for the development of soil conditioners.

The tryptophan story seems to come around at regular intervals. I got involved early in my career measuring free and bound plasma tryptophan with a home-made apparatus of your designing for which I gave you no thanks at the time. It only cost a few pence to make and one of the interesting things even now is how frontier research can still be done with very simple bits of apparatus – a great deal of the high-powered genes work, for instance, uses very simple technology. But anyway, there have been various reports of lowering of levels and then there is the tryptophan depletion drinks story. What does it all mean?

Very early on we did some work on plasma tryptophan in depression and found that it was low but the results were what I call significant but not *significant*. It was statistically significant but mean values were not so low that one could imagine it being a major causal influence in depression. Nevertheless, over the years the great majority of people who have reported on this have found statistically significantly lowered values.

Is this because they would not have reported it if they hadn't?

That's an argument that can be made against any positive finding. Initially there were some mixed findings and this kind of equivocal stage is often followed by a fizzling out of the whole story. But this hasn't happened and the balance of papers strongly indicates low levels. Is it due to increased HPA activity or to the fact that depressives tend to have poor appetites and therefore take in less tryptophan? Perhaps a combination of these factors.

An important recent paper by Holsboer et al. is relevant to the HPA/tryptophan story. They used a pepped-up version of the dexamethasone test where it is given followed by CRF so that the increases in cortisol are magnified. Very high increases occurred in depression, and first-degree relatives of depressed subjects who were psychiatrically normal but with a strong familial component of affective illness had increases mid-way between the depressed and control groups. This might suggest that a tendency to high HPA activity does not confer depression per se but vulnerability to a critical further increase of activity in stressful circumstances and hence vulnerability to depression. Our rat experiments in which chronic corticosterone treatment caused decreased behavioural responsiveness of 5HT receptors could be relevant here.

Another important result as well as that from Holsboer was from Simon Young's lab at McGill, where the tryptophan depletion procedure you mention was applied to ordinary normals and normal first-order relatives of depressives. Only the second group showed a lowering of mood. These findings taken together suggest that both low 5HT function and high HPA activity are causally linked and confer a vulnerability to depression rather than that low 5HT equals depression. For most depressives, their moderately low tryptophan availability may not be causally very important but within the depressive population there may be a subgroup in which basal 5HT function is on the low side of normal so that moderate tryptophan deficits, whether due to stress or low food intake, could have pathological consequences. There is also the question of whether tryptophan is an antidepressant – in general it doesn't seem to be an effective antidepressant but some patients do apparently respond – perhaps they are the ones with a brain tryptophan deficit.

An interesting but arduous study might be to combine the Holsboer and Young experiments on a single group of subjects.

In terms of the 1950s, who were the key figures?

In the 1950s I was in my twenties and very much on the periphery and knew none of the key figures personally. I remember hearing Blaschko talking about monoamine oxidase in 1949, during my first year as a PhD student, at the First International Biochemical Congress at Cambridge, a meeting attended, as far as I can remember, by something like 200 people. A few years later Dick Pratt managed to get me into a small select meeting on biological psychiatry at the CIBA foundation. I remember thinking that I was the only person there who had never been heard of. So when trying to answer your question, all of this has to be borne in mind. Many people who appeared prominent in the 1950s did not turn out later to have been influential. Others were. For example, Axelrod, Brodie, Udenfriend et al. at NIH, Blaschko, Feldberg, Gaddum, Richter, Vogt in Britain. But a decade is a long time in 20th century science history and many who are now already part of the history of neuroscience – what the Japanese would call 'living human treasures' – had hardly got going then.

In the 1950s there seems to have been some feeling among the grandees of the field, Gaddtum and people like, that the chemistry of the brain was not likely to be very important, that chemical neurotransmission might happen in the periphery but not in the brain. Did this debate impinge on you at all?

In those days I was not all that aware of the neurochemical implications of neurotransmission. In fact, it only gradually sank in to me that brain chemistry had essential differences from the chemistry of other organs. I remember very early on I gave a paper on brain 5HT metabolism and during the discussion someone said, 'What about compartmentation?' I'm afraid I hadn't thought about receptors and I hadn't thought about compartmentation. My approach involved the unvoiced assumption that the brain was a kind of soup with active chemicals in it. I don't think the penny really dropped about compartmentation until the histochemical fluorescence method came out and one could actually see that neurotransmitters were in specific tracts. As for the multiplicity of central transmitters I remember in the early days many of the neurologists here were sceptical about anything other than acetylcholine being a neurotransmitter.

That kind of thinking could still be picked up in the late 1970s.

Yes, you are right. Criteria for a substance to be a neurotransmitter which had been defined largely through acetylcholine research had all to be obeyed and the gaps we had in our knowledge of other substances meant that they were referred to at best as putative neurotransmitters. I certainly used the word 'putative' in self-defence until quite late. A personal problem I had was that confidence when talking to Queen Square clinicians only came to me slowly. I began as a chemist – a northern chemist in the fullest sense of the word in that while certain people at Oxford and Cambridge are rather pejoratively called northern chemists, I was a northern chemist who went to a local grammar school and did my degree in the north – at Leeds, my home town. When I came to Queen Square, I was the only postdoc non-medical person here and surrounded by public school, ancient university products with that characteristically confident way of speaking. This was intensified by the fact that they were clinicians. After all, what the patient wants is the confident statement, 'You have X disease. I will treat you in the following way.' So it took me a long time to stand up intellectually to them. Things have changed a lot over the years but there was an enormous gulf then between clinicians and non-clinicians.

Somewhere in the 1960s, the field of the biochemistry of the mood disorders began to take off. Why? Was it the work of Ashcroft and others?

The really critical stages were the opposite behavioural effects of reserpine which was known to deplete brain transmitters and of monoamine oxidase inhibitors which elevated them.

The reserpine story caused such controversy in the early days. Was depression due to low 5HT or due to low catecholamines? It now seems more likely that depression may be mediated by more than one neurochemical mechanism and that antidepressant drugs mostly increase the availability to receptors of 5HT or noradrenaline (or dopamine). I suspect that 10–20 years from now the standard antidepressants will be drugs acting on specific postsynaptic 5HT and catecholamine receptors instead of by presynaptic mechanisms, which is how most of the present ones act.

Most of my interests have centred on 5HT as such rather than specifically on depression and I have gradually shifted from a purely chemical attitude to a more interdisciplinary approach.

What is a purely chemical attitude and what has the change been in your attitude – is it a move towards more systems-based thinking?

I eventually decided to try to focus not so much on brain chemistry in isolation but on relationships between neurochemistry and behaviour. I then started to try to look at non-drug-induced variations of transmitter metabolism and its correlation with behaviour but only limited progress was possible with the existing technology. Monitoring techniques like in vivo voltammetry or microdialysis were not yet available. Also, I knew nothing about animal behaviour in those days. What I have since learnt was largely taught by the people who came to work in my lab.

At that time it was my impression that too many drugs had come along that turned out to be less selective than first appeared and I felt cautious about using drugs as research tools which might turn out later not only to affect 5-HT function but also other things that had never been suspected initially. So I was resistant to novel pharmacological tools until made to realise their value by my collaborators.

At this stage I had a big interest in the effect of feeding on brain 5HT metabolism as brain 5HT synthesis requires tryptophan, and as this was an essential amino acid it had to come from food. Charles Marsden had recently been studying tryptamine synthesis in my lab and there had recently been some work in Canada on tryptamine as a possible neuromodulator for 5HT. Colin Dourish then arrived in the lab from Canada, where he had been working on behavioural effects of tryptamine. So I suggested to Colin that he should investigate the effects of injecting 5HT into the brain with different amounts of tryptamine but he favoured using the new $5HT_{1A}$ agonist 8OH-DPAT. This went against my reluctance to use new drugs but Colin Dourish and Peter Hutson tried it out on a few rats left over from another experiment. As soon as the rats were given 8-OH-DPAT they started to eat. Colin and Peter said, 'As we are interested in the effect of feeding on 5HT, why not combine this with the effect of 5HTergic drugs on feeding?' It was one of those productive intellectual interactions. I had set the problem and they had made a creative jump from it. Peter Hutson, who was a first class observer, noted that the rats were eating more and in a very short time he and Colin had done a lot of experiments and Colin had produced a draft paper on the effects of $5HT_{1A}$ agonists on feeding. This started us off on effects of drugs acting at specific 5HT receptors on feeding.

In these studies, Guy Kennett found that activation of $5HT_{2C}$ receptors suppressed feeding – we were probably the first group to show a behavioural effect of activating these sites. I then went to a meeting in the USA at which I heard that a group at NIH were producing anxiety in humans by giving them the drug mCPP. As this was the substance we had been using to activate $5\text{-}HT_{2c}$ sites, I came back from the meeting and said, 'Let's see if MCPP has an anxiogenic effect in rats and if this is due to 2C activation.' That's how another strand of our 5HT work started.

Did the rats become anxious?

Insofar as one could tell. I tend to be cautious and write 'anxiety-like' behaviour. They responded appropriately to established rat anxiety models like the elevated plus maze and the social interaction test. That arm of the work is being developed by Guy Kennett who is now at SmithKline Beecham and involved in the study of a series of selective $5HT_{2c}$ antagonists as potential anxiolytic drugs. That's been quite pleasing – to have something that began in my lab being developed possible for clinical application. At the moment, it is not entirely clear whether they oppose anxiety via $5HT_{2C}$ or $5HT_{2B}$ receptors. However, evidence that activation of $5HT_{2C}$ sites suppresses feeding appears to be more conclusive.

Has the 5HT and feeding story been finally sorted out yet?

Hardly, though we now know quite a lot about relationships between feeding 5HT and appetite. Because of my early aim of avoiding drug experiments, much of our work started from a study in which Michael Joseph and Peter Knott were involved in which we tried to decrease brain tryptophan and hence 5HT synthesis by a physiological mechanism, i.e. by withdrawing food (and hence dietary supplies of tryptophan) for one day. To our surprise, brain tryptophan didn't decrease – it increased. Similarly, when Dick Wurtman and his colleagues at MIT gave rats a high-carbohydrate, zero-protein meal, brain tryptophan increased. George Sarna later confirmed this in my lab. These seemingly paradoxical findings are now readily explained. To my mind they imply that adequate supplies of tryptophan for 5HT synthesis are normally effectively ensured in acute deficiency of dietary tryptophan. Wurtman's emphasis has been different – that is, that the effect of feeding on 5HT synthesis has physiologically important consequences for appetite. In my opinion, this idea is largely based on pharmacological/physiological borderland experiments involving very high carbohydrate or very high protein meals. They could well be relevant in extreme cases. For example, those rats that live in sugar cane plantations. However, almost all of our meals are more complex. Even the so-called carbohydrate snacks which are causally implicated in obesity are usually carbohydrate/fat snacks. However, it is an attractive idea that dietary effects on 5HT could in some subjects influence appetite whether in an appropriate or inappropriate direction. In the latter case, the result could be a disorder of appetite. Certainly, our work on 8-OH-DPAT and mCPP indicates that 5HTergic drugs affect food intake. Indeed, dexfenfluramine, the principal clinically used appetite suppressant, can release 5HT though recent work both in Italy and in my own lab strongly suggests that a direct action on a 5HT receptor is more likely to explain its effect on appetite.

You said that your approach was initially chemical but became more integrated. This seems to be the paradigm of the emergence of neuroscience – people working in disparate areas who at some point in the 1980s became neuroscientists.

I guess it was in the 1980s or thereabouts that I started thinking of myself as a neuroscientist though it was my impression that many people got there about ten years before.

Other than the institute run by Francis Schmidt, I am only aware of the neuroscience concept appearing with any regularity at some point in the mid-1980s.

This is a somewhat etymological issue. The first people calling themselves neuroscientists were mostly not so much neurotransmitter-centred neuro-chemists/neuropharmacologists like me but neurophysiologists and neuroanatomists. But these classifications are becoming less important.

Why? Science normally seems to proceed by breaking things up but for some strange reason in the neurosciences we seem in one sense to be putting things back together again.

Well, subjects as previously taught in universities were based on the convenience for teaching purposes of having, for example, one set of lecturers, text books, degrees etc. for physics and another for chemistry and so on. But the problems nature sets us are not easily solved by means of these tidy academic subjects in isolation.

When were you aware that the field seemed to be developing into a neuroscience field?

My own development in that direction began about 20 years ago soon after I got my first MRC programme grant. I decided to try to study behaviour as well as brain chemistry so I asked the MRC for a supplementary grant to buy an activity meter. They went to the trouble of sending a very distinguished behavioural scientist with an FRS to see whether it was justifiable to give a neurochemist £1000 for a piece of behavioural equipment. I by no means convinced him. In fact he tore me apart! Not too difficult because I knew almost nothing about behaviour at that time. Finally, he said, 'What will happen if I say you shouldn't have this £1000?' I replied that I would continue doing neurochemistry and not try to relate it to behaviour and that this would be a pity. In the end we got the activity meter. I soon realised its limitations but it did get us started on trying to assess behaviour though I didn't get heavily involved until we started to work on serotonergic drugs and feeding. Although much of the stimulus for my research has come from thinking about human psychiatric illness, most of it has not been on human material. The psychiatry department here was small with few patients and they often tended to be complicated cases who were not good subjects for research. Round about the 1970s there was a report on medical education advising that teaching neurology and psychiatry in London should be on one site. But the Maudsley people didn't want to join with Queen Square and the Queen Square people didn't want to join with the Maudsley. My research would have probably had a larger clinical component if the integration had taken place.

Moving to the organisational framework in which you have worked, what were the societies in which you were involved in the 1950s, for instance?

A lot of my early papers were in the *Biochemical Journal*. These were on something I haven't mentioned, the enzyme kinetics of plasma caeruloplasmin, the copper protein deficient in Wilson's disease, which was a big interest of John Cumings, the head of the Chem. Path. Dept. of which I was then a member. This was very enjoyable and intellectually stimulating and formed much of any research apprenticeship but it was not neurochemistry. Then I began to do work that was published in journals with 'neuro-' or 'psycho-' or 'pharmaco-' in their titles. Quite a lot went to the *Journal of Neurochemistry* because that was an appropriate place for our work on feeding and brain 5HT synthesis. More recently much of the work on effects of drugs on 5HT function was published in the British and the European journals of pharmacology. Some of the early papers (with Richard Green, for instance) also went to the *British Journal of Pharmacology*.

I am probably trying to avoid answering your question because, apart from editorial work, my time on the MRC Neuroscience Board and occasionally helping to organise a session at a meeting, my involvement with organisational aspects of neuroscience has not been great. I do not look on myself as a good committee man. Different scientists divide their time up in different ways, which is probably a good thing. To misquote the Bible: 'In the scientific kingdom there are many mansions.' I must say though that I had not appreciated how much effort some other scientists have put into the service of the profession until I became the historian/archivist of the International Society for Neurochemistry (ISN) and started to go through its archives.

Were you involved in the Brain Research Society?

I went to some meetings in the early years when it was a rather small informal society. Nowadays, most meetings that are of interest to me have a big pharmacological component and I also go to most ISN meetings, partly because being the historian of the society I try to organise sessions with a historical component. But I find that more and more papers given at purely neurochemical meetings are outside my area of interest and knowledge, whereas psychopharmacology meetings are becoming of more interest to me.

When did you get interested in the history of neuroscience?

It didn't come from an interest in the history of science as such. In fact when I was younger, I was rather scornful about scientists getting interested in the history of their subject as they got older. In my case it started from a more general interest in history during which I became particularly attracted to the approach of the French Annales group of historians who were to apply numerical methods to economic and social history – people like Braudel, Le Roy Ladurie, and Duby. I felt that if there is one area of history to which numerical methods might be applied it was the history of science. I also became interested in numerical applications of the citation index. About 12 years ago I wrote to Brian Ansell, then the secretary of the ISN, putting forward my thoughts about these things. He handed on my letter to Henry McIlwain, who was the ISN historian. I was invited to give a historical paper at the next meeting of the society. Eventually, Henry proposed that I should succeed him as the historian.

My work on the history of the subject has shifted over the years. The first historical paper I did was essentially non-quantitative. It was about one particular incident, the identification of the structure of tryptophan by the great Frederick Gowland Hopkins. Then I did an analysis of the history of the development of research on reserpine and chlorpromazine using a quantitative approach based on citations. The time courses of their citations turned out to follow very different patterns. Reserpine had what you might call a normal pattern – after one or two key papers the citation rate increased rapidly and then slowly came down again. But in the case of chlorpromazine, the initial discoveries were followed by many years with very few citations and then suddenly the citations zoom up. This raised questions about the different patterns. The answer has probably taken us back to the point I made earlier which was that neurochemists were initially not very interested in receptors even though they were aware of their existence. Thus, reserpine, which acted presynaptically, was easily understandable but a drug which acted on a postsynaptic site didn't spark off much scientific interest until many years later, even though clinically it was extensively used. The next history paper I did was completely quantitative. It was an analysis of the history of neurochemistry as revealed by changing contents of the *Journal of Neurochemistry* over 30 years. I guess the idea for it came from one of the Annales approaches – what they called 'the history of the long duration'. That is, the revelation of trends only apparent from analysis of long spans of time.

How do you read the interest in history in the field? It always seems less to me than it should be, particularly for psychiatry which lives by its ability to take history.

There certainly have been psychiatrists who were distinguished historians of their subject. For example, Richard Hunter, who with Ida MacAlpine did the study on which Alan Bennett's play *The Madness of George III* was based. Hugh Freeman, a recent chief editor of the *British Journal of Psychiatry*, has published important work. But, in general, historical knowledge among psychiatrists seems not very apparent. Recently the *Lancet* published a – in my opinion – magisterial article on Freud which led to a large correspondence that exhibited powerful preconceptions but little historical knowledge. One might have thought that there would have been letters from serious students of the history of psychiatry.

When I came here in 1952 I knew essentially nothing about psychiatry and was surprised to find that many psychiatrists were largely dismissive of psychoanalysis. This was when educated laymen mostly saw psychoanalysis as having scientific validity. This attitude is now fading away though one still gets involved in dinner table discussions in which people insist that analytical methods are highly successful and also have a kind of higher authority than the methods of biological psychiatry. Ideas take a long time to die!

It is a pity that scientists tend to get interested in the history of their subject only as they approach retirement. I would be pleased if a neurochemist who was still in the thick of active research but with an interest in the history of the subject would take on the job of ISN historian from me in a few years. I don't want it just to be a hobby for retired scientists.

What can be done to change that?

Perhaps if there was more of a historical component in the way the subject was taught – more on the development of ideas – then more younger scientists would became interested. But I am not too hopeful, one doesn't expect many explorers to be interested in the history of exploration.

The field has grown old enough for people to reinvent your ideas about tryptophan and cortisol and be unaware that this was all there 30 years before. Are you aware of this?

Yes, I am, though I don't know about it having been *all* there! I am afraid that once papers and reviews especially don't quote the early literature it becomes buried and more deeply so when early papers are not accessible by electronic methods. Long ago when the literature was much smaller, scientists would often browse in the early journals. I read somewhere about organic chemists browsing through all the back numbers of Leibig's Annalen as part of their education. This kind of thing would be out of the question now.

Nothing that happened before 1966 exists anymore.

That's true, things are reinvented every 15–20 years although often they are reinvented in a rather more sophisticated way, aren't they? There are two images of progress in science: the linear ideal and the more realistic circular or rather the upwardly helical one.

You've mentioned Charles Marsden, Guy Kennett, Colin Dourish, Richard Green, many who've gone on to make substantial names for themselves. Is there anyone else?

I have been very fortunate in the people who came to my lab. I started with a degree in chemistry and most of what I've learned about biological science has been from colleagues who were trained in different subjects. Richard Green, my second PhD student's findings on the idea that HPA activity influenced

5HT metabolism, produced some high-profile papers so that the lab became more prominent and other good workers were attracted to it, including Peter Hutson, Michael Joseph, Simon Young, Mark Tricklebank as well as those you have mentioned. They are now leading figures and it is gratifying that, on the whole, they have remained in research and in the field of adjacent fields.

One idea I've always had is that psychopharmacology is not the kind of science that proceeds by the hypothetical-deductive method that is so beloved of places like Oxford, Cambridge and the Maudsley. It seems to me that the technology leads us. A new drug throws up observations that theory has to accommodate rather than the other way around.

Medawar has written a paper on this called 'The scientific paper is a fraud' which says that science doesn't proceed in the way we were taught at school – hypothesis, experiment and then deduction. Certainly, in psychopharmacology, a great deal has come from accidental observations. Also, intuition and daydreams play a part – the famous example is Kekule's vision of the snake biting its tail, from which he derived the structure of benzene. My own ideas often come when my mind is drifting – for example, in the morning while shaving. As for technology leading us, this has been true in the past – the availability of paper chromatography in the late 1940s permitted advances that would otherwise have been impossible – Sanger's determination of the structure of insulin, for example. But I wonder whether technology is starting to offer an embarrassment of riches. I remember Krebs saying about 20 years ago that we will one day be able to measure anything in everything so that the problem will be to decide what is most worth measuring. But this does not discount the influence on neuropharmacology in recent years of the development of techniques like HPLC which have enabled us to monitor transmitter concentrations in the extracellular spaces of the brain.

But to come back to ACh, it's a good case in point in that from being the pre-eminent neurotransmitter because we haven't had the methods to detect it the way we have had for the catecholamines or serotonin it's withered on the vine, it hasn't found a niche even though clearly many of the drugs we use affect it even more than they do the other neurotransmitters.

Well yes. Merton Sandler has often said the reason there is so much research on catecholamines and 5HT is because they have been more measurable than other transmitters and unlike, for example, glutamate they occur only in neurones and not elsewhere in the brain.

So in a sense we're still fiddling at the margins, we're playing around with the easy problems.

I wouldn't quite say that! We are looking at a landscape. Parts of it are obscured by clouds – our ignorance, our preconceptions, unspoken assumptions. Parts of it are too far away. But there is no reason to assume that the parts we know about are less important than those we don't know about. Nevertheless, if you ask me 'Will we ever completely understand the brain?' then I really have no idea. Is the brain complicated in the way that, let's say, a one inch to the mile map of the British Isles is complicated? That is, while there is no great difficult principle involved, it's just damned complicated, there are a lot of roads and rivers and hills and footpaths and while any part of it is easily understandable, no one person can take in the whole map. Or is the brain something that we can learn things about but the overall understanding of it is simply beyond the capacity of the human brain? Some philosophers have said that as we are ourselves part of nature, there is no intrinsic reason why our minds should be constructed in such a way that we are capable of understanding all of the concepts on which nature is based. There's a cartoon by Gary Larson, showing dog scientists in their laboratory. One of the dogs is describing a diagram of a doorknob to students. Another is dissecting, a doorknob. A third is looking at a doorknob down a microscope. The caption says, 'The dog scientists know that if they could only solve the doorknob problem it would benefit dogs all over the world.' They are obviously not going to solve the doorknob problem. There may be more subtle doorknob problems that even human minds are simply not up to.

This is not a negative point of view. There is still much that we know or can learn about the brain. For example, that a drug has a particular influence on mood and that this is mediated by a particular neurochemical change. But if I try to think how a chemical change can alter mood, consciousness or awareness then I'm up against a blank wall. Dennett wrote a book called *Consciousness Explained* but others have called it 'Consciousness Ignored' or 'Consciousness not Explained' and I tend to agree with them.

But isn't the interesting thing how with very selective probes like LSD or ketamine in very small doses you can radically alter self-awareness?

Small doses but lots of molecules! That a chemical substance could alter mood had a great impact. Many people found it repellent. They would say, 'Do you mean that the brain is just so much chemistry?' I don't find it too difficult that actions of transmitters at receptors can, for example, influence movement by neuromuscular links. How they can affect mood, consciousness or awareness is beyond me.

The next ISN session with a historical component that I hope to organise (with Susan Greenfield) is called 'The neuroscience of consciousness: Past, present and future'. A great interest in consciousness has developed in recent years. Philosophers used to say that it can't be defined and that if it can't be defined it can't be studied. But now many of them are trying to study it as are any number of basic scientists from different disciplines, such as Francis Crick and Roger Penrose. There is also the hard data we are learning from PET scanning and so forth about what parts of the brain are activated by different kinds of thinking.

Coming back to the LSD story – when I first came to Queen Square to work with Dick Pratt in 1953, part of our project was for him to give psychiatric patients mescaline or LSD and record their mood changes while I would look for associated changes in urinary indolic and phenolic substances.

There are great problems giving anything like that these days.

Yes, a lot of early work on effects of psychotropic drugs on normal humans was financed by the US military in ethically dubious ways for ethically dubious purposes.

I'm sure that's influenced attitudes since. There's a certain lingering suspicion as to why anyone would want to do this kind of thing. But in contrast almost, when you began the idea of taking a biochemical approach to these intimate areas of human functioning, would have seemed to many people in the street almost Satanic yet now we're in the era of the designer drug and Prozac is a topic of coffee table conversation and people are quite unfazed by all of this. What's happened?

Perhaps the coffee table conversations you have are at a more knowledgeable level than some of those I have. If one says, 'A chemical can affect how we feel about ourselves', people still often say, 'Oh, but what about the soul?' Or if one speaks about brain *mechanisms*, they say, 'Do you mean its just a mechanism?' They often don't have the concept or the vocabulary to realise that whatever's going on up there is occurring through a mechanism of some kind or other. They tend to think of mechanisms in terms of clockwork toys from Woolworths. I suffer a great deal from the things that educated non-scientists say about the brain. You must have had this one: 'Can you really learn anything about the human brain from work on animals?' Well not everything but quite a lot!

But the change in culture is actually quite striking, isn't it?

Yes, I agree that the advent of drugs like Prozac is shifting attitudes. But there is a lot of suspicion about drugs that affect the brain – some of it justified of course, but there is also a tendency to lump all drugs that affect the brain together with cocaine and heroin. There is a tendency also to see effects of drugs on mood etc. as diminishing our self-hood or self-esteem, which is strange because, after all, the effects of alcohol or a good meal on mood have been known for thousands of years. However, in our society, substances perceived as drugs that affect behaviour and mood are looked on with suspicion though other societies may be more accepting.

Not in the same way.

I suppose it depends on the preconceptions of the particular society. If one believes the Gods have given us the gift of the mescal cactus or the hallucinogenic mushroom through which we can experience a reality that is normally hidden then one's attitude is going to be different but, on the whole, Western religions haven't involved the use of chemical substances – being unpleasant to yourself in various ways perhaps to attempt to attain union with the divine or punish yourself for your sins but not interventions with chemical substances. Alcohol, in particular in the form of wine, is used but not to produce intoxication.

Who have been the important people in the field? Who have been the potential Nobel laureates?

Arvid Carlsson was one, when you consider his involvement in the recognition of the behavioural importance of brain dopamine. It would have been reasonable for him and Hornykiewicz to have got a joint Nobel Prize. Snyder also for his pioneering work in receptorology. But a problem nowadays with the Nobel Prize is that it is getting more and more difficult to ascribe major findings to individuals. Even Newton said, 'I have stood on the shoulders of giants.' Scientific papers around the turn of the century had one or two authors, three was very rare. Now the number of names on biological science papers is going up all the time. The one-author paper is essentially unknown, the two is rare, the average in neurochemistry is somewhere between three and four so it's very hard to say who is 'the' person anymore. Indeed, not only is the average numbers of authors/paper rising but also the number of laboratories, even countries per paper. I have heard someone say, 'He got the Nobel Prize and it was a *good* Nobel Prize', meaning that it was unusual in that one individual was definitely responsible for the important finding. The age of the lone worker looking down the microscope has largely faded away and labs are getting to be more like small factories. Perhaps the big prizes should be awarded to laboratories rather than individuals.

What about Brodie, should he have got one? Did you know him?

I went to meetings that he was present at and we might have said a few words to each other but I wouldn't say I knew him personally. A Nobel would have been completely appropriate for Brodie but there's only a limited number of Nobels and only a fraction of the scientists who might reasonably have got one do get one. Consider the enormous increase in the number of working scientists since the Prizes began.

But it's rare that there isn't some pedigree to ideas.

Well, it depends what you mean by 'pedigree'. In the case of Carlsson and Hornykiewicz, there was a well-defined idea that dopamine was a transmitter, not merely a noradrenaline precursor, and that it was deficient in Parkinson's disease, that its precursor dopa had therapeutic effect and that there was a very satisfactory link-up with the classical neuropathology of the disease. These certainly were tremendously influential findings and altered neurologists' attitudes. I remember in my early years at Queen Square a distinguished neurologist saying that pharmacology had little to offer the neurologist. There was a meeting here at which I said, 'Hornykiewicz in Vienna finds that Parkinson's disease is due to a defect in dopamine.' A great eminence stood up and said through clenched teeth, 'If Dr Curzon had ever seen a parkinsonian brain, he would know that this disease is *nothing* to do with chemistry.' Indeed, I hadn't seen a parkinsonian brain and I felt too crushed to say that chemistry has something to do with *everything* that goes on in the brain. Anyway, years later, Hornykiewicz came to give a lecture at Queen Square and I had the pleasure of using the story when I introduced him.

Select bibliography

Curzon C (1987). Hopkins and the discovery of tryptophan. In *Progress in Tryptophan and Serotonin Research*. Walter de Gruyter & Co., Berlin, pp 29–38.

Curzon G (1990). How reserpine and chlorpromazine act: the impact of key discoveries on the history of psychopharmacology. *Trends in Pharmacological Sciences*, **11**, 61–63.

Curzon G (1993). The history of neurochemistry as revealed by the *Journal of Neurochemistry*, **61**, 780–786.

Tallis RC (1996). Burying Freud. *Lancet*, **347**, 669–671 with letters 1039–1041.

15 Leslie Iversen

Neuroscience and drug development

You went to Julie Axelrod's lab in the mid-1960s. What was it like to go from Britain to the NIMH in the 1960s?

It was a completely mind-blowing experience for a young English scientist, brought up to be very economical with running expenses and not having all that much access to equipment, although in Cambridge, when I was doing my PhD, I was very lucky in a number of respects. I had absolutely committed myself to doing brain research by the time I graduated in biochemistry in Cambridge. I was obsessed with plants and botany as a sixth former and got a scholarship to come to Cambridge on the grounds of my performance in botany. But the classical botany taught in Cambridge in the late 1950s soon proved boring, and I rapidly became enthused by biochemistry, which was a much more glamorous subject. I ended up specialising in biochemistry at an enormously exciting time for biochemistry in general and biochemistry in Cambridge in particular, because this was only a few years after Crick and Watson had made their dramatic discovery about DNA. I became fascinated by brain research, largely because I read a couple of books by Aldous Huxley called *The Doors of Perception* and *Heaven and Hell*, which related his experiences of taking mescaline and then later taking lysergic acid. These books were absolutely fascinating, among the most influential I ever read. The mystery which Huxley describes so beautifully was, how is it that taking a minute amount of chemical substance can so totally alter your perception, your consciousness and your view of the world even to the extent of believing that you have had a visionary experience? I found that absolutely fascinating – and I still do. It's a mystery that still hasn't been solved. But that's what triggered my interest and also brain research at the time was beginning to take off as a growth area in biology.

My problem in Cambridge was that there was no one in the Biochemistry Department doing anything remotely concerned with brain research and I wanted to be a biochemist and to do brain research. My great stroke of luck was to find a supervisor in Gordon Whitby when I was about to start my PhD. He had just come back to Biochemistry in Cambridge from a year in Axelrod's lab at the NIH and he had been among the first to use radioactively labelled noradrenaline to demonstrate the concept that noradrenaline was disposed of in the body not only by metabolism but also by an uptake mechanism mediating recapture into sympathetic nerves, which was then a totally novel concept. So I was extremely fortunate in having Gordon Whitby, as a supervisor, which allowed me to do neurochemistry research in a very early stage of what proved to be an exciting branch of neurochemistry and neuropharmacology, and to use the techniques that he had just learnt in one of the world's top laboratories.[1]

The other stroke of good luck was that we had one of the first radioactive scintillation counters in Cambridge, although in those days we had to reuse the glass bottles that we put each sample in, wash them out at night and reuse them the next day. One of the things about going to the National Institute of Health was that you didn't have to be quite that economical! I went to the Axelrod lab, of course, because my mentor in Cambridge had trained there and I had that introduction. I was very fortunate to be there at a fairly early stage of the Axelrod lab, as you know from your interview with Julie. He was what you might call a late starter. He didn't get his PhD until he was in his forties and he was in his late forties before he was put in charge of his own laboratory for the first time. Since then he has never looked back. He was enormously productive but when I went there he was still at a relatively early stage. He had had a number of foreign visitors and postdocs but we were still among the first generation of those.

It was a great time. From the point of view of the area I was in, catecholamine research, things were booming. There were so many things to be discovered still with radioactively labelled noradrenaline and other catecholamines. It was like ripe fruit ready to be picked. Jacques Glowinski, a French visitor, and I worked together very closely during that year in Julie's lab, capitalising on work that he had already started before I came. The project was based on the idea that you could study catecholamine metabolism and drug effects in the brain by using radioactive catecholamines. But they had to be injected directly into the brain because they wouldn't pass the blood–brain barrier. Jacques had devised a technique of injecting radioactive amine into the ventricular system in the rat brain and we did hundreds of experiments. Thousands of scintillation vials were stacked up outside the door each day and we worked from morning to night. It was a really intense period with great encouragement from Julie Axelrod, who was, on the one hand, a source of more ideas than you could possibly handle, and on the other hand, he let young people do their own thing with an extraordinary degree of freedom. He was a wonderful teacher.

During that time the National Institute of Health was in an enormous boom period. One reason for this was that the best of the output of American medical schools had decided quite reasonably that a couple of years' research at the NIH was probably preferable to going to the jungles of Vietnam and

---

[1]Axelrod J (1996). The discovery of amine reuptake. In *The Psychopharmacologists*, Vol I, pp 29–50.

being a soldier doctor. Instead they fought each other to get into the NIH to do their military service in that way and the NIH had the pick of the most talented young doctors. There were some extraordinarily bright people, who stayed for a short time and left. Unfortunately I think the NIH has since become much more ossified and is no longer the intellectual powerhouse that it used to be.

So even something like the Vietnam War can in some respects be a good thing?

I think that's right! But it was a period in any case, despite the Vietnam War, of immense optimism about medical research and its ability to discover the secrets of human disease and eventually to treat them. All of us had that naive optimism that we could understand even mental illnesses and treat them far better than had been done previously. Remember at that time, in the early 1960s, we were seeing the enormous benefits to mentally ill people that had come from the introduction in rapid succession of new drugs for treating psychiatric disease, monoamine oxidase inhibitors, tricyclic antidepressants, the neuroleptics, chlorpromazine and all the others after it, for treating schizophrenic illness and the benzodiazepine tranquillisers. That all happened in a remarkably short space of time and I suppose we felt that it was going to go on happening like that and we would understand more and more and have rational grounds for developing centrally acting drugs. In retrospect we didn't realise that those were the big CNS drugs of the 20th century. What's happened since has been far less spectacular on the whole. But anyway it was great and it was in a log-growth period, and it's always fun to be in a lab which is in a growth phase and in a field that's optimistic and full of ideas, so that was a very influential time for me.

What about the other people? Some of the older stars were still there, people like Brodie, but his star was probably starting to wane ...

Well, Bernard Brodie was there but for some reason, which I never really understood at that time, the Axelrod lab were not really on speaking terms with the Brodie lab. Perhaps because Brodie resented the fact that his pupil, Axelrod, had become so spectacularly successful. I don't know why but we were not really close to them at all so we never got to see people like Costa, Udenfriend and Brodie. We knew that they were somewhere in the same building – we just never visited. We saw them at seminars but we really didn't have much relationship and that's something I regret. I came to know some of those people later. Mimo Costa, for example, is someone I have grown to respect and like as the years went by. At that time, particularly Jacques Glowinski would have stand-up debates with Mimo Costa, who was famous for his Latin temperament and was prone to get carried away in public debate. Jacques Glowinski also has something of the Latin in him and they would sometimes have very spectacular arguments at public conferences.

So we first got to know Costa in that way, but I have got to know him since as a friend and a colleague and admire his continuing ability to come up with original ideas, some of which don't work out but some of which do. He's that sort of person – he has no inhibitions about telling you what his latest idea is and why it's important. On the other hand he's a very intelligent, ingenious and inventive person and has contributed a great deal to the field of neurochemistry and neuropharmacology and still does. In his seventies, he lost his job with the Fidia Research Laboratory in Georgetown, Washington, because the company went bankrupt, but Mimo then got himself a new job and a new career in Chicago. Even though he is in his seventies he was recently appointed as a full tenure professor in the University of Illinois. You have to admire someone who can keep going like that and keep wanting to do research and having good ideas.

At the other end, there were people who were just beginning to come into the system, people like Sol Snyder.

Sol was beginning his research career as you say in the Axelrod lab. We didn't actually work together. Sol was doing his own thing, which was somewhat different from the catecholamine research that Jacques and I were doing. But Sol and I were very close then and have been close friends ever since, and I've followed his subsequent research in great detail and with great admiration. Again a person of extraordinary intellect and originality, with the ability to know when to jump into a field and when to move on also, which is equally important. He would tell you, I think, that he owes a great deal of that way of doing research to Julie Axelrod, who also is a fountain of sheer creativity and originality. As you know, Julie's saying was, 'Don't read the literature because it will only confuse you.' You should just get on and do your own thing and have your own ideas about what the problem is and how to solve it. That's very much been Sol's way of doing things – with great success. He has not only contributed enormously through his own ideas but he's trained a whole group of people in the United States who have gone into American academic life and many of them occupy important and senior positions. So he has been very much a mentor also in his way, teaching that way of doing research.

After the NIH?

I had a year in Harvard, which was also very influential for me. The years I spent in America were enormously important, because I gained contacts in the North American research community, which is so huge and productive and important. At Harvard I met a different sort of scientist. They were much more neurobiology and cell biology oriented and less biochemistry and pharmacology oriented than the Axelrod group. To be in Steve Kuffler's Department of Neurobiology for a year was a great privilege and a joy. I worked with the biochemist in that lab, Ed Kravitz. I was the first postdoc that he had ever had, and he and I got on very well and I got introduced to many new areas of neurochemistry and neurobiology.

In particular I got to work on the aminoacid inhibitory transmitter, GABA, for the first time. I was again lucky enough to be in the right place at the right time because the Harvard group had spent years of detailed, meticulous research pinpointing the role of GABA as the inhibitory transmitter for nerve–muscle transmission in lobster and other crustacea. In such animals, the muscle fibres are innervated not only by excitatory motor fibres that create contraction in the muscle but each muscle also receives an inhibitory fibre. This is quite unlike what goes on in mammals, where all the inhibition takes place in the central nervous system. So you had these two rather large axons innervating each bundle of muscle fibres and they had very good circumstantial evidence for the role of GABA as the inhibitory transmitter.

We developed a project to demonstrate finally that it was GABA by showing that when you stimulated the inhibitory nerve electrically, you could demonstrate the release of GABA into the surrounding fluid. A classic Otto Loewi type experiment if you like. There was every reason to think that it would work if only we could work out how to do it. The problem we faced, Ed Kravitz and I and Masanori Otsuka, the Japanese neurophysiologist who was responsible for that side of the work, was how to do the experiment on a suitable muscle. One of the unwritten rules of the lab was that you shouldn't work on edible parts of the lobster, so preferably you worked on the walking leg or something like that. And secondly, more importantly, was how to measure the minute amount of GABA that was likely to be released from nerves. This came out in seawater which is 0.5 molar sodium chloride, so we had to pick up this minute trace of amino acid in a highly saline fluid. Those were just technical problems but they took almost a year to solve and we ended up violating the lab rule – by using one of the large crusher claws of the animal. The whole muscle weighing several grammes is innervated by a single nerve fibre and Otsuka could find it, pick it up and stimulate it and Ed Kravitz and I collected the seawater that was dripping over it. Lo and behold, in the last few weeks before I had to go back to England, we did show GABA release from that preparation. It was a first ever demonstration and it nailed down the idea that GABA was a neurotransmitter, which I then went on to work on in mammalian CNS. Now everybody believes that GABA is the main inhibitory transmitter in the brain. But those were heady days because this was pioneering in a relatively new field at the time and in a great lab. I was exposed not just to biochemistry but to all the other disciplines in neurobiology. At that time the Harvard Neurobiology Department was one of the first neuroscience departments anywhere, the idea, which subsequently really took off, that neuroscience is a discipline in its own right but it embraces all sort of methodologies and principles.

Was this anything to do with Francis Schmitt?

He was also a great influence on me later when I became an Associate of the Neuroscience Research Program at MIT but not at the time. I didn't know Frank Schmitt when I was in Harvard at all, although he was at MIT. He had already started his remarkable 'Invisible University of the Brain', as it was sometimes called – the Neuroscience Research Program at MIT, which was funded by NIH money. It brought together groups of experts in many disciplines from crystallography through to psychology and made them sit in a small room and talk about brain research problems. But Steve Kuffler was the moving force behind the Harvard lab.

Who was Steve Kuffler?

He was a neurophysiologist of extraordinary talent, technically and intellectually, who had brought together a group of very able people in Harvard. He had this genius for choosing the right people and knowing the right sort of preparation to work on to solve a particular problem. He would come up with some extraordinary organisms and extraordinary preparations to look at problems.

At the time I was there, for example, he was interested in glial cells and he came up with the optic nerve of the mud-puppy as a suitable preparation. It's a sort of amphibian, a very exotic thing and it just happens that the optic nerves have these giant glial cells that are big enough for a neurophysiologist to impale and record from directly and then stimulate the optic nerve and see what happens. Everyone at the time saw the glial cells as non-functional, just a supporting cell that held the nervous system together somehow. But Kuffler and his colleagues were among the first to show that if you did record from them they undergo potential changes as the nerves are active and subsequently of course we now know that glial cells have all sorts of pharmacology, they have receptors for a variety of neurotransmitters and peptides. But none of that was known at the time.

Kuffler had this gift of going out into the animal kingdom and finding the most suitable prep and then finding brilliant people. At the time I was there, for example, Hubel and Wiesel were working in the visual system and making their dramatic discoveries about single cells in visual cortex that recognise direction of the stimulus and orientation and so on, which blossomed later into a hugely important area of neuroscience research. So those were exciting times and for me a great experience – an entry into the neuroscience world which I wasn't really familiar with and entry into a new area of neuropharmacology which I subsequently continued to be involved in.

You returned to Cambridge and later joined the MRC in Cambridge. For most of us the MRC/LMB complex is the closest thing outside the US to what the NIH must have been when you went to it.

That's an interesting perception, yes. The MRC labs on the hospital site in Cambridge were a very important set of resources for the Medical Research Council. I must say my own unit, the Neurochemical Pharmacology Unit, didn't have that much contact with the Laboratory for Molecular Biology. We were fairly self-contained in the Department of Pharmacology next door to the LMB but not actually part of it.

I worked for the MRC for 12 years and it was a terrific time. I have been lucky throughout my career in being in places where there was a growth phase of development and the MRC was in such a phase in the 1970s. It wasn't exactly an era when money grew on trees, but the MRC budget was growing at a healthy rate, about 10% a year, and they were setting up new units and the neuroscience area was flourishing. I was lucky to get my own unit at quite a young age. And the MRC in those days had a wonderful policy of letting you do your own thing. I can hardly believe in retrospect how much freedom we had. We had, of course, to talk to people in Head Office in MRC but we had friendly relations with them. One had to write a progress report but only once every 3 years; there was a site visit once every 6 years. When I think what it was like subsequently working in a company, where you had to write a report every week of the year, this was really a luxury. We didn't have an enormous budget but we had enough to do most of the things we wanted to do and I was lucky to have a constant stream of wonderful young people as graduate students and postdoctoral visitors from all over the world. We had a really fantastic time during the 1970s and the science was also developing apace. We were still very optimistic at that time about the ability of neurochemistry and neuroscience to crack some of the remaining problems like schizophrenia, which is just one of the areas that we concentrated a good deal of effort on.

You moved into the dopamine field. Do you want to take me through that?

I was very much influenced by a particular event. It was at a meeting organised by the Neuroscience Research Program at MIT, by which time I was an Associate of that and a regular attender at his meetings. It was a great opportunity for me to go to the States two or three times a year and meet top neuroscientists and maintain contacts. One of the things the Neuroscience Research Program used to do was to have large summer school meetings in the Rocky Mountains in Boulder, Colorado that used to last 3 weeks at a time. They would invite students from all over the world and have a high-level faculty teaching – the whole of neuroscience in 3 weeks, basically. A very grand concept, nobody would ever find the money to do it now.

At one of those events in 1972 Sol Snyder gave a lecture on the dopamine theory of schizophrenia and reviewed the evidence which was coming together at that time, which said, 'Dopamine release is how amphetamines cause psychosis, antipsychotic drugs work by blocking dopamine, and this is what it's all about.' Sol's lecture was a wonderful synthesis and it really triggered my enthusiasm for that area. I was lucky shortly after that to get into dopamine research through the discovery made originally by Paul Greengard in Yale and John Kebabian, his graduate student, of a biochemical model for the dopamine receptor in brain, which relied on the measurement of dopamine-stimulated cyclic AMP formation in brain homogenate.

This was before radiolabelling?

Yes, this was before anybody had a way of labelling the receptors. Many people believed that the dopamine receptor in brain was the target for antischizophrenic drugs but nobody had the biochemical tools to prove that. Richard Miller, who was an outstanding graduate student, started his thesis work with me in Cambridge on the dopamine-stimulated cyclic AMP system that

Greengard had described originally in retina. We were able to show in the brain, much to our delight, that a number of antischizophrenic drugs inhibited responses to dopamine in this system and they did so in a rank order of potency which fitted their clinical effects. For example, compounds in the phenothiazine series that were not clinically active did not block, so we thought we had discovered the target for antischizophrenic drugs, although there were some warning signs that should have told us that we were wrong. A whole group of drugs, the butyrophenones, haloperidol-type drugs, simply did not work in this system and we knew of course that they were very powerful antischizophrenic drugs. Shortly after that it became apparent, when Sol Snyder's lab in Baltimore and Phil Seeman's lab in Canada finally got the right radioligand to label the dopamine receptor, that what they were labelling was a different dopamine receptor from the one that we had been studying. We had been studying what is now known as the D1 receptor and the key target for antipsychotic drugs act is the D2. Of course we didn't know that at the time.

When the Snyder work developed did you make the jump to the idea that there must be a D1 receptor there or how did the D1 receptor ...

Well I guess at the time the Snyder and Seaman work came out, we were out of that field. Richard Miller had gone on to do other things in the US. But we had actually come to the conclusion that there must be more than one dopamine receptor because the butyrophenones didn't work on the adenylate cyclase model.

Instead of further work on dopamine receptors I decided to pursue the dopamine hypothesis by trying to collect postmortem brain from patients dying of schizophrenic illness. I developed a major project with Angus MacKay, who was a young psychiatrist training in research in my laboratory, and with Ted Bird, an enormously enthusiastic and energetic American visitor who had the idea of setting up a brain tissue bank in the MRC Unit in Cambridge. I think we were one of the first anywhere in the world to start a systematic collection of frozen postmortem human brain, carefully dissected into particular regions and stored and made available to the academic researchers around the world. Ted Bird and I were surprised really at how many things you could do with such tissue specimens. Biochemists are brought up to believe that you have got to remove tissue from the organism as soon as the animal is dead, and you have got to freeze it quickly otherwise it is not going to be of any value. It turns out that that isn't true for neurotransmitters and neuropeptide systems in brain. The biochemical systems associated with neurotransmitters, the enzymes, the uptake sites, the various receptor proteins are remarkably stable post mortem and can be measured even under the normal conditions of postmortem collection and storage.

So we set up, among other things, to test the dopamine hypothesis of schizophrenia, which at first sight might seem quite straightforward. But, of course, we hit many problems en route. The results were initially encouraging because we were able to show that you can indeed measure increased levels of dopamine and increased densities of dopamine receptors using the then available radioligand binding assays. But, of course, the interpretation of these data was not simple because it was becoming apparent from animal studies that treatment with antischizophrenic drugs for any length of time leads to adaptive changes in brain chemistry – including increased dopamine levels and increased densities of dopamine receptors – as some sort of compensation to the receptor blockage. So the results remained ambiguous and I think to this day it is unclear whether the postmortem findings mean anything in terms of the dopamine hypothesis. Like others we tried to find drug naive subjects, but they are few and far between in developed countries. So this remains a set of findings which we were quite pleased with but really in the long run I don't think they helped us understand the illness all that much.

This area has I suppose been taken over by the in vivo brain imaging people but while it lasted one or two of the key figures trained with you – Gavin Reynolds.

Yes, although brain imaging of dopamine receptors in schizophrenics has also given conflicting results. Gavin was in Cambridge as a visitor and he has continued with great dedication to work in this area, in which he continues to make important contributions, but I think he would admit like anyone else that this field of study is fraught with many problems of interpretation. The finding that he has made which I find very intriguing is the observation of increased dopamine levels on one side of the brain in schizophrenia, in the amygdala. That is important for some of the other neurobiological ideas about the nature of schizophrenic illness, what goes wrong in the brain. Maybe some day, we will put our finger on a neurochemical abnormality in the dopamine system in schizophrenia, but so far I think we have to admit that it's eluded us.

One of the other things we did on catecholamines was to pursue the use of 6-hydroxydopamine as a tool for probing catecholamine systems in the brain. This was around 1970, and a young American postdoctoral fellow, Norman Uretsky, from Chicago got onto this project. Hans Thoenen and his colleagues in Switzerland had shown the remarkable ability of 6-hydroxydopamine to destroy selectively sympathetic nerve endings in the periphery. It is a remarkably selective neurotoxin, a catecholamine derivative that is taken up and concentrated by the uptake mechanism in sympathetic nerves, and then by means of a cytotoxic free radical mechanism it kills the nerve. Nobody had used it at that time in the brain and Norman Uretsky was able to show that if you gave the compound directly into the brain – you can't deliver it by other routes because it doesn't get through the blood–brain barrier – it causes a very selective distruction of both noradrenergic and dopamine systems. Later on that became refined by us and by many others to show that if one administered minute local micro-injections of 6-hydroxydopamine into one area of the brain, it would cause selective damage to one particular dopamine adrenergic system. You could if you injected into just one side of the basal ganglia, for example, as Ungerstedt and his colleagues showed, produce an animal with a hemi-parkinsonism syndrome. Such animals when stimulated with dopaminergic drugs would rotate in one particular direction or another. That became a whole industry of its own in neuropharmacology – the rotating rat. This was exciting stuff and again we were lucky enough to be in at the very early stages of it.

Personally the most rewarding area to get into during that period in the 1970s was to get involved in neuropeptide research, which was for me an entirely new area. We started quite early in the 1970s with research on substance P, which I continue to be fascinated by as a neuropeptide. The structure of the peptide had only just been announced by Susan Lehman in 1970 as an 11-amino acid peptide. In those days it wasn't that easy to make peptides synthetically but a lab at the Merck Institute in the US had made large amounts of substance P. Ralph Hirschman, the head of the chemistry group there at that time, generously enough gave me a substantial amount (50 mg) of the peptide, which kept us going for years. We started a whole programme of research around that 50 mg of synthetic peptide. It was enough to make antibodies with, and an Argentinian visitor, Claudio Coello, used the antibodies to immunohistochemically map substance P systems in the brain. We were also able to measure substance P release from isolated fragments of brain or spinal cord using a radioimmunoassay. Tom Jessell did some of that work and was able to show for the first time that the release of substance P from the sensory endings in the brain stem was inhibited by morphine and other opiates. That suggested a mechanism to explain one of the ways in which morphine controls the input of pain information into the CNS, an idea which became quite widely accepted.

In the mid 1970s, there was something of a sea-change happening with research – it became less inclined to be seen as pure research. There was a very famous LMB episode with Caesar Milstein where they discovered monoclonal antibodies and hinted that there might be quite a lot of money to be made out of all this, but the MRC failed to get a patent on it. This is often seen since as a key episode where the old attitudes were seen as being wonderful but not suited to the modern world. You were in there when all of this was going on. Did things seem to be changing to you?

Not then, although it certainly has since. I think you are right to say that the particular episode, when the MRC failed to recognise the importance of monoclonal antibodies, was one of the events that later helped to crystallise thinking in this area, and explains why attitudes now are so different 20 years on.

There has been a sea-change in the attitude of university people. Academic people and MRC scientists now think about their work in commercial terms whereas we never paid any attention to that whatsoever. During the entire period that I worked for the MRC it never crossed our mind at all that anything we were doing might have any commercial value, nor did it cross the mind of any of our administrators at the MRC Head Office, as far as I could see. It wasn't the way we thought about science. Now I think the pendulum has swung almost too far the other way. Scientists are looking over their shoulder at their lawyer to ask whether they are allowed to talk about what they are doing and this is one of the frustrating aspects of modern science, this requirement for confidentiality, imposed on scientists by the pressure for commercialisation. I think it's had a lot more effect in the United States than it has in Britain. In the US it's almost the norm for my academic colleagues to be involved somehow in one or other small company, whereas that's still very uncommon here.

When I came to Cambridge at the end of 1985, the impact of your leaving was still quite substantial. There was a remarkable amount of surprise but on the other hand both you and John Hughes, for instance, in the early 1980s, were making a move from academia to industry.

I can't understand to this day why people were so surprised. It's not as if I or Humphrey Rang (going to Sandoz) or John Hughes (to Parke Davies),[2] were the first academics ever to move to the pharmaceutical industry . There is a long tradition in Britain, starting with Sir Henry Dale, who went to the Wellcome labs at the turn of the century and revolutionised their research programmes. Then he went back to academia. John Vane went to Wellcome and came back to academia. Sir James Black went from industry to academia and then back to industry. There has been a fairly healthy interchange in Britian and this is one of the reasons, I think, why Britain has done so well in the pharmaceutical research area. We have, for example, in the British Pharmacological Society, as many members from industry as we do from academia.

During the 1960s and 1970s was it as respectable as it is now?

Well I suppose it's become more so. Attitudes have changed greatly in the last 50 years. In America, it was only after the Second World War that pharmacologists working in industry were allowed to join the American Pharmacological Society. They were taboo; they were not allowed in because what they were doing in industry wasn't good science. So the US had similar snooty attitudes.

Why did I become involved with the Merck project? Merck came to Britain as part of its global expansion plan. The company was expanding in all directions and quite rightly felt that they should expand their research and make it more international. They picked on Britain as one of their European centres and they picked on neuroscience as an area that was blossoming in Britain and they were looking for someone to direct their new laboratory. I was initially involved with this project as an advisor and as I got more involved I could see what an exciting large project it was. I could see that the people from Merck were serious about what they intended to do. They were willing to spend money, they were willing to take a long-term view of what came out of the lab and I liked the people I was dealing with.

When they set this up, it was probably the strongest neuroscience research facility in the UK, stronger than any university departments.

Well, it flourished. We were treated very generously and were able to construct a wonderful modern building which is one of the most delightful places I have ever worked in. I think people's work is influenced by the surroundings they

---

[2]Hughes J (1996). The discovery of the opioid peptides. In *The Psychopharmacologists*, Vol I, pp 539–564.

336 The Psychopharmacologists II

work in and this was a wonderful place, done with great care and quality down to the last detail. There was an opportunity to start completely from scratch because Merck had no research operation in neuroscience in Europe at all. We were able to go out and recruit the best people we could find and at that time there were, fortunately for us, quite a number of good people around looking for jobs. We hired some very talented people in pharmacology, chemistry, biochemistry and behavioural science and built up to somewhere around 200 scientists when we got to our peak capacity, with another 100 support staff. So it was another period of log-growth which I enjoyed being in. It was a terrific privilege to have that opportunity.

Partly by serendipity, partly by opportunism, we got into some very exciting areas of science quite quickly – most notably into the glutamate area of pharmacology, which was a completely new one for me, although it was expanding during the 1980s quite rapidly. We got into this through a Merck compound, which is called MK-801.

This is one of those compounds like 3-PPP, or 8-OH-DPAT, whose codes are highly significant for psychopharmacologists but which aren't known by the public at large.

Yes, this is one of those code numbers that are well known to scientists all around the world. MK-801 was developed by Merck in a sort of old-fashioned way. It was picked up through random screening of organic chemicals as a powerful anticonvulsant. It has extraordinary effectiveness at very low doses in animal models of epilepsy. It was orally active and brain penetrant – so active that Merck decided to develop it as a potential antiepileptic drug. They had got quite far into development by the time I joined the company and started the Harlow Neuroscience Research Centre. Indeed Merck was about ready to go into the clinic with this new chemical but they didn't have the faintest idea how it worked. It was simply an anticonvulsant with an unknown mechanism, and they thought, quite rightly, we should try and find out how it worked and determine whether we could build a better second-generation compound.

We took that challenge on and fortunately we made very quick progress, following the Sol Snyder paradigm, which by then, thanks to his pioneering work, was the obvious thing to do, i.e. to radiolabel MK-801 and then see if we could find a binding site for the drug in brain homogenates. Eric Wong, who had just joined the lab as a PhD scientist, was rapidly able to do this. He found a nanomolar afinity binding site which had a unique distribution in brain, which was displaced by various analogues of MK-801 with the right rank order of potency according to their anticonvulsant activities. We knew that we had the pharmacologically relevant site but we still didn't know what it was. So we again used the Sol Snyder technique, which is to grab hold of the Sigma catalogue and tick off all the things you can think of and throw them into your binding assay to see if they interfere. But we still didn't find the answer. Even though we put in glutamate and N-methyl-aspartic acid, nothing happened. In retrospect we know why that had happened – because there is so much glutamate present in the brain homogenate that adding a bit more doesn't make any difference, it's already occupying the sites and doesn't have any further effects.

In any case the drug doesn't bind to the glutamate recognition site; it binds to some other part of the receptor. So that didn't work.

The only compounds that Eric Wong found that worked in displacing radiolabelled MK-801 were phencyclidine and ketamine. Were it not for another piece of good luck, that wouldn't have helped us either, because nobody really knew how they worked. They were anaesthetics of unknown mechanisms and that didn't help. However, David Lodge, a neurophysiologist and neuropharmacologist, fortunately for us had just published at this time some observations on phencyclidine and ketamine, involving classical neurophysiology-type experiments, recording from single neurones in the brain of an anaesthetised animal then applying glutamate, phencyclidine or ketamine and finding that these anaesthetics were quite good glutamate antagonists. Not only that but they appeared to be NMDA subtype selective. So that gave us a clue and then John Kemp, who ran the neurophysiology lab in the Merck Neuroscience Research Centre, went on to show in brain slices, and later in brain cells in culture, that indeed MK-801 was an extraordinarily potent noncompetitive NMDA receptor blocker.

So that gave us a mechanism and we were, almost unwittingly, plunged into a rapidly expanding area of neuropharmacology with an extraordinary tool. We did a lot of work on MK-801. Epilepsy wasn't the big indication. The big prize was neuroprotection: the idea that you could protect the brain against damage after a stroke or a head injury where there is a lot of free glutamate floating around doing damage. The NMDA receptor, which MK-801 targetted, seemed to be the key toxic mechanism. We were able to show, thanks to good work done with Jim McCulloch in Glasgow, who is a real expert on animal models of stroke, that MK-801 was highly protective. It reduced the volume of damage in animal models of stroke by a quite spectacular degree. Not only that, it was effective even when given some time after the initial insult to the brain. We thought we were really onto something quite exciting. Many other companies rushed into that field all with the same objective. Even now we don't know the answer as to whether this is going to work in the clinic, although some companies are now quite well advanced into clinical studies.

Merck, however, much to my disappointment at the time, decided to pull out of the area for a number of commercially sound reasons. MK-801 had a number of grey clouds floating over it. Apart from the very positive results that we had in animal models of neuroprotection, there was also the question of whether it might not be a psychotomimetic drug like phencyclidine, and indeed clinical experience now with other compounds does indeed show that it is very likely that most NMDA blockers will be phencyclidine-like psychotomimetics, when given to people. Whether that is a sufficient no-go area to prevent you using it, especially after strokes, I think is still debatable.

There is a curious ethical issue there – do you stop the production of these kinds of drugs because they will leak out on to the street?

That was one of the worries of course. Merck is a highly successful company and very much aware of not doing anything that might damage its excellent image in the medical community. That's one of the reasons why it behaves somewhat cautiously and conservatively. That was only one of the issues. There were a number of other question marks. One was a very practical one. MK-801 causes, among other things, an increased autonomic outflow which leads to a quite substantial rise in blood pressure and heart rate both in animals and in people. This, we knew from volunteer studies, was likely to occur within the range of doses that we were going to have to use. So if you think about that – there's a patient who has had a stroke and you are about to give a drug that's likely to give a surge in blood pressure, a normal thrombo-embolic stroke might be converted into a haemorrhagic one, which you can't do anything about. This was regarded as a rather high-risk side-effect, even though it was probably one that could be controlled by suitable co-medication.

But it's that kind of situation, where high risks are worth taking.

Well, there's a balance of risk and reward in most drug development projects. But really the final straw that led to the company's withdrawal was a paper published by John Olney in *Science* in 1989. He made the surprising observation that when you give a single dose of MK-801 or phencyclidine to animals and look carefully in the brain for histological changes, in some areas of the cortex most of the large neurones became honeycombed – full of fluid-filled vesicles. The neurones became swollen and they looked like Swiss cheese. He described this as a neuropathology associated with these drugs, although even in the first paper he showed it was reversible – within a few hours it disappeared again. And he also showed that if you gave a second dose of MK-801 you didn't get the reaction a second time around. Nevertheless, it created a large problem because, if Merck is cautious, the FDA in America are even more cautious.

They convened a special meeting of experts to discuss this new set of findings. I had to go there as an expert witness for Merck and make our submission. We ourselves, of course, began to study this phenomenon intensely. We found that this was very largely a reversible pathology. On the other hand, if you gave a very large dose of MK-801 you did show a tiny percentage of neurones dying in these areas of brain. We were faced with this problem – here we had a drug that under extreme conditions of dosage might conceivably cause the death of a very small number of brain cells, while on the other hand it could potentially rescue a thousand million other brain cells. After some years have passed the balance of opinion now is that this isn't a no-go issue – drug companies are being allowed to develop NMDA antagonists which have similar pathology. We understand the phenomenon and that makes the FDA more comfortable with it, but at the time they set a number of rather stringent conditions for Merck and the other companies involved. Merck decided not to proceed with the development of MK-801. It was a commercial decision, probably correct at the time, but obviously disappointing to me and to the other scientists involved.

We continued to work in the area, trying to get a better version of MK-801 and trying to target another aspect of the NMDA receptor, the glycine modulatory site. But so far that hasn't come to fruition, although there are now compounds around from a number of companies in trial for the acute treatment of stroke, using this NMDA mechanism, and we are all waiting to see how it's going to develop.

One of the other areas you moved into in this period was the neuropeptide area. Now you recently wrote a piece called 'Neuropeptides – promise unfulfilled?'

Right. That proved to be a field again like the dopamine theory of schizophrenia, if you like, of great optimism, which somehow wasn't fulfilled in the sense that we still don't understand the basis of schizophrenia even though I think we now understand how antischizophrenic drugs work, which is a step forward. With peptides, we understand a great deal about how they are made, where they are and how they are released. We are now beginning in the 1990s to have a whole pharmacology based on a series of novel non-peptide organic drug molecules that target peptide receptors, which is a tremendous step forward. But we still don't understand what the neuropeptides are all about and why they are there. It remains as good a mystery as it was when we started working in the area. That doesn't mean that we didn't have a lot of fun on the way and make some interesting discoveries.

Substance P was the focus of that activity in the Merck labs as it was in my Cambridge lab. We had a substantial chemistry programme aimed at the rational design of an antagonist, based on looking at substance P and trying to make confirmationally restrained analogues of it. Brian Williams and others in the Chemistry Department at Merck did a wonderful job in making such compounds. We also tried the other Merck traditional approach, which is natural product screening. Merck had a large programme of screening micro-organism fermentation products and looking for, not just antibiotics, but for all sorts of drugs. That programme over the years has been very successful.

For another neuropeptide, for example, cholecystokinin, Merck in the States discovered the first non-peptide drugs that antagonised CCK receptors from a natural product lead, asperlicin. We did quite a lot of work on the CCK antagonists to try and support the idea that they might have some therapeutic utility in the treatment of panic and anxiety states. That actually never came to anything. If you inject CCK peptide into people it induces a panic state that lasts for a few minutes. It's very unpleasant and you can obtain a dose–response curve for panic versus dose of CCK and that could be blocked with the Merck antagonist, so we thought we were really onto something quite interesting. But when the antagonist drug was given to patients who normally experienced panic attacks at regular intervals, it didn't do anything. They continued to have their panic attacks with the same frequency and the same severity. So all we ended up proving was that we didn't understand the basic rules of logic. The premise was that 'CCK causes panic' but you can see that the implication that therefore 'panic is caused by CCK' is a non-sequitur.

We spent a lot of effort on substance P without getting very far. We didn't find anything in the natural product screening programme and we gave up on the programme for a few years until 1991, when scientists from Pfizer published the first paper on a non-peptide drug that targetted substance P receptors. This was a very important discovery and got us back into the area. That one discovery was enough to trigger drug companies all over the world to create a multiplicity of new substance P receptor antagonists all based on the original starting point from Pfizer.

There's a public perception that being natural has to be better but in actual fact when you compare, for instance, TPA versus streptokinase, the artificial compound comes out superior to the natural one. It's curious isn't it?

Well, I don't go along with this natural approach. Certainly for brain peptides you're not going to make much progress that way because the peptides don't get across the blood–brain barrier. In retrospect we would never have found a substance P antagonist by using substance P as the starting point for our chemistry, which is what we were trying to do. The newly discovered antagonist drugs actually bind to a different part of the receptor from the site where substance P binds and they bear little structural resemblance to substance P. It's not like another key that fits the same lock, it's a different key that fits a different part of the lock. We could have spent a hundred years modelling substance P and you would never have discovered these new drug molecules. But now you have got one agent and you can model from that with computer modelling techniques and come up with 101 other antagonists.

I am looking forward to seeing how some of these stories play out. The NMDA story is still wide open in terms of whether it is going to have any therapeutic utility, and the substance P story is coming to that stage now. There are a number of very powerful substance P antagonist drugs from different companies in different stages of development for a variety of indications. For example, substance P is involved in the vagal emesis reflex circuit and substance P antagonists have proved to be broad-spectrum antiemetics in animals. They work against a wider range of emetic stimuli than the recently introduced 5HT$_3$ blocking drugs which have proved very succesful both medically and commercial.

Shortly after you moved over to the industry, I was aware that a few of your colleagues such as Roger Pinder and Brian Leonard saw a potential clash ahead, which was that you were going to Merck for the opportunity to move science forward while Merck made drugs – there was a clash potentially there, they felt, and they weren't sure how it would play out. How did it play?

Well, when I moved to Merck, certainly one of the attractions was having a brand new lab, the ability to recruit a whole cohort of talented scientists, a lot of freedom to choose what sort of scientists we felt we needed and the ability to choose more or less what we wanted to do as targets, although we knew right from day one that this was a drug discovery lab. It wasn't like some of the research labs that had been set up by companies, which were essentially public relations exercises, like the Roche Institute for Molecular Biology in

Nutley, New Jersey, for example, or the Roche Institute for Immunology in Basel – pure blue sky science and not related to the company. The Merck Neuroscience Research Center was never like that, and I knew it was not going to be. It had, right from day one, taken over the responsibility of inventing new drugs in the CNS area for the company world wide. Merck dispersed the small CNS group they had previously had in the States. So we were out there on our own and if we didn't get CNS drugs we knew that the company only had one set of people to blame and that was us.

Fortunately for us, the company was going through an extremely success-ful period commercially and they could afford to take a long-term view, which they did. I have got no complaints at all about the way that Merck treated me or the other scientists at the Neuroscience Research Center. They gave us very generous support and we had a great deal of freedom in choos-ing projects to work on. We wanted as badly as anyone else to make drugs for the company. On the whole I think our track record was not bad in that respect. Discovering drugs and developing them is a highly risky business. Not more than one in 10 of the ones that are recommended by the basic research lab actually make it all the way through development and into the clinic and get registered. There are many, many ways of losing compounds and, over the years, we discovered several of them!

So we did achieve some of the things that we set out to do but we also lost some good-looking projects and some good-looking compounds. You've heard about MK-801. We also got into a very fruitful collaboration very early on with a small Danish company called Ferrosan and a very talented group of drug dis-covery scientists from whom we learnt a great deal. We worked with them on partial agonist benzodiazepines with the idea that a benzodiazepine that didn't have the full agonist profile of diazepam might have some advantages as an antianxiety compound but lacking the sedation and lacking the dependence properties of some of the classical benzodiazepines. That was a good idea, although nobody has actually pulled it off successfully in the clinic as yet, despite many attempts. Abecarnil is on the market now and it's the closest to a partial BZ agonist but not a perfect one. Anyway, we got into this collaboration and within a few years of starting the Neuroscience Research Center we had development compounds from that, which looked very promising in animals. Unfortunately all the development compounds were lost through toxicology in animals for various reasons and never got through to being given to patients.

At the time, Merck and Glaxo were the two largest players and both were making a big deal about the fact that they were science driven. It had become the respectable thing to be into 'rational drug development'. How much is that mythology?

That was not mythology from Merck's point of view. Merck is a very unusual company in being science led. I think it has been since the time of George Merck in the 1930s, who was among the first to recognise that if you want to be suc-cessful in pharmaceutical research you have got to go out and attract top-quality scientists and give them a working environment that they find attractive. You have got to allow them to publish. Merck did that at an early period, before the Second World War, when other companies weren't behaving like that and Merck continues to have science as its driving force. After all, Roy Vagelos went from being an academic research scientist, to Head of Research and Development in Merck and then to being Chief Executive Officer of the company and one of the American business community's hero figures of the 1980s and 1990s.

What was he like?

As you'd expect, he's a charismatic figure. He drove the cholestrol-lowering programme and also the angiotensin converting enzyme inhibitor programme at Merck, both of which when the company started on them were speculative. Nobody could have predicted that blocking angiotensin synthesis would prove to be of universal benefit in all people with high blood pressure and of enormous benefit to people with heart failure. But Roy Vagelos drove that programme with enormous energy and, of course, he brought in the idea of a cholestrol-lowering programme and led that. It was a long programme that took nearly 20 years to reach fruition. So yes, he deserves all the credit.

Did you encounter any problems at Merck?

I think one disadvantage we had in the Neuroscience Research Center was not being on the headquarters site, so we lacked that day-to-day contact with the rest of the company. Another disadvantage was that Merck had nothing else going in the CNS area. The only major CNS product when I joined the company was Sinemet, a combination of L-dopa and carbidopa for Parkinson's disease, which was a very successful product. It dominated the world market for Parkinson's disease for many years. But the research on Sinemet had been done long before I joined. None of the development people had had any experience of developing a CNS drug. Nor had any of the senior management, who sit around the high table in Merck and make the decisions about what goes forward and what doesn't.

Merck had hit the doldrums in the CNS for a number of years. That was one of the reasons why they set up the Neuroscience Center. So we had the disadvantage that we were talking to people to whom you had to explain everything from the beginning and that wasn't so easy sometimes in a company that deals with anti-infective agents, cholesterol-lowering agents and cardiovascular agents, where you've got nice clear endpoints. You can measure blood pressure, that's easy; you can measure whether you treat the bacterial infection; you can measure cholesterol, but if you go into the development of CNS drugs you're talking about clinical trials where many of the patients get better on placebo anyway and you are looking for some small change on top of that, and how do you measure depression or anxiety?

One of the interviews I read with great interest in your first volume was by Peter Waldmeier at Ciba-Geigy.[3] I share some of the obvious agonies that he

[3]Waldmeier P (1996). From mental illness to neurodegeneration. In *The Psychopharmacologists*, Vol I, pp 565–586.

went through in a long career, of having what he thought were really excellent projects turned down by senior management, or if not turned down at least not supported, which is almost the same thing. In order to get something through to the end in a drug company, you have to have people who really believe in it and champion it, otherwise, they just look for reasons to stop it, which is what you could see from that account that he gave you. I knew Peter Waldemeir very well and Laurent Maitre, his boss, from a period in the 1970s when I acted as a consultant to that group. They had what appeared to me very good ideas. They were working on 5HT uptake inhibitors long before anybody had thought about them, at least at the same time as Arvid Carlsson was, but this was never followed up by the company.

Talking about 5HT uptake inhibitors, I can tell you a little about zimelidine. One of my first exposures to drug development and how complicated the whole process is was within a few weeks after joining Merck, in 1983. I went to visit the clinical research group in the US, a large group, headed by Marv Jaffe. They had a small CNS team there which had been working with Astra on zimelidine, because Merck has a deal with Astra, which gives them access to any Astra product for development in North America. They had completed the Phase III trials for zimelidine in the USA and Canada and they were overjoyed because clearly the drug was working as well as amitriptyline, and it was far less toxic. They were over the moon. They were having a party to celebrate the loading of the truck that was going to go down to Washington with the registration file in it. I saw it in this room and it impacted on me just how complicated it all was – to see a room full of volumes of data going from floor to ceiling in several large piles, 200 or more volumes of data. If it had gone through, zimelidine would have been registered probably a year before Prozac in the States. It was already on the market in Europe, by Astra. But no sooner did the truck get to Washington, than serious adverse effects began to crop up in Europe, at a rate of about one in 100,000. This is the nightmare that any drug company has. It doesn't matter how well you have done the clinical research. You can have 3000 patients in a Phase III trial and never pick up a rare serious complication.

Of course, the reason Prozac has done so well to some extent has been because Lilly is a US company and the Americans are going to home-buy but if Merck had been pushing zimelidine, would Prozac have ever been heard of?

We could have had a part of that market. From my point of view the story has some extra appeal because I started in reseach working on amine uptake. We knew how antidepressants worked very early on. As soon as the uptake mechanisms for 5HT and noradrenaline were characterised, it was apparent that the conventional tricyclic antidepressants acted as amine uptake inhibitors. One could ask, why didn't the major companies like Merck and Ciba-Geigy get right back in there and make better uptake inhibitors as soon as they knew about it? Merck had amitriptyline but the main thing wrong with amitriptyline was its powerful cholinergic effects, which makes it toxic. We could have had a 'son of amitriptyline' but we didn't get there. We didn't even think about working on zimelidine in the neuroscience lab in Merck because we thought that story was all over. But it's strange to think how a mechanism that we already knew about for the conventional antidepressants could suddenly become overnight a block-buster with Prozac selling $2000 million a year and portrayed as a totally new development in psychopharmacology, which basically it isn't. The 5HT uptake inhibitors have some advantages but their main one is that you cannot commit suicide by overdosing because they are not that toxic.

Let me hop to another emblematic scene in which you have had connections with all the players. Another Merck drug, a D4 antagonist, failed. Merck put a lot of money into try-ing to test this out clinically – on the back I guess of claims by Phil Seeman. Now, often claims made on the back of sometimes flimsy data or thin arguments seem to catch the field and one of those who are caught are the drug companies. You could say they're possibly naive to move so fast on the back of these claims but on the other hand companies are the only people who can actually test some of these claims out. Another player in all this, who worked with you previously, Gavin Reynolds, did perhaps more than anyone else to kill the D4 story.

Well, the dopamine D4 antagonist as a novel CNS drug discovery target is a beautiful example of how powerful the techniques of molecular biology are and what impact they now have on drug discovery in CNS, as in every other area. What motivated us to start a project for D4 wasn't really the Phil Seeman paper claiming large increases in D4 receptors in the brains of schizophrenics, it was the original paper published in *Nature* by Seeman's group – by van Tol et al., who first described the discovery of this dopamine receptor. It was not only novel but it also had unusual pharmacology in the sense that clozapine had a preferential affinity for this site. Now clozapine somehow holds the clue about how to make better antipsychotics. If you could only understand how clozapine worked, you might have a way of making 'son of clozapine', which would be the next generation of antischizophrenic drugs. So we were always alert to anything that had to do with clozapine and we came across this paper. My boss in Merck, Ed Scolnick, who is very molecular biology-oriented in his thinking, said, 'This is it, go for it.' And that was all it took, that one letter in *Nature*, and we went for it. The Merck chemistry team in Harlow did a mag-nificent job in coming up with a highly selective, high-affinity dopamine D4 antagonist in a very short space of time. We got a development project in place and we carried it right through and it was completed after I left, but we now know that in the clinical trial the patients didn't show any improvement, in fact there was a tendency for them to get worse (Kramer et al. 1996, *Psychopharmacology Bulletin*, 32: 467). They couldn't tell whether they had the active drug or the placebo. But this was a nice example, I think, of what a big company can do. You can have an idea, but to put it into practice is quite another thing and to put it into practice quickly, so you could have some com-petitive commercial advantage, you have got to move quite fast and you have to be willing to put in a significant resource. I couldn't tell you how many dol-lars or pounds were spent on that particular project but it was a significant effort. Not just one chemist in a back room but a whole team.

At first sight it was very good news for us that having chosen to do a D4 antagonist project and put all this effort in, a paper comes out almost the next day from Phil Seeman claiming a seven-fold increase in this receptor in schizophrenia. We thought this was great, but then we looked at the paper more closely and tried to replicate it and I talked to Gavin Reynolds and we realised clearly that it was a very contentious claim. There's something about schizophrenia research that impels people to make extraordinary claims. If you look over the history of schizophrenia research, it is littered with the skeletons of chemical hypotheses.

There's an art to these claims. There has to be good marketing copy to the claim. One person who has been able to do this awfully well whom you liaised with in Cambridge was Tim Crow. The idea of type 1 and type 2 or positive and negative schizophrenia and the progression from one to the other was an extraordinarily influential claim, which in some respects ran in the face of all the evidence, but it was a good marketing concept and I think marketing plays more of a part in academia than many people would like to concede.

Like other aspects of life, it's one thing to have an idea, it's another thing whether you can convince other people that your idea has any merit, and some people are better at this than others. Sol Synder is a very good exponent of this art. Merton Sandler is a wonderfully persuasive talker. Mimo Costa is another person who could get up and give you an outrageous hypothesis and you would find it very plausible because of the way he delivered it. I don't think I'd put myself in that category of being a proponent of hypotheses. My way of doing things is usually more opportunistic. If something looks good I am willing to take it up and run with it at a very early stage if I have the feeling that it's ready for development.

In addition to having worked with Sol Snyder you also did some work with what at the time must have been a fairly young Sol Langer..

Sol Langer and I worked together briefly in the 1960s in Cambridge when he came as a visiting scientist to Marthe Vogt. We were not in the same department. Marthe Vogt worked with Gaddum at Babraham. She was the first person to describe the existence of noradrenaline in the brain in the 1950s. It took some effort to persuade people to think about chemical transmitters in the brain in those days. She was one of that generation of scientists who basically never give up research and just go on going into the lab every day. Feldberg was another example, who should perhaps have been stopped but nobody had the temerity to tell him so. Actually, when I was planning to do a PhD in Cambridge in 1961 one of the people I had talked to was Marthe Vogt and I had seriously thought about going there to do a PhD with her.

What was she like then?

She was a fairly austere lady in many ways. It was quite difficult to get on friendly terms with her although eventually I did. She was very open, always willing to tell you about her research. She was trained in a classical mode of pharmacology, which I don't think would have suited me very much as I was trained in biochemical techniques. But she did what she did with great ability and continued to make contributions for many years. So that's how I got to know Sol Langer. Sol and I had been friends before that because when I was a postdoc in the neurobiology lab at Harvard he was a postdoc in the Department of Pharmacology, just a few floors up in the same building, and we used to see each other there. He is one of those people who went into industry and continued to do original research of his own. I don't know how he managed it.

If you had stayed with reuptake mechanisms when you were working on it and wrote the monograph on it, you would have had the chance to market yourself as the creator of this generation of drugs to some extent ...

It would have been incredibly boring scientifically. I suppose it's a weakness but I can't stick with one area of science for ever. There are so many exciting things happening all the time in our field that you'd like to be part of. Right now if I was given the chance to do new research, a lab and new work, I would learn about molecular genetics and get into research on the genetic risk factors in psychiatric illness, which I think is the big project for the future in psychiatry. It's where we are going to see, hopefully, very soon, the really big discoveries being made, whereas you could say psychopharmacology research has been spinning its wheels for the last 30 or 40 years, since the really major discoveries were made in the 1950s and 1960s.

But are the molecular genetic projects not going to spell trouble for the industry in that they are going to break down the monolithic concepts like schizophrenia, which means the market is not going to look as attractive?

That's a very perceptive comment, I think. It's true not just for psychiatry but for any illness with a polygenic basis. You can see it happening in diabetes research, for example. There won't be a single gene for diabetes, there will be 10 or 12 risk factor genes for diabetes. And then you have a single disease turned into 12 different genetically based entities and how you are going to treat each one of those fragments, whereas you can treat them all with insulin and you can treat all schizophrenics with chlorpromazine? So, you're right but we don't have to think about everything in terms of whether it's good for the pharmaceutical industry, we have to take a broader picture. Whether it's good for us as a species to understand schizophrenic illnesses, I have no doubt at all. It's going to be probably by small advances that we will suddenly realise that we have made a major insight. You can see it happening already in Alzheimer's disease in the last 5 years. There are now four different genes identified as risk factors and many more no doubt will be coming. It will give us a totally new way of looking at these diseases and in the long run it must give us a totally new way of thinking about how you might prescribe therapy.

Was there ever at any point, working within the industry, when you felt that people just aren't grateful for what the industry does? You find the drugs which cure the infectious diseases that kill their children and they're very grateful for a short time, but then everybody forgets about that pretty quickly and just thinks about the nasty pharmaceutical industry again.

That was one of the striking things about moving from academia to industry. You go from a profession in academic research which isn't particularly liked by the community at large but it isn't particularly disliked either, it's sort of neutral. People think about scientists as some strange creatures but they don't necessarily hate them. Then you go to be a scientist in industry and you are universally hated and reviled.

It's curious, isn't it, when you think of all the benefits that derive from pharmaceutical research. Just look at the reduced risk now for cardiovascular disease, which is seen because of the new pharmacological treatments but somehow it goes over people's heads. The other thing in the pharmaceutical industry that I find very strange is that you are always being asked for perfection – you have to have a drug which is totally safe and totally effective with no side-effects . This is what is expected of you, whereas as a surgeon if I wanted to invent a new surgical procedure which had a mortality rate of 10%, I could go ahead and do that. I might even say that my operation was wonderful because it had a 90% success rate! Look at the early history of heart transplant surgery where everyone died quite soon after the operation, but everybody thought that this was a great advance and the surgeon a great hero. It's very difficult to understand.

I suppose at the back of it is the fact that drug companies make a lot of money. Maybe surgeons make a lot of money too but not on the same scale. It's the idea that you can profit from the sick that sticks in the gullet of many people. Personally, I don't have any problem with that. I think that the pharmaceutical industry may have been guilty of considerable excesses in the last few decades, finding it too easy to make money and having too high a profit margin and being somewhat self-indulgent about the way that it spent money. But on the whole the free enterprise system has created far more drugs than any other system that you could think of. Look at the Soviet system, producing virtually no new pharmaceutical discoveries at all in the last 50-odd years. Here we are in the capitalist system with companies competing against each other for commercial advantage and that's one of the ways of getting things done and getting them done in a hurry. But there are limits to this. You might ask, why do we need seven different angiotensin converting enzyme inhibitors, wouldn't two be enough? And the industry is thinning itself out on these lines. You won't have seven drugs of the same type any more because it won't be commercially viable to do it.

You left Merck and moved back into academia. How's that going?

To go out on Monday morning and not to have to think about getting on the airplane to Rahway, New Jersey has some attractions! I've got some new interests now. I'm interested in positron emission temography, or PET imaging, and I have a link with the MRC Cyclotron Unit at the Hammersmith Hospital – one of the pioneering labs in this area. The reason I find it fascinating as a pharmacologist is that this is the only way in which you can look at drug receptor binding phenomena in the living patient. You can look inside the brain and you can even see dopamine receptor ligands binding dopamine receptors in the brain and you can do all sorts of things with that. I find that very exciting, so I am working with them to help inject more pharmacology into the way they do things.

Do you see yourself as a neuroscientist or a psychopharmacologist?

I think of myself really more as a neuroscientist than a psychopharmacologist. Clinical psychopharmacology has never really excited me much, I am sorry to say. If I have a choice of meetings to go to, I will go to the Society of Neuroscience in the USA rather than to the ACNP, although I have been many times to the ACNP and CINP meetings. I find the ACNP and even more so the CINP have a sort of old boys' club feeling about them. They tend to be dominated by cohorts of people who have been around for a long time and they have this special relationship with one another and with certain pharmaceutical companies, and it's all very cosy. I don't find it particularly attractive.

Wouldn't you get any of that in the Society of Neuroscience?

No, it's not like that. It's a very democratically run and dynamic society. They've had a remarkable success in building a society in only 20 years. The Neuroscience Research Programme had a great deal to do with that. A lot of people who were in the NRP ended up as presidents of the Society for Neuroscience. Frank Schmitt's NRP group was not a fixed group of people, there was turnover there, and a lot of people went through the NRP in that way. I was an Associate for about 10 years. NRP had a great influence on the development of American neuroscience in the 1960s and 1970s. The society grew out of that and has become phenomenally successful. Too successful, some would say. There are more than 25,000 members and I am going to a meeting next month (November 1996) where 24,000 people will register.

And will they all be there for serious business, as opposed to people who go to the APA meetings where most people are there on a junket ...

They're not going to be out on the beach in Washington in November. They are there to listen to science and it's on a big scale and very efficiently run. Maybe a little bit overpowering; it takes you a few days to recover from an event like that. I find the depressing thing about going to a big meeting like that is that you realise just how insignificant you are. I gave a lecture there a few years ago on MK-801 and you go into auditorium built like an aircraft hanger and you can't even see the back row of seats from the stage. It was an intimidating experience. The experience of attending these mega meetings is like going out into a field on a dark winter night and looking up at the stars in the sky. If you do that for a few minutes you realise how utterly insignificant you are. If you fell under a bus tomorrow it wouldn't make the slightest bit of difference.

What about Frank Schmitt?

Frank was very much the guru figure of the NRP. He was a very forceful person. I grew to like him more over the years than I did initially. Initially to an English person who has been brought up to be fairly reticent, Frank was overwhelming. He was always telling you how wonderful things were and how important the contributions of NRP were. This was it – the NRP, in that little room, was probably the centre of the entire brain research universe. And he had this almost grandiose vision of how this organisation ought to operate. On first exposure I found that a very un-European way of doing things. The NRP used to have meetings where they would have verbatim transcripts on a meeting that went on for 2 days. Every word was harvested in case some gems of wisdom were uttered. But I got to like and respect Frank a lot more over the years. He had this knack of identifying an interesting subject and then bringing in people who had never thought about it before. He brought in nuclear physicists or electrical engineers or people who write electronic circuit diagrams and made them think about the brain.

In the foreword to Volume 1 of these interviews I mentioned that someone had put it to me that if I really wanted to find out about the history of the field, I should interview the wives of these eminent pharmacologists – but in your case your wife is an equally eminent psychopharmacologist.

Yes, Susan was with me during the 2 years of postdoc in the States in the 1960s. In Harvard, when we were there, she worked in Peter Dew's lab in the Department of Pharmacology, the same building in which I was in Neurobiology. At that time she got involved in psychopharmacology and in behavioural studies and she got so enthusiastic about that field that she stayed with it and has done ever since in her research career. When I moved to the Merck lab she moved shortly afterwards to become Head of the Behavioural group there and set up a behavioural psychopharmacology lab. She has made her own important contributions in the study of peptides in brain and particularly in the study of brain dopamine using 6-hydroxydopamine as a tool, which we developed as a way of lesioning the specific catecholamine pathways in brain. This allowed her to show conclusively that amphetamine owes most of its psychostimulant properties in animals to its ability to interact with the dopamine pathways. We have worked very closely on many projects.

It must have been an extraordinary marriage because she hasn't just been the quiet wife tagging along after her husband because she's been a President of the BAP and is now Professor of Psychology here in Oxford.

Yes, she is particularly enjoying her present job as Chairman of the Department of Experimental Psychology in Oxford. The person who had that job before, Larry Weiskrantz, was her PhD mentor in Cambridge in the 1960s. She's been closely attached to the department in Oxford for many years and is now enjoying her new role. She is, I think, the sixth woman professor in

Oxford against some 280 men professors, so there is still a bit of gender bias in the selection process.

Select bibliography

Iversen LL (1967). *The Uptake and Storage of Noradrenaline in Sympathetic Nerves.* Cambridge University Press, Cambridge.

Iversen SD, Iversen LL (1975, 1981). *Behavioural Pharmacology.* Oxford University Press, Oxford.

Iversen LL, Iversen SD, Snyder SH (1975–1988). *Handbook of Psychopharmacology* vols 1–20. Plenum Press, New York.

Iversen LL, Kravitz EA, Otsuka M (1968). Release of gamma-aminobutyric acid (GABA) from lobster inhibitory neurones. *Journal of Physiology*, **188**, 21–22P.

16 *Jeff Watkins*

Excitatory amino acids: from basic science to therapeutic applications

How did you get into the field?

Well, I was a chemist, a 'pure' chemist, interested in chemistry for its own sake. I didn't have the opportunity to go to medical school in Australia, in Perth. It didn't have a medical school but in any case I doubt if I would have been attracted to medicine. I did science because all my friends did science and I also liked mixing things up in the lab. So I ended up as a chemist and then the thing to do was a PhD. Luckily I got a scholarship to Cambridge, and then what many people did in those days was to go to America. In the mid-1950s, you could usually get a postdoc position just by writing to whoever you wanted to work with. I went to Yale for a couple of years. All this was automatic, before I really started to think what I ultimately wanted to do or be.

I wasn't exactly 'mixed up' but I wasn't quite certain what I wanted to do with my life. I was reading everything – philosophy, religion, that sort of thing – and it just came to me, rather 'Eureka-fashion', in the middle of the night, that you couldn't know anything fundamental about oneself until you knew something about the brain. Young people think in these terms – what constitutes 'I'? 'I' do this, 'I' do that – but what is 'I'? Basically what came to me was that the sense of self can only be in the brain, somewhere. Not very original, you might say, but new to me, to be thinking in those terms. So that was quite a conclusion to come to – that I was actually interested in the brain itself – how it worked, not in just using it for some purpose or other like doing chemistry, for its own sake, for example. Of course, LSD was around at the time and this was a drug that altered 'perception', that is how people, I mean, how their *brain* interpreted the sensations they received – how it produced in itself the experience of what they saw, heard, felt, etc., and that made me think that there must be chemical elements at work there. What was known about the chemistry of the brain at that time? Virtually nothing! Nothing anyway that overtly related to the special functions that the brain performed and the mechanisms underlying such activity.

Glutamate curiously had been mentioned – long before noradrenaline or 5HT. There was a report from Derek Richter about glutamate and schizophrenia in the 1950s which seems early and prescient.

I worked in his unit later on. I think the evidence underlying this speculation was pretty flimsy and quite probably irrelevant – but I would need to look at those reports again. Even before that, in the late 1940s, Heinrich Waelsch and others in the States were looking at glutamate as a possible cognitive enhancer. They thought it increased intelligence in mentally handicapped children. So glutamate was already in the field but I believe that was just coincidental and whether or not it has any relevance to what is known about glutamate today is debatable, but shouldn't be dismissed.

Were they in any way thinking about it as a neutransmitter at the time?

No. Except for Hayashi. At that stage the idea of chemical transmission wasn't even universally accepted for the brain. It was generally accepted for the peripheral nervous system and some people said that if neuromuscular transmission worked like that then probably synaptic transmission also worked like that in the brain, and bit by bit, between the 1920s and early 1950s, everybody came over to the chemical theory for brain synaptic transmission except the chap I went to work for eventually – JC Eccles.

It wasn't glutamate that interested me at that time, it was chemistry of the brain in general. Now, luckily enough, in Yale I was living in a medical school hall of residence, and even though I went to the chemistry department on the other side of town every day, I was actually living with medics. When I got the idea I would like to do something on the chemistry of the brain, one of my medical friends said, 'Well, you ought to write to this chap Eccles in Australia and tell him', which I did. I wrote to him and said, 'Look, I know it's a bit ridiculous, I know nothing about the brain, or any physiology or even biochemistry, nothing biological at all, let alone neurophysiology', but, I said, 'Surely the brain is made up of chemicals.'

Not the man to say this to.

Well, he was by that stage, 1956, although he was almost the last man to have come across from stout adherence to the electrical transmission theory, except for a chap called Lloyd. He did that in the early 1950s, as I recall.

But then he managed to make it look like he had discovered the whole idea of chemical transmission.

Well, there's nothing like a convert for enthusiasm. He had to prove it to himself scientifically and he did this by being the first person to record intracellularly in neurones in the brain. The spinal cord, actually, because it was easier there but he correctly surmised that what happened in the spinal cord would happen in the brain as well. When he found that stimulating the nerves from antagonistic muscles produced a different postsynaptic potential change, one depolarising, the other hyperpolarising, in the same spinal motoneurone, he said, well, obviously, it can't all be done by the same *electrical* influence of one cell on another, so, overnight, he said it must be done *chemically,* a complete volte-face. The different pathways stimulated must result in the release of different transmitters, one excitatory and one inhibitory, producing opposite potential changes in the neuronal membrane of the same motoneurone. He had just done all this three or four years before my letter arrived saying 'Surely you must have a place for a chemist.' His reply bounced back saying that it couldn't be more appropriate to have a chemist in the department at this stage and that I must come and work with a young chap there who was just completing his PhD called David Curtis. Even though he, David Curtis, had no real chemistry background, he had recently been trying – or thinking about trying – to extract chemicals from the brain. He suggested we should work together, which we subsequently did. I began there in January 1958.

The idea was that I should take over from David and try to extract transmitters from the brain. I said, 'Well, there must be a thousand compounds at least in the brain and they're all mixed up in there. To get any one out individually will be difficult and how are you, David, going to test each of them to see if they might be transmitters?' He said, 'I'll put each one in these little micro-electrodes and pass them out electrophoretically on to single neurones in the spinal cord and monitor the electrical activity of that particular neurone.' I said, 'But if I'm taking a chemical from the brain, and you're testing it on just a single cell in the spinal cord, how will you know you're testing it on the same sort of cell that it might act on as a transmitter in the brain? Can you provide me with a broader screening system?' He said, 'Well, there's the isolated toad spinal cord that some Japanese have used, and also Eccles a few years ago. He said we could take the spinal cord out of the Queensland toad – an enormous thing – bathe the cord in artificial CSF and then just wash in all my compounds or crude extracts and if we see any gross activity, as reflected in recordings from ventral roots, we can then test them further, and in more detail with the micro-electrophoretic method in mammalian spinal cord. The toad spinal cord will allow us to monitor the activity of a large number of neurones simultaneously, and it is likely that neurones in the spinal cord, and their transmitters, will be similar to those in the brain. Although the toad spinal cord will obviously have differences from the mammalian spinal cord, there is a good chance that there will be many similarities as well.'

This was fairly early to be doing micro-electrophoresis.

He was not the pioneer of the technique itself but he was the first to use it in the CNS. Rose Eccles, his daughter, and David Curtis, did it first I think, on Renshaw cells in the spinal cord because they surmised that the synapse formed between motoneurone axon collaterals and Renshaw cells was likely to be a cholinergic system. Fatt and Katz had used the technique in the neuromuscular junction, a couple of years before. I'm not sure but I think Nastuk or Del Castillo and Katz actually pioneered the method.

This early work was in Australia?

Yes. Eccles had been at Oxford with Sherrington but he moved back to the Antipodes and after a couple of prior posts in Sydney and Dunedin, I think, ultimately took the Chair in the Physiology Department of the new John Curtin School of Medical Research at the Australian National University, which had been created and generously endowed by the government to be a place of excellence. Conditions were extremely good and Eccles attracted people from everywhere. It really was the most intellectually exciting period of my life because there were all these good young people coming to work with Eccles. I was working down the end of the same corridor and I knew enough at this stage to know that this work of his really was at the very forefront of brain research.

What was he like, Eccles?

He had one overriding interest and that was his research. He didn't really want to talk much about anything else actually – at least, that was my impression at the time. In retrospect, I'm sure he would have talked enthusiastically about 'consciousness' and the nature of 'mind'. I didn't get to talk to him very much because I wasn't one of his group. I virtually only saw him at seminars and in the tea room or corridor and whatnot. He obviously had a very sharp mind and dominated all the seminars – most of which he gave personally. It was nice to meet him again in 1993, after 28 years, on the occasion of his 90th birthday celebration.[1] He was still working more or less until about 4 or 5 years ago, mainly on philosophical topics and has written a number of books – none of which I've read yet, I'm afraid. I did read a very early book, *The Neurophysiological Basis of Mind*, based on a series of lectures he gave at Oxford in the mid-1950s. The last chapter, as I recall, was on the nature of mind and I remember a neurophysiologist I was friendly with saying that the book was very good except for the last chapter. But I must say I enjoyed this chapter most of all, though I'm not sure I accepted all his assertions.

Everyone in his group was well organised. His students could be there at 3 in the morning but they were nevertheless expected to be there again at 9 a.m. or before, on the next day, to process the results of the night before. The students I think also prepared the animal for each experiment and on those days Eccles himself would come into the lab about 11 a.m. to take charge of the experiment. The students took notes, I believe, while Eccles manipulated the microelectrodes.

He was keen on 'wholesome' activities such as square dancing, 'social' tennis – he had a tennis court – and walking. I was invited only once for Sunday afternoon tennis. Partnering Lady Eccles in doubles I let rip one of my erratic cannon-ball services which whistled dangerously past her ear. She displayed considerable nervousness thereafter. Also, my performance seemed not to fit

---

[1] He died on 2 May 1997.

the description of 'social'. To make matters worse, at that time I smoked. That was definitely unwholesome. My further participation was not requested.

I can tell you a story about 'the Nobel Prize that wasn't'. We all used to work at nights. One night a reporter on the *Canberra Times* rang up to say that it had just come over on the 7 p.m. BBC news, from London, that Eccles had won the Nobel Prize. She then came to see him in the lab. Aged about 18 she said, 'Could you tell me, Sir John, what exactly *is* the Nobel Prize?' Somewhat incredulously he replied, 'Young lady, if you don't know that you had better go back and send someone who does!' I went off to purchase suitable celebratory beverages, returning well stocked. Eccles – virtually a teetotaller – allowed himself half a glass of sherry, then went off home to celebrate with family and friends there. At 9 p.m. the BBC repeated the report, and the party at the lab gathered steam. By 11 p.m. most experiments had been abandoned. But in the 11 p.m. news the BBC corrected the error. Another Australian, not Eccles, but Macfarlane Burnet of Melbourne, had won the Nobel Prize, shared with Medawar. Eccles immediately came back to the lab to resurrect what he could of the experiments, staying presumably till 3 or 4 a.m. as was customary. The next day, by chance, the real winner of the Nobel Prize turned up in Canberra while Eccles, David Curtis and I were having lunch together. Eccles leapt out of his chair, rushed over to the chap, congratulated him warmly, indeed most effusively, and showed none of the great disappointment and embarrassment he must have been suffering. Luckily he did win the Nobel Prize two years later, which he shared with Hodgkin and Huxley.

There are lots of other little anecdotes. One of the biochemists at the tea break one day said, 'I am finding it difficult to keep up with the literature these days. How do you cope, Sir John?' Eccles replied that 'People tend to send me reprints if they want me to know of their work. If they don't send me reprints they don't deserve to be read!' These were unsolicited reprints of course. An Eccles tea break usually consisted of two cups of tea, swamped with cold milk, the quicker to be able to consume them. Both cups were gulped down while still standing at the counter, giving a total tea break of approx. 15 secs plus travel time to and from his lab, one floor up. If you wanted to talk to him you had to chase after him as he left the tea room and complete your discussion, often from two paces behind, before he got back to the lab.

What gave you the feeling it was a breakthrough area, because the oddity is that all the fuss had been about the catecholamines and 5HT. The glutamate story has been a slow burner, as it were.

Well, the slow take-off of the glutamate story was because we were somewhat negative in the first paper we wrote about the possibility of it being a transmitter. This was understandable in the light of what we knew at the time. We had got onto glutamate because I had said that I wasn't keen to go to the great trouble of extracting brain to get all of these compounds out individually when I could get some of them, already in pure form, straight from the laboratory shelf. There was a big bottle of glutamate up there and I knew that glu-

356 The Psychopharmacologists II

tamate was one of the main chemicals in the brain, so I said let's try this first and we did. In a sense, our discovery of its excitatory activity came *too easily* for us to regard glutamate as the transmitter we were mentally prepared to spend years searching for. And its action was shared by several structurally related compounds, some endogenous, others not. We tested many other known brain constituents as well but it was the excitatory amino acids, and also the inhibitory ones, related to GABA, that had the most obvious effects, so we concentrated on those.

Following a paper on GABA by Curtis and John Phillis, his PhD student, published in *Nature* in 1958, we published a letter in *Nature* on glutamate in 1959, and a full paper in the *Journal of Physiology* in 1960, but we unfortunately slanted it that, although these were extremely interesting effects, glutamate wasn't likely to be a transmitter for a long list of reasons: for example, because it had important other roles as a protein constituent and as a metabolite involved in energy metabolism and there's so much of it there, whereas you don't need much if it's a transmitter. Its overall concentration in the brain is about 10 millimolar, which is a huge concentration compared, for instance, to acetylcholine which is there in only nanomolar concentrations. Also there was one crucial experiment from which the wrong conclusion was drawn, an experiment to see if the reversal potential for glutamate was the same as the reversal potential for the natural transmitter when you stimulated the pathway to the particular neurone under observation which was responding to glutamate. The 'wrong' answer was obtained mainly because the techniques weren't developed enough at the time. Our feeling then was that, whatever the mechanism of this interesting action of glutamate, it seemed to be different from that of the excitatory transmitter to this particular neurone because the reversal potentials for glutamate and the natural transmitter appeared to be different. Therefore glutamate probably wasn't a transmitter. It was to be another 10–15 years before techniques were improved sufficiently for others to show that in fact the reversal potentials are indeed similar.

What was David Curtis' background?

I think he was originally a neurosurgeon who decided he would rather do neurophysiological research than practise medicine. If I remember correctly, he got a scholarship in Eccles' department, did a PhD with Eccles and then more or less went off on his own projects. I arrived at that point and my background nicely complemented his chemical interests. I stayed for 7 years and we got a nice series of papers out. Also there in Canberra at this time was Kris Krnjevic, who was a postdoc I think at that stage, and he and David's student John Phillis later got together in England, at Babraham, and took the view that the Canberra attitude to glutamate was possibly overly negative. Eccles himself felt that glutamate looked promising despite the 'contraindications'. Krnjevic and Phillis repeated in the cerebral cortex everything we had done in the spinal cord and got more or less the same answers – not exactly the same, which is interesting now, in retrospect, with the range of different receptor types that have recently been recognised. As I recall, they also failed to show a reversal potential for glutamate similar to that of natural excitatory postsynaptic potentials.

I did a little cartoon a few years ago in the form of a schematic electrophysiological response to illustrate the history of the glutamate story. There was an initial burst of interest – 'excitation' – followed immediately by 'inhibition', which kept the field depressed. Not many people were interested for 20 years or so after our initial discovery of the excitatory action, mainly I suppose because of our initial pessimism. Then there was a series of 'spikes' in the 1980s following the discovery of antagonists and the excitation has continued since then with the recent breakthroughs in molecular biology. The early period of 'inhibition' was due to all sorts of factors. The main one was this thing about the wrong reversal potential but the other major prejudice was that there's 'too much' glutamate in the brain and it obviously had other roles and why would a transmitter need to have other roles? And people became more interested, as you say, in 5HT, noradrenaline and dopamine – all the Americans went off in that direction and there was just a few of us left interested in glutamate.

Who was left interested – you and ...

David Curtis kept it up after I left in 1965 with a younger colleague, Graham Johnston, a chemist like myself. Later – about 1968 – there was Hugh McLennan in Vancouver. In the mid 1960s there was also a spattering of interest elsewhere: Krnjevic, of course, in Babraham and then Montreal, and Takeuchi and Takeuchi in Japan, working on crayfish muscle, following the pioneering work in this tissue by Robbins in the USA, and later Usherwood in England with his proposal that glutamate was the transmitter at the insect neuromuscular junction. McIlwain pioneered some combined electrophysiological–biochemical studies on brain slices. But there were only a few of us consistently involved from the electrophysiological angle over a period of 20 years or thereabouts – 1960–80 – certainly as far as the mammalian CNS was concerned. Krnjevic remained active for a while in the 1970s but his interests were broader and the definitive pharmacological tools had not yet been developed. Donald Straughan, a colleague of Krnjevic in Babraham, also maintained an interest for a while, though I think he was more interested in amines. John Davies of course began collaborating with me in 1970, as did Tim Biscoe and Dick Evans in 1973. David Lodge joined David Curtis in 1974 having done his PhD with Tim Biscoe, an ex-Krnjevic associate at Babraham, who had later also spent a year at Canberra with David Curtis. Lodge has been a stalwart in the field ever since. Other people publishing in this area between 1970 and 1980 included Shinozaki, who introduced kainic acid and continues to make a major contribution to the present day, Barker and Nicoll, Zieglgansberger, Engberg, Stone, Macdonald, Nistri and Constanti, and later on Krogsgaard-Larsen with Curtis, but there weren't many, to be sure. Throughout the 1970s, however, an increasing band of neurochemists became interested – Aprison, Bradford, Cotman, Balazs, Roberts, Fonnum, Cuenod, the McGeers, Wenthold and others.

But how does this fit with the point you made earlier that you had felt that this was break-through stuff?

Eccles, of course, with his straight neurophysiology, elucidating the electrical responses of neurones rather than the chemistry of these responses, was involved in major advances in understanding of the excitatory and inhibitory synaptic activity and connections in spinal cord and brain. I'm not sure I really thought our work was necessarily 'breakthrough stuff', because we were lacking the definitive evidence of its real importance. The reason it went so quiet was because there were no antagonists. You couldn't tell one way or the other if the glutamate action was important. You just made up your mind on the basis of other factors. But I, personally, not being trained in neurophysiology, was restricted to a chemical approach so I kept on doing chemistry related to glutamate. Luckily the MRC here supported me from 1973 on to make new compounds until we eventually did get some antagonists. Only then was I able to convince myself that there might be something in the glutamate transmitter theory. I wasn't trying to prove people wrong or anything, I just didn't know myself whether glutamate was or was not a transmitter and I did not want to give up until I knew, one way or the other.

How did the NMDA angle come into the picture?

Curtis and Johnston had something to do with that, following a lead from one of David Curtis' students called Arthur Duggan and before them Hugh McLennan. They looked at the relative potencies in the brain of a few amino acids and saw they were different depending on which cell and in which region of the CNS they were tested, and they thought, therefore, that there might be more than one glutamate receptor. That was in the late 1960s–early 1970s.

Had you made NMDA before that?

Yes, I made it 10 years before that. I made NMDA in order to see if there was any difference in stereoisomers. In the spinal cord there wasn't much difference in potency between D- and L-glutamate or between D- and L-aspartate and for a receptor you'd expect there to be marked enantiomeric differences. So I thought maybe if you introduced larger groups at the asymmetric carbon atom, steric differences might show up better, and they did. That was in the early 1960s.

What did you think you had produced though when you made NMDA – just another chemical?

Yes, to begin with, but it proved to be by far the most potent agonist we had tested at that stage and very interesting just from that point of view. We didn't know why it was so potent but originally assumed that it had a higher affinity for the receptor than glutamate. Now we know the NMDA potency is actually due to its lack of rapid uptake. This knowledge is due mainly to Graham Johnston and his student Vladimir Balcar. Glutamate is taken up by the cells when you try to test it, and therefore you don't see the full effect at the receptors, whereas the NMDA isn't taken up, so you do get the full effect. But we didn't know that in 1960, we just knew that in some tests NMDA was up to a thousand times more potent than glutamate. We now, of course, know that glutamate is actually about ten-fold more potent than NMDA at the receptor level. Harry Olverman in my group showed that in the mid 1980s. Of course, we were only thinking of a single glutamate receptor at the time I first made NMDA.

Was there any feeling at the time that there might have been any commercial applications for NMDA?

No, not really. It was of peripheral interest to investigators of a murder in Sydney. A couple of well-known scientists suddenly and mysteriously died after a party and one of their friends clutching at straws rang me up asking whether NMDA could have caused their deaths. I said it wasn't likely to have been that, whatever it was, because NMDA wouldn't be likely to cross the blood–brain barrier sufficiently – according to our tests on mice. The murders are still unsolved, I think. No, there wasn't any immediate commercial interest and we weren't interested to search for any possible commercial application.

How did McLennan get involved? Did he have any links with the original group?

No. It was quite independent work, as far as I know. He was one of the original GABA investigators, working with Florey on factor I. I think it was after he saw our results that he swapped over to glutamate. I believe he was working on the crayfish stretch receptor with regard to GABA actions. Robbins in the States had independently published similar results to ours on the actions of excitatory amino acids on crustacean neuromuscular junctions, so I think McLennan came via those two areas, deciding to look at these substances also in the mammalian CNS. This was the mid 1960s but once he was in the field he stayed in until he retired about 7 or 8 years ago. It was he who first got the idea at the end of the 1960s that there was more than one glutamate receptor.

Three things came together in the multiple receptor story. First there was McLennan suggesting it. Then Arthur Duggan, a PhD student of Curtis', on his own initiative, looked at glutamate and aspartate potencies on Renshaw and other interneurones in the spinal cord and found they were different, suggesting to him the possible existence of two different types of receptor – maybe a 'glutamate' and maybe an 'aspartate' receptor. Finally Curtis and Johnston said, 'Well, if that's the case, some bulkier molecules might show this better and they chose NMDA and kainate to test on the same types of interneurones as Duggan had used and did indeed get bigger differences, so they supported the idea of two different receptors, one more sensitive to NMDA, and one more sensitive to kainate.

At this stage, I was making substances that were beginning to look like they might be antagonists. In view of the multiple receptor possibility, I decided to test them on a range of agonists. I soon found that my first antagonists were all NMDA selective and didn't touch some amino acid agonists at all. That led me to propose the NMDA receptor as one easily identifiable receptor type in the late 1970s.

Did you run into the problems that the monamine receptor people ran into, which was a certain scepticism about whether these had functional relevance, whether they were any more than binding sites?

No, because we had started on the functional side. There was scepticism in relation to whether they had a functional synaptic role, but they clearly could influence synaptic activity. Harry Olverman introduced binding here, in Bristol, later, and gratifyingly got parallel results to those I had obtained in our electrophysiological systems. I would usually be more swayed by the electrophysiological–functional tests rather than the binding data if only one set of results were available – except where uptake or enzyme degradation may be expected to obscure the electrophysiological effect. It is like the present-day situation with cloned receptors. We can differentiate several different subtypes of EAA receptors in our functional assays and sometimes get activity with compounds that don't seem to have any action on some of the cloned receptors.

When we pass our compounds on to our electrophysiological colleagues, Graham Collingridge here, and Tom Salt previously here and now at the Institute of Ophthalmology in London, to see what our compounds do in the hippocampus or the thalamus, respectively they find that the same compounds also usually work in those areas similarly to their actions in the spinal cord. So we believe in our functional receptors. I don't necessarily believe the importance of everything you find from a neurochemical or binding assay or even from studies on cloned receptors but one needs evidence from as many sources as possible of course.

Is there a sense in which the whole NMDA field compared to the monoamine field has always remained more functional? With the monoamines in the mid-1970s when people were beginning to radiolabel these receptors for the first time, the field had a choice between electrophysiological work showing that the antidepressants improved signal-to-noise ratios and changes in receptor number. The scientific market-place, as it were, took a view that receptors rather than electrophysiology were the way forward.

I haven't kept up with the monoamine field very well but there was a lot of work in the mid-1960s finding out where these monoamines were active in the brain and then later with labelling the neurones containing the amines, and finding out where there were concentrations of monoamine receptors via binding studies. I think there is probably a fair amount of functional correlation for dopamine, 5HT, noradrenaline, etc., as regards location of receptors and behavioural effects so I'm not quite sure I agree with you that the two have been divorced, except with regard to demonstrable effects at single synapses or on discrete populations of neurones. I think in the drug development field they just want to screen as many compounds as possible, as quickly as possible, with the screens that have previously thrown up successful drugs, albeit somewhat empirically. As to the benefit of looking in the brain to see exactly what's going on, synaptic effects of amines for example and the possible function of such effects, the drug companies seem to have been less interested but between receptor binding studies and the behavioural effects there seems to be quite a good correlation. I think all the required conceptual connections will be made in due course – you get shifts in emphasis don't you? It would in any case be well nigh impossible to screen all new compounds produced by pharmaceutical companies for electrophysiological effects of functional relevance in brain.

You proposed the NMDA receptor idea in 1977. Had the field begun to pick-up speed at that stage or was it still a small field?

It had picked up a bit but was still a relatively small field. Once we'd produced specific antagonists things changed. The first antagonists were just longer molecular-chain glutamate analogues such as D-α-aminoadipate, the 'unnatural' form of the next higher acidic amino acid homologue to glutamate, which was something McLennan indirectly first got onto as a possible antagonist but without reference to possible selectivity. At this stage we already had similar compounds and by then already knew of their selective actions. When I saw McLennan's results, I felt I knew in advance what D-α-aminoadipate would do in our system and could confidently predict that it would be selective. We had already made a range of similar compounds and McLennan didn't have the D-form of α-aminoadipate, having made his logical prediction of the glutamate/aspartate antagonist activity of the D-form on the basis of the activity of the DL- and L-forms. I made the D-form of α-aminoadipate and found that it was NMDA selective like our earlier compounds and that convinced me of the existence of a specific NMDA receptor. Then I made many more related compounds and there were other types of NMDA antagonist as well, such as magnesium and HA-966, which we had actually characterised as selective NMDA antagonists prior to the D-α-aminoadipate group. They all had a similar spectrum of antagonist action against the same range of agonists.

Did they all come on stream at the same time, and how did magnesium appear?

Yes, they did. Magnesium had been used at the neuromuscular junction to block transmission on the basis that it inhibited calcium influx into presynaptic terminals. We tried it for this purpose in the frog spinal cord and then found unexpectedly that the presence of magnesium had a differential antagonist effect against a range of exogenous excitatory amino acid agonists. It so happens that the medium that you use for frog spinal cord preparations in vitro doesn't have magnesium in it, and that was lucky because it meant our preparations were very sensitive to NMDA agonists and antagonists. When we added magnesium to the medium, in quite low concentrations, much lower than needed for presynaptic depression of transmitter release, we got both a strong depression of synaptic activity as well as this selective depression of excitatory amino acid agonist actions. The depression produced by magnesium turned out to be similar to that which we saw a little later with organic compounds. So it looked as though magnesium was involved in the activity of this new receptor type that we were identifying as the NMDA receptor, and importantly, that this receptor had functional significance, since transmission and NMDA receptor activity were reduced in parallel by low concentrations of magnesium.

About the same time we also had our similar results with this other compound known as HA-966 – later it was found by Lodge to be an antagonist at the glycine site of the NMDA receptor, after this had been described by Ascher in the late 1980s, but we didn't know that in the late 1970s. This was the first glutamate/aspartate antagonist we had got onto in the early 1970s when I first began working with my colleague John Davies. We didn't know how or why but when we got the new antagonists later in the 1970s we found that HA-966 had a similar spectrum or activity – they were all acting at the same receptor.

How did you get onto HA-966 and how did John Davies come into the picture?

John and I first got together in early 1970. I'll tell you later how this came about and also the beginnings of the HA-966 story. The background is that I had left Canberra to try my luck in England in 1965, to broaden my horizons, so to speak. I didn't do any further electrophysiological work on glutamate for a few years. I went to Babraham and worked for a while on liposomes. The head of the institute when I went there was one of the foremost cholinergic pharmacologists, John Gaddum.

I actually went to Babaham first on sabbatical leave from Canberra in1963/64 as a trial for a possible future longer-term move. I went there to work on model membranes. I thought, why do all this work on animals when you might be able to do it on model membranes? They were doing lipid membrane work there and I thought I'd like to try it out. I became involved with Alec Bangham in the development of liposomes.

How did liposomes come into the picture?

Well, I was interested in the interaction of amino acids with neuronal membranes, and biological cell membranes were considered to be protein-coated bimolecular lipid layers, so that's how I got involved. I had written rather a speculative paper that had proved popular on the possible involvement of bimolecular lipid/protein membranes in glutamate/GABA action. Liposomes were just coming into the picture. I was originally more interested in the Mueller–Rudin bimolecular 'black film' that you get when you take a plastic beaker, poke a hole in the side of it, immerse it in an aqueous fluid and paint a solution of phospholipids over it, whereupon, if you're lucky, it forms a bimolecular film over the hole with the lipid parts of the molecules meeting in the middle of the film and the polar parts extending in the fluid on each side of the hole. So you can have an 'internal' medium and an 'external' medium and can find what happens to electrical potentials created between the two with different solutions on either side. That's what I was interested in doing but Alec Bangham was more interested in the structure and permeability of liposomes per se. The liposomes were also easier to work with and so I spent three years doing that eventually. I did try GABA and glutamate on liposomes – with some vaguely encouraging results – but not very seriously.

Was there any feeling at the time that some of the compounds you were using were membrane stabilising in some sense?

Membrane active but not membrane stabilising, more membrane destabilising really. The receptor idea took root because of the differences in the actions of a range of molecules of different shapes. If they were all just dissolving in the membrane, you wouldn't expect such big differences. But we had found that even a single methyl group on glutamate, for example, could practically abolish activity altogether. The question was, were these receptors just chance orientations of groups on extracellular proteins or whatnot, coating the lipid core? Just chance, without functional meaning. Pure coincidence. I mean, if you threw glutamate onto the floor you might find some wood, sand or clay particles that would absorb it 'specifically' just because the shape of parts of the molecular surface of some of the component substances just happened to be complementary to the acidic and basic parts of the amino acid molecules.

That's not a receptor idea?

It would be a 'receptor' in the sense of an arrangement of atoms on the surface of a macromolecule that is complementary to a pattern of atomic sites on the foreign molecule. It doesn't mean to say its a functional receptor in any sense. It is certainly a molecular entity, but only fortuitously resembling a so-called physiological or pharmacological receptor. We would now say our compounds are acting on a functional glutamate receptor. By this we would mean part of a macromolecule that plays a specific physiological role, in this case being specifically located within synapses, and playing a discrete role in transmission. The active sites of the protein interact with complementary sites on the glutamate molecule so as to induce a change in the conformation of the protein and allow ions in or out of the cell that wouldn't normally be able to get in or out so easily and so change the electrochemical potential across the cell membrane. If the protein was serving some other purpose, for instance, as a structural component of the membrane matrix, the glutamate action could be regarded as an interesting pharmacological phenomenon but not necessarily related to synaptic physiology. When we eventually obtained the antagonists and were able to antagonise both the synaptic event and the glutamate event and show that the pharmacology was the same, that's when people began to believe that the glutamate receptor was indeed involved in synaptic transmission.

John Davies unfortunately died about 5 years ago, a great loss to the field. As mentioned earlier, in the late 1960s I was working on model membranes. This was more a fundamental biophysical than a truly physiological project and I felt I would like to get back to working on neurotransmission. First I left Babraham to work in Richter's MRC Neuropsychiatry Unit at Carshalton, where I began working again on amino acids, but mainly on the metabolic side. I subsequently arranged to go back to Canberra for three months and I took a few compounds with me and worked with David Curtis for three weeks at the beginning of 1970. David felt I was somewhat 'wasted' working on model membranes and metabolism and that I should work preferably with someone like Donald Straughan, Professor of Pharmacology, at the School of Pharmacy, London, who had worked with Krnjevic at Babraham and who was doing micro-electrophoresis. I got in touch with Donald Straughan, who said he had a young lecturer in the department, John Davies, and suggested they both come over to Carshalton to talk about the possibility of collaborating. They came over, John got interested, and it began from there.

At this stage, when I was working in Richter's unit at Carshalton, I was looking at amino acid and energy metabolism as influenced by the actions of extracellular glutamate and other excitatory amino acids. Richter wasn't particularly happy with what I was doing and neither was I. So we agreed I could spend 1 day a week at the School of Pharmacy working with John. I went in with a lot of speculative compounds to test, the third one of which was HA-966. We got onto that fairly quickly since I had seen a brief report on its central action and thought it had an 'amino acid-like' structure related to glycine, which turned out to be an important factor. It proved to be a glutamate/aspartate antagonist, and we got a note into *Nature*, which was very nice. Iversen wrote a little note in the 'News and Views' section hailing the discovery and emphasising its possible importance. John Davies' appetite for that sort of work was truly whetted, such that we then worked together for another 20 years, even though we were geographically separated for most of that time.

When that association first developed, David Curtis wrote to me and suggested that John Davies should come out and work with him for a while to learn more about the electrophoretic technique. John went out for two years from 1972 to 1974. David Lodge also went out there about the same time. That was a continuation of a Bristol/Canberra link which began with Tim Biscoe, who had been at Babraham working in association with both Krnjevic and Straughan. Biscoe wrote to David Curtis, after he had become interested in this sort of work through Krnjevic and Straughan, and subsequently worked with him in Canberra for a while. Then when Biscoe came to Bristol, the Professor of Physiology here at the time was Arthur Buller, who had also worked with Eccles in Canberra – so there's a long connection between Canberra and Bristol. Buller had worked on nerve–muscle interactions. There were slow muscles and fast muscles and what Eccles and Buller did, as I recall, was to cross the nerves to these muscles over, whereafter fast muscles became slower and slow muscles became faster, correlating with corresponding changes in the activity of motoneurones. That was all going on in Canberra when I was there. Then Arthur Buller came back to England and eventually got the Chair here in Bristol and when Tim Biscoe came back from Australia he also came to work here, eventually succeeding Buller as Professor. Biscoe had two students – Max Headley, who worked in Canberra later with Duggan and who is back here again now, as a Professor in the Physiology Department, and David Lodge, who became Professor of Veterinary Physiology in London and is now a Research Director with Lilly.

So John Davies was out there at the same time and on his return we resumed our collaboration. He became a long-term colleague. John did the really crucial experiment that finally convinced me, after 20 years, that gluta-mate receptors were indeed involved in neurotransmission in the CNS. He showed that D-α-aminoadipate, the specific NMDA receptor antagonist, selec-tively blocked transmission through non-cholinergic pathways to Renshaw cells, for which no previous antagonist was known, while nicotinic-type acetylcholine antagonists selectively blocked cholinergic activation of the same cell through the motoneurone axon collateral pathway. This was the real turn-ing point in the field.

At this stage I must also mention Dick Evans. When I came to Bristol it was with the idea of collaborating with Tim Biscoe in the Department of Physiology by supplying substances to him for testing micro-electrophoreti-cally in spinal cord in vivo, as in Canberra and London. We did this – David Lodge, Max Headley, Mike Martin and I – for several months but, as in Canberra and London, progress was very slow. Dick Evans, a relatively young lecturer in the Department of Pharmacology at the time, expressed a keenness to collaborate and, thinking of less labour-intensive techniques, suggested we try the isolated spinal cord of the local frog *(R. temporaria or R. pipiens)* as a screening method, as the Queensland toad spinal cord had proved so useful in Australia. This was in 1974. The system worked very well and we made a lot of our original discoveries on magnesium, HA-966 and diaminopimelate, leading on to D-α-aminoadipate, using it. Later, Dick adapted the isolated spinal cord of the neonatal rat as described first by Konishi and Otsuka in 1974 and this had several advantages over the frog spinal cord. It was mammalian; it gave a more elaborate dorsal root-evoked ventral root potential which could be differentiated into several components. It also responded to more endogenous transmitter candidates – acetylcholine, amines, peptides. We are still working with this technique today, and much credit must go to Dick for providing us both with his electrophysiological expertise and a magnificently useful screen-ing preparation. We definitely could not have made the advances we have done without his crucial input.

You were still a small group at this time? What kind of impact did you have at scientific meetings at the time – were there any symposia on glutamate?

Our 'group' at that time comprised just Dick Evans, a chemical technician, Dan Oakes, and myself. In 1975 this was expanded with MRC help to include a pharmacological technician, Alison Francis, and later a postdoctoral chemist Keith Hunt, who was succeeded in 1978 by Arwel Jones. Arwel was with us for 6 years and was involved in our big leap forward with competitive antagonists.

No, there were no glutamate symposia then. The first glutamate sympo-sium as distinct from general amino acid symposia was in 1979. Neuroactive amino acid symposia actually began in the late 1950s. They were then mainly about GABA with glutamate sometimes thrown in. The glutamate component in later symposia grew gradually throughout the 1970s and the first specifical-ly glutamate symposium was co-organised by Graham Johnston from Canberra and yet another chap originally from Bristol, Peter Roberts, who is also back here now as a Professor of Pharmacology, working on the neuro-chemistry of excitatory amino acids. He was here as a PhD student when I first arrived here, working on excitatory amino acids under James Mitchell, anoth-er ex Babraham man, who had originally been mainly interested in acetyl-choline. Peter is one of the originators of the binding technique as applied to excitatory amino acids and he also published early neurochemical results sug-gestive of metabotropic glutamate receptors.

The room Peter and Graham had arranged, in Jerusalem, would have taken at most about 30 to 40 people, I would say. It was a session within a Meeting of the International Society for Neurochemistry, a fairly big affair, but not one that we thought would have necessarily attracted many people who were inter-ested in glutamate. But we greatly underestimated the number. The room was full and overflowing, with standing in the aisles and doorways. This was very encouraging. Even so, it has since developed much beyond what we could ever have imagined. You only have to look at the abstracts for the Society for Neuroscience now – there are 20-odd sessions that are somehow related to glutamate, through epilepsy, neurodegeneration, and all that, not to mention psychology and psychiatric conditions in addition to basic neurophysiology and neuropharmacology.

Did it take 2 or 3 years more for the next symposium?

Yes, the next one I can recall was on Excitotoxicity in Stockholm in 1982. For a while they continued to be linked to those on GABA but by the mid to late 1980s they became increasingly resticted to excitatory amino acids as a topic in its own right.

Somewhere in the early 1980s, the MK-801 story began to impact as it became clear that this drug also acted on the NMDA receptor. How important was that?

Well, it was important in advancing the ketamine/PCP story and the recogni-tion and elucidation of the channel-blocking mechanism. The ketamine story began in the early 1980s through the work of David Lodge, and later, also Max Headley here. MK-801 was the most potent compound showing a similar action, identified as such by Iversen and colleagues at Merck, Sharpe & Dohme in the mid-1980s.

Did you have any feeling before 1980 that ketamine was acting through the NMDA receptor?

No, in fact at that stage I knew nothing about ketamine. It was David Lodge who found that out. He's a vet and I believe it had a use in veterinary medi-cine. He tested many known medical and veterinary drugs for actions in excitatory amino acid systems and found several correlations. Interestingly, we had earlier, in 1977, found that chlorpromazine and diazepam in rela-tively high concentrations had NMDA-selective depressant actions. These have never been further investigated but are quite probably channel-block-ing effects.

How did the ketamine angle get missed then? Was it because there were so few people working in the area?

Yes, there weren't many people at that stage thinking that they should test clinically used CNS drugs on glutamate receptors. It just didn't figure in people's thinking until the early to mid-1980s. Remember the NMDA receptor had been recognised as a functional glutamate receptor only a short while before. Lodge's work on ketamine and PCP was the first to establish the principle and then the work on MK801 followed.

What impact did David's work have on you here?

Not much, really. Its mechanism of action was originally problematical, though it was clearly non-competitive. Harry Olverman, within our group, found it did not displace labelled AP5 from brain membranes. David was interested in it, I think, mainly because it was clinically effective. But its molecular structure didn't fit into our previously elucidated structure–activity relations for competitive NMDA antagonists and I didn't really want to get involved with a more complicated phenomenon shown by a range of chemically disparate substances. All these channel-blockers as they ultimately turned out to be were a problem 'structure–activity-wise' because they all had different molecular shapes. And we had our hands full already with competitive antagonists.

Did the sheer complexity of the NMDA receptor hold things back? It's such a complicated beast with glycine sites and all that.

No, it didn't. We weren't originally aware that it was so complicated. We were able to make very potent NMDA receptor antagonists, which were competitive and completely conventional, pharmacologically. I got involved with Sandoz on this and helped develop a compound that may mitigate brain damage in cerebral ischaemia. Such conventional antagonists were all developed before we knew about glycine and the channel-blocking story, or the spermine–spermidine modulatory site on the NMDA receptor or the various subtypes of NMDA receptor that have since emerged. We didn't know about this complexity. If we had done we might have been a little put off, though I don't think so, really. At the time it all seemed rather simple. You take an amino acid molecule a bit longer than glutamate, put a phosphonate group on the end, bend it round a bit forming various cyclic groups, arrange for the amino acid end to be of the D configuration – in the earliest antagonists, anyway – and you ought to have a good NMDA antagonist. That much was easy, and although somewhat simplistic, produced many a good new NMDA receptor antagonist.

Other things weren't so easy. Similarly specific and potent antagonists for kainate and AMPA were not as readily developed. You could get compounds that were somewhat active although they weren't very potent or selective. But they did depress the synaptic responses which weren't depressed by pure NMDA antagonists. That was important because it implicated non-NMDA receptors also in synaptic transmission. But, no, ketamine didn't make too much impact on me, although I'm sure it impacted more on anyone involved in clinical medicine and on the drug companies, who were also looking at other ways of getting at the NMDA receptor. Ketamine is one of the few substances in the field that passes the blood–brain barrier readily.

When did the long-term potentiation story, the LTP story, impact?

The LTP story, pharmacologically speaking, started here in Bristol as well, in a sense – Graham Collingridge was one of our first pharmacology students here. He came out of the second year that the course was run, graduating in 1977. It was a famous year. He and Mark Mayer, now at NIH, and two others all got firsts. In fact there was a fifth one who should have got a first but the external examiner said we can't possibly have five out of nine getting firsts. After completing his first degree here, Graham went to work with John Davies as a PhD student and then to Hugh McLennan in Vancouver as a postdoc. It was when he was working with Hugh McLennan that he decided to see if this LTP phenomenon was susceptible to modification with excitatory amino acid agonists or antagonists. That led him to the discovery that the NMDA antagonists were able to prevent the generation of LTP. He came back here as a Lecturer, then went off to Birmingham for a while but came back here again 2 or 3 years ago as Professor in Anatomy.

LTP has become a subject in its own right now. You could almost be an LTP-ologist. It has become one of those central phenomena that pulls things into it.

Yes, his MRC programme grant is simply for investigating LTP now. The original findings pulled in Richard Morris, an experimental psychologist, who I guess was originally interested in any pharmacology that related to memory and learning. He tried some of these compounds behaviourally, testing them on memory and learning, and found that there a specific deficit developed if you put NMDA antagonists directly into the hippocampus – the rats couldn't learn as well as control animals how to get to a submerged platform under the influence of the drug.

We gave ketamine to healthy volunteers recently with a rationale that it was going to affect frontal lobe function and that it would mimic schizophrenic psychoses but the biggest effects showed up in memory.

To my way of thinking it is surprising when some functions aren't affected with these drugs because the NMDA receptor appears to be involved in practically all central synaptic events. Quite probably it is just that some forms of memory acquisition are particularly sensitive rather than uniquely affected.

Synaptic plasticity is one of the things that fall out of the NMDA story but this is not part of the usual lock-and-key way of viewing things.

But that's getting all tied up now with increasing knowledge of the involvement of the metabotropic glutamate receptors in longer-term effects. That's one of our main interests now, in collaboration with Graham Collingridge.

How did the metabotropic idea come on stream?

I can't claim anything to do with the beginnings of that except that we had probably the first specific agonist without knowing it, which was the phosphonic acid analogue of glutamate – what we called L-AP4. It is just glutamate with a phosphonic acid group rather than a carboxyl group at the end of the molecule. Our first group of NMDA antagonists were all the D-forms of glutamate analogues. Normally, we made racemic forms and separated the D and L forms, so we ended up with both. We tried the D-form of AP4 and it was a weak NMDA antagonist but not very selective. The next longer one, the equivalent of D-α-aminoadipate but with a terminal phosphonic acid group, has become the standard specific NMDA receptor antagonist now – D-AP5.

Carl Cotman, who has also been in the excitatory amino acid field for a long time, some 30 years or so now, and was one of the first people to work on hippocampal pharmacology, wanted some of this compound and I sent some of both forms to him, D- and L-AP4. He wrote back and asked if we had the labels mixed up because they found L-AP4 to be much more potent than the D-form at depressing synaptic transmission in the perforant path of the hippocampus. We had expected the D-form to be the most active, based on EAA receptor antagonism. He sent the sample back and we checked and said no, we hadn't got them mixed up. At about the same time we were finding that L-AP4 was unexpectedly depressing monosynaptic transmission in the spinal cord. This was mainly Dick Evans' discovery using his in vitro preparation, but John Davies confirmed it also in vivo. We didn't know how it caused this depression. It didn't fit in with any of our – by now – quite neat structure–activity relationships for excitatory amino acid antagonists. In fact it didn't antagonise any of our excitatory amino acid agonists -NMDA, quisqualate or kainate – at all but it still depressed transmission.

We now know that its action is via a metabotropic effect. At the time we thought it was probably working presynaptically because it wasn't working postsynaptically on any known excitatory amino acid receptors. Cotman and colleagues did some elegant work on miniature excitatory postsynaptic potentials that definitely suggested the L-AP4 effect was presynaptic, but we didn't know the exact mechanism. Now we know its action fits into those of Group 3 metabotropic glutamate receptors, mGluRs. Indeed, this activation characterised Group Ill mGluRs. They are activated by L-AP4 and some of them at least mediate depression of synaptic transmitter release. Their action is associated with a depression of cyclic AMP synthesis.

But when did the metabotropic idea emerge?

From the mid-1980s, via neurochemistry, glutamate-stimulated inositol phosphate formation from phosphatidyl inositol initially. These results led up to the idea that there was a particular kind of glutamate receptor that caused metabolic changes. Nicolletti, Costa and colleagues were the original proponents. As I recall, it wasn't till late 1987 that Sugiyama, a Japanese neuroscientist, actually showed an electrophysiological effect of such receptors in oocytes. They expressed a cloned receptor in oocytes that was coupled to a G-protein, and associated with glutamate-induced effects on certain channel currents. They suggested that these receptors be called metabotropic because they were obviously coupled to metabolic changes. This idea was already prevalent for amines.

But the word metabotropic isn't used in the amine field.

No.   I think the Sugiyama group suggested it to differentiate the function of these EAA receptors from the ionotropic actions of the amino acids at certain receptors. I am not sure whether there are purely ionotropic receptors for amines. Possibly all are of the metabotropic type.

When did the implication take hold that one was neurotransmission related and the others were metabolic related with longer-term effects on synaptic efficacy?

Well, I suppose the implication was there from the mid-1980s, when people were working with brain slices and getting significant neurochemical effects that were initiated by glutamate and a restricted number of analogues, but not by the standard excitatory amino acid agonists, NMDA, kainate or AMPA, and not antagonised by any of the usual antagonists of the then known transmission-related glutamate receptor subtypes. The molecular biologists began to clone all the different ionotropic and metabotrophic receptors and characterised a range of subtypes within each major group in the late 1980s and early 1990s. Then Collingridge showed the involvement of one particular group of mGluRs in the generation of hippocampal LTP, while Salt showed a particular association with the transmission of pain responses in the lateral thalamus. I suppose the Collingridge work in the early 1990s brought the possible role of mGluRs in longer-term electrophysiological effects to the fore though metabolic cascade effects would probably imply that mGluRs participate in longer-term changes than the rapidly reversible ionic effects induced by ionotropic receptors.

Before we leave the Japanese completely, some credit for kicking off the area seems owing to another Japanese – Hayashi. He had a first report on glutamate in 1954. Who was he?

His first important publication in English was in 1954, as far as I know, but there were earlier reports in Japanese. I think he was doing his work mainly in the late 1940s and early 1950s.

Was this an isolated effort?

If you mean was Hayashi alone in investigating glutamate as a neuro-excitatory agent well, yes, I believe so, but he had a number of students working with him. He seems to have been the first one to cotton on that glutamate was a convulsant substance. He tested a whole series of both glutamate-related and glutamate-unrelated compounds. His work was mostly reported in Japanese until he wrote a book in the late 1950s on amino acids related to glutamate and their possible role in epilepsy. He was the first one to put his finger on the excitatory action of glutamate but the mechanism was not clear. You could, of course, cause convulsions by putting any number of substances into the brain, so the glutamate action couldn't necessarily be assumed to be caused by a direct synaptic effect.

I think he died in the late 1950s. He was an experimental neurologist, I think, who had these interesting ideas of endogenous convulsant substances and put students to work on them. There are all sorts of little bits in the abstracts of meetings in Japan in the early 1950s. But he gets the credit quite rightly for being the first one to report the excitatory action of glutamate as manifested in convulsions, and his speculation that this might be due to an effect on sodium permeability proved essentially correct, though based on ion fluxes occurring during electrical conduction in nerve fibres as elucidated by Hodgkin and Huxley, rather than on known synaptic events.

When did John Olney's name begin to come into the frame?

In the late 1950s there was a paper by Lucas and Newhouse who found some neurodegenerative effects in retina when they injected large quantities of glutamate subcutaneously, I think. It seemed to be destroying retinal cells. Olney picked this up in the late 1960s. I believe he began his work completely independently of our results, originally, and only later became aware of our earlier work on excitatory amino acids in general. I know he did write to David Curtis in the early 1970s and got some compounds from him. Irrespective of how and when he came across our series of amino acids, his series turned out to be practically identical, potency-wise, in its ability to cause neuronal damage when given in excess, as we had found to be excitatory. It fitted in very nicely. The excitotoxic story, though obviously related to excitatory amino acid actions, is a separate story and deserves recognition as such. He tells the story that the first time he postulated at a conference that endogenous glutamate may cause the degeneration seen in certain medical conditions, the hall guffawed with scornful laughter. I'm sure his ideas are taken more seriously now.

He halted MK-801 when he reported on the vacuolation following its use.

You can see why. I don't know the full story but if you do find things like that in drugs that are in the clinical trial stage, I think you're duty-bound to report it.

When did you become aware of interest from either the clinical people or the drug companies?

Well, I first became aware of this unexpectedly and in a rather unfortunate manner. I was never interested in those sorts of things. I was only interested in finding out how the central nervous system worked. But, anyway, I developed these phosphonic acid compounds and I would talk to anybody about them. To cut a long story short, some unpublished results of ours were seized upon by others, developed along the lines we were already following, and patents applied for.

This told me that some people were keen to take out patents in this area, so I had better be more careful in future. The next time I had a good compound I got in touch with the British Technology Group, which was a government department at the time – since privatized – and the appropriate authority for

taking inventions in universities and getting patents on them. That culminated in the drug that Sandoz is now developing. Because of all that, however, we
were held up with publications on that compound and on related analogues
and we didn't get into press until some four years later and then with a lot of
extra names on the paper, relative to our initial group. By then we were experiencing competition from Ciba, and not long after by Lilly, Parke-Davis and
others. But the early to mid-1980s was the time when people began to think
there might be some drug potential in the area.

The clinical indications were ...?

As anticonvulsants first and antispastics. But with Olney and other 'excitoxicol-
ogists' coming in and stressing all the brain damage that could be caused by glutamate and analogues, it became obvious that antagonists might also be useful
to prevent or alleviate the progress of some neurodegenerative conditions. This
idea came out of excitatory amino acid meetings in the early 1980s. I wasn't all
that drawn in this direction myself, and was somewhat sceptical. When the
research director of a large continental drug firm got in touch with me and
asked if they should be looking towards excitatory amino acids as possible drugs
to prevent brain damage, in stroke, heart failure, or head injury, for example, I
said quite honestly I doubt whether there's any future in it. If you antagonise
the main transmitter receptors in brain, God knows what's going to happen.
They dropped the idea and did something else. They probably saved a lot of
money because that was 15 years ago and there's nothing on the market yet. But
traumatic head and spinal injuries are the best current indications since the anticonvulsant possibility went by the board due to unacceptable side-effects.
Neuroprotection via glutamate antagonists looks a better possibility now.

What about schizophrenia and nervous conditions generally?

I wouldn't have thought so yet. But with all the subtypes of amino acid receptor now known there's bound to be some that are more involved in particular
medical conditions than others. Huntingdon's chorea and ALS are possibilities. Maybe some aspects of Alzheimer's. Parkinson's too – L-dopa for instance
is an excitatory amino acid. There are, of course, any number of neurological
and psychiatric syndromes in which there may be some particular involvement
of the NMDA or other glutamate receptor system susceptible to drug modification. Maybe even in schizophrenia.

I'll tell you something I just learned two days ago. David Lodge is now
Research Director at Lilly's lab in Windlesham. In an open lecture a couple of
days ago he told us about this new compound they have, which is a potent agonist at one of the metabotropic glutamate receptor subtypes. It passes the
blood–brain barrier well, which is unusual for these compounds. It turned out
to be quite potent at the cloned receptor level but they didn't know what to
look for in terms of therapeutic usefulness, so they put it through a whole
range of behavioural tests and it turned out to be anxiolytic. It was as potent as
the benzodiazepines but it was without the benzodiazepine side-effects. So I

think it is only a matter of time now before glutamate receptor agonists and antagonists make it to the clinic. If you can find a substance with a discrete action at a specific type of amino acid receptor, I think a drug use will be found for it eventually, provided it can be got to the target site, one way or another.

Curiously the glutamate field has evolved in a completely different way from the monoamine field, which grew up in order to explain the effects of drugs we already had and as a means of producing more. The amino acid area has grown without much input from clinical compounds, other than ketamine, PCP and MK-801, and with relatively little support from the companies originally.

Yes, it has been more oriented towards fundamental research. All the compounds you've mentioned clearly had their side-effects which made them generally unsuitable clinically. But there was big debate whether the side-effects had anything to do with NMDA receptor antagonism. Unfortunately, the early Phase I clinical studies with pure competitive antagonists also brought on these effects. In epileptic patients they came on at much lower doses. As they were nice pure drugs which acted on very little else, it definitely looked like the NMDA receptor was involved in the unwanted side-effects, although there are so many NMDA receptor subtypes that we may eventually be able to control for some of these effects by developing more subtype-specific drugs.

How many years before there will be an impact clinically?

Maybe even within the next couple of years. I have a feeling that it will soon take off. Maybe not for five years, but it's only a matter of time. The trouble with these drugs is the difficulty getting most of them through the blood–brain barrier. If that can be overcome – ketamine gets through quickly and this latest anxiolytic one also – it will be interesting. So far none of them have much effect on the peripheral nervous system, or on the major physiological systems, so even if only a small proportion of a drug gets through, you could afford to give a large dose in order to get a therapeutic dose.

It's a unique position to have been associated with the development of a field.

I've been lucky, that's the first thing to say – lucky in being at the right place at the right time and being able to contribute an expertise that had been largely lacking in the field at that time. Profoundly lucky also in the people I have worked with over the past 40 years in Canberra, London and Bristol, not to mention many other outstanding collaborators in other institutions. The second thing to say is that the field has now grown beyond the point where I feel I can continue to contribute much to it. It's gone well beyond my ability even to keep up with the literature. In fact I don't even try now. I still have a programme grant which goes on for another 12 months but I decided a couple of years ago that I would now begin to retire. I don't feel the need to stay personally active in the field. I'm confident that my present team under David Jane will continue to make a major contribution – they are an excellent group.

I gave up talking about the subject 3 or 4 years ago. I'm happy to have done my bit. I wanted to make a contribution. More than anything I had wanted to find out something about how the brain worked and I've accumulated enough knowledge about that now – poor as this is in relation to what remains unknown – to be able to begin to think about its relationship to the phenomenon of mind and the idea of 'self', which was the original motivation. Maybe I'll do this in retirement but I suspect that I will not be able to contribute anything new or original.

Has the area got the recognition it deserves in terms of honours etc.?

Pretty well. Who contributed what in the past is difficult to disentangle, but modern advances are less confused. I've had three international awards in the last few years, each shared with other people, which is quite right. Olney, Choi and I shared a Wakeman Award, for contributions towards the treatment of spinal injury. Another was the Dana Award for pioneering achievements in health. This one was shared with Olney again, and with Philippe Ascher, for his glycine and magnesium contribution. The last one was a Bristol-Myers Squibb Award for outstanding achievement in neuroscience which I shared with the molecular biologists Heinemann and Nakanishi, who had cloned, expressed and characterised glutamate receptor subtypes. There will probably be many more awards in the field in due course. One problem has been the rather slow build-up and the number of individual discoveries made that contributed to our present understanding. It is difficult to single out individual people or individual papers. There are so many people who have made or are currently making important contributions. My particular contribution has always been as part of a team. Indeed our collaborators have done much more with our compounds than we could have ourselves, to characterise their actions and demonstrate their potential usefulness in the field. People like Graham Collingridge, Mark Mayer, Carl Cotman, Dan Monahan, Shigedada Nakanishi, Tom Salt, Peter Roberts, Brian Meldrum and Astrid Chapman, Peter Cook and many others, Harry Bradford, Martin Croucher, Richard and Robert Miller and all their colleagues, not to forget our industrial associates.

A lot of people wouldn't see it the same way. In science clearly there can be the co-operative approach, which you seem to have, but there is also the competitive approach which many people have.

Well, while I felt there was nobody else interested, I was more open but once people began to patent compounds based on our discoveries it changes one's attitude. It was more fun in the early days. I'm obviously not against the development of compounds which will be of a therapeutic benefit, and these would seem to be on the way now, I'm glad to think. But the commercial element changes the field and, for the academically orientated person, not for the better. Despite this there is still plenty of scope for co-operation since neuroscience is multi-disciplinary by nature and any one group will probably not progress as fast as they could without combining forces with other groups with complementary disciplines. I personally derive more satisfaction from such a collaborative approach and I feel our work has benefited greatly from it.

Select bibliography

Watkins JC (1986). Twenty-five years of excitatory amino acid research. In (Roberts PJ, Strom-Mathisen J, Bradford HF, eds). Macmillan Press, London, pp 1–39.

Watkins, JC (1994) The NMDA receptor concept: origins and development. In: The NMDA Receptor. (Collingridge G, Watkins JC, eds). Oxford University Press, Oxford, pp 1–30.

17 Irving Gottesman

Predisposed towards predispositions

How did you end up in the field? What's your primary training and where did you do it?

My primary training is as a child and adult clinical psychologist. I went into training in 1956, just as the chlorpromazine era hit the United States full force. I started in the US Navy as an Ensign in cryptography during the Korean War. I had enough time in the combat zone to get the GI Bill which then financed my graduate education. I originally went to the University of Minnesota, which I had carefully researched, because they had the clinical psychology training programme that was most oriented towards biology, genetics and an objective assessment of personality. In fact they were on the map of psychopathology because that was the home of the famous MMPI, Minnesota Multiphasic Personality Inventory. The inventor of it, Starke Hathaway, was a very active professor there in the medical school, Department of Psychiatry, and he became one of my mentors along with Paul Meehl.

A very famous name.

Paul Meehl ended up on my dissertation committee, which I will come to shortly. I also went there because it was the only place that was trying to train child clinical psychologists and I featured myself as doing that initially. The person in charge of that was Robert Wirt. He's known to some psychopharmacologists because he was involved with one of the very first controlled trials of chlorpromazine which they matched against reserpine and placebo for chronic schizophrenics in the Veterans Administration Hospital of Minneapolis, which is where I did my 1-year internship at the end of my training. In those days you could actually get through if you were organised, in 4 years, and that would include a 1-year full-time psychiatric internship. So I had 3 years of course work, during which time I also worked half time in a child guidance clinic under the supervision of a Freudian analyst, Hyman Lippman MD, someone who had actually been analysed by Anna Freud in Vienna.

You say you picked your course because of its biological underpinning. Why this orientation so early, can you remember?

I was always interested in the possibilities of becoming a physician but I didn't pursue that line because I joined the service after World War II. I had always been fascinated by biology and chemistry and was a collector of dead animals and interested in bird watching, collecting birds' eggs and things like that. I even went so far as to acquire hearts and eyes from the family butcher in order to take them into school to my biology teacher so we could have hands-on dissection experience. So that was rather enterprising and fun. I think I would have become some kind of physician. As it is I ended up being very much a neuroscientist anyway. Also I was impressed by Sinclair Lewis' book *Arrowsmith* and I think that set me in the direction of realising these kinds of things could be done for a living.

For a dissertation topic, it seemed to me that I should try to combine the knowledge and skills I had acquired about personality assessment, especially using the MMPI, the home instrument. Then I had learned in a course on the psychology of individual differences about the research that had been done on twins who suffered from schizophrenia. I especially noted the studies of Kallmann, who was an immigrant to the United States from Germany and Slater at the Maudsley, the Institute of Psychiatry. I had the fantasy that it would be nice to do something like that but I realised it was impossible because of the difficulty of obtaining twins who had schizophrenia and getting enough of them.

While I was taking course work, I took a course in genetics from a well-known *Drosophila* geneticist named Sheldon Reed. He had already by that time left *Drosophila* and gone into family studies of mental retardation and psychosis. He actually completed a huge family study of mental retardation in the old-fashioned way, using one of our state hospitals in Minnesota. The study was very well conducted because Minnesota was one of the very first states to apply IQ tests to children, so they had reservoirs of psychological test data on individuals who could be family members of the mentally retarded and they used these data to make some advance guesses about the genetic aspects of mental retardation. Now this man was very interested in trying to recruit a psychologist to be interested in the genetics of behaviour. He, himself, had done the genetics of *Drosophila* behaviour and thought that there was so much there that American psychology wasn't paying attention to and he was actually correct. It just appealed to me. I said that I would like to do a twin study with personality. The last time that had been done in the States was in 1937. He thought it was a marvellous idea and he helped me to organise it and in the process I learned more and more about human genetics.

I carried off this study using the adolescent twins of both Minneapolis and St Paul – known as the Twin Cities – and I had very good co-operation. I did not get co-operation from the religious private schools because they were offended by the personal nature of the items on the questionnaire. So I made do with the public school children and established the fact that the MMPI was a better test for assessing personality than the tests used by Newman, Freeman and Holzinger in 1937. Rather than getting ambiguous results as they had, I got very positive results showing that for most of the standard scales, and using them in the normal range – because these were not patients, they were normal kids – the heritability was in the neighbourhood of 0.5, 0.6, which made personality traits as genetically influenced as intellectual ability. That came as a surprise to the Faculty at the university, who thought that it might come out that way, but they didn't think that anybody could actually prove it. I published my dissertation by 1963. It was rejected by the journal I sent it to the first time. I sent it in as a monograph and it was rejected out of hand as being irrelevant to psychology. They said that the nature versus nurture battle had already been settled and that nurture had won. So there was no point in bringing it up again.

Wow!

So I talked to my professors, who were well connected. Paul Meehl was one of these. Gardner Lindzey was another. This was before Paul Meehl had got into schizotypy. I finished and left Minnesota in 1960. My work was a novelty and attracted some attention from people like Franz Kallmann, who at that time was a kind of a hero. I didn't know enough about him to know that there was a dark side as well to his personality and his research.

Do you want to comment on that further, because that's been made something of by the anti-genes lobby?

I was dealing with second-hand information about Kallmann at the time – the way the textbooks wrote it up, the way the journals wrote it up. It was only later that I got to meet him personally after he had written about my results asking for permission to cite some of the tables. I also then met his younger research associates Nikki Erlenmeyer-Kimling, who is a well known behavioural geneticist, still doing schizophrenia research and I'm a consultant on her projects, and his other research associate Arthur Falek, who is a human biologist, interested in basic processes, cytogenetics and drug abuse. They changed my view about Kallmann. Kallmann himself changed my view, which had been acquired second hand. I got to appreciate that he was perhaps over-selling the field of psychiatric genetics and in the process he was making more enemies than friends. He was very confrontational and would not abide by psychoanalytic interpretations of psychopathology, even though one of his good friends, Sandor Rado, was one of Freud's direct disciples. My views of Kallmann have continued to evolve in a positive direction. I keep learning more about him in connection with recent publications about Nazi Germany and the 50th anniversary of the Nuremberg War Crimes Trials.

Going back to Meehl, it turned out that he had two analyses, one by a Freudian who happened to be my mentor in the child guidance clinic during the 2 years I was there. Then later he decided he would have another analysis and this time he picked a Radovian analysis. It was Rado who had picked up on the idea of schizotypy from Kallmann. Kallmann, of course, got it from the rest of European Psychiatry, especially the people around Munich, who were interested in ways of characterising the not quite normal relatives, sometimes pretty far away from normal but not psychotic relatives, of schizophrenics. So they used this term and Meehl got a lot of mileage out of it. It became a growth industry in the States. Later it was picked up by the Danish American adoption studies of schizophrenia, Kety and Rosenthal, and they made more of it and it ended up having an effect on DSM-III.[1]

Now we are around 1963, which must be close to the time when you came to the Maudsley.

I should say that when I left Minnesota in 1960, my first job was at Harvard University, a difficult post to get, but they were interested in somebody different. They thought anybody interested in or a defender of genetics was different and they thought I couldn't do too much damage because they had a set policy that you could only be there for 3 years and then you moved on. There was almost no promotion from within.

I was in the Department of Social Relations, which was very famous because it was a first attempt to combine the disciplines of sociology, anthropology and social/clinical psychology. They managed to pull that off for a postwar generation, in competition with 'proper' psychology under Skinner and SS Stevens in the Department of Psychology over the road. The people involved were Harry Murray – he was the inventor of the TAT, thematic apperception test; Gordon Allport, who single-handedly invented personality theory in the United States. His 1937 book was influential – on me as well. Clive Kluckhohn was the cultural anthropologist. Another person well known in his own field was the sociologist, Talcott Parsons. So there was quite a heady environment. My immediate boss was David McCelland. He is known for his work on the need for achievement and his use of projective tests like the TAT to measure these things. So I was an odd duck advocating the use of this objective personality test, the MMPI, with its roots in Kraepelinian psychiatry.

They had an initial effort to socialise the new boys. My first teaching job was to co-teach a course on personality with Harry Murrray and then during the second half of that first year I co-taught the next version of the course with Gordon Allport. So here I was in the beginning of my career and I was sitting next to rather than at the feet of these two famous men after having been exposed to Paul Meehl and Starke Hathaway at Minnesota. I was lucky to get such a solid start.

As a result of my dissertation I was invited, at the expense of the American Society for Human Genetics via a travel grant, to go to the Second International Congress on Human Genetics in 1961 in Rome. Because of my close association with Sheldon Reed, who was really my closest mentor in regard to the genetics in human behaviour – we were both learning at the same time – I was introduced there to, among other people, Kallmann and Eliot Slater. I knew about Eliot's work and I went to hear his talk. I went up to him afterwards and said it would be nice if some time in the future I could come over and be a postdoctoral fellow and I was sure that there was something that I could find that would be interesting to both of us. He said, well, if you ever get a chance, come

---

[1]See Claridge G, Healy D (1996). *The Psychopharmacologists*, Vol I.

along. At that time I didn't know that his brother was a psychologist and later on I realised that was part of the reason he was so friendly to me.

During my last year at Harvard, I applied to the US Public Health Service to have a full-time fellowship abroad and it just so happened that at that time there was a big push to try to get people trained in one discipline to obtain training in another and one of the fields they were encouraging was genetics. They were also encouraging ethology and physiology and things like that. So I applied and, based largely on my dissertation, as I had been publishing a few things from it, I got the fellowship. I worked it out with Slater that I would come to his MRC Unit in Psychiatric Genetics and do one of two or three things. One of the things on my wish list was to do a study just like his, the genetics of schizophrenia, using the twins that he had accumulated from the register that he had set up in 1948.

After the War he realised that his own twin study was not ideal because of the sample ascertainment which was just from resident chronic cases in the old traditional hospitals, around London. So he set up a register at the Maudsley and the Bethlem Royal, and in the emergency units of nearby hospitals in Camberwell. He set up a face-sheet in all those places, so that all the intake workers had to ask whether or not you were one of a pair of twins and he managed to get a different kind of register from anything in the literature – consecutive admissions to both in- and outpatient services. This would allow you, for example, to get a case of schizophrenia that had never had inpatient treatment. When I came over and started work, some of the twins on the register had never had an inpatient contact, but because of the nature of schizophrenia it is virtually impossible to stay as an outpatient for your whole life, and by the end of our study every one of the patients had put in time as an inpatient. I was very lucky that Eliot agreed that I could do this. It was such a precious resource. It gave me tremendous advantage in my career to be able to do something this important 3 years out of my degree.

He set me up to work with Jerry Shields. I knew Jerry Shields from the literature because of his world-renowned study on identical twins reared apart. What I didn't know was that Shields was confined to a wheelchair because he was one of the last adults to get polio in the UK and that his formal training was as a social worker. The vaccine when it first arrived was given to children here and then to adults and it didn't get to him on time. We were a very complementary team.

Can I ask you more about the personal impact people like Eliot Slater and Jerry Shields made on you?

Eliot was my senior by a number of years. He was a very good mentor. He was pretty much a hands-off kind of person. He wasn't interested in micromanaging. He was interested in the grand scheme. I told him what I wanted to do. He said Mr Shields will help you acomplish this. I know you will like him. I explained my scheme to Jerry Shields and we implemented it. What I proposed was to give the MMPI, based on my sympathies with Paul Meehl, to try to assess whether schizotypy was on a continuous dimension. We right away rejected the so-called medical model and shifted towards a model for dealing with chronic diseases like heart disease and diabetes. I was a strange kind of psychologist to be talking like this but this was the way I had been trained by Sheldon Reed to appreciate complex traits from plant and animal genetics work.

I also said that I was going to tape record my semi-structured interviews, which were designed again to get a dimensional appreciation of mental illness. They said, well, Englishmen aren't going to let you come into their house and turn on that machine and tape record the interviews. They also probably won't be too happy to fill in the questionnaire asking them about their sex lives and their religion among other things – that will take a good 45 minutes to an hour. I said, well let me try it and I'll see. I went out and I was very lucky initially and that gave me confidence to go ahead even when I obtained resistance. The path had been smoothed by the research assistants in the old genetic hut. This was the MRC Psychiatric Genetics Unit and that was my point of attachment. Eliot provided me with a room there. It was a small wartime hut but it contained Eliot most days of the week, Jerry Shields and Valerie Cowie.

Can I ask you about Valerie Cowie, because if you read the interview by Alec Coppen, he says that she was probably the brightest woman he had ever met. Is this right?

She was extremely bright. She was kind of a favourite child of Eliot. He brought her along quite quickly in her career. She had the good sense to take his advice and obtain a PhD in genetics after she had trained as a psychiatrist. She took a PhD in genetics with Lionel Penrose. Now Penrose and Slater were never friends, they were antagonistic about each other. Penrose had a very poor opinion of psychiatric genetics, or of psychiatry in general, even though I believe he served as a psychiatrist both in Canada and in the UK. At any rate Valerie got along famously with Penrose and she got along famously with Eliot.

I was there from 1963 to 1964 and came back the following year for 3 months and then I came back every year for 25 years for 2–3 weeks just to work with Shields and sometimes directly with Slater on the data analysis and the writing of the papers and the book, which told it all. The book was published in 1972. In 1971, I had published with Shields the edited and collected papers of Slater. We thought we better do that while he was still around to appreciate it. So we stood down work on our own book and pulled together the best of his papers in all the areas that he had worked in.

It is clear from what you have told me about him and from what he writes in the book that he was reluctant to get involved in this experiment of committing his thoughts to posterity in this form. What sort of a man was he and how do you estimate his contribution?

He is one of the major figures in 20th century psychopathology. He had the abilities, both technical and personological, to pick important topics and to approach them in a classical British empirical manner and, to add to this, a genetic orientation. His own genetic orientation he acquired almost by chance.

In the early 1930s, when he arrived at the Maudsley, his mentor, the one who eased him in, was Aubrey Lewis. Aubrey Lewis was well connected on an international basis. Among the many possibilities that Eliot expressed interest in, Aubrey recommended that he pursue genetics, as a postdoctoral fellow. He had to organise so that he could obtain a Rockefeller Fellowship just as Aubrey himself had obtained a Rockefeller Fellowship to do anthropology, when he still lived in Australia.

Eliot went over to Munich at a very obnoxious time in German history. Hitler had just taken over in 1933. Academia was trying to go on as usual but there were splits as he described them to me, which I talked him into writing for the book – splits between the sensible academic Germans, who were disinterested in politics, and those who worked along with the Nazi overlords and the inclination to abuse both genetics and psychiatry for political purposes. He wrote some very emotional papers after he returned from Germany. While he was there he also met Lydia Pasternak, the sister of Boris, and married her and that's the mother of his children. He also was very keen on art and poetry. He wrote poetry which he published privately. He became a very good Sunday painter. I am flattered that in his will he gave only two people paintings: one was Martin Roth and the other was myself. We did become close personal friends, even though there was a big difference in our ages. I think he looked on me as another one of his sons.

He was quite willing to challenge received wisdom and took a great deal of pleasure in it. It got him into difficulties with Lewis, got him into difficulties with the Washington Univerity school of thought, where I later spent part of my career. They got into a big fight on the topic of hysteria. Eliot thought of it as an iatrogenic disorder and in his own work involved with follow-up of patients from Queens Square, he was able to show that the vast majority of these people who had a diagnosis, usually of conversion hysteria, later on had something wrong with their brain and he could show it. They had a different view at Washington University. At any rate he spent a lot of energy without having an empire. It is very unlike research enterprises today, where people need a lot of money and they need a lot of associates. He was able to organise himself and Jerry Shields and maybe one other field worker and acomplish incredible amounts of work, of very high quality, and then see it through to publication. During the time that I was here he was also the first editor of the *British Journal of Psychiatry* – under its new name.

How important was that to the field? He obviously had the discretion to accept articles on the genetics of psychiatry, at a time when you might have found it hard to get them published elsewhere and having him there must have encouraged people to think about doing this kind of work.

Yes, you're absolutely right. And he had this ability to give advice without being threatening. His letters of acceptance were usually lessons administered in a way that you had no reluctance to accept all of the advice and make it a much better paper – especially knowing that it was going to be accepted. Many papers that had been rejected by American journals, especially, came his way. He shaped those up and they were published in the BJP. Our first paper on the results of schizophrenia in this new sample of twins was published in 1966 in the BJP in the very same issue that he published results of the first adoption study of schizophrenia by Leonard Heston.

It's interesting to bring in Leonard Heston to the story because Heston was a young registrar when he first communicated with me – we were born a couple of weeks apart in 1930. He heard that I had spent a year here and he wondered whether or not there was any point in him disrupting his life, the way I had disrupted mine to come over to work with Eliot and Jerry Shields. I told him – absolutely yes. So he, on my advice, came over to work with and have his work shaped by both Eliot and Jerry and ended up with his adoption study on the offspring of schizophrenic mothers being published. So 1966 was a momentous year for us with the publication of these two brand new approaches. Ours was new because as I've already mentioned I used the MMPI to get continuous indicators of psychopathology and I used tape-recorded interviews, but another thing we did was to not allow ourselves to be the diagnosticians, given the criticism that both Slater and Kallmann and the earlier investigators had received. They had diagnosed both members of the twin pair, so there was no way for them to be blind, as to whether they were diagnosing identical or fraternal twins. So if they had a genetic bias, an unhealthy one rather than a healthy one, they could make the results look more genetical than they were. We avoided that by involving a blindfolded panel of six judges to whom we gave extensive case history material, MMPI profiles and verbatim interview material from my semi-structured interview. At the time I was using my own purpose-built semi-structured interview, John Wing working next door to us in the social psychiatry hut was working on the PSE. That period 1963–1965 was a very important time for me to be here.

You then went back – to Minnesota?

I went back to the States. I was recruited while I was here by the University of North Carolina to the Psychiatry Department by George Ham, who most people have never heard of. He had become very impressed with the part that genetics might play in psychiatry and he looked around for possibilities but there weren't many people who had the proper training or background. He heard about me and tried to recruit me. I had no other opportunities and so I was happy to take up the post in the Psychiatry Department, after I had guaranteed that I could also be appointed in Genetics. Also I didn't want to lose my contact with psychology and the Psychology Department there was very happy to have me as a member. I worked in North Carolina Medical School for just over 2 years, as it turned out. George Ham left his post as the Chair and the person who replaced him was not interested in supporting this area.

About that time, I got a call back to Minnesota saying that they were hoping to get a National Institute of Health grant that would allow for the training of people like the person I had become, trained in both psychopathology and in human genetics. They thought if I worked there, they could pull it off and I would be the co-director of this programme with Sheldon Reed. It would be housed initially in the psychology department because people like Paul Meehl were all enthusiastic about it. So I went back to Minnesota in 1966 and stayed there until 1980 when I got the call to go to Washington University, where that Psychiatry Department wanted to build up genetics as a major rather than as a minor part of their offerings. In Minnesota I was a full member of the Departments of Psychiatry, Genetics and Cell Biology and Psychology. I was coming to enjoy being somebody who wasn't typecast but who could operate freely in this larger area that requires an integation of areas. I did a lot of work during my time in Minnesota. For the 14 years there I was mentoring personally two PhDs per annum in the areas of behavioural genetics or clinical psychology and they in turn have produced students and it's snowballed in that fashion. So I have had an influence via my original students who stayed in the area and then very gifted postdoctoral students such as Peter McGuffin and his wife, Ann Farmer, who came to St Louis partly because I was there and they knew of my connection to Slater and Shields.

When did the concept of Behavioral Genetics begin to crystallise out and who coined the phrase?

Up until 1960, the area that became known as behavioural genetics usually went by such labels as the Nature versus Nuture controversy. In fact, it grew out of the area of the psychology of individual differences, which has a very German tradition. It goes back to World War I. The Germans were very interested in measuring individual differences in intelligence and personality. It had a military application, as part of their effort to select the best people to do the most difficult jobs, or to decide which enlisted men should become officers. That quickly spread to other countries like the UK and the United States. So there was a big testing tradition behind behavioural genetics. In 1960, the first book was published that actually had the title *Behavioural Genetics*, and that was the coining of the phrase that stuck. That was by John Fuller, who was a zoologist and an expert in dog behaviour, and William Thompson, a Canadian psychologist who brain drained to the States – he was an expert in mouse behaviour genetics. The two of them compiled the literature going back to the time of Galton, put it together in this book and it became the bible for the field. It had chapters on psychopathology. The Slater and Cowie book was the first that dealt specifically with psychopathology but that didn't come out until 1971.

When you were in Minnesota at this point, Travis Thompson was also there.

Travis Thompson was a colleague of mine. We both graduated the same year. We didn't know each other too much in graduate school but afterwards when we were trained, especially when I returned to Minnesota we were good friends. He was my house neighbour. Our families were good friends. Travis wasn't interested particularly in genetics but he realised that pharmacology was a new area that psychologists should be involved in and he became very influential in a short time, training both the MDs and PhDs in behavioural pharmacology. He had been a go-ahead straightforward Skinnerian, trained by Kenneth McCorquodale, who was Meehl's closest friend. So all these things seem to keep weaving in and out and linking.

Skinner himself had been there during the 1930s with Bill Estes, wasn't he, and Howard Hunt was there at one point, and then he went to Chicago?

Right, they were all there and they all fitted in to the Minnesota scheme, which was pejoratively called dustbowl empiricism. They eschewed theory because theory was considered to be kind of fatuous. They were never a talking club. They didn't want psychology to be near philosophy, which was part of its roots. They wanted it to be nearer to biology, mathematics and the harder sciences which acquired the most money for research from the federal government and from foundations. They weren't going to support the philosopy of X and Y or chitchat but they were going to support empirical research, the result of which could be put to use to improve the lot of mankind. Most of the funds came from the National Institute of Mental Health, which started up right after World War II.

Was there any reason why Travis was so successful in being able to pull people into the field? What kind of personality was he?

I would say it was his sincerity, his strength of purpose and his dedication to empiricism. Behavioural psychopharmacology was completely new to American psychology but also a natural evolution as the field of psychology after World War II divided up into specialities. This became one of the specialities that was highly regarded by the Federal Government and the granting authorities. It immediately attracted the attention of the pharmaceutical industry so that Travis quickly acquired an empire. He was always in the Medical School at Minnesota for his major base of operations. I was a full Professor eventually in the Medical School but my base was in the Psychology Department. Meehl split himself between psychology and psychiatry. Hathaway was full-time psychiatry.

Minnesota was an unusual place in that there was no internecine warfare or tension at that time – it's changed a lot since then, but at that time there was a kind of continuous love affair between psychology and psychiatry. There was no prejudice shown on either side. The Department of Psychiatry had a huge contingent of clinical psychologists, many of them trained by Hathaway and the psychiatrists at that time. Don Hastings was the Head of Psychiatry after the war and he was a very close personal friend of Hathaway. He trusted him completely and allowed Hathaway to, in effect, be the executive administrator of the Psychiatry Department, even though he had no formal medical qualifications. He was extremely knowledgable about psychiatry and psychosomatic medicine and he was also an equipment buff. He was interested in psychophysiology. He had written the first book of physiological psychology, published in the same series as Skinner's *The Behavior of Organisms*.

How did you get involved in the Danish twin studies?

During the time I was a Public Health Fellow at the Maudsley, I took a study tour at Eliot's suggestion. Through him I was able to go to Sweden and meet Erik Essen-Möller. I liked him and he liked me obviously. I got him to agree to be a blindfolded diagnostician for every one of our twins. This was the beginning of our multi-judge blindfolded panel that got away from the criticisms of the earlier twin studies. He was in his retirement and welcomed the opportunity to have a go at this. Then after that I went to Denmark to visit with another of Eliot's friends, Erik Strömgren, who was at Riskov, north of Aarhus. There he introduced me to a young psychiatrist who was doing a twin study of schizophrenia, Margot Fisher. We became quick friends because of our overlapping interests even though Shields and I were way ahead of her in terms of getting the job done on our sample. I also then went to Copenhagen to visit a friend of mine, Brendan Maher, who like myself was at Harvard in the early 60s and through Maher I met Sarnoff Mednick and Fini Schulsinger. I then spent more time chatting with and communicating with Mednick. From then things sort of went into hibernation.

Then in 1967 there was this famous meeting in Puerto Rico, the Dorado Beach Conference, organised by Seymour Kety and David Rosenthal and financed by the Foundations' Fund for Research in Psychiatry, which had as its goal bringing together in a confrontational manner all of the world experts on schizophrenia whether they be on the far psycho-analytic side or on the far genetical biological side. Because of my normal twin work plus my schizophrenia work, both Kety and Rosenthal knew what I was up to. So they invited not only Slater, of course, and Shields but also me and Leonard Heston. By that time Heston had also had a postdoctoral year at the Maudsley in Slater's unit and he and I had become very close friends. As it turned out he was the best man at my wedding and his wife was godmother to my younger son. So that's where I got together again with Mednick and Schulsinger and the Danes that had been involved in the adoption studies. I had no idea at that time that I would take my next sabbatical, on a Guggenheim Fellowship to Denmark, which I did in 1972/73.

What was the Puerto Rico conference like? You say that they set this confrontational meeting up – how confrontational did it turn out to be?

Well, nobody came to blows. I think everybody was moved forward toward somebody else's position. They didn't relinquish their own position but they moderated within the direction of, let's say, a multi-factorial approach. Some moved more than others. Some made pseudo-moves during the week and then quickly reverted to their original positions, such as Professor Lidz, and he certainly was confrontational. The people who believed in schizophrenogenic mothers were there defending their positions and they listened politely. There seemed to be kind of a sleeper effect because later on some of those people approached us on the genetic end of the spectrum and asked for and took advice about new research they got involved with. One conspicuous example was Pekka Tienari, the Finnish psychiatrist. He had been working on his own twin study for schizophrenia which he interpreted initially to completely support the environmental psycho-dynamic position. He was very much under the influence of Alanen, who was very much under the influence of Lidz. There are a lot of these pedigrees that you can see in the history of this field. Lyman Wynne was there along with Margaret Singer talking about constructs, which in Britain would be called EE, expressed emotion. They were talking about such things as communication deviance and affective style. Right now Pekka Tienari and Lyman Wynne are doing a new adoption study of schizophrenia and I am one of their genetics consultants along with Ken Kendler and they are using the MMPI. So that goes all the way back to 1967 ...

So it was a good thing, that meeting?

Well it was a landmark meeting and the book out of it is a landmark book which is not fully appreciated by the field. The proceedings of the meeting actually included a fair amount of the table talk, which was recorded. A lot of the slightly cleaned-up confrontation was published by David Rosenthal in the book as discussion.

How do you credit the contribution of Kety or Rosenthal in getting all of that off the ground plus their role in the adoption work at the time?

The motivation behind the meeting was to disseminate their major findings, which they knew would shake up the world although they hadn't appreciated that Leonard Heston was doing something similar on a small one-man scale and with a sample size of 47 in his experimental and 50 in his control group of children with normal mothers adopted away. But they invited Heston to present his updated results and then they, with great pride, deservedly, presented their three strategies. These were presented for the first time at this meeting. It was saved for the end of the week after everybody else had done their thing. Then comes the big surprise, major findings. They were and they are.

I think everybody was very impressed. We all knew that we were present at a major event in the history of psychopathology. To have present at the meeting Manfred Bleuter – he was then near retirement. I guess he was about 68 or so. Eliot Slater also about the same age. Lidz, Lyman Wynne were there, as was another pioneer of behavioural genetics, Nikki Erlenmeyer-Kimling. Sociologists like Clausen and Rosler were there, who were very interested in rural/urban differences and the impact of sociological things on the incidence of schizophrenia. All of these things were put on the plate at one time, so you could see that they each had a role to play and you couldn't reject any completely. But you could now be in a position of assigning informed weights to these factors and clearly genetics came out way ahead and for the first time genetic studies were not vulnerable to the kind of criticisms of the past. Einar Kringlen was there from Norway with his newish twin study of schizophrenia. It was just an accident that five of us started and completed new twin studies of schizophrenia at about the same time – Tienari in Finland, Kringlen in Norway, Fisher in Denmark and you had me and Shields working with Slater in the UK, all of them coming to fruition around 1966, give or take a year. So you had all these laid out and no one could say then that Kallmann's findings were spurious, the result of a hereditarian attitude or that Slater's results were genetically influenced because he obviously had an axe to grind and so forth.

Then you had the twin studies backed up with these new adoption studies. The strategy that Heston had initiated at the same time as Rosenthal and Kety involved looking at the adopted away children of schizophrenic mothers. Rosenthal did it by looking at the children of adopted-away mothers or fathers who had schizophrenia. Then Kety's strategy was a study with adopted-away children who grew up to be schizophrenic – he then went back and using the assets of the Danish mental health system tracked down the biological parents and relatives and the adoptive parents and relatives of these adoptees. There was one further strategy which necessarily had a small sample size and this was called the cross-fostering strategy. The lead on that was Paul Wender, the child psychiatrist, who was not particularly interested in genetics but was drawn in because he was a young man working at the NIMH at the time and was very valued by both Kety and Rosenthal. There they looked at children who were born to normal parents, adopted away into the homes of parents who later developed schizophrenia. All of these findings pushed towards a genetical explanation, as the major but not the exclusive explanation for the data. I think everybody was impressed, no matter what their stance. Those people who didn't put much weight on genetic factors could not possibly avoid them after this meeting.

There are one or two kinds of ambiguities there that you may wish to comment on. One was, at the time, the Americans would have been very soft in their diagnosis of schizophrenia but, on the other hand, some of the Danes may have been over-diagnosing manic-depressive disorder because of the influence of lithium. How did that fit in?

There were so many different diagnostic orientations – this is a whole treatise by itself. Bob Kendell's book is a case in point. The diagnoses that Shields and I used were a mix of all these schools of thought because among the blindfolded judges we had Essen-Möller. We had Americans like Loren Mosher. We had a number of British psychiatrists but each of them were of different persuasions. We had Jim Birley, for instance, who was a Schneiderian with a catego S+ point of view, making diagnoses. We had Paul Meehl, who was very generous in his diagnosing of schizotypal personality. All these people together allowed us to play an empirical game of picking out the abnormal from the normals. We didn't throw out anybody's information – we used all the information and in our own case we reached the conclusion, that a middle of the road diagnosis was the most meaningful one – something that wasn't too generous in diagnosing odd personalities as being schizophrenia-related but would be generous on the other end and not require just a catego S+ person to be a schizophrenic.

Kringlen was using diagnoses that were influenced by Langfeld and Strömgren because at that time Strömgren was the only one who had a *Textbook of Psychiatry* and that served all of the Scandinavian countries. Later on there were others, including Kringlen's own textbook and Welner and Schulsinger's textbook. The Danish adoption-related diagnoses were mainly influenced by the Americans, so when they had a panel of judges perhaps only one of three would be Danish and that individual was usually more westernised so to speak and some distance from the Strömgren school of diagnosis. It was only later, after the work presented at Puerto Rico, that you could see this influence of what we might now call over-diagnosing of a manic-depressive illness because of the enthusiasm in the use of lithium in the Schou and Strömgren school of thought. They were very close friends and aided and abetted each other's advocacy of biological psychiatry and a special brand of social psychiatry that's very much influenced by biological psychiatry and pharmacology.

Later you ended up participating in the Danish twin work yourself. How did that come about?

The advantage of going to Denmark was so obvious to me that I was willing to disrupt my life and go abroad again for a full year. This time I could do it from a secure base rather than being between jobs. I was lucky to win a Guggenhein Fellowship, which freed me up to do what I wanted to do. I arranged with Mednick to be a guest worker in his institute where the adoption studies of criminality and schizophrenia were being conducted as well as his prospective, longitudinal high-risk studies of the offspring of schizophrenics.

Can you tell me some more about Mednick?

Sarnof Mednick is a famous entrepreneur who has this ability to gather funds for novel research strategies. He recognised the crucial importance of the Danish system in providing you access to carefully diagnosed unbiased samples of individuals and their relatives. He has the advantage of working in a country that has a national psychiatric register that is now computerised, where there is a national twin register that dates back to 1870, as well as a national police register and a national adoption register which was formalised using the American funds that he helped bring to Denmark via Kety and Rosenthal. Kety and Rosenthal needed their contacts with Mednick and Schulsinger to pull off all this work that has brought them fame in the field.

When I went there in 1972 it was with the idea that I would be working with Margit Fisher in Aarhus on a different project, a new project where we were interested in the offspring born to two psychiatric inpatients. Given the Danish resources we could pull off this extremely rare and difficult strategy. It had been tried in Germany in the 1920s and 1930s to advantage but those results were lost and they have never been translated into English. It was clearly a very powerful strategy that would inform both taxonomy and genetics. She started collecting data and then I came over and joined her. I brought over American money, from the Scottish Rite Foundation, on which Board

Seymour Kety sat and helped promote our research. We began that project in earnest and that work is still on going with Aksel Bertelsen because a little bit later unfortunately Fisher committed suicide.

When she did that, it left another of her projects unfinished. This was the project that she published in its initial form in 1971. She was looking at the psychiatric status of children born to the twins as a function of whether or not both twins were schizophrenic or only one in the pair was schizophrenic. This gave you the terrific power to show what became of children of normal individuals who happened to be the MZ or DZ co-twins of a schizophrenic. After her death I then was partnered up, with Strömgren's help, with Aksel Bertelsen. With him I have been continuing the work on the offspring of dual matings, as we called that project, and we finalised the study of the offspring of concordant and discordant identical and fraternal twins to see who has schizophrenia and what that meant. We didn't publish that paper until 1989. It appeared in the *Archives of General Psychiatry* and brought us a lot of attention, as it should have. It also led to Fisher posthumously and Bertelsen and myself getting the Kurt Schneider Prize – the first time it was given to non-Germans.

There were other connections with the Danish high-risk studies. The high-risk studies were separate projects of Mednick and Schulsinger and Fini Schulsinger's spouse Hanna and that is famous in its own right and a major contribution to this field.

Were they the first to conceive of the idea of a high-risk strategy or did that idea come from elsewhere and they just happened to be the ones who were first to implement it?

The idea came from elsewhere, actually from Minnesota. In a paper published in about 1958, it was suggested as a strategy by a psychologist John Pearson who was a Minnesota-trained person influenced by Meehl and his co-worker Irene Kley. Having been influenced by Kallmann's research on schizophrenia, they proposed that the way to get results in a hurry and not have these results be confounded by the effects of hospitalisation and so forth was to look at the children of schizophrenics, while they were normal and then follow them until the 'fated' 10% or so would develop schizophrenia. They couldn't do the work themselves. Mednick noticed this and realised he could implement this in Denmark given all these national resources. So he got a good head start on everybody else. Other people jumped on that band wagon and tried to do it but they were doing it in countries that did not lend itself so well as did the Danish system. So Mednick's findings were the most mature, followed by the Erlenmeyer–Kimling findings which are now appearing in the literature in final form.

The strength of these studies converge in showing that children of schizophrenics raised by them develop schizophrenia at the same old high rate – between 10% and 15% or so. But in addition because of the emphasis on schizophrenia spectrum disorder, schizotypal personality, schizoid personality and so forth, the number of disordered children have grown proportionately so now we realised that many more than this core group are disadvantaged. The strategy of the high-risk design allows you to detect abnormalities or deviance from normality on the way toward development of schizophrenia and allows you to do this economically because you only have to study 100 children in order to get say 15 schizophrenics, whereas ordinarily in order to get 15 schizophrenics you would have to study 2000 individuals from birth till aged 55–60. The results of both of these strategies are very encouraging and these findings will be tied to the next generation of genetic studies where molecular genetics will be linked to these traits that feed into the development of schizoprhenia proper, but which by themselves can be seen as departures from normality that need not necessarily have pathological overtones.

Was Mednick just being opportunistic about all this or did he have a personal vision of some sort? Did he come into this kind of work with any prior beliefs about the outcomes?

He had established a reputation for himself as a well-trained experimental clinical psychologist, interested in learning theory as it might pertain to schizophrenia. He also was becoming very interested in psychophysiology, especially the psycho-physiology of the autonomic nervous system, as it might be an indicator of the schizophrenic state itself either in an episode or in remission. And he was curious about what the children of schizophrenics looked like on these dimensions that were relevant to Pavlovian conditioning as well as American style learning theory. So that's how he entered. He was not interested in genetics per se, but he quickly acquired an interest in it.

And Fini Schulsinger?

Fini Schulsinger was the Chief Psychiatrist at the then Community (Kommune) Psychiatric Hospital in the centre of Copenhagen. They were personal friends. Fini was the one who greased the skids into the Danish National Health system for Sarnoff. Then the two of them together were able to put together a very impressive grant request to the National Institute of Health and quickly obtained the funds to mount the field studies which led, among other things, to the training of an entire cohort of Danish psychologists and psychiatrists in these new techniques of psychophysiology, learning theory and epidemiology of mental illness.

Danish and possibly Scandinavian psychiatry has always been very biologically oriented. Do you think this work has had a part to play in that, because it must be very hard to be a Danish mental health researcher and not be influenced by all this?

Right. The people who are of a strong psychodynamic, psychoanalytical persuasion are a real minority and not a big influence. It's because of the general values of the people working in the Danish mental health system that so much of this work has been able to be done so efficiently without resistance.

What are the values? Because it's odd in a sense that they were so close to Germany and yet all of this has been perfectly acceptable and virtually no problem at all in Denmark.

The Danes were among the very first countries to pass laws that authorised health services to sterilise individuals if they had a severe mental retardation or a severe mental illness but it was never done in a coercive atmosphere which was what distinguished the Nazi approach, from the time Hitler took over in 1933. The Danes had passed these laws, as had the Swedes earlier, but with a panel of ombudspersons to guarantee civil rights for individuals, not to let the wrong people get into the act. Danish psychiatry was very much influenced by biology and by a German tradition of phenomenological psychiatry. As I said, almost all the knowledge came out of one textbook written by Strömgren. Strömgren was very influenced by German traditions and like Slater had gone to Germany and had the same reactions – it was a good place to learn about psychiatric genetics, but it was also appalling to see the abuse of civil rights and the going along with the Nazi government of these scientists in order to maintain their empires – which is the main charge laid against Rudin. Other people chose to leave, especially if they were Jews and they came to the UK or the United States to carry on the way Kallmann did. Some people became apolitical and got away with it. They included Bruno Schulz, the real mentor of both Slater and Strömgren. Schulz was somebody who just kept his nose to the grindstone, didn't get involved in politics and was extremely talented mathematically. Slater, I think, only met Rudin once or twice and then just in passing. Same with Strömgren.

It's still odd that given what happened in Germany after the war – the whole eclipse of this area of research – that one of the strongest places where it then re-emerged was in a place so close to Germany. The Danes perhaps have a funny relationship with the Germans.

There is no love lost but there is an admiration of their science and of their culture. But the Danish tradition in psychiatry always had a very large, almost dominant role for genetic factors and this can be attributed to Strömgren and the people that he has influenced in the modern generation, like Rafaelsen, Juel-Nielsen, Bertelsen and Fisher, and slightly before her Joseph Welner, who was the clinician in the Danish adoption studies. He was the one who actually did the interviews. He was a direct disciple of Strömgren although they went their own ways and he became much more interested in psychotherapy. He was a good friend of mine while I was there and afterwards. He was an extremely gifted clinician. He also became a judge on our Maudsley twins with Essen-Möller.

You came to Washington University at a time when they were maturing, I guess. The first group of people had actually left or were leaving. People like the late George Winokur had gone to Iowa although the links were still there, I guess.

George had left and Don Goodwin had left. The links are still there and form a kind of visible college, not invisible college. Some of the individuals who came out of Washington University training went on to become Chairs of departments: Paula Clayton is the Chair at Minnesota, Don Goodwin went to the Chair in Kansas, George went to Chair Iowa.

And they see themselves, I guess, as being seminal within the US context.

394   The Psychopharmacologists II

Yes, they see themselves as having been responsible for the development of DSM-III with its criteria-based diagnoses because it depended in part on the scheme that had evolved at Washington University, known as the Feighner criteria. It was paradoxical that it should be known by that name because Feighner was a registrar at the time and he was just assigned the writing up of the paper, so he was the first of a long string of authors that included Sam Guze and Eli Robins.

So it ought to really be the Robins criteria, you think?

It should be the Robins–Guze criteria, if you want to give it a name. Feighner is inappropriate; he was trenchant and a good worker but he has gone off now to a non-academic career doing drug trials. The other people involved, like Guze, Winokur and Robins, were all outstanding clinical researchers – not theoreticians. The theoreticians came later, like Ted Reich and Bob Cloninger. The general attitude in Washington University before and after I arrived, in 1979, was that in fact they had more gas chromatograph pieces of apparatus than they had clinical psychiatrists. They had no special spot reserved for training of their residents in psychotherapy and especially not in psychoanalysis. They always had one psychoanalyst around who would come in and try to bell the cats and some people acquired those skills but they were a real minority. It essentially was a stronghold of biological psychiatrists who then in a natural way branched into psychiatric genetics.

Guze and Robins had the foresight to take people out of service at a great cost to the cash flow of the department and allow them to go away for up to 2 years for postdoctoral training at the expense of the Department of Psychiatry, to be properly trained as geneticists. So Ted Reich came to the UK and worked in Falconer's unit in Edinburgh to learn quantitative genetics as it applied to medical genetics and as he would then apply it to psychiatric genetics. Bob Cloninger was allowed the luxury for any doctor or psychiatrist to go to Hawaii for more than a year to work with Newton Morton, who was the man who devised contemporary linkage strategies on which he had published as early as 1955. Newton Morton was a direct contact with the holy men of population genetics – RA Fisher, Sewell Wright, James Crow and T Dobzhansky. Newton Morton has since become interested in psychiatric genetics. I worked with him via DC Rao, who is another one of these catches for Washington University. He is a biostatistician and a geneticist, who the Psychiatry Department in Washington University went way out of their way to recruit and to make it possible financially. They have done that repeatedly, most recently with Alison Goate.

They did it with me when I was in Minnesota. I had met them socially and professionally at meetings and committtees and they made it worth my while to come and have the title of Professor of Psychiatric Genetics – nobody else had that title. I fitted right in to the team approach and I facilitated getting very large grants at a time when the government was not sure whether they were better off to fund individual researchers or to fund what we call Clinical Research Centres. They took the middle of the road position when they decided to fund both the CRCs and individual researchers but the money that was deliverd to CRCs was a very large drain on funding individual researchers. There was a sort of recognition of the fact that you could not do all research on a solo basis. You had to have Manhattan project-like teams and Washington University was eminently successful in getting not one CRC but multiple CRCs because of the people that they had brought together. A large proportion of the people were basic scientists rather than MDs but Robins and then after him Guze used their own authority and because it was a private university not subject to public oversights, they could say 'How about this?' and they would get it. They would go out on a limb but they managed to be very successful. They were prepared to go in a hole in order to do that and hope to make it up later on. It does make Washington University nearer to being a mini-NIMH where under one roof you could have MDs and PhDs of all sorts working together on projects. The nearest would be UCLA and New York State Psychiatric Institute.

Where did the Washington University ideal come from? Was it down to Eli Robins and if so where did he get it from?

It can be attributed to Eli Robins and to Sam Guze following him. Their orientation to psychiatry is really from internal medicine and via the aristocracy of American medical schools, namely Harvard and Johns Hopkins. Both of them were internists at heart who then became psychiatrists and other things. But Eli Robins was specially influenced by O Lowry, who was a discoverer of adenylate cyclase and that's where he acquired his enthusiasm for laboratory approaches to psychopathology. He saw psychopathology as just one more branch of medicine whereas the rest of the American psychiatry, influenced by Freudian and other psychodynamic schools of thought, stayed separate from the other parts of the medical school – sometimes going so far as be in separate buildings a few miles away from the main medical school.

Washington University for a long time were outside the mainstream – they were doing something that was seen to be quite idiosyncratic but yet it ended up being the winning side. The Feighner criteria were the basis for the DSM-III criteria etc. How much though did it take the contributions of someone like Klerman, who was part of the East Coast kind of establishment, very well connected politically to bring the Washington University project to fruition?

The distribution of large funds for research that I mentioned before was tilting towards CRCs and collaborative projects, which would often involve four or five different medical centres. Washington University took the lead in the first collaborative study of depression which meant pharmacology. Klerman was involved in a number of ways with this project. I was involved accidentally. When it first came in for funding I was on the committee that was overseeing all grants that were worth a million dollars or more. At that time a million dollars was thought to be a lot of money, nowadays it's not. On the committee at the same time were Seymour Kety, Neal Miller, Ed Sachar and Barbara Fish. I am not sure of the sequence here, but because Klerman was the director of NIMH, he got to call a lot of shots and influence a lot of things. The way they talk about it is that we need to have the right stocks in our portfolio – stock being a research programme that will make science better, but also will make Congress happier and the medical establishment happier that there are such enterprises going on. So they could decide, for example, to have a project on the use of dialysis for the treatment of schizophrenia but they wouldn't do it unless there were a lot of smart people behind the idea. The depression project has had a very long life, it still involves Washington University and is still producing results. It was divided up into a basic and a clinical part. The basic part had to do with basic pharmacology and the clinical part involved people like Myrna Weissman who became Klerman's spouse.

Were you at the Williamsburg Virginia Conference in 1969, which seems to have been the key forum, because out of that came an awful lot of the agenda that ultimately led to DSM-III.

That was before my connections to any of those people. I was involved in DSM-III as a consultant on the schizophrenia section and that could be attributed to my having been at the Maudsley and having been connected to Slater and European psychiatry generally – because they were not keen to have very many psychologists on those committees. It was completely dominated by establishment psychiatry. I was on the task-force for schizophrenia.

I guess schizophrenia wasn't really the controversial area in DSM-III. Depression was really where the livelihoods were going to be won and lost. But can I switch and ask you about the hostility to genetic research? There is a very trenchantly argued book which came out 10/12 years ago called Not in Your Genes by Steven Rose, Leon Kamin and Richard Lewontin in which they use the ad hominen argument extensively picking out whatever faults there were in the early research that was done by Eliot Slater and Franz Kallmann to tar the whole enterprise. The word determinism tends to recur. Then more recently there have been the conferences on the Genetics of Aggression and Violence which have been picketed, pilloried and otherwise abused. How do you see it?

Well, it's a continuation of general hostility toward anything that can be seen as doing away with free will – anything that is seen as a personal threat to your own self-expression. If you think, or come to believe, that the drive for self-xpression can be compromised by some kind of wiring diagram in your brain, in your neurotransmitter system, then that is perceived by some individuals, a small group, as threatening and something that should not be encouarged. It is very clear if you read the preface to the book, *Not in Your Genes*, that it is a political and ideological argument that is about to be vented. The authors all admit to their ideological Marxistic associations in the preface. Most people don't read the preface of books. They jump right in and think these are scientists, speaking as scientists. They are scientists but they are speaking as ideologues in that particular book and in many of their other writings, all of which I find generally offensive to those of us who have no such evil intent but who are interested in the welfare of our species.

I know Lewontin and Kamin personally through various encounters, sometimes pleasant, sometimes unpleasant. I am lucky in that I am seldom the focus of their hostility and criticism. I think it's because I'm careful in my work not to go beyond my data but also because they know me personally so they can't imagine me as being an evil person, affiliated with the Nazis or the racists and so forth. This constant use of the theme of determinism is political. As I was saying in my talk here at the Royal College, all of us are probabilists – none of us are determinists. We go way out of our way to find and to use any evidence that suggests that experience and environment in the physical sense are contributing to the variation in the individual's liability to developing any of these major mental disorders or even personality disorders such as antisocial personality. When you get in the same room with them, which I have done, they back off when you show them data. Although when they have the freedom to preach from their pulpit, as they do in the book which is as we all recognise an un-refereed document, they can insult anybody they want, in any way they want, short of the libel laws of the country. Libel laws almost never come into play to protect scientists from their politicised critics.

They have some good points and it's worth bringing out that most of us in this business have not until lately gone out of our way to worry about bio-ethical issues or think ahead to the implications for health insurance and the prejudice that accrues to anyone who is either a mental patient or a relative of a mental patient, if someone else has data to show that those disorders have an important genetic component. In fact when we now go about our business of genotyping relatives, we acquire information which would be very valuable to an insurance company but I would think you would be culpable of some kind of negligence if you allowed an insurance company to get information about genotyping that was an accurate indication of somebody's liability for developing schizophrenia or bipolar disorder. Lewontin and Kamin and their colleagues, especially in the Cambridge, Massachusetts area, have made a crusade out of this kind of genetic discrimination, as they call it. That's a good name for it and once those of us who are doing the work are aware of it, then we are very happy to join them in their cause but they don't give us the opportunity to because they are so busy attacking us on the assumption that we are evil and that we are producing evil with our data.

A lot of the hostility stems from the old nature/nurture wars with regard to the issue of intelligence. This is associated almost straightaway with racism and race prejudice, which was a big thing in the United States. It's probably liable to be a big thing in the UK as individuals with various ethnic backgrounds increase their frequency in the UK population. There are always rightist forces that are interested in maintaining the status quo and they will use anything that comes their way in their own defence. Unfortunately a lot of the data produced by individuals like myself can be misused in the service of these racist purposes. Then we have the burden of going out of our way to deny them the use of our data for their own purposes and point out how they have distorted our findings. This is also a point made in passing by Lewontin, Kamin and Rose and their colleagues but they very quickly get emotional in talking and writing about these things and I find that is very dangerous. When I find myself becoming emotional I realise that I'd better stop and sort things out and try to mount a reasonable defence against the prosecution knowing that I am likely to win when we go with the data rather than with assumptions of evil on our part.

In the US this is particularly tricky at the moment. I understand there was a major NIMH conference that was supposed to be held some years back that got put off because of concern about the reaction. It was aimed at looking at genetic inputs to social problems.

Yes, this was directly related to proposals to study the biology and the genetics of violence. Violence being a code word for all kinds of legal offences but especially in our country murder and drug dealing, which is correlated 1.0 with murder. I had been involved with this particular controversy from the beginning. It began through the curiosity of a political philosopher, David Wasserman at the University of Maryland. He was intrigued by all of the lack of resolution of issues and by the controversy surrounding the then Director of the NIMH, Fred Goodwin, a well-known psychiatric pharmacologist and author of the major treatise on manic-depressive disorder with Kay Jamison, when he spoke in an off-hand manner about the utility of analogising pharmacological and animal research on primates with regard to aggression. He spoke as if this was a model for life in the inner city, inner city being a code word in our country for African-Americans. He was set upon by the media and by black members of our Congress – so that anything that he touched was poison. Now he was interested in supporting this meeting, I believe, he saw it as something useful. That of course meant that it could not go forward.

In the meantime a very ideological, psychiatrically trained physician, named Peter Breggin, volunteered to go on one of the cable television channels aimed at blacks – Black Entertainment Television – to explain to the black audience that this meeting was going forward and that the motivation for the meeting included such things as the detection of future law breakers in the black school children population which would lead to them being incarcerated preventatively. It would lead to the development of pharmacology that would be used as a chemical straight-jacket, as he likes to talk about in his various books even before this time. This brought it to the attention of Dr Sullivan, an African-American, who was the Head of the Department of Health and Human Services, which was the overriding authority for NIH and NIMH at that time. Mr Sullivan convened a panel to look into this matter to see if it was dangerous, inflammatory, forbidden knowledge that was being generated. The panel was quite clearly prejudiced against letting this go forward and they came to the conclusion that it should not go forward. This meant a withdrawal of funds, which had already been appropriated by a peer review committee at the NIMH. I had already been told to buy my plane ticket for the meeting and then I received a phone call telling me to forget about it, that it had been cancelled.

It went into a deep freeze. The more Wasserman and the authorities at his university thought about it, the more they realised that this was a gross encroachment on academic freedom and freedom of speech, which is a very big deal in our country – it's guaranteed by the Bill of Rights. They mounted a counterattack, which by then was being presented to a different set of administrators.

Fred Goodwin in effect had been fired from his job. Mr Sullivan had gone back into the private sector and there were new people to be talked to. They agreed that if the programme, as originally formulated, would be opened up so as to invite as many people there who were against the idea of genetic involvement in aggression as there were for it, they could see going ahead with it.

Almost in a sense to replicate the meeting that Seymour Kety had put on in Puerto Rico?

Yes, very much like that. Although here we were involving political scientists and certain people in public sectors, involved in the criminal justice system and in the welfare system – all these things are, from my point of view, outside the realm of science. In order to be safe and not allow for unauthorised people to disrupt the meeting, they decided to not have it in the University of Maryland proper but instead to have it in the eastern part of the State of Maryland at an out of the way spot, so we could have a free and easy debate with papers being presented. I was invited to give the keynote address for the entire 2½-day session which meant that I was the only one authorised to speak for 1 hour. All the rest were given 20 minutes. I did my keynote address and I was severely criticised by members of the invited audience for going too far, for using concepts like heritability, without warning everybody that this was a toxic kind of statistic and so forth – even though I knew I had gone way out of my way to get a balanced presentation. I got through my talk and felt that I had been wounded by these unsympathetic listeners but figured all was fair in war and proper science and the meeting continued.

A lot of the people at the meeting were involved with the group in Boston and with individuals connected to them who wanted to associate anything we did in this area with eugenics. Their definition of eugenics was always Nazi-eugenics. There is a good side to eugenics, believe it or not, which nowadays we call genetic counselling. And that's done without a lot of hassle. But some time during the course of this meeting, someone had organised a disruption. The meeting was disrupted by a group of shouting men and women, some of them youngish college age, waving flags. Some of them carried the red banner of Marxism and declared themselves to be members of the Communist Party. I didn't know we still had one in America, but I guess we do. Others claimed themselves to be the victims of the pharmaceutical industry and psychiatry – that they were the ones who were wearing the chemical straight-jackets and they would have no more of this infringement of their civil rights. They objected to other things in loud voices using their own battery-powered microphone system. They completely dominated the meeting and brought it to a halt.

All of this was done in front of the television cameras. CNN had been authorised to cover the entire meeting from front to end, which meant 25 hours of video coverage from two different camera angles. They had promised Dr Wasserman that they would produce a documentary of the meeting and they more or less promised that they would end up with 2 hours of good video tape to be broadcast on CNN. Because of their presence they were authorised to be the video feed for the other national television systems – ABC, CBS and

NBC. These people, who interrupted the meeting, knew that they might make national television that evening but none of us appreciated that that would be the only thing that would be on national television. That's the way it turned out. None of the science, either by the pro or the con school of thoughts, made it, other than as very small soundbites. The majority of the coverage about 5 out of 6 minutes was about the disruption, the shouting, the ranting and the raving, with brief interviews from scientists who were in the camp of Lewontin and Kamin. They said to the press, who would speak to them, and the TV cameras about how this would lead to a revival of Nazi-eugenics, a seeking out of the people that have genetic potential for violence and aggression, and either their preventive incarceration or something related to sterilisation. They poisoned the whole atmosphere. It was a very disagreeable 2½ days . Nothing was accomplished. It was not like Puerto Rico. Nobody moved from their position towards some centre position. They ended up hating each other more than before.

Can you put a date on this?

October 1995. I still hear about this because people in the media hear about it who weren't around at the time and they want to re-awaken the interest. I have been asked to appear on television debating with people like Peter Breggin. I refused to do it. I don't want to inflame the situation. I don't want to give him any credibility by allowing him to appear with a scientist.

That brings me back to the work with Mednick. You have also done some work, not just on the genetics of schizophrenia but on the heritability of criminal behaviour.

Correct. This was one of the by-products of my Guggenheim year in Denmark. Through Mednick, I met this marvellous sociologist and lawyer, Karl Otto Christiansen, one of my heroes now. He had started the Danish twin study of criminality using all these wonderful resources. He was completely naive about anything genetic. His interest in doing the project was to show how unimportant genetic factors were compared to their alleged importance based on the old German literature from before World War II. Much of this literature was produced by people financed by the Nazi system. There was very much of a Nazi tinge or taint to some of this early work. The Nazis were very interested in minimising the effects of criminality and they had a premature biological and genetical view of this, to say the least. In the process they did some twin studies which suggested that criminality was a genetically influenced trait. But because they were naive in those days, they wanted to associate that with some simple Mendelian form of disease such as holds for Huntington's disease. There was no way for it to be that kind of disorder or condition. They also forgot the fact that the phenotype defined by the criminal justice system of the day was not anything like the phenotype that we would have among the mental disorders, where the criteria are spelled out by ICD-10 or DSM-IV. The law changes from time to time. At one time it was a severe offence to be a black person sitting in the front of a bus in the United States but that went by the board with civil rights legislation.

Anyway, through Mednick, I was introduced to Christiansen and quickly became his partner when he wanted to get a genetic angle into it. He was a very open person and he realised that there might be something there, even though he had always been pushing for a sociological explanation for crime. He also realised that you had to really do sommersaults to criticise the twin data up to that time, plus his own initial results were the strongest evidence in the literature that genetic factors could be importantly involved in felony offending in a country where there is no racial prejudice and no ability to blame a lot of it on poverty because of the system of socialism that had evolved with its social support networks and so forth.

By being involved with Karl Otto Christiansen I was able to write some important papers, one of which was a theoretical paper which I wrote with Ted Reich and Bob Cloninger in Washington University, using the techniques that Ted Reich and I had acquired from Douglas Falconer. Douglas Falconer is a famous British geneticist, still alive in Edinburgh, whose life has been spent developing statistics that go with analysing agricultural features and then he generalised that information to congenital malformations. He did this just at the time when Shields and I were analysing our data on schizophrenia in 1965. When I read the article the month it came out in the *Annals of Human Genetics*, I said to Jerry, 'Let's go and talk to the man, he's only in Edinburgh.' That was Jerry Shields' home town, born and raised. But he said, 'Oh no, he's an important man, he doesn't want to talk to us about schizophrenia.' I said, 'Let's give it a go.' So we communicated with him and he was very eager to see how we had applied his theory and model to the genetics of schizophrenia. He was very warm and welcoming. He thought that we had made some improvements in his model actually, which we did accidentally, not by design, but he incorporated those suggestions in his next version. So we were in on the ground floor, using this new system for converting qualitative data, plus or minus, into quantitative information to allow us to talk about the liability to developing a disease like schizophrenia or bipolar disorder in a quantitative manner. That further encouraged me to think quantitatively about this rather than in terms of single major genes. Because of this, I became with Shields a leader in the movement to think about these major mental disorders as the result of gene systems rather than the previous tradition of monogenic theories which had also been used by Eliot Slater to account for the origin of schizophrenia.

So Christiansen knew about my work on schizophrenia. He had already quoted it. He didn't expect to meet me and I never expected to meet him. I had heard about his work but I was not interested in criminality at the time, although I have always been interested in antisocial personality and aggressive behaviour on a continuum, since my work on normal adolescent twins way back in the 1950s. So it came full circle. Here I was involved again in antisocial behaviour and enjoying it and realising this is a very dangerous explosive thing to get involved with. Everybody thinks they know about it and you have such polarised opinions about the role of society and discrimination and poverty, homelessness and so forth but nobody had really tried to sort out what was cause and what was effect. Here we were in a position to be able to do it in a solid manner with a twin study, at the same time that Mednick and Barry Hutchings, an expatriate Welsh psychologist, were carrying out an adoption study of crime in Denmark.

We used the same field workers to look through the national criminal register and to identify all of these individuals through the Danish national address register. I learned at the time, because I had better connections to the genetic side of things than Christiansen who didn't have any connections, that he had missed out on a lot of subjects who were in the Danish twin register. He was not aware they existed until I brought in this information from colleagues in the genetic world – Harvald and Hauge. The work went forward but unfortunately Christiansen died while he was a visiting Professor at the University of Minnesota, working with me to finalise the data. It is one of the tragedies of my research career that this study has not yet been finished. I am hoping some day to return to it but it became politicised within Denmark. Some of the other people involved were not so open-minded as Christiansen and after his death they used that as an excuse to close down the project. We still managed to report the final results in chapters that I had written with Cloninger in a book edited by Mednick and in the context of chapters that I have written with Peter McGuffin for Michael Rutter's *Handbook* and with other American colleagues for other books. The data show that there is a clear genetic contribution to the liability to committing a felony offence, but especially to recidivist felony offences. This is the same as the results in the Danish adoption study of criminality, which uses a different strategy but one that complements the twin strategy

Is it over-simplistic then to say that there will be genes for antisocial personality disorder and they will be possibly discoverable soon?

I don't think it's a gross over-simplification. It's the way you would put it if you were applying for funds to the MRC or the NIH and you'd be found credible based on these data and studies that are already in the literature. The secret to it, as I see it, is to reduce the phenotype to endo-phenotypic components which are more manageable and which are less subject to the unreliability of psychiatric diagnosis. You can do this by taking the symptoms that feed into a diagnosis, whether it be ICD or DSM, and let the symptoms be the variable of interest rather than the phenotype at the higher level. With these traits then you are in a better position, not only to analogise to research we have conducted with mice and dogs, but also to get a piece of the total genetic picture with individual genes. My hope is that it will come about perhaps more rapidly with antisocial personality than with schizophrenia or bipolar disorder because the genes involved in neurotransmitters such as serotonin and dopamine are already identified and some of these have functional polymorphisms with an already known effect on parameters of CNS functioning and metabolism.

Where does Lee Robins' antisocial personality disorder construct come into this? There is an interesting story behind that: I understand she discovered all these records in a locked room or something.

Lee Robins has her PhD in sociology and ASP the topic of her dissertation, which was later published as a book – *Deviant Children Grown Up*. She made use of the cases brought to child guidance clinics in St Louis and then followed up many years later. She was not interested in genetics or biology. She was a traditional sociologist. But because of her work and her expertise on what we now would call conduct disorders and ADHD, or sociopathy, as it was called at the time she was doing her work, and partly because she was the spouse of Eli Robins, she became involved in the DSM-III committees. She used her dissertation results as the source for the symptoms that would become the criteria. As a result she has a huge influence on the American way of making a diagnosis of ASP, in that even now a gateway to receive a diagnosis requires that you meet the criteria for conduct disorder before the age of 15. Now it's clear that when you are making a diagnosis of conduct disorder in somebody who is aged 25 or 30, you are depending on retrospective information, subject to all kinds of distortion. Nobody ever asks the question for any of the structured interviews whether they are telling the truth to the interviewer. In fact it is only the MMPI that detects an untruth using some covert devices. So her role is significant but it may be a role which has to be modified in DSM-V and ICD-11 in order to take account of some things that are of current interest, involving say psychophysiology or some non-criminally related components such as cold-bloodedness. I bypass the problem in my own work by focusing on the symptoms themselves instead of on the formal diagnosis.

There is a further St Louis input there. Bob Cloninger's work heads more toward the symptom area and dimensional spectrums of symptomatology. How do you see that?

I was present during the entire pregnancy, delivery and childhood of Cloninger's ideas and was able to influence him to pay attention to the psychological roots of his evolving ideas. What Cloninger has done is to improve upon and embellish the ideas of Hans Eysenck and Raymond Cattell with some input from the MMPI via this other instrument that is competitive now with the Cloninger test called the Multi-dimensional Personality Questionnaire (Tellegen). Cloninger is the only psychiatrist who has paid attention to the whole realm of personality disorders. He rightfully saw it as the vacuum within the field and he has been able to capture a lot of the best that was already in personality psychology and bring it in to psychopathology, via his model. In the latest version of it he maintains that there are seven factors to be derived via factor analysis, whereas Eysenck only worked with three.

One feels that perhaps this is the way it has to go but with the profusion of axes one gets a slight Ptolemaic feel – extra universes are being added in to cope with the discrepancies.

I am sure that the next step will be for someone to come along and administer all these inventories to the same sample, conduct a great big factor analysis and see what they have and then do a secondary factor analysis to see what they really ought to have. But it may be that this is just keeping us busy while waiting for the pharmacologists and the molecular geneticists to tell us what we really ought to be including – which are the functional polymorphisms. In other words Cloninger is using the top-down approach, which is completely legitimate but with the techniques that we now have available we can work from the bottom up and do it more efficiently. We are bound to meet in the middle. We already are via the findings on DRD4 and some of these measures of novelty seeking and sensation seeking. Those initial findings may turn out to be flukes that cannot be cross-validated but something will come with these approaches.

It feels as though we are on the cusp of change?

I think we are. As we get so many scientists who need to publish or perish and so many gene markers and such easy access to automation of these tedious procedures, we are going to have rapid advances in the next few years. The prediction is that the human genome project will give us all the genes in humans by the year 2005. It actually may be earlier, 2004, if we have more automation coming on-line. All this is being driven by the pharmaceutical industry because of the huge profit that lies there waiting to be captured by the people who get to these functional polymorphisms first, because then that will lead to reverse genetics, which should lead to improved pharmacological treatment of these disorders.

Will it? In the case of disorders like peptic ulcers and tuberculosis, there's a genetic component to the heritabilty but this is a susceptibility component.

Correct. From the neighbourhood of 5% compared to the rest, a small heritable component compared to the real cause.

Sure, but even so, susceptibility is one way into the trap which is a disease. The way out of the trap, however, may not be back the same path through which you have come in. It could be but I can conceive of certain forms of rapid cycling manic-depressive disorder where there might be a thyroid axis component and perhaps the best way out of that is to put right what has gone wrong in the endocrine axis. And often in terms of disease the ultimate way out is surgical, which isn't the way anyone got into the problem but it can work pretty well. So while from an aetiological and theoretical point of view, there is a very compelling argument that the genetic route is the way forward, if one looks at medicine and how it works, it tends to be much more pragmatic. We don't really care at the end of the day about aetiology, we go with what works. There's clinical validity but also clinical utility.

But this is an advance on the simple form of empiricism because it's driven by the specificity of the genes involved in the gene to phenotype pathway. There's a big difference, as I see it, between the use of aspirin for reducing fever versus the use of an antibiotic for getting rid of the bacterial infection of a certain source. It is that difference.

But the antibiotic again will work across bacterial infections.

Correct, but for some there is less of a wide spectrum and more of a narrow spectrum approach and it is the narrow spectrum that I am hoping will come out of this wedding of molecular genetics with clinical psychiatry. There are no guarantees but it seems reasonable that it will be a short cut to looking for something else less like aspirin would be for schizophrenia.

What access do companies have to genetic material to use in drug development programmes?

There is another aspect of my work, which is not directly related to genetics, it is just my general interest in various forms of psychopathology. As a result of my having been on an Oversight Committee for the Institute of Medicine, which is part of the National Academy of Sciences, which is commissioned by our Congress to be a consultant to the Congress, I was involved in the committee that looked into the effects of the Vietnam War on the Vietnam Vet. Part of this was a concern about the alleged effect of Agent Orange, which was an ingredient in the chemical defoliants sprayed in Vietnam to improve the visibility of the ground for combat reasons.

Before I got involved with that committee, I had been consulted by the Veterans Administration to help them solve the problem of how you decide whether or not these numerous claims from veterans were legitimate compensable disorders or diseases. I suggested to them that they use the classical twin method with some modifications. Because of the number of men involved in the war, we would have access to twins where one had been exposed to combat and defoliant agents and the other one would have been, say, stationed in West Germany. They thought that it was a marvellous idea. They had never heard about twins being used like this. They went ahead and formulated a twin register for the Vietnam War. Meantime, parallel to this there was a study of a larger sample of men who are not twins to see whether or not there is anything different about them neuropsychiatrically or in other somatic domains. We looked at such things as sperm count, for example. Dermatologists looked for chloracne, which was the only pay-off in this area, and then we had oncologists looking for unusual incidences of cancers earlier than they should have appeared in this population.

None of these things worked out. But because of all the data collected, using psychological testing, including at my suggestion the MMPI, we had a huge battery of neuropsychological and psychological tests on thousands of men and even on some women, who were nurses there exposed to extremely stressful conditions. I am now in the process of analysing these data with my graduate students in clinical or other branches of psychology to make a secondary usage, because the data were very under-analysed once they reached the political decision to pay out all claims and not worry about whether Agent Orange did something to the individual. Now we are seeing a repeat of all this in the Gulf War syndrome, with similar questions being raised, and I have already made the suggestion that we now find all twins who served in the Gulf

War and the control twins who were in at the same time, to control for age and so forth, who were stationed someplace else. Without sounding like a broken record I see all kinds of continued use being made of this method.

Now in NIMH it was decided during the era of Lew Judd, who succeeded Fred Goodwin, who was also both biologically and non-biologically oriented – a man for all seasons – to invest heavily in collaborative research that would give us a head start over any other country in finding the genes for schizophrenia, bipolar disorder and Alzheimer's disease. At the same time another institute was interested in doing this for alcoholism. So there were four major initiatives, as they called them, launched. For the schizophrenia dataset, now that the original investigators have had a go at them, it is realised by the current management of NIH, Dr Varmus, that these data are too precious to just be kept under cover and to be used in the relatively amateurish fashion that we do in academia. So he has decided, and it has been agreed, that these data will be made available to any qualified scientist or scientific organisation and that included very specifically the pharmaceutical industry, not only that of the United States but in Europe as well. As soon as this was decided, they needed to have people who would vet the applications – Richard Wyatt and myself were designated as the people to review the applications for schizophrenia and the very first applications that came in were from the pharmaceutical industries.

So they really think that this is the way forward?

They really think it's the way forward and they are getting all these millions of dollars worth of information at no cost to them other than a trivial amount.

How did you say it was collected in the first place?

It was collected by a co-operative agreement among nine universities, including Washington University, of course, and NIMH itself with a group led by Elliott Gershon. These 10 sites collected the families, mainly affected sib-pairs. They collected the blood for DNA and they divided it into cell lines and stored it at a facility, the Coriell Institute in Camden, New Jersey. They then, under contract from our government, made available the DNA for $50 a shot per individual. With that comes all the diagnostic information collected and structured interviews and so forth.

There's another variation of the genetic input to pharmacology: pharmacogenetics or the genetics of individual responses to particular drugs. Is that another way forward? In addition to trying to find the best drug for the condition, we can find the best drug for you with this condition, as opposed to me. What might suit you, might not suit me.

Correct. This is a very important strategy and it's an area that is slowly gaining attention and qualified people but it was explored many years ago by Kalow, who has a book out.

It was also looked at by Linford Rees and Michael Pare, who showed that there were a group of people who were depressed who would respond to any antidepressants but there were some people who were depressed who only responded to MAOIs and some people who only responded to tricylics and that liability tended to run in families.

There are lot of those ideas and they came from the British system. I remember that one of our twin pairs was a subject of a case study where one twin was treated systematically with chlorpromazine and the other identical twin, who was also a schizophrenic, was treated systematically with reserpine. They found that chlorpromazine worked and reserpine didn't and they crossed over the other twin and she, indeed, responded. So, this tells you that this is a very important stategy for finding a family's medication. But that leads immediately to questions about possible racism because one of the things that you are bound to find here, as has already been found with some agents, is that they are very bad for some races and very good for others. This then brings to awareness that races are indeed genetically different, although many people would argue there is no such thing as race. In a certain sense they are correct. Race is something that's defined socially and race doesn't mean anything nowadays when there are so many mixtures of individuals. But still you find that some drugs are lethal for some individuals with certain racial backgrounds and for others they appear to be therapeutic.

How long do you think it is going to before we begin to get into the area of having blood tests to predict which antidepressant you should take, for instance?

I think it's almost immediate – because of the risk of liability involved.

Select bibliography
Gottesman II (1963). Heritability of personality: a demonstration. *Psychological Monographs*, **77**(9) 1-21.
Rosenthal D, Kety S (1968). The transmission of schizophrenia. *Journal of Psychiatric Research*, 6 suppl 1.
Slater E (1971). Autobiographical Sketch. In *Man, Mind and Heredity. Selected Papers of Eliot Slater*, (Shields J, Gottesman I, eds). Johns Hopkins Press, Baltimore.
Gottesman II, Shields J (1972). *Schizophrenia and Genetics: A Twin Study Vantage Point.* Academic Press, New York.
Gottesman II (1991). *Schizophrenia Genesis: The Origins of Madness.* Freeman, New York.
Torrey EF, Bowler AE, Taylor EH, Gottesman II (1994). *Schizophrenia and Manic-Depressive Disorder: The Biological Roots of Mental Illness as Revealed by a Landmark Study of Identical Twins.* Basic Books, New York.
Gottesman II, McGuffin P (1996). Eliot Slater and the birth of psychiatric genetics in Great Britain. In *150 Years of British Psychiatry* Vol 2. Athlone Press, London.
Gottesman II, Bertelsen A (1996). Legacy of German psychiatric genetics. Hindsight is always 20/20. *American Journal of Medical Genetics*, **67**, 317–322.
Faraone SV, Gottesman II, Tsuang MT (1997). Fifty years of the Nuremberg Code: a time for retrospection and introspection. *American Journal of Medical Genetics*, **74**, 345–347.

18 Juan Lopez-Ibor

Personality, disease and psychopharmacology

I often ask people why they went into psychiatry but in your case I wonder would it have been possible not to have gone into it – there's a certain history in the family isn't there?

Of course, my father was a psychiatrist. He had a brother who also practised psychiatry. My mother has a brother who practises psychiatry and I have two cousins who are also psychiatrists. Furthermore, I am the eldest of 12 brothers and sisters, of whom six are physicians and of those four are psychiatrists. I have a sister who is a psychologist and two daughters in the medical field, so it seems like a genetic disease in my family. There are other families like this. There is a Spanish family of physicians in the *Guinness Book of Records* because for more than a hundred years there has been a physician with the same name in succeeding generations.

Extraordinary. Is there a reason why this should happen more in Spain?

I have looked with my students at the question of why somebody becomes a doctor. Now it's more difficult to say because we have examinations which limit the entrance into medical schools so it means that you are not as free to choose as we were in the past. In the past, you freely decided whatever you wanted to do and usually physicians in Spain came from families where a lot of people were either physicians or teachers in schools or professors in the universities – professions devoted to the service to people. So I think that this was something that you saw at home when you were young. Then our families have stronger links than in other parts of Europe – we live with our families a longer time than the UK, for instance, and this also plays a role.

So when did you go into medicine?

I went into medicine in 1957. But I was not so much interested in psychiatry in the beginning. I was more interested in basic research. I think that is something which every physician has gone through – the possibility of fascinating research in biological science. Before I went to medical school, in fact, I thought about doing physics but it was not the right choice in a country like Spain. I also thought about archeology; I am a failed Egyptologist like many people in this world. Then suddenly I was fascinated by the CNS and I started neurology but I very quickly jumped to psychiatry.

How did the field look then?

It looked very complicated. I finished my studies in 1965. I was fortunate in one sense, which is that I had very extraordinary teachers in the medical school. At this time academic careers in Spain ended in Madrid. Every good professor had gone to one or two other universities and then ended his or her life in Madrid. So in Madrid we had the top-level professors in the country. It was a generation of physicians who had gone through the Civil War, had been characterised by their endurance and by big efforts to renew their own speciality. So although we were very large groups of students, even if the contact with the professor was not very intense, the spectacle of such a group of people was enough to give a big impact on yourself. I was glad of that. When I finished I went to Germany and there I was happy to find that my training has been as good as what you would expect from a country that was much more developed in this sense, as Germany was at these times. This was especially so on the theoretical rather than the practical aspect but if you wanted you could find time to develop practical skills in the hospitals with patients.

What was the primary orientation at the time in Spanish psychiatry? The European countries tend to split between those who were psychodynamically oriented and those that were more biologically oriented. Spain is interesting in that you have always had a tradition of biological research from Cajal and people like that ...

Well, in medical school we had two disciplines related to psychiatry. One was medical psychology which was taught in the pre-clinical years, as a basic science for medicine, and then psychiatry, as the specialty of psychiatry for all physicians. There was a great impact, I would say, from humanistic medicine, more than biological psychiatry. Most of the professors of psychiatry in this field at the time had had some training in Germany and were very much influenced by the German anthropological psychiatry – phenomenologically oriented and related to existential philosophy. This gave a very strong philosophical background for the speciality. This was seen as the goal of the training. It was very much linked to clinical activities and was quite a way from any reductionistic perspective, be it purely psychodynamic or purely biological.

Ramon-y-Cajal was not a psychiatrist, he was a prominent neuroscientist. He never showed any interest in psychiatry. In his memoirs, Kraepelin tells about a trip to Spain, where he wanted to meet Ramon-y-Cajal. He mentions that he was astonished by the ignorance Ramon-y-Cajal had of the developments in psychiatry in central Europe – he was not interested at all. He was primarily interested in neuroscience and histological research. He became a model for a generation of Spanish physicians in the sense that he was the scientist who brought science into Spanish medicine or even more into Spanish culture but he did not have much direct impact on psychiatry.

I'm Irish and, coming from a Catholic background, there was a certain feeling in the 1960s that brain chemicals were not something that people really wanted to think about closely. The fact that the brain might be just a bunch of chemicals didn't seem to fit very well with a spiritual view of man. Did that apply at all to Spain?

Not in Spain. No. My family has a strong Catholic background, actually my father gave advice to the Holy See on issues of marriage annulment, where he took a very liberal view, and birth control, where his view was more traditional, and both he and I have written on the interface between religion and psychopathology.

But the strong clinical background I described led some people in Spain, especially my father who started a very prominent school of thought, in the late 1940s, to the notion that neurotic disorders were not of psychodynamic origin – that psychoanalysis could not explain neurotic disorders. If dynamic factors are not the explanation, some biological background must be involved. At first he thought it was only some of the neurotic disorders that this applied to but his research led him eventually to say that in every neurotic disorder there is a biological element, which can be treated with psychotropic drugs. So he tried drugs and other kinds of biological treatments, such as sleep, ECT, and a minor form of ECT – acetycholine shocks which were used by Fiambertti in Italy to treat depression. This was a mild form of shock where the patient did not lose consciousness. It worked. Then when psychotropic drugs became available, especially the tricyclic antidepressants and MAO inhibitors, he started using them and these, in a sense, confirmed his ideas that some biological element was present and that this biological element could be treated.

How acceptable would that have been generally in Spain, at that time?

In general it became very widely accepted. But you have to add in another element, at this time – the late 1960s, which is that social psychiatry, political psychiatry, anti-psychiatry in Spain was also linked with the last years of the period of Franco's regime. This led to struggles in psychiatry, which were very difficult, in the sense that people in academia were seen often as people who had some kind of commitment to Franco's regime. It was not usually like that – in the case of my father, he was deported once because of some writings against Franco after the war. I think the university was quite independent from the influence of the regime – I think this was because Franco never thought that the university was a danger. Intellectual life was really unimportant for a Big General.

Perhaps he was right.

Yes it's peanuts – these people can speak and write but real power is something different. Nevertheless, a group of psychiatrists were not very happy with the regime and they politicized very much the discipline. This was in the period of anti-psychiatry and it led to very strong commitments and an important struggle, as happened in other countries. This was when biological psychiatry was born, as a reaction against political anti-psychiatry, in many countries.

In a place like Holland, someone like Herman van Praag had to have a police escort because there was a feeling that what he was doing was in league with Satan. This was not Christian.

This never happened in Spain. We were not, I was going to say so violent – except when we go to Civil War – but I think it was not this kind of problem. There were struggles in the media, in congresses, in meetings and in scientific journals. There was a lot of lobbying but it never became confrontational in the way it did here in Holland. Nobody lost his or her job, because of those kinds of things.

In the late 1960s, I was planning a double-blind comparative study on intravenous nialamide, an MAOI, with placebo or tryptophan. In order to test its tolerability we did a few cases. The first one was a lady from Seville who had been depressed for 11 years. The third day of treatment with 500 mg of nialamide and 6 g of tryptophan, she came to my office requesting to be discharged as she had no symptoms. She stayed four more days. She was discharged and the following day she phoned to tell that at a precise spot on the train back to Seville, the symptoms had reappeared in full severity. I told her to come back, which she did. I went through the treatment and I saw that for the last two days tryptophan had not been given to her because, being prepared in small amounts by the hospital pharmacist, it was reserved for patients who might need it more.

We discussed the case at the big weekly round. At the time the antipsychiatric atmosphere was intense and the majority stressed the influence of psychogenic factors and the fact of relapsing while she was going back to a home with many difficulties. In spite of all this, I decided to go back to the full treatment and see what happened. The third day came with no change – a difficult day for those of us who believed in biological psychiatry and serotonin but fortunately the day after the patient came to say that she was again relieved. She was discharged with nialamide and tryptophan and was followed up for three years with no reappearance of the symptoms.

You began to practise clinically in the mid-1960s. Fairly early on you were involved in one of the developments which have been seminal really – the work with clomipramine and OCD. How did you come to that?

This was following very much in my father's thoughts on biological treatment for neurotic disorders. This meant that every new biological treatment was tried in not only depression or whatever but also in other disorders. I had heard at the time that clomipramine could be used intravenously. Now, we had in our clinic very severe cases from all over the country and some from abroad. I told my father that a man called Sigwald in France had been giving clomipramine intravenously and that we should use it for our severe patients and for other patients and so we started with this. Very soon we saw that in obsessive patients it worked and people started to get better. Not in the sense that the obsessions disappeared but the patient became more able to resist the obsessions.

This effect of clomipramine is very different from its effect in depression and that is why we thought it was something specific. Just as any other anti-depressant, clomipramine washes away the symptoms of depression as an analgesic produces relief of pain. But in obsessive patients, it is different because the obsessions may remain very long, while the patient gains control over them. The first patient was a young man who would not touch some-thing that had been touched by another human being. He had long-standing washing routines. One day after hearing from him that his condition had not improved at all I saw him playing table tennis and I told him that I wondered if was not better as he was able to hold the racket that had been touched by other players. He said no, he was still washing. A few days later, I saw him after playing and he did not go immediately to wash his hands. Again, he insisted that the obsession remained the same but as the following game between two patients was so interesting, he decided to postpone his washing. A day later he admitted he had gained a lot of control over his obsessions.

That's how we started with clomipramine, then we did a double-blind comparing intravenous with oral but the person who had the codes suddenly died and we were never able to find the codes for these patients, which was a big disappointment. But what we described in this period still holds today, even though they were open studies which today isn't considered sufficient for any development of new ideas, but the proof of the pudding is in the eating. Just recently I have finished a double-blind study comparing clomipramine with one of the new antiserotonergic antidepressants and clomipramine seems to work a little bit better.

When you began to see this happening first, how did you explain it? At the time it was thought that most of those who had OCD were also depressed and many people would have thought an antidepressant was working on that component of the picture.

No. To us it was very clear that neurotic disorders were related to depression but they were different disorders. It was not that OCD was a form of depres-sion or something like that. At this period of time my main work was not in this area in fact, it was in the area of masked depression and I published a book on masked depression, but there was nothing about OCD in this book. It was very clear that the anxiety disorders, obsessive disorders, phobic disorders and so on were different from depression, were different nosological entities and the treatment was different. Also we didn't have an explanation why clomipramine worked so well and why the other antidepressants didn't. It was Yayuria-Tobias, an Argentinian, who said that it was probably the serotonergic aspect of its action that was important. At this time I was also working with serotonin – we had done a replication of some of the early Coppen work adding tryptophan and later 5-hydroxytryptophan to an MAO inhibitor and this worked very well but the idea of serotonin involvement in OCD was Yayuria-Tobias'.

At the time when you were using clomipramine for OCD, the impression I get is that Geigy weren't awfully interested in the drug, it was ...

I think they were interested in the drug but they were even more interested in masked depression. Actually the concept of masked depression, in some countries like Germany, became in the end not so interesting because the promotion of drugs to be used across fields went almost too wide, so that everything which could be treated with antidepressants became masked depression. This expanded the market but with little credibility in the end.

Where did you get your ideas on masked depression from in the first place?

Well, when I did my PhD, my father gave me the suggestion to do research in this field. Actually he had described in his work with neurotic disorders not only the psychological symptoms but also the somatic manifestations of anxiety, and he thought that there were also many somatic manifestations of depression and that these could be or should be well described because patients would not look for the psychiatrist as a first option in these cases – they would go to other physicians. That's how this whole field started for me. I started selecting patients from different parts and looking at them, their symptoms, how the symptoms changed, which ones remained, how they were combined with each other and so on – what were the tools for diagnosis. Geigy were interested in this because of their interest in the field of antidepressants. They had promoted a group, called the Committee for Diagnosis, Prevention and Treatment of Depression. This was a group set up by Kielholz and supported by Ciba-Geigy for many years. Now this group is supported by Eli Lilly. It's the group which started the teaching of depression for general practitioners.

An early Defeat Depression campaign?

Yes, it was around 1971/72. Now the World Psychiatric Association has joined efforts with them to develop a new educational programme in this area. It was supported by Ciba-Geigy for many years and some people in the company were extremely interested in this area of knowledge. They were less interested in OCD in the sense that OCD was considered to be a very rare disease. But I think they were interested in this drug for a period of time.

Have we gone too far in the recognition of depression in the sense that in the 1960s when people looked out at the range of nervous disorders there were in the community it wasn't obvious that these were all people who were depressed? A lot of them were thought of as being anxious but now everybody's seen as depressed and you rarely hear of a primary diagnosis of an anxiety disorder.

Well, there are several things involved with this. One is there is an overlapping of symptoms between the anxiety and depressive disorders. Second, patients with anxiety tend to develop in their evolution depressive symptoms. I think these symptoms should be considered more often than not a secondary depression. This happens in OCD, it is very clear, but it also happens in panic disorders. We have done a follow-up of anxiety disorder for many years. I have seen that they in the end have developed depressive symptoms, and somatising symptoms also. For a physician to use a drug which is called an antidepressant, although they could be called something else because they are not only antidepressants – they do other things – it's easier to justify if there is an underlying diagnosis of depressive disorders.

Indeed, but how do you rationalise the fact that these drugs work on more than one illness? What are they really working on? Clomipramine clearly works on mood disorders. It also works on people with OCD and ...

Well, the drug works on serotonin, which is clearly a very important neurotransmitter to modulate mood and behaviour. Second, most of these drugs, especially the tricyclics, are not clean drugs, they have multiple effects. Usually this is seen as not very desirable because of side-effects but sometimes it may be good because the influence on a number of different symptoms may help the individual to reach a better balance of function. In the past, the fact that there was a very striking modification of a severe disorder, major depression with melancholia, with a drug was a very impressive clinical development and this took precedence accordingly.

OK. Working on 5HT is one thing but is there some common psychological element that these drugs work on, some antecedent for both affective and neurotic disorders. Would it in any way make sense to say that Esquirol in 1838 made a mistake when he split off the affective disorders as something separate – that they are actually downstream from something else?

I don't like the expression affective disorders because affect is something more restrictive than mood. Mood can mean many things. The concept of mood in German for instance, Gemüt, sometimes refers to the whole of psychological life. Kant, the philosopher, uses it this way. He said that 'Geisteskrankheiten sind Gemütskrankheiten', which means that mental disorders were mood disorders in this sense. That's why I like the expression mood disorders as in ICD-10 and DSM-IV, with the affective in brackets – I don't think the word affective describes all mood disorders.

Another thing is that when you look into schizophrenia or other disorders, you always find some kind of abnormal mood in many of the symptoms or manifestations of these disorders. But even so these are different disorders, from an evolutionary or genetic point of view or from the point of view of their manifestations. The schizophrenic disorders, depressive disorders and anxiety disorders are distinct but always there may be some overlapping of symptoms. There may be some common mechanisms for these symptoms and in some cases it may be difficult to make a diagnosis of depression, for instance, but I think it is better to keep them as separate disorders. I am not very much in favour of the single psychosis, as Janzarik and others, such as Llopis in Spain and others have suggested.

There is a middle European concept which you don't find in the UK or in the US, which I have found it hard to get anyone to explain to me in a way I can understand – this is the concept of vegetative dystonia. What kind of relationship, if any, did that have to masked depression?

This has more to do with masked anxiety. In the work of my father with anxiety and neurotic disorders, this was one of the core issues. My father had spent some time with Hess in Switzerland and studied the hypothalamus and had correspondence with him on the areas which later McLean called the triune brain. It is also related to the studies of stress by Selye, the whole system which maintains our internal stability, our homeostasis. Sometimes the system does not work properly or over-reacts. Disorders of stress can kill the person because the reaction against stress becomes more important than external aggression and the individual may be killed not by the external agent but by their internal reactions. The corticoids are 'cell tranquillisers'. The other side of the coin is anxiety and anxiolytics. Bakan, a psychologist in Chicago, who migrated to Israel, wrote a book on the parallelism between Freud's and Selye's thinking, between psychological and physical homeostasis and the self-destructive mechanism in psychological homeostasis which Federn called thanatos. It is so destructive that it is called the death instinct. All this is related to the vegetative side of the anxiety disorders. Vegetative dystonia may be the expression of a masked anxiety but also of an abnormal stress reaction.

Is it a somatisation issue then?

Yes. It's the somatic correlates of anxiety. Every affective state has somatic correlates – tachycardia, sweats, movement, whatever you want. The philosopher Sartre interpreted the role of emotions as a need of the individual to survive in a world where rational interpretation is not possible anymore and the vegetative correlates of every emotion are the serious part of them. This implies that when an individual has to face the loss of a loved one, for instance, or an overwhelming threat, mechanisms appear to allow him/her to survive both at the psychophysiological and psychological levels – in the first case, the withdrawal from a world which has no meaning without the loved one; in the other, a preparation for fight or flight. It is always like that and the whole theory of psychosomatic medicine was born around this concept. My father studied this closely because as a clinician the somatic aspects of anxiety were very important to him. In this school of thought it is not only aspects of the psychodynamic state that can cause a problem. Psychosomatic medicine held that there were some states, some vicious circles which created and maintained the symptoms of what is called anxiety or stress in Anglo-Saxon words or nervous diseases in the old English tradition or neurasthenia or other concepts such as vegetative dystonia in the German-speaking world.

At one point Geigy marketed Opripramol for this – Insidon. Did it actually work for these conditions – neither the drug or the conditions ever got to the UK or the US.

It was very good and very widely used for people with minor anxiety symptoms. I can tell you an anecdote. Once a healer came to me who wanted his wife treated. She had a mild depression and I told him, 'You know very well how to deal with this – I am sure you see lots of these people.' He said, 'Yes and I also know which things work and which things don't work but with things that I usually have success these have not worked with my wife, that's why I come here.' So I asked him what he did with his people and he said, 'Well, I tell them what they have or I tell them what they have to do to get better and then I give them Insidon.'

This popular healer had very quickly learnt that this drug worked for states of anxiety and mixed anxiety and depression with a lot of somatic manifestations. It is very interesting that when you look at DSM and ICD-10, in anxiety there is always the mention of the importance of somatic symptoms but this is much less the case in depression.

This is where your work is interesting because you have always emphasised the somatic and vegetative symptoms of the mood disorders as well, but I'm still finding it hard in my own mind to tease these apart from the vegetative components of anxiety.

Well, there is an overlapping of anxiety and depression. But essentially they are different because most of the symptoms of anxiety show a hyper-reactivity to external stimuli, the body is hyper-responsive, while in depression the main characteristic probably is inhibition – dry skin, dry hair, constipation, pain – everything which has to do with inhibition.

Is Insidon an antidepressant or an anxiolytic?

I don't know. It was marketed very quickly with very few studies. The idea was a very funny one because Insidon has the structure both of an antidepressant like imipramine and an antipsychotic like chlorpromazine. It wanted to be a drug which worked for depression and for schizophrenia at the same time but it did not work for severe depression or for schizophrenia. It was marketed and it worked for these mild anxiety symptoms.

Is there a certain sense that during the 1960s you had a range of compounds, such as amitriptyline, clomipramine and Insidon, all of which were similar in some respects, but which have turned out to be rather different clinically and perhaps we are just beginning to appreciate more today how different they are to each other? But in the 1960s, the companies in order to get a market had to decide on the compounds fitting into one or two groups. They were either antipsychotics or antidepressants. There was no room for anything else.

No, we had room for something in between. We had Insidon, we had Melitracen, which was a drug which was marketed in Germany. You had some groups of drugs which were used for mild psychiatric conditions but all of these disappeared when the benzodiazepines came to the market. There were others like meprobamate which were used for minor psychiatric disorders and which were also called minor tranquillisers. All these vanished when Librium and Valium came on the market but these conditions and agents existed and should not be forgotten about.

Let me move into another area where there is overlap and confusion. In your ECNP plenary lecture yesterday you addressed the topic of the personality disorders. When did you begin to move into that area?

Personality disorders may be linked to the anxiety disorders and masked depression as there are behavioural masked depressions, which are quite common in childhood and adolescence. The mood disturbance is expressed, not as a complaint of mood disturbance or as vegetative symptoms but as behaviour, which is unexplained. Second, when you treat patients with psychiatric disorders, where you have also some kind of personality disturbance and this changes also during the treatment, you have to postulate that they have something in common. A third point is that dualism remains very much present in psychopathology. Kurt Schneider, for instance, in his description of personality disorders and neurotic disorders, was dualistic and this has created many difficulties in this area.

My father and I published in 1974 a book on the *Experience of the Body*, which has some philosophical aspects to it – it was influenced by the German anthropological approach. It covered body image, body experience and so on. One of the chapters was about the limits of dualism. From this point of view it followed that it was necessary to look into the biological substrate of personality, the way we are shaped. We are not shaped in two parts but in one part. From this came my scientific interest in this field. We then went on to some studies with CSF in depressed patients, using serotonergic probes – such as fenfluramine. We were interested in suicide and we did some studies trying to look at suicides in subjects who were not depressed. These people did not fit the criteria for depression – that was an exclusion criterion – but they all could get a diagnosis of personality disorder. In a sense it was a waste basket diagnosis when you take away psychosis and depression but these people are something – most of them were borderline, some were hysterical and the findings were interesting.

Then gambling started in Spain. After the death of Franco, casinos slowly opened and people started gambling and, of course, some after a few years became gambling addicts, pathological gamblers. I have been interested for many years in this because a behaviour like gambling is like an addiction without the drug. It seemed a good model to study this kind of behaviour, without the influence of the drugs. Dr Saiz in my unit and I became very interested in this group and we set up a programme for pathological gamblers with psychological and biological treatments. One day we decided to compare these with more 'normal behaviours' in bullfighters and explosives experts, who also take risks but in their professions. This study was done with Drs Carrasco and Saiz who had done his PhD many years before correlating personality variables and biological findings in normal subjects. So the idea of studying the biological aspects of non-major psychiatric patients had been present in our group for some time.

Explosive experts did extremely well on the psychological tests. They proved to be highly controlled, low in sensation or novelty seeking and very rational people. This was natural if we remember that these individuals have been selected through a strict procedure and intensively trained. Bullfighters, on the contrary, were high in sensation and novelty-seeking and extroversion. The controls were in the middle but the gamblers performed even higher than the bullfighters on sensation and novelty-seeking.

The results from platelet MAO activity were very interesting as pathological gamblers had the lowest activity and as a group the smallest variance. The rest had higher levels of activity distributed under a wide bell-shaped curve. In the three non-patient groups there was a correlation between MAO activity and novelty and sensation seeking. We interpreted this as a consequence of two phenomena – a dimensional model that could be applied to non-patients with a correlation between biological and psychological measurements and categorical differences between healthy subjects and pathological gamblers.

Some time later I became a member of the Royal Academy of Medicine in Spain, a very important and honourable institution in our country. When you are elected, you have to make a speech, usually of a historical value and devoted to a consideration of a specific topic. I thought that the most challenging would be to describe this area, so I devoted some time to put in order my ideas and to fit the pieces of our research together. That's how the interest developed. It has really been a fascinating group of people because they have been very neglected. They are very difficult to study because they are very difficult patients to relate to, they create a lot of problems in the doctor–patient relationship, they are difficult to follow in the lab and so on, but in the end they are a group who suffer a lot because of this disorder of personality.

When you began to move into that area were you aware of any one else working in the area?

Yes, of course. I was very much aware of Eysenck's work. I had been at the Maudsley, so I met him in some of his sessions and lectures. I still remember one day when he came in and said that now for the first time we have data which show that behaviour therapy is better than phenelzine. He was elated by this. But he had an interest in correlating traits with biological variables and he had a very good statistical approach to this work and I was very much aware of this. More recently I was aware of the work of Zuckerman, who helped to open up this field and then of course the work of Cloninger, Siever and Davies. I was also aware of the studies of suicide and impulsivity by Cocarro, Marie Åsberg and others. I was also very struck by the study of Brown in the States, who showed in a population of non-patients, men in the Army, that there was a correlation between violence, impulsivity and low 5HIAA, the metabolite of 5HT in the CSF. It was the first time that such a strong correlation was found in people who could not be considered as patients.

In one sense you are saying, it would appear to me, that one of the conclusions you can draw from all this is that biological research on the psychoses is doomed if we are not controlling for personality.

In a sense, yes. You could say that genetic research, for instance, is more related to personality – i.e. in the vulnerability hypothesis of schizophrenia. In the Danish study on schizophrenia, the genetic element is manifested in schizotypal personality disorder, which may or may not become a schizophrenia, depending on some other external circumstances. So perhaps in this sense, the genetics of the personality is more important than the genetics of the disorder.

In one sense that has to be true when you think about it but we don't think about it that way now, which raises a range of other questions. When I suggested to you earlier that someone like van Praag was seen as being in league with Satan when he was looking at the biology of the major disorders, there is almost a deeper problem it seems with the biology of personality and temperament where people have felt there are Nazi connections or something like that. Irv Gottesman or Markku Linnoila working on this in the US have to be very very careful what they say to which groups when, because it is seen as having a right wing agenda of some sort. You must be even more aware of this than I am.

The States is a very strange country in this context. When you look at the discussions between the creationists and the evolutionists – it's actually a ridiculous discussion from every point of view, scientific and religious. They tend to take the part for the whole of things. They have a very narrow scope sometimes . The fact of being biological does not mean that something is inherited genetically. The best research on this question or hints about what can happen are the studies of Sapolsky, which I learned about because of our studies on this group of violent suicidal people. We found in this group not only a blunted endocrine response after challenges but also a very strange pattern of cortisol secretion. Compared to controls at baseline, they have a high cortisol and when challenged this cortisol did not increase, while the controls had lower baseline concentrations which after a challenge increased significantly.

I looked everywhere to find an interpretation of this and similar findings. I found it, a little bit by chance, in one of the studies of Sapolsky, who studied endocrine variables and social status. As this is very difficult to do in human beings, he went to the Serengeti National Park in Kenya to study the baboons. There he found that baboons high in the hierarchy, in normal conditions, had low baseline cortisol concentrations in blood and high testosterone concentrations. Those lower in the hierarchy had the opposite – high cortisol with low testosterone. Under stress those high in cortisol increased slightly or not at all whereas those who were low went high. These latter had a good adaptation to stress but those with high cortisol were clearly chronically stressed and they could not react to another external stress – they were working at the ceiling of their possibilities.

You might think that some baboons are born maladapted and that's why they go higher, but that's not true because sometimes baboons organise revolutions just as human beings do and in the revolution everybody has high cortisol and low testosterone. I often say that the hippies were right when they said make love and not war, because you cannot have high cortisol and high testosterone at the same time. After the revolution the same patterns reappear but this pattern was independent from the pattern that the same baboon had before. So social rank has an impact on the pattern of secretion of cortisol and testosterone. Sapolsky developed this looking into CRF and other mechanisms and established that this is a brain mechanism. So there is a biological background to how individuals respond to stressful situations but according to social rank.

Now in our studies, the controls were mostly medical students and young physicians, who are very privileged people in society, which protects them, teaches them, puts them in big hospitals with the best teachers. They are very high in terms of social privileges, compared with the people who are unable to face frustration, which means unable to cope with some external stressor – these were the ones who were admitted to hospital because of impulsive suicide attempts. So although we have biological findings, the origin may be social. It's not fate that you are born like that and you will be like that necessarily.

But in order to understand these issues, you think we must understand the biology?

Yes of course.

Why has the study of temperament been so underplayed in the last 40 years? Is it because of the Nazi programme or is it because the drugs, when they came out, in contrast to what Eysenck's theories would have predicted, which is that we would find drugs which would alter personality, in actual fact the drugs were agents to treat specific diseases or at least they were sold that way. Is it because it has seemed easier to go down the disease route that we have neglected the biology of temperament so much? In the mid-1950s, it was very respectable to look at constitutions, at body build and things like that, but all of that's gone out of the window, at least at the moment. What's the reason for this eclipse?

Well, there are difficulties with this kind of research. It is very easy in a sense to work with somebody who is a patient now who was not a patient a few months ago and then when you give treatment and see a change and the person becomes what he or she was before the illness, you can take a measure and you can study a lot of things. But in the area of personality it is very difficult and this has to do very much with the notion of dimensions of personalities and traits. Traits are present everywhere. We all share the same traits with a little bit of variation but this is not stable. It may change with the time of the year, the time of the day or the environment. So work in this area is very difficult to do and that's why Sapolsky went to do it in baboons, because it's much more simple.

It's also very difficult to put boundaries into these issues. One of the outcomes of our studies is the notion that dimensions are present in everyday life but you have a categorical difference when you jump into the pathological field. Coming back to the study of bullfighters and explosives experts, when I presented this at an APA meeting somebody said, 'Now you have a treatment for these bloody bastard bullfighters who cause such suffering to these poor bulls; are you going to give them fluoxetine?' I think the answer to this is that fluoxetine may help a pathological gambler or may help an impulsively suicidal patient but it will never make out of a bullfighter an explosives expert. That's the difference.

What drugs do is to control some tendencies and what you see in diseases is that all these things which are a little bit more or less in us sometimes become autonomous, to use the expression of the English psychiatrist, Gillespie – he talked about the autonomy of these states as in autonomous depression. This means that we all react to the environment with sadness on occasions but sometimes this sadness becomes autonomous and then it's a vicious circle, which is difficult to get out of. When you treat personalities with drugs, what you see is that some of these traits which have become too autonomous, too conflicting, are reduced and the person is able to find a new balance – a balance within himself or herself or in a relationship with other people. This is not the same as getting relief from a well-characterised symptom.

How do you read the fluoxetine phenomenon? Because this, in one sense, could be seen as the return of the repressed idea that maybe drugs could act on the personality rather than on a disease.

Yes, *Listening to Prozac* was a very unfortunate book, in the sense that based on real descriptions of things that everybody has, Kramer expanded these points to a theory that personality can change, which means that human beings can change and the world can change because of a single drug – that we will be able to influence creativity and that people will never be the same again, which is nonsense. But the fact is that we can take away certain traits of personality when they are present in an extensive and dominant way in people. Now this can be considered as a disorder of the personality but treatment will not change the whole personality of an individual.

In your lecture yesterday you mentioned that in recent years there has been a migration of certain personality disorders from being seen as Axis II disorders to Axis I disorders. When did this begin to happen and has it been happening because the drugs have begun clearly to have an effect on what have seemed to be personality disorders – like the RIMAs for avoidant personality disorder – giving people the feeling that personality disorders perhaps are treatable entities?

There is another issue we should touch on first, which is the distinction between personality disorders and variants of personality. This is often confused and it is confused in DSM-IV and this I think is an error from the conceptual point of view. There are difficulties present but this does not mean that we should not try to identify a group of people who have disorders of the personality, which are not just a little bit different from the norm, as we all are from each other. This confusion is what leads to the kind of generalisation in Kramer's book. When you don't make this distinction and you find that some personality disorders have a biological pattern or respond to some kind of treatment, what happens? People say, well, these were not personality disorders after all. They are something else. So that is why certain personality disorders have been moved over to the illness axis.

My approach to this would be to keep these disorders in the personality disorders group, and say that they have a biological pattern which can be treated just as the major psychiatric disorders can. I have nothing against having schizotypal personality disorder either as a personality disorder in DSM-IV or as schizotypal disorders within the spectrum of schizophrenia as it is in ICD-10. I don't mind having epileptic personality or organic personality disorders within the chapter of personality disorders. You could have cyclothymic personality, or dysthymic personality instead of dysthymia or cyclothymia, provided you explain what these are and how they can be treated, how they can be diagnosed and so on. There is also avoidant personality, which is becoming one of the anxiety disorders. But I think this migration is bad. In the end there will appear to be no personality disorders but I think we will come back to Kurt Schneider's expression 'personality disorders are dead, long live personality disorders'.

Did he actually say that?

He says that every generation tries to kill the concept of personality disorders.

You find within psychiatry that people react viscerally against the term personality disorder. Many people feel you are doing patients a great disservice to label them as personality disordered.

In DSM you are forced to label people when you give them an Axis II diagnosis. You don't have this in ICD-10 in this sense because in the multi-axial version you have Axis III, where you have environmental conditions and life-style, you can always tell the person his or her life-style makes them vulnerable for certain disorders or problems. This is not a diagnosis. Type A behaviour, for instance, this is not an illness or a personality disorder, it is a life-style. You can discuss why some people have this life-style and others have another but this is not a clinical diagnosis. But where do you put type A behaviour in DSM? – either you cannot put it anywhere or you put is as a personality disorder, which it is not and this is really not a very good approach.

As I've said, the whole area of personality is one that people haven't wanted to talk about for 10–20 years, but is the vulnerability hypothesis in one sense the politically correct language for referring to this area?

Well, yes. You have personality disorders and variants of personalities and of those some are relevant for medicine, some are irrelevant. Those which are relevant for medicine are relevant because they imply a certain vulnerability or they are often associated with disorders and you will have to manage these aspects of the case when you are dealing with risk factors or dealing with the rehabilitation of patients and that's why some are relevant and others are not. But it depends on what you are doing. If you have to lead a team, all kinds of personalities come in – they are relevant for your work but they are not personality disorders. I think we have to make the distinction very clearly between these personality traits which may look abnormal and pathological but not to the degree of the higher psychiatric disorders. They are limited to this aspect of a situation, they are different from other personalities, they may be very awkward or very different but nevertheless they are not pathological.

Now, despite working in an area that is politically tricky and despite coming from Spain, you have been very influential on the world psychiatric stage. You are involved in the WPA. You were involved in ICD-10, which along with DSM is one the major political blocs in psychiatry.

I have been one of many persons in a very large task-force. Secondly ICD-10 is very much influenced by DSM-III, which is is quite natural. The change from DSM-II to DSM-III was the important change, a change of historical proportion. DSM-IIIR, IV and ICD-10 are improvements but the real change was from DSM-II to III. Nevertheless, there are some differences which are important, which came about because the task-force for ICD-10 was much more international. Many different schools of thoughts had to be accepted – the clinical psychopathological tradition of Europe is more present in ICD-10 than in DSM but if you look at the task-force of ICD 10, the largest number are people who were involved came from the United States. This was very natural and it should not be seen as opposing blocks. In ordinary clinical conditions, it is irrelevant whether you use one or the other. The differences are minimal and really only present in situations where we have no data to make a decision. There are some other cases such as neurasthenia, which is not in DSM because nobody uses the term neurasthesia in the States but it is in ICD-10 because in some parts of the world it is used.

There are two main differences: one has to do with this personality issue, which is tricky and difficult. It is difficult to produce research to convince people and it is difficult to say that one perspective has more advantages than the other. This remains open for dicussion. Another one has to do with the degree of disability, which is important for making a diagnosis in DSM but not in ICD-10. This is because disability is related to the environment and this may change from one country to the other, so it is more difficult to establish a criterion for disability. In the States, if you don't have either suffering or disablement, the symptoms count for nothing because they don't want to be accused of making a disease of a social condition. For instance, when does shyness become social phobia? – is it when it produces a lot of suffering to the person, or when it produces a significant disability for the performance of a job? This question of disability as a criterion for diagnosis is not taken up in ICD-10 but both points of view have good reasons to exist. We are are in a transitional period for some years and we will need to find a good solution to solve this.

Can I ask you about Gerald Klerman? He was one of the key driving forces behind DSM-III. What did you make of the man and his approach. He was very Kraepelinian in one sense.

Klerman was a very intelligent psychiatrist, very knowledgeable, very interested in everything and with very large views. I see him as one of the most European Americans in this context, no doubt. But the idea that all research had to be done based on symptoms etc. I would describe more as the Robert Spitzer style than the Klerman style.

You were involved as well in the alprazolam studies for panic disorder, which were set up by Klerman. What did you make of all that, because the disability issue comes in there as well?

Sure. I was involved in that. It was a period that was very bad in Spain, there was very little money for research. Things had changed with the death of Franco and nobody knew where research was going, we were in a bit of disarray, so it was an opportunity to do a large study with a very large international group with opportunities to travel, to meet people, and this study was therefore a very important experience for many of us in Spain. The study was disappointing, however, for a number of reasons because it did not show any important advantage for alprazolam over imipramine and the follow-up was not encouraging. The placebo response was also very big in this study, which of course is something you would expect in this kind of patient given that there was a lot of interaction with doctors. When a patient went through this study, he had gone through more hours with the doctor than in most kinds of psychotherapy. It was more than 5 hours per week. Of course I would say nothing negative about the skills of a psychotherapist but there is the question of personal contact as much as the question of the actual skills to do all this. I mean, the patients will need to be reassured and so on. It was very funny to see that this placebo response was different from one unit to the other and from one country to the other, which showed very clearly how patients were recruited and treated in each country, or how humane was the group treating the patient or how rigid and less humane.

On the question of disability, panic disorder is a very disabling condition and Klerman's studies proved the degree of disability and the suicidal risk. This appeared in the study and it appeared in all the countries involved. Societies are human constructs, what people believe about themselves and the world, and the nature of the world plays a role but certainly this disorder was very similar across the world regardless of the setting.

That's kind of surprising, I guess.

Not if you really think this is a disease. Yes, if you think that it is a human condition, in which the social side plays the primary role.

What did you make of the controversies that grew up between Klerman and Isaac Marks and the correspondence in the British Journal of Psychiatry? There isn't anything else quite like it in the psychiatric literature.

I was sitting with Marks when Klerman presented the studies at the APA meeting and we were discussing these things. Marks, I think, was in a period of positive disappointment. All his studies of behaviour therapy with OCD were in a period where the serotonin bandwagon was begining to roll, so his research and the other things they had in OCD were not so attractive for many people in this period. So, he was trying to protect his position in the field. He is a real fighter and a very knowledgeable person and I think he was able to pull out of himself the best of himself to make a critique of these studies, although I think he went a little bit too far. The results of the study were clear and evident – they were not as promising as Upjohn had hoped, although they were solid and important and relevant. People are now using alprazolam to treat panic all over the place. One has to think of the setting and whether the patients are suited. Every general practitioner in the country can treat panic disorder with alprazolam or maybe with some of the antidepressants but in most parts of the world, even in the United Kingdom, there are not many units, like Mark's unit, to do behaviour therapy.

Secondly, we are in period of time where we are starting to realise that behaviour therapy as such does not exist. Biological psychiatry as such does not exist either. It is specific drugs for specific diseases. Specific techniques for specific problems of specific disorders and this kind of specificity lead to the notion that what works in OCD does not work in phobias and what works in phobias does not work in depression. The development of techniques which will be better applied for different disorders and should be available in the training of physicians is coming but we are not yet at this stage. So there was the scientific discussion of panic on the one hand and the other aspect was what is relevant to medical practice in many parts of the world.

Coming back to the international perspective, the ICD-10 meetings have to have been rather extraordinary in that you had the input from all different traditions in the world. The Chinese, for instance, have more neurasthetics than all the patients we have got in Europe put together probably.

Very much so and then I was also present in meetings to discuss DSM-IV and ICD-10 – to find some consensus. That was also very interesting because you learn very quickly where the limits of our knowledge are and where we need more knowledge. ICD-10 and DSM are different because we don't, for instance, have the knowledge to decide whether 2 years' or 2 months' worth of symptoms are needed to make a diagnosis or whether we need three symptoms out of ten or five out of fifteen or whichever. All these differences are there because the problem has not been subjected to enough research but it will be clarified in the future, I hope.

Can you fill me in on your involvement in the World Psychiatric Association and what you perceive its role to be in world psychiatry?

Well, the World Psychiatric Association began in 1950 as the society to organise World Congresses in Psychiatry. The first one was in Paris and it was a Congress of Reconciliation between German and French psychiatry after the war. Then it grew up in a very important way during the period of Cold War confrontation with the dissidents issue. This consumed a lot of energies and money from the WPA. Once it was solved the WPA was ready to play a role in education and in facing new challenges.

One challenge has to do with the common diagnostic language all over the world. Another has to do with trying to promote the exchange of information around the world. Another has to do with increasing the ethical standards of the profession. A concern with the ethical issues began in the 1970s with the Hawaii Declaration, which was born in the period of the political abuse of psychiatry. Now this has almost disappeared and all over the world the foremost issue is the discrimination and stigmatisation of patients which is addressed in the Madrid Declaration. This is a more refined Declaration. Discrimination against psychiatric patients is present all over the world and the Declaration raises the status of the patient with psychiatric disorders to an equal partner of the psychiatrist, which is a very important concept and very well formulated.

This was put out at the recent (1996) World Psychiatric Congress in Madrid?

Yes, that's why it's called the Madrid Declaration. The WPA has an Ethics Committee who looks at these issues, who is concerned with challenges for the profession. Each time Ethics Committee members are appointed, they change every 6 years, they start afresh and look at what are the issues and that's how this Ethics Committee produced this Declaration.

There were issues which were not present in the Hawaii Declaration, such as organ transplant, sex change, and addressing these led them to consider how they might find a more general formulation. The original resolution was born from a group who had very much the notion of political abuse in psychiatry but this could change and when new people came in the Ethics Committee changed very much. In the first version psychiatry was seen as an agent of social control but in the second the status of mental patients was considered in a more positive way. So it was with all this in mind and all this background, that the Madrid Declaration was born.

One of the critiques you could raise about groups like the WPA is the potential for diagnostic imperialism. The people who can put the resources into an education campaign, at present, are the drug companies who are wedded to a Kraepelinian model which is working very well for them and their compounds at the moment. Are you going to educate the world to suit the industry?

Well, the WPA is better prepared than many other international institutions and the reason is that we are an association of member societies, which may be less easy to influence than a single large organisation. But in the case of many of these member societies, their interests go beyond what has to do with drug treatments for psychiatric disorders. They have other interests and they have other views. Then you have a lot of sections in the WPA and most of them deal in topics which are not relevant to biological psychiatry, nor for psychopharmacology – the place of women in psychiatry, forensic psychiatry, social psychiatry, victims of abuse , epidemiology and many other things. So we are less prone to the kind of influence you mentioned – the idea that there are specific disorders, which should be treated by a specific drug, which happens to be produced by a specific drug company.

The WPA had produced guidelines to address specific issues for which we need sponsorship, which companies could help sponsor. But, for instance, at the World Congress we had CME credits for the American participants and we had to produce conflict of interest declarations regarding sponsorship following the standards of the American Medical Association. The application of these standards may not be perfect but still there are some standards that address this issue. In the Congress in Madrid we tried to identify very clearly which were the industry-sponsored symposia, which were industry supported and we are going along this path as much as we can. We have to be independent from all these pressures and I think we are better than many other associations. For instance, if you look at the composition of the WPA Executive Committee you will find more often than not people who have not been involved in drug research or in psychopharmacology and the same happens with the leadership of most of our member societies – the Royal College of the UK, the APA in the States, or the Royal Australian College of Psychiatrists ...

In the case of this ECNP meeting here, there seems to be a disease model-oriented form of psychiatry, very Kraepelinian in one sense, more than in any other society I can think of really; there's a greater focus on the disease entity and the drug treatment of the disease and much less on, for instance, the basic sciences input.

Well, the ECNP is a neuropsychopharmacology association like the CINP or ACNP. There is perhaps less focus on diseases in ACNP because if you compare the huge amount of basic research done in the States with the amount done in Europe then you can understand why the impact of basic research is very important in ACNP, much more so than in ECNP. The drug company presence could be as large here but drug companies in the States are doing more research compared to the research in the central nervous system in the European companies, and so you can understand why many people who work in the laboratories of drugs companies in the States go to ACNP, but for many laboratories working in the central nervous system in Europe they are probably all here but you cannot see them.

Second, those are associations which are in the field of neuropsychopharmacology, which is about the rational application of and the development of drugs for treatment of disorders, and I think that the concept of specificity is very important to do with disorders. If you don't have a diagnosis, you have the

Kramer approach. We need a diagnosis. We are not like psychoanalysts or psychiatrists who don't need a diagnosis, who think that a diagnosis may harm the patient and who just apply psychoanalysis to everybody who is willing to come and pay money. That's not the approach of medicine. The approach of medicine always is related to specificity, to the notion of morbid species. So I don't see a real problem in this. I see a discussion on how psychotropic drugs should be applied to the treatment of schizophrenia or depression or panic disorder because it is essential in clinical trials to compare drugs and to ask whether drug A is a better drug than drug B. In order to get an answer you have to ask for what condition or for what symptoms of what condition we are talking about. So I don't see that specificity by itself is bad. It may be abused but that's a risk.

One of the things that hits me about that is that there have been clearly a lot of people from the Spanish-speaking world who have been working fairly intensively in psychopharmacology but the credits for some of these developments don't go to people who have published in Spanish. You mentioned Yayuria-Tobias earlier.

Well, one reason for this was the conditions to do the work, which were much more difficult. In my academic career I had to move several times. I am now on my fourth place, and in the first three I had to start my department from zero – no staff, no facilities, nothing. So it took a lot of time to create something and then once it was created I moved. There was that lack of stability. This has changed. Our country is very different from what it was 30 years ago but this created problems for anyone who wanted to do research of sufficient quality to be accepted. Then many things were published in Spanish and while we think the Spanish language is a very important one, not everybody thinks the same thing or reads Spanish.

In one respect it may be the most important language in that probably there are more people actually practising psychopharmacology in Spanish, but it has been the Anglo-Saxon and German influence that seems to control the organs of publication and things like that. This is relevant here in that when you go into the history of biological psychiatry for many of the developments, such as sleep treatments, ECT, psychosurgery, the earliest use of the phenothiazine nucleus by giving methylene blue in affective disorders, you can usually find a Spaniard or Italian who has done the first work in the area but they usually don't get the credit. In addition, among the founder members of the CINP there were quite a few people who were from the Spanish-speaking world. Who for you have been the key thinkers?

In psychopharmacology, biological psychiatry or in psychiatry in general, I would prefer to speak of groups. For instance first in South America, you have in Chile a group of very good thinkers, in psychiatry and in psychopathology. In Chile they have very good medical schools and the training of physicians is excellent and they are good in other specialities as well. In Buenos Aires, which is the city where you find the greatest variety of psychiatrists, you have also an important group of people. It is not Spanish speaking but in Sao Paulo there is a group of people oriented in biological psychiatry also. So there are several groups. There is not one person now. We are not any more in the period of sin-

gle personalities, it is a matter of groups and I would say that these four cities
have groups of people, who do a lot of work and who are becoming and need
to become more and more important.

You have to remember that South America has gone through an extremely
difficult economic situation – political and economic. In some countries for
some years you could not import books. So this has produced certain drawbacks in say books, equipment for research or opportunities to travel, for
instance. This is changing very quickly, I think, but it will take a few years and
I think the situation will change very much in future. And of course in the case
of Spain, we are now part of Europe.

*There's one way in which Spain hasn't been part of northern Europe – the regulation of
the pharmaceutical industry in Spain has been different from that in the US and UK; it's
been somewhat easier and more flexible. Drugs have been available over the counter that
haven't been available in northern Europe. Now you find these witch hunts happening
with the benzodiazepines in northern Europe, but do you have them in Spain?*

No, on the contrary. With regard to the consumption of benzodiazepines this
was relatively low compared to the UK or France up to 10 years ago, even
though the prescription and the availability were much more liberal. Now regulations tend to be more strict.

But, for instance, if you want to identify a problem I would say that the prescription by a non-psychiatrist of non benzodiazepines in Spain will become
an issue of importance. The prescription of drugs which are supposed to be
antidepressant and are not proven to be antidepressants but which are marketed and prescribed by general practitioners is extremely high. We also still have
drugs on the market which have never been proven to work or combinations
of drugs some of which have been ineffective or have very low doses in them
and some are combined with a vitamin. These will disappear soon – not from
one day to the other because it will mean closing some companies and putting
more jobless people on the streets, but I think this will change.

*Is this always a good thing though? Because one of the things you hear in this part of the
world is that the reason we haven't had the breakthroughs in recent years compared with
situation between 1957 and 1962 is that it is so hard to get the compounds on to the markets here in this part of the world and the thing that actually generates discovery is the range
of compounds on the markets, people noticing something different the way you once did
with clomipramine and OCD.*

I think in Europe the drug industry was very much harmed by the anti-psy-
chiatric movement. They moved away from the central nervous system. They
wanted to work in other fields which are more acceptable to our social groups,
like cardiology or cancer or whatever you want. At the same time some
American companies, following the spirit of the Decade of the Brain, concentrated in the central nervous system and that's why now they have a lead.
European companies are beginning to come back. For the first time in a while
I see a stand by Hoechst here, which is very good. Lundbeck is here and

although it's a small company compared to others it's 100% devoted to CNS. Others are getting more interested. So, that's why the lead comes in a great part from the United States – they have kept doing research and the Decade of the Brain also created a movement and that has helped their image.

It seems to me that impulsivity, for instance, is a very European concept really and while there is some work done by the US researchers on it, it's still the kind of concept that one associates with people like yourself and Herman van Praag rather than with the Americans. Is there some reason why concepts like that occur over here much more than over there?

I think in Europe we have more a tradition of psychopathology. In the States this never existed in the same way. The best example is again DSM, which is atheoretical and non-psychopathological. Even the word psychopathology is not well understood in the States but psychopathology is the science that leads to an interest in anxiety, impulsivity and in other modes of behaviour or psychopathological conditions.

But there is an area here where the public, I guess, feels a bit unsure. When people are deluded clearly they're crazy but when someone's impulses are out of order there is the almost unresolvable question of whether they are bad or mad.

But I think here one should apply the principle which is essential, in forensic psychiatry, which is first you make the diagnosis and for this you have to study the psychopathology. First you need a diagnosis and then you study the responsibility of the patient. The clinical diagnosis is always the first step. If there is no diagnosis the boundaries are different. It's the same with the rest of medicine. You have to put some limits.

There has been a change clearly and we have moved people out of the mental hospitals and there's a perception that we are dealing with disease entities more effectively than we were before. But if you begin to look closely at what actually happened when you ask some people what is going on often the kind of message is that clozapine, for instance, is a good treatment but it is not so much a great treatment for schizophrenia as a very good anti-aggressive agent and in some respects it could be argued that what psychiatrists do in practice comes down to the management of impulsivity and aggression and things like that. Now we couldn't let the public know that that's what we do. We have to say that we're treating disease entities.

Clozapine is a very good example to mention. Clozapine is not an antischizophrenic drug. There are no antischizophrenic drugs. Schizophrenia is a very complicated disease and clozapine is an antipsychotic that relieves some of the symptoms. It works in hallucinations and with delusions and for some behavioural problems related to the psychotic symptoms. Clozapine may alleviate the impulsivity from psychotic symptoms which a schizophrenic patient might have but if you give clozapine to suicidal patients who have aggressivity against themselves or for the impulsivity or aggression that goes with sexual abuse cases it does not work. So first you need a diagnosis and then you treat the specific problem within this diagnosis. In the same way a serotonergic agent may work in some impulse control disorders, in bulimia for instance, but it will not work in the impulsivity of a schizophrenic, which is different.

OK, but there are ambiguities it seems to me in that to some extent you and I know they are not the treatment for schizophrenia but the public has to be told they are a magic bullet for the entity that is schizophrenia.

No. You have to tell the truth, that's why you have to speak the same language, and the truth is that while you cannot treat schizophrenia without drugs the drugs are not the only treatment for schizophrenia. Schizophrenia is a severe disease which needs treatment for many years and a lot of effort from the patient, from the doctor, from the family and so on. There is no easy answer, just like there is no cure for cancer. You know that there are still things that you can do – but this is a common situation in medicine.

I think that psychiatry now is at a very important turning point. At the World Congress, I had at the end to do an interview on television and they asked me to make a summary of the Congress. I said, well, I can make it around the theme of one world, one language and what this means. It means first that we psychiatrists should speak the same diagnostic language among ourselves, we should have the same protocols for interventions, the same outcome measures and so on. We are a single community dealing with the same problems. Secondly, we have to speak the same language as the rest of medicine, which means we have to learn the language of primary medicine and we have to teach our language to the rest and this is very important. Third, we have to learn to speak the same language as science. We are part of neuroscience and I always like to say this in the singular. Fourth, we have to speak the same language as our patients and I think the Madrid Declaration is a good example of what can be done. And fifth, we have to speak the same language as society in general – we have to open our doors as much as we can and we have to have an impact in the press. We had a big impact in Madrid and I was impressed by two editorials 6 days apart in one of the big Spanish journals. The first day of the Congress the title was 'Psychiatry from mental hospitals to science'. It described the perception of society and the changes we have actually achieved. On the last day the same journal had another editorial on the Congress entitled 'Psychiatry opens its doors'. I think that this is a really big change in our profession.

When you made the point about psychiatry and neuroscience sharing a common language, do you see psychiatrists evolving into clinical neuroscientists?

No. I put the example of research in neuroscience in the statement but neuroscience is also changing. When you study the molecular genetics of behaviour or the field of social biology, neuroscience is not only concerned with what is happening within the central nervous system but with an individual in their environment and within this larger scope the interests of different disciplines come together to the study of brain and behaviour in disease and under normal conditions. But in this sense I was thinking more as a clinician, that we have to open the door to the lab and to those who want to do field research and sociological research.

As a symbol though would it help if we were to become clinical neuroscientists rather than psychiatrists? Psychiatrists are always going to be soul doctors in some sense and what you're saying really is we need to be more effectively treating medical problems rather than disorders of the soul.

I think that we should defend our medical identity and that we are dealing with an important part of medicine – we are not magicians. What is the soul? I don't know but I know where I have to find how the soul works – the mind is the brain in action. I think we should define ourselves as physicians first because there is so much to give our patients and that's our basic mission – to treat patients. To treat patients and to try to help them to get some of what they are missing in this world. I see myself as a physician first even though I do many other things – I teach, I do research, I am a member of the Board of a Health Insurance Company – but the bottom line is that I am a physician. All these other things I think interest me because of issues which play a role in our profession. We are not politicians. We are not sociologists. We should not lose our identity as clinicians. That's why I like the WPA very much because it is an association of clinicians. You have everything there but the bottom line is that we are clinicians. I see patients and I like to see patients.

Listening to two lectures recently, one of which was yours and the other from the director of what is called a medium secure unit in Britain, I had a fantasy which had to do with the period around the 1820s/40s when the first asylums were built. They were built in part because of public concern about dangerous lunatics at large in the community but this was allied with concern that there were people in jail who were more appropriately seen as being ill and in need of treatment. When the first asylums opened there were some who were keen on a moral/behavioural approach but others who felt that it was obvious that the conditions were medical and that we would only really have the answers when we had treatments that targetted the biological bases of the conditions. Very quickly, however, the demand for beds outstripped the supply and things began to fall apart.

Now recently in my clinical practice, I seem to be deluged with referrals of angry young men. It seems that there is some shift to seeing these problems as medical even though conventional diagnostic frameworks don't handle these cases very satisfactorily. In Britain a new generation of asylums seems to be growing up – the medium secure units I've mentioned above – and while these services were set up in the first instance for a restricted number of deluded criminals these other patients inevitably get referred to the forensic services and already demand greatly outstrips supply. Is this history repeating itself and will the cycle have to be as long this time, or do you think we will have learnt anything from what we've been through?

Actually the first institution for mental patients based on a humanitarian approach was founded in Valencia in 1411 by a priest called Jofré, who after watching children in the streets throwing stones at a lunatic, preached in favour of such institutions the same day during Mass. At the end several merchants offered him the money for this institution under the condition that it should be run independently from the King, the nobles and the Church. Before the end of the 15th century, several Spanish cities, Seville and Zaragoza, had hospitals and early in the 16th century, less than 50 years after Columbus' first trip to America, the first hospital was built in Mexico City, two centuries before an institution of this kind was created in English-speaking America.

Now the boundaries between psychiatric and normal behaviour and deliquency and crime are not always clear and there is a group of individuals who create problems for both the health care system and the judicial and prison system. The fact that most prisons in developed countries provide the inmates with mental health care in a sense helps to solve this issue without confronting it. In Spain, now we are in the opposite situation; a new penal code takes a position against the discrimination against prisoners and transfers their care to the health care system. This creates confusion about the origin of dangerousness. All of this is forcing the psychiatric community to look for methods of care which will not transform every psychiatric unit into a high security unit and to differentiate the psychiatric and non-psychiatric aspects of aggressivity. In this context drugs of abuse are an important problem in parts of our country, especially against a background of high unemployment rates and a loss of traditional family values. My feeling is that in Spain we are going to follow the British model. Whether we will avoid an abuse of this or not I don't know. I think an external commission to supervise treatment and rehabilitation will be essential.

Select bibliography

Fernández Córdoba E, López-Ibor Aliño JJ (1967). La monoclorimipramina en enfermos psiquiátricos resistentes a otros tratamientos. *Actas Luso-ospañolas de Neurología Y Psiquiatría*, **26**, 119–147.

Lopez-Ibor JJ Jr (1969). Intravenous perfusions of monochlorimipramine. Technique and results. In *The Present Status of Psychotropic Drugs* (Cerletti A, Boye FJ, eds). Excerpta Medica, Amsterdam, pp 519–521.

Moreno I, Saiz-Ruiz J, López-Ibor JJ Jr (1991). Serotonin and gambling dependence. *Human Psychopharmacology*, **6**, 9–12.

López-Ibor JJ Jr (1992). Masked depression under the light of the new biological and nosological research. *L'Encephale*, **18**, 35–40.

López-Ibor JJ Jr (1993). *La Personalidad en Medicine Y sus Trastornos. Discurso de ingreso a la Real Academia Nacional de Medicina Instituto de España*. Real Academia Nacional de Medicina, Madrid, Octubre.

Carrasco, JL, Sáiz-Ruíz, J, Hollander E, César J, López-Ibor JJ Jr (1994).Low platelet monoamine oxidase activity in pathological gambling. *Acta Psychiatrica Scandinavica*, **90**, 427–43.

López-Ibor JJ Jr, Saiz Ruíz J, López-Ibor Alcocer MI, Viñas Pifarre, R (1995) Trastorno obsesivo-compulsivo y depresión. *Actas Luso-Españolas de Neurología, Psiquiatría Y Ciencias Afines*, **23**, 97–113.

Lopez-Ibor JJ Jr (1997). The concept and boundaries of personality disorder. *American Journal of Psychiatry*, **154**, suppl. 21–25.

See also interview with George Beaumont in *The Psychopharmacologists* Vol 1.

19 Oakley Ray

A psychologist in American neuropsychopharmacology

You began in 1958 doing clinical psychology.

When I went to graduate school at Pittsburgh I insisted that I go into clinical. The people there said, 'All your scores would suggest you would do better in research.' I said 'No' and got my degree in clinical psychology. But at that time when you took a PhD in psychology everyone took the same course work; the only difference between clinical and experimental was what you did in the afternoon – if you were clinical you went to a clinic, if you were experimental you went into a lab. When I finished my dissertation I had half a year to go before I got my degree and I was bored to tears with clinical work. I was at a VA mental hygiene clinic. You went in at 8 o'clock and had coffee and dough-nuts and then at 9 o'clock you saw a patient until about 10.30 and by that time it was almost time to go to lunch and so on. I said I've got to get out of here and see if I can get some human research. At that time the only person in a VA hospital in Pittsburgh doing research was Larry Stein but he was doing animal research. I went and talked with him. His first reaction was, well there's no place for a clinical psychologist here, but since I had all the experimental course work I could talk about Kenneth Spence and Hull and their theories, he said, OK why don't you come in. I joined the lab and fell in love with animal research. Larry didn't like organising the lab, the nitty-gritty things which I can do in my sleep and so within three or four weeks I was running the routine things in the lab. I felt if I could take some of the worry with technicians and this and that, which would help him, and besides it was a good experience for me. At that time back in 1958, 59, 60, if you wanted electrodes for brain stimulation you made them – you couldn't go out and buy them. Just about anything we did we had to do with our hands. Larry was the person who introduced me to physiological psychology.

By physiological in this context you mean what? It's a term that has slipped out of use.

It just means looking at the biological basis of behaviour. At that time, that would range all the way from the electrical stimulation of the brain and the chemical stimulation of the brain that Alan Fisher was doing at University of Pittsburgh. Alan had gone to McGill to talk with Donald Hebb and the story is that he said, I want to become rich and famous like Jim Olds – what can I do? Hebb scratched his head apparently and said, 'Well, Jim is doing electrical stimulation of the brain, why don't you do chemical stimulation?' And so then he started tracking down the cholinergic system in the brain and he would have gone on to really good things except for his untimely death. But that's what I mean by physiological psychology. It goes back to Lashley and the ablation studies and other things he did, which are still very germane.

Anyway I started with Larry and really found a home in his lab. Larry had started his postdoctoral research with Joe Brady, who came out of the University of Chicago to the Walter Reed Research Institute and set up a behavioural lab with Murray Sidman. It was a golden time for experimental psychology because it was during the Korean War and all these bright people who were graduating didn't want to go to Korea and so they became Privates in the army at Walter Reed and did research there. They had, it seems now, almost unlimited funds. David Rioch was there, the neuroanatomist, and Murray Sidman, and Peter Calton and Eliott Hearst as well as Larry Stein and many others. Irv Geller was there as a technician but people told him he was wasting his time and he ought to get a PhD etc. and come back. It was through Larry and his connections that I got to know anybody at all in psychopharmacology.

At the time we were linked to Amadeo Marrazzi, who had done very early drug stimulation of the brain. He was the first person, I believe, to show the activity of a drug on an actual living brain using a transcallosal preparation. His problem was that he got hooked on the technique and that's usually a kiss of death in a fast-moving research area. It was certainly his kiss of death because he had a great set-up with lots of money – back in 1958 he had a budget of over $100,000 to run a lab. Ross Hart, who was a pharmacologist, was there and Mel Gluckman, a biochemist, and Larry Stein and he had a neurosurgeon to do transcallosal preparations. I got a chance to learn some biochemistry and pharmacology and neuroanatomy that I hadn't learned before. It was a good place to interact. The problem was that if Amadeo had a choice of either helping you or hurting you or leaving you alone, he would hurt you because he had a belief, it seemed, that the further down he pushed you the higher up he seemed to be. As a result almost everybody who went through his labs saved most of their good material and didn't publish it while they were there because he insisted that his name was on it. He drove all of us away ultimately and there was a scandal because of the way he was using Japanese doctorates and not paying them even a living wage. He treated me very well even though I didn't publish a whole bunch because I saved it like everybody else.

Back in those days I gave papers at the Mid Western Psychological Association, the Eastern Psychological Association and the ASPET meetings, as well as the American Psychological and FASEB meetings – five meetings per year. We had a big enough lab that you could turn out different papers for each of those. In the process of that I got to know Irv Geller who was then at Wyeth running a lab. He came to Pittsburgh to see if I was interested in a job. I remember Irv, his boss, Larry and me were in East Liberty in a restaurant having dinner. I told Larry I wasn't interested because my wife was teaching, my kids were beginning to come along and we were happy bunnies in Pittsburgh. I had already turned down an offer to go to the Neuropsychiatric Institute at UCLA, which was run by Ted Magoon. He came to visit Marrazzi's lab because they were old buddies. I was really tempted because Jim Olds and Keith Killam were there and it was an exciting time but my wife was teaching and finishing up her degrees, and it was close to my family and her family. Who wants to go across the country and never see anybody again? So Larry said do you care if I apply for the job and, in fact, they ended up offering Larry a job – a different and even better position.

Larry left and Amadeo wanted to get someone else in with the kind of reputation that Larry Stein had. So he called everybody in the world – Gordon Bowers and Joe Brady and others – but he couldn't find anybody. Finally he offered me the job. It was exactly what I wanted because I could stay in Pittsburgh and I was running the lab anyway. Marrazzi's problem was that he could never spend his money. The fiscal year ended at the end of June – so he would call me about the last week of May and say, 'Oakley, can you spend $20,000 in the next two weeks?' I could always spend $20,000. So we bought equipment like crazy and I tripled the size of the lab. As far as that went everything was fine and I had enough hard-working graduate and undergraduate students from Chatham College where I was also teaching in addition to the University of Pittsburgh.

About 1959 when I had finished my VA internships, I went on an NIMH postdoctoral programme for 2 years and then I was put on staff in the VA. A while later a fellow called Elston Hooper came by from the VA central office in Washington. He was in charge of the VA Psychology Research Program. He said, 'Well Oakley, you've got a nice operation here, anytime you want a lab of your own let me know.' I grabbed him by the arm and said, 'I'm letting you know.' We were at Leech Farm VA Hospital where Marrazzi had the whole top floor of building number 1. We started the machinations and after about six months I set up my lab in the same hospital but in a different building – in the old insulin shock therapy ward. One of my animal labs over there was in the hydrotherapy room when they had taken out the tubs. So I moved across with VA and NIMH money and Child Health and Human Development money and NSF money for the summer educational programmes for high school science teachers.

I was very happy there and with what I was doing when in 1969 I got a letter from Vanderbilt University asking if I had any students ready to be a distinguished associate professor. I wrote back and said I didn't know any distinguished associate professors but I like to travel and talk and I'd be glad to look at the job myself. They explained to me that they needed somebody to take over the multi-disciplinary graduate training programme in psychopharmacology and to be an associate professor in the Department of Psychology. I gave a talk to the psychology people and the following weekend I gave a different talk in the Medical School to Allen Bass' Department of Pharmacology, and before the weekend was out they offered me a job as a tenured professor. My wife and I thought about it and we decided we would move. So I picked up the phone and called Dick Fowler, who was then in charge of research in the VA in Washington, and said, 'Dick, I'm not going to be putting in my request for VA funding for next year because I am going to leave the VA and go and be an academician.' I could move the other grants but not that one. He said, 'Don't do anything for three days and I'll call you back.' In fact he did call me back on Friday and he said, 'I want you to think about the possibility of moving your whole lab to Nashville and staying in the VA and being Chief of the Psychology Service at the VA hospital there as well Professor of Psychology and Associate Professor in Pharmacology.'

The VA in Nashville didn't have a psychology service there then. As in many places, they had a psychiatry service and psychology was a section of it. That didn't sit very well with the people in Washington and they were not about to put one of their prime research people into a psychiatry service. But since I was a clinician and had my licence and had become President of the Pennsylvania Psychological Association, when I went down to Nashville the people in the VA said, yes we are willing to set up a Psychology Service, and they did. So I essentially ended up with the best of all worlds.

Can we hop back to what you were researching?

One of the things that happened while I was in Pittsburgh is that there were a couple of guys, Zivic and Miller, who wanted to start an animal breeding colony and they started breeding faster than they could sell the animals. So I bought animals from them at 25 or 50 cents a piece when they were typically going for maybe 3 or 4 dollars each. This meant that we could do a whole bunch of studies that required large numbers just because we could afford to do it – nobody else could. Partly because of that we got into genetic studies. Because I was looking at mechanisms of learning, I wanted to try animals from different breeders etc. We ran one study which we wanted to replicate but we couldn't. We scratched our heads and looked at everything – the time of the year, was it hot, was it cold? – we tried to control everything. I finally called the people, not Zivic and Miller, where we bought the animals and said, tell me how you pick the animals that you ship out to researchers. What happened, it turned out, is that the way that they pick their animals was not really as random as they thought. Incidentally, they changed the system because of our study. For example, now if I wanted 60-day-old males, they would take five from colony A, five from colony B etc. but what had happened the first time was that the only place they had 60-day-old males was from one colony. So I got a unique genetic population and because of this we couldn't replicate our data which led us to study genetic effects on learning and performance.

I was also running LSD, psilocybin and mescaline studies in rats but then Sandoz decided to get out of that business. Back then, if you wanted LSD for your research, you picked up the phone and called Rudi Bircher at Sandoz and say, 'Rudi, I need 100 ampoules of LSD.' He'd send you them or whatever else you wanted if Sandoz produced it. When they got out of the business, you could still get what you needed from the government but it meant a lot of paperwork and it wasn't worth it. So I scratched that whole line of research.

Another research area was anxiety paradigms in animals. I had come up with three different paradigms – one was conditioned suppression, another was conditioned avoidance and the third was a conflict paradigm. Each had a built-in control for motor effects. The three classes of drugs at the time were the tranquillisers, reserpine, the phenothiazines and meprobamate and each of these worked in one paradigm and not the others. I never really trained with a neurophysiologist or a biochemist – I just picked up enough to be dangerous. Actually we probably did one of the very first brain biochemistry behaviour studies. We used two different breeds of rats, which under normal conditions couldn't be told apart, but when you shocked them one became hyperactive but the other didn't. So we did the brain assays on these two species and showed nice differences. I made a decision at the time that that's the wave of the future but I didn't want to be a biochemist. So when I moved from Pittsburgh to Vanderbilt, I took Bob Barrett with me as a postdoc, who was also a behaviourist who does lots of sophisticated brain–behaviour studies, and when I went into administration I gave the lab to him and he has done awfully well.

When I took over the clinical service in the Nashville VA, my agreement was that I hired clinicians to do the clinical work and I could oversee them if need be, but I never hired anybody who wasn't better at their job than I was. I hired really good clinicians and they did it very well and that was fine. I worked in the lab meanwhile and went to the hospital once a week. Then the Chief of Staff, the head professional person in the hospital, left and we had a new Chief of Staff, who got into an argument with the Chief of Psychiatry in the VA Hospital. The Chief of Psychiatry made the fatal mistake of telling veterans and their families that the Vanderbilt psychiatrists were in the VA hospital to do research and to train residents because the VA was a steady source of funding. Not one word about taking care of sick folk. Bad form. There was much acrimonious discussion between the Chief of Staff and the psychiatrists, with the result that all of the pychiatrists were pulled out of the VA hospital. Amazingly the Dean of the Medical School didn't pick up the phone and tell the Chair of Psychiatry that he couldn't disaffiliate because the affiliation was not with him, it was with the Medical School. So as a result here's an affiliated VA Hospital in which psychiatry has pulled out. Walt Gobbel, the Chief of Staff, picked up the phone, called me and said, 'Oakley, I need to talk to you. You're the senior mental health person here, you've got to make it work.'

So I put together the first, the only, mental health and behavioural sciences unit in the VA system in the United States. At first it was headed by a psychiatrist because they felt that was the only way it would be acceptable but finally the psychiatrist said, 'Walt, Oakley's running the unit. Let's make him chief.' That didn't sit too well with a lot of people because psychiatrists are supposed to run things, not psychologists. It was interesting because the Joint Commission on Accreditation of Hospitals came and they'd meet the Chief of Mental Health and realise that I was a psychologist and say, well there is no way we can accredit you. But every time when they walked out after 2 or 3 days evaluating the programme and said, its the best unit we've ever seen, they gave us full accreditation every time. It was one of the best units in the whole country and the reason for that was because everybody knew it was a unique situation. All the psychologists worked like hell, and so did the clinical nurse specialists, the social workers and the attendants. It was a happy family really.

When I hired staff, I told them, look we are going to hire psychiatrists and they won't know as much as you do but they are going to make a lot more money than you do and the reason for that is because they are MDs. If that's going to bother you, don't come. Now the reason we did that was because no top psychiatrist would want to come and work in that situation and be alienated from the Department of Psychiatry at Vanderbilt. We had a bunch of foreign medical graduates who had finished their residency in psychiatry, who were good but they weren't mainstream. They were just really on their way to some type of a private practice.

When we ran the mental hygiene program, everyone had to take call. Because I lived 29 miles out of Nashville, I would take call Friday night and sleep in my office. We finally worked out with the Chief of Medicine that when somebody came in to the Emergency Room, medical residents would screen them no matter what the psychiatric problem was. If they thought the patient was medically OK, we'd assume responsibility. I did not want non-physicians to see somebody, do a psychiatric evaluation then find out he's got some basic medical problems that nobody had looked at. There was a lot of hemming and hawing in the beginning but it worked very well.

One of the reasons why the arrangement worked was because Tennessee, like some rural states in the United States, had a rule that a licensed clinical psychologist can commit somebody if you can't locate a psychiatrist. This was really made for the rural area where there is nobody around. We just translated it to say, look we can't get a psychiatrist because, even though they are across the street at Vanderbilt, they aren't about to come over here and evaluate this individual. So I decide I'm going to commit you and we're going to send you off to Murfeesboro VA Hospital. When the individual arrived there, the MOD would usually say, 'They sent you down here on commitment papers and if I commit you then you're going to be here in the hospital for a significant period of time because in order for you to get out of the hospital we have to go before a judge and show him it's OK to release you. But if you come into hospital voluntarily, I won't have to commit you and that will make it much easier for us to release you when we think you are ready.' And 999 times out of a 1000 the individual would agree. But I signed many commitment papers and sent them off – it was just one of those situations.

You also have to go back and see how the world was in the early 1970s here in the States. We had people who would drop kids who were high on drugs off at an ER and you would sometimes have a technician in the ER who would then call the police and turn the person in. I was teaching a drugs course at Vanderbilt with 200–300 students and one of the things I would say throughout the semester was, look if you have any problems at all with drugs call me day or night – you've got my home number in the syllabus. In the early 1970s I would get maybe four, five or six calls in a semester but I haven't had a call now in 4 years. People who are doing drugs are smarter about drug use and if they have problems they aren't afraid to go to the ER or clinics.

Running the mental health unit became my life in the late 1970s and that's when I left the lab. I essentially left research then and have done only a few minor things since then. I have put more time into writing and conceptualising. Another one of my characteristics is I'm a dilettante. I will never be the world's authority on anything because I never want to know everything about one thing – I don't have that kind of personality.

I go back to an old Kurt Koffka phrase, 'multa, non multum' – much, not many. If you know two things and how they relate that's better than if you know 20 things that are just separate facts. Call it wisdom if you want. Trying to get people to put things together rather than just pile up facts. This is one of the reasons why I have never once regretted not continuing research. I was turning out good blocks in the wall of science, I had a big lab and so much money I turned back grants in Nashville because I couldn't spend it. The lab could have turned out a publishable study a month. Would any of them have been keystones or giant leaps forward? – probably not. That's not good or bad – most people don't turn out keystones. A few do and those are the people that we need to support and foster.

On that point, around this time you brought out your book Drugs, Society and Human Behavior, *which went into hundreds of thousands of copies. What was the philosophy behind it?*

A simple thing. You've got to remember where the world was in 1970. Everyone was doing drugs. Being one of the few people who knew about drugs, and a psychologist who could put two or three words together, I did a lot of talking and travelling in the 1960s. I gave a workshop for psychologists at the American Psychological Association meeting in Miami – a 1-day workshop on everything you needed to know about drugs. At lunchtime Dick Davis, an Editor for Mosby, grabbed me and said, that's really interesting stuff, why don't you put it into a book? I think the world is ready for a book on society, drugs and psychopharmacology. I said, piece of cake – I'll turn it out in no time at all. A bad mistake. From the time I decided to do it, I literally did nothing else. I was still in the lab and I had people scurrying off to the libraries to get me stuff. When I went home I would write until about midnight before getting up at six for work. All day Saturday, all day Sunday – the only time that I took off was Christmas Day.

I got caught up in trying to make it a good book and to do this I got taken up by the history and other things that a lot of other people might have learned when they were first-year medical or graduate students but it was brand new to me because I didn't have that kind of a background. What I did was try to put together an honest rational book that integrated science, history and society. I turned it out in nine months. Its in its seventh edition. It took off because it was a book that John Doe, psychologist, could pick up and teach from. It was his course all laid out – from the introductions to drugs and society and the nervous system etc. Another reason was the fact that it was neither pro nor con on drug use – when the government did stupid things I would say, 'Even my mother would laugh at that.' I can go back now and read things that I wrote in the first edition and I'm still saying the same stuff today. It hasn't changed because the government is still doing the same stupid things and the rational position, and proposals in the final chapter in the 1972 edition is still a rational position in 1997 when it comes to drugs.

Because of the book I started travelling a lot around the country, talking on drug education and drug programmes. A fellow came through and met me in my lab in Nashville and wondered if I might be interested in a job in Washington in SAODAP, the Special Action Office on Drug Abuse Prevention, as the head of education. I didn't know but it was exciting enough to look at it. That was the first time I met Jerry Jaffe, who was the drug czar for President Nixon. At that time Jaffe went back and forth to Vietnam many times and when he went there they treated him like he was a Four-Star General. When he said something Nixon listened and you pay attention to people like that if you're in the military. Anyway we met and Jerry talked about what they were trying to do then, which was to cut down on inner-city drug use, which means black heroin use. They were going to try to do that with many approaches, including footprints, so that they could make sure that you don't come to get your methadone from me and then go over there and get it from another guy etc. Well, it became clear to me that they weren't primarily interested in educational programmes. It also became very clear to Jerry, I'm sure, that I was not the kind of person who was going to do for them what they needed to have done. So in five minutes we knew that we were not made for each other.

One of the reasons why I have never been well loved in Washington is that my solutions are realistic long-term, not political solutions. You can do all the interdiction you want but you aren't going to keep drugs out. A lot of people say that but I go a step further – if you really want to have an impact on drug use then you need to start in the home. Nobody wants to hear that because in this country you don't go fiddling with people's homes and their families, although we're switching a little bit now.

Anyway the book took off and I was having a fine time keeping up with everything and then in 1986 I had a bout of lymphoma and the publisher picked a co-author for me. I send him things and he drafts the first version and we kick it around. It's not as much of a fun book for me now even to teach from but that's because students have changed too. Students don't want the history unless it's really cutesy history.

Why?

It's too complicated to explain fully here but beginning about 1971 I started giving a talk to freshmen in my introductory psychology course – a classroom of about 480. It got to be enough of a classic that it became one of the essentials of the overall freshmen orientation. I ended up titling it 'Welcome to Vanderbilt – Try the Salad Bar'. The idea was to take a splattering of everything, don't just zero in on your major subject. Back in the mid-1970s, students in the United States had as one of their major reasons for going to college developing a philosophy of life. By the time I stopped giving that lecture in the early 1990s – by mutual agreement – I was unhappy with the way the students were receiving it and they were unhappy with what I would say. They had changed. Originally most of them wanted to develop a philosophy of life and values and fewer were concerned about making a living. But it had switched by the early 1990s. They weren't interested in history as a broad-based liberal education. In the 1960s, I used to tell people that when I got tired of being a psychologist I was going to start a real career as a historian because that's where the answers to many social problems are. Many of the things that I would talk about in class were in the earlier editions of the book but they aren't in there any more. The world doesn't care about that kind of thing and the students certainly don't. They just want you to tell them what they need to know to pass the exam. The book is much better now but I'm less happy with it. The book has kept up with the world and I haven't but that's the way it goes. I'm in the process of updating a whole bunch of things and trying to branch out because there are not too many people who are talking good sense about drug use in today's world, I think.

What are they saying and what ought they to be saying?

Well, what they ought to be saying is that in fact drug use is always going to be with us and what you need to do is not just engage in harm reduction or interdiction but to see what some of the causes are. When I got into drug abuse prevention they would design programmes to educate people about drugs and what they would find is that in fact drug use increased after a drug education programme in the schools. Why? If I tell you the dangers of mainlining heroin then I'm also telling you how you can use heroin more safely and so safe drug use goes up. I used to tell parent–teacher and state groups all over the country – do you realise that if you put in a drug education programme what you may very well get is an increase in drug use. What you're not going to do is change values very much. But they always said let's put the programme in. That's because parents don't want to talk about things like sex and drugs to their kids – the kids know more than they do and it's embarrassing. What the parents wanted to do was absolve themselves of having to deal with any of that but I think we need to appreciate the fact that there's a role for the home, for the schools and for the community as well as for the government in drug abuse prevention.

I used to give a talk called 'Vanderbilt as Midwife' on Parents' Weekend. The basic thesis was that Vanderbilt is not a miracle worker. If you send us your child and he's a klutz, we'll educate him and he'll be an educated klutz. We're not going to unklutz him. Parents don't like to hear that too much but it's true and this is why by the time a child is six you can make some pretty good predictions about whether they are going to use drugs inappropriately and so on. I tell my students the best drug education programme never even mentions drugs. What it does is gives people a reason not to do drugs. We know what is not effective. It's not things like DARE, drug abuse resistance education. Herb

Kleber told me at a meeting we were at in September 1996 that the DARE programme specifically doesn't work with middle class kids. It may work better,
but not very well, with lower class kids but that's because it's uniformed
policemen who are doing the whole thing.

I think the President and the people in Washington don't want to bite the
bullet. The bullet you've got to bite is to tell parents this is what has to be done,
and if you're not going to do it then we'll do it for you. One of the things
Lyndon Johnson did back in the 1960s, which has now fallen by the wayside,
is he took middle class mothers and sent them into the inner city to teach
inner-city mothers how to be better mothers. In this country everyone wants
to talk black/white but that's not the problem; the problem is socio-economic
class and the attitudes that go along with that. But we are so hung up on the
black/white thing that people don't pay attention to the data. A study came out
recently in Atlanta where the preschool children of welfare mothers were
shown to be already 1 to 2 years behind their peers – these are 3–5 years old so
that's a big lag. Well, you know what's going to happen if you come in to school
and you're not ready – you're always behind, the teacher doesn't like you
because you're a chore, the other kids wonder why you're dumb and you never
catch up. If you want to train people to be drop-outs that's exactly the way you
do it. The family is sancrosanct in the United States. It looks even as though
OJ Simpson will get custody of his kids because we have this unbelievable idea
that blood is thicker than water and so if he wants his kids he should get them.

*There seems to be something peculiar about social attitudes to drug use. It's almost like VD
– a hidden dirty area. What's involved? Why do we react this way?*

It's interesting why we identify drug users as different and why we think we
can treat it differently than teenage mothers, or delinquents. I think the reason
is that people believe more so with drug use than anything else that you made
a conscious decision to become a bad person and use drugs and you have to
live with the consequences. Another aspect is that you would not have made
that decision if we'd kept the drugs away from you and this is why the focus is
on the supply side rather than on the demand side. We are going to cut off the
supply and that will solve the drug problem, and of course it never will. How
do you change attitudes? I try to change attitudes in part by talking facts but I
always tell people that information never changed behaviour except when the
information is within a value context.

Values determine the limits within which information can be used in order
to select what we think is the best of all options for our personal selves. This
is why if I tell you at 16 that if you smoke cigarettes it's going to kill you it
doesn't mean a damn thing. Any statement at that age that has to do with anything beyond the age of 25 has no meaning. You need to plug information into
some value system that you have and this is why it makes a lot more sense to
talk about the effect cigarette smoking is going to have on your relationship
with that girl or guy. You're not going to smoke because she not going to kiss
somebody who tastes of tobacco and tars. So the value system is the important
thing. My argument always is you've got to give people a reason not to do

drugs. I got onto that back in the 1970s after a study they did in Mississippi on alcohol abusers. They were asked why did you drink so much and the answer was 'Why not?' There was no reason not to get drunk.

Let's come back to Nashville and your running the mental health service. That has to have caused a considerable amount of paranoia among the brethren.

Oh yes, a lot of paranoia. It was interesting. I don't think it's quite as bad in Europe between PhDs and MDs as it is in this country. Here it's really bad. I remember the Chief of Medicine in the Nashville VA, Roger Duprez, came over to see me in my lab once and we talked research and it became very clear to me that the reason why I was acceptable to him was because my research credentials were every bit as good as his and the people whom he respected. If I hadn't had that I would have been nothing, even though I was Chief of the Psychology Services.

I hired the very first PharmD in the VA system. You talk about paranoia. All the service Chiefs for Medicine and Surgery were sitting around and I said, 'I'm going to hire a PharmD.' They said, 'You're going to do what? What's a PharmD going to do?' I said, 'He's going to write prescriptions.' 'Is he a doctor?' 'Yes.' 'Is he an MD?' 'No.' Of course what happens is they run him on a protocol and a 'real' doctor signs off and says OK; no problem, once he feels comfortable and the PharmD goes on and does his thing. Now there are many PharmDs in the VA system and in the world; the place couldn't function without them. But I hired the very first one and he's still there, Dave Shepherd. He's superb and everybody loves him but not only did the VA staff worry about him, the Nashville Association of Physicians sent Alan Bass to talk to me and I can still hear him: 'Oakley, what is it you're going to do with this PharmD?' But we did everything right.

I survived in that situation by doing what I did well. I never once told a physician how to treat somebody. I never once suggested, why not use this drug rather than that one. You're the MD so whatever you say, that's it. If I think you're doing really bad work then I'll put you in a situation where you can't screw up too many things. It's one of the reasons why I've survived in ACNP. I keep my hands off the things that I think the secretary should not be involved in. I've got the nominating process set up now so that if you were to become chairman of the nominating committee I hand you about 12 pages and I say, here's the procedure and I'm out of it. In this kind of position too many people would say, 'Oakley's a king-maker.' I don't even vote in the ACNP election. I don't touch the damn thing because I don't think anybody should. I set up procedures in just that way for anything I can, so if I get run over by a trailer truck ACNP could go without a secretary for 2 years.

This leads onto the issue of prescribing rights for psychologists. Can I take you through the history of this? Where did the issue come from?

This started up as a move by Pat DeLeon who was in Senator Inouye's office – he was his legislative aide. He's an important gun in the American Psychological Association. He started to push prescribing privileges for psychologists in the late 1980s and so they set up a Blue Ribbon Panel which included people from both APAs and the government. About the same time Dick Shader, who had been involved in that, said we need to put together a statement from the ACNP. That was the first move but I hit the idea of calling them Council Consensus Statements – it's not a statement by the ACNP because we don't vote on it and could never get an acceptable statement from the diverse ACNP members, but it is something that Council has discussed widely and agreed to so it's a Council Consensus Statement. We publish them in the journal. We have probably four or five of them now – there's one on Clozaril and things like that.

In the Council Consensus Statement on non-physicians prescribing, the basic idea was that the ACNP has no problem at all with anybody prescribing medications providing they have the appropriate background and training. Well, since we had that statement out there and the Department of Defense was moving ahead with setting up a programme, they decided one of the things that they had to do was get somebody to evaluate it. Well, you can't have the American Psychological or the American Psychiatric. The one group that would have some kind of credibility to all groups was ACNP. We know about drugs and we've got psychiatrists and psychologists. Dave Engelhart and I wrote a proposal which was approved by the ACNP Council to evaluate the DoD programme. It was accepted by the DoD and it's been continued ever since. We had three board certified psychiatrists and three licensed clinical psychologists doing the evaluation visits and we've done marvellous things for the rigour of the programme. One of the things that's happened is that some of the psychologists who were for the programme in the beginning are now against it, and some of the psychiatrists who were against it are now for it.

Let me come back to my own personal feeling about medical training. Give me a bright high school graduate well motivated for 1 year and they can handle about 90% of the stuff that walks through the GP's door. So why do they need 4 years of college and 4 years of medical school and 3 years of residency – it's that other 10%. Much of the stuff is pretty Mickey Mouse and as a matter of fact, most of what comes to a first-level physician doesn't even have something physically wrong with them – 17% may have something physically wrong with them. So that's where I come from.

Now on this programme, sometimes the supervision was as casual as 'I'm a prescribing psychologist and you're my supervisory psychiatrist and I pass you in the hall and say I saw this guy and I did this and you say fine, that sounds pretty reasonable, and maybe we sit down once every week or two.' Or it can be somebody who is just sitting there all the time saying you didn't dot the i or this and that. Now the last report that I wrote, after we evaluated these graduates, which all of the committee agreed with was that none of us were ready to say these guys, who had really good training, were ready to go out and be independent practitioners in the real world. We stated it that way even though within a military setting they could probably be independent practitioners –

because who do you deal with, you deal with 18, 19, 20, 30-year-olds who are basically healthy people and almost anybody could handle that. Indeed one of the problems we are having is that they don't see a broad enough spectrum of problems.

The problem is they might miss some of the medical problems. Now I know psychiatrists are going to miss a medical problem. The DoD fellows are doing physicals maybe two a week – how many of the psychiatrists here have done a physical recently and if they have how good were they? But all of this gets caught up in the whole bit as to what's good medicine, what's legally safe and all these things go back and forth. If you screw up, no problem, you're an MD and you had an error in judgement – they're not going to hang you for it. If a practising prescribing psychologist screws up there is no precedent for it – who would want to write the insurance for that? Things are changing in this country and I'm hoping that none of the programmes that are out there now get developed because they are not nearly as rigorous as the one that we have helped shape in the DOD.

Another interesting thing is that PsyDs who do not have a solid science background have been quite successful in the medical school course work.

So one of the things that I have become convinced about, which a lot of people have a suspicion about, is that many things we put up are hurdles. We just want to make sure that if you're good enough to get through biochemistry, then that means you are conscientious enough and maybe you'll make a good physician. It's not quite that open and shut but you don't need all this science background in order to get through the classes in medical school. Would I send these prescribing psychologists out into the community? – no I wouldn't, even though many of the psychiatrists who train them say, 'Hey, I would send my mother to them, that's how much I trust them.'

You're also interested in the area of neuroendocrinology.

Yes, I'm really interested in what I call psychoendoneuroimmunology – PENI-ology to make it easy. I've got a book written on it which I'm trying to get published. What I'm interested in are things like the impact of thoughts on these systems. We learned about these systems separately and way back they didn't supposedly talk to each other but then we began to realise they interact with each other. We are beginning to appreciate that all three systems turn out messengers and they can all talk back and forth.

Now I'm not a philosopher but for as many years as I have been teaching I have been asking what is the mind, what are thoughts ? – they're actions in the brain. What are actions in the brain? – it's got to be neurotransmitters and so why should it surprise you that if you think certain kinds of thoughts it's going to change your biochemistry? That shouldn't surprise anybody. Why wouldn't you expect that? One of the things I'm interested in now is the extent to which individuals have a will to live. There are good data out there that talk about people delaying or speeding up the time at which they die just by their belief systems. That's an important thing for people to know. Another one of them is you're only as old as you think you are. One of the things that amazes physicians even is the fact that an independent predictor of when a person's going to die is just to ask the person a simple sloppy question: 'For your age, how do you feel?' That's a pretty good independent predictor.

I got into this whole thing way back in the 1960s when I heard Tom Holmes talk on Critical Life Events and he just blew me away. I had him come and talk in Pennsylvania and Nashville. In Nashville, Roger Duprez, the Chief of Medicine, and his people were there and he categorically rejected it – that's not possible, it's a different realm. It's these kinds of attitudes that we need to change. I think the pharmaceutical companies are finally now beginning to jump on it, realising that there are other things out there that influence behaviour and mood than the nervous system. One of the big things is the endocrine system and in time we're going to begin to realise that the immune system also has some impact. As everybody says since Selye, one of the things that happens when people get sick is they don't feel good. We're getting to the point where we're going to understand what it is that the immune system does to the nervous system and to the endocrine system that makes us not feel good. Why can't you be sick, fight infection, and still feel good?

We are also going to have compounds that will slow down ageing. What is ageing? We can agree that it's probably a biochemical process and if it's a biochemical process then we can find out which knobs and whistles you adjust and you're going to be able to slow it down or stop it, which would be interesting. We've got to think about this. Suppose you could put something in the water and just stop everybody from ageing right now – you may think that would be great but suppose you have a 4-year-old child, do you want to have a 4-year-old child running around your house for the rest of eternity – probably not. Or suppose we have something that will only stop the ageing process for 20 years when do you want it to happen – when you're 20 years old in the physical prime of your life, or would you rather it be 40 or 60? If somebody wants to live to be 100 today and they're under the age of 30 we know what they've got to do to make that very probable. Whether or not you want to live that way is another issue.

I think nootopics are on their way but then there's all kinds of problems about how you handle it. We've had smart drugs for a long time – we used to do things with smart rats and dumb rats. Everybody always had the idea that if you give them all a smart drug, then all animals would improve their learning, but that's not what happens. What happens is the dumb rats become as smart as the smart rats. Now in the United States the one legal basis on which you can discriminate against people is intelligence. Because you're bright, we're going to send you to medical school and you get an opportunity for a much more affluent life than being a garbage truck driver. Well, suppose everyone is equally bright, how do we pick who gets those chances? The women's revolution, the black revolution, are going to be nothing compared to the intelligence revolution.

What about your role in ACNP?

As regards ACNP, the tradition has been that you serve as Secretary and go on to be President. They've stopped asking me if I want to be nominated for President because I can't think of a worse job for me. I'm more interested in the nuts and bolts and developing projects. I would have been a great Chief of Staff for a General or a President because I like making things happen. If somebody says we'll sit and think about great thoughts I can probably do that as well as most people but President of the ACNP is not a place to think great thoughts. This is one of the things we're going to talk about tomorrow – should the ACNP President be for more than one year? I think we will reject it out of hand because if we are going to run two people and we are not going to pick them for the honour then you have to select them for a reason. That means you need to have a platform and know what the ACNP should be doing over the next two years if you are elected. I think it would destroy ACNP – we're not that kind of organisation.

In 1981 Don Klein became President and he said, I think we need to be involved in Washington. So we went and got ourselves a Washington lawyer and we started going and visiting the Hill and did all of those things. Maybe that was good or maybe it wasn't – with most politicking and lobbying it's never a yes or no clean thing. Tom Detre came along in 1994 and said, I don't think there is any point in this. Now the world had changed and you know great men have a way of saying things that fit in with the zeitgeist, which is what makes them great I guess. So we got rid of our Washington lawyer and we never visited the Hill anymore. We also tried, without great success so far, to get a grass-roots movement going.

We're about to move into an explosion of electronic publishing. At ACNP we are in the process of re-doing all of our contracts with the journal people and the Fourth Generation of Neuropsychopharmacology publishers. We want to control all of the intellectual content and be able to do with it what we want. Can you imagine if we could take the Fourth Generation and put it on-line? We've got to figure out how to finance it. That is what everyone is concerned about. But if you put it on line, everybody all over the world is going to have immediate access to the very best information. What's more, if you've written a chapter on SSRIs and there's a new finding you can change paragraph 3 instantly. Material can be continually updated – we are talking about updating on at least a quarterly basis. We already have an ACNP web site, as well as CD-ROMs for both the journal and Fourth Generation. This organisation has people who are unbelievably brilliant, like Stan Watson or Floyd Bloom, to point the directions. I make things happen, I'm a doer.

*In recent years one hears that ACNP is the most professional psychopharmacology associ-
ation and puts on one of the best scientific meetings in the world. However, one hears from
Tom Ban and others that Arthur Koestler was a guest at one of the earlier meetings and
commented on the apparent shambles. Does this transformation coincide with your arrival
on the scene?*

I agree with your comments about what it is and I would be ecstatic if someone could show that I was responsible for ACNP being what it is, but I have
no delusions. I was in the right place at the right time and I have helped to
shape the college. But you have to remember several very important facts. First
the membership consists of the very best brain–behaviour–drug researchers in
the world and membership has always been very competitive. In the beginning
it was limited to 180 Members and Fellows, not counting Life Fellows and
Past-Presidents, and it was almost true that someone had to die before new
people could become members. Currently we take about 30 new scientific
Members per year and the bottom line for the membership committee continues to be research excellence, creativity and productivity.

The second fact is that the ACNP meeting is closed – non-members can
come by invitation only. This has two effects – it keeps the meeting small and
thus you have opportunities to really talk to other scientists. Second, if you get
on the programme, you know that the best in the field will be in the audience
and so people save their best data for the ACNP meeting.

Each year we elect a new president. Between being president elect, president and past-president for two years, this gives that person an opportunity to
accomplish certain objectives and they use the Secretariat for this. But elec-
tions for Council and officers are based on scientific stature and personality –
there are no statements about plans or agendas and no campaigns before the
election. The Secretariat is now organised to take over all the mundane things
to do with membership selection and programme development, leaving the
members free to focus on what they do best, which is pick the best of the nom-
inees for membership or the best symposia for the programme. Finally we
have had excellent support from the pharmaceutical industry. As the programme has gotten better the pharmaceutical companies want to support it
and that makes the programme even better but the organisation is non-com-
mercial and we don't have exhibits, or sponsored programmes and the
Secretariat works hard to be industry-neutral.

*Unlike the secretary for CINP or BAP, you've been the Secretary for ACNP since the
early 1980s. I'm sure it's made for stability having one person like you there but all the
organisations seem to be facing change – ACNP at the moment seems reasonably stable
but you threw off the ASCP there recently.*[1]

That was because I think the ACNP was not responsive. I have tried for a long
time without success to get Council to do the kinds of things that ASCP is

---

[1]See Klein D (1996). *The Psychopharmacologists*, Vol I.

doing but they weren't interested. Now they're starting to do it by having regional meetings, spreading the word out to the 'heathen' out there rather than just talking among ourselves, which is what the annual meeting is. Tom Detre a few years back talked about ACNP as a one time a year organisation but now we're moving toward a year round organisation with regional meetings and a bunch of other things that will keep us busy year round interacting with and educating people. Our honorific President system means that people come and go and this has some obvious disadvantages.

I'm not sure what will happen down the road but with the people we've had recently we've been able to upgrade our whole computer systems and move into the electronic era. Most people see the strong point of ACNP now as the annual meeting. You hear all the time that it's the best meeting in the world and it probably is for the kinds of things that we're after. I'd like to push people to support our extension into an annual update on the CD-ROM and into the World Wide Web because what we are really good at is creating and communicating information. If we can do this I think we'll do well.

As regards CINP, it's been pushed by ECNP. Remember when the ECNP started not too long ago it was going to fill in the gaps every other year and then they were making so much money they decided they might as well do it every year and now they have so much money it's obscene. One of the things that I have talked to Lew Judd and Claude de Montigny and others about is finding a new niche for the CINP. The ECNP has taken over Europe and it's expanding and getting more people in from Asia and they offer a good meeting. If they can just keep it from being swallowed up by pharmaceutical companies then ...

Do you think this is a problem?

Well, if you look at the kinds of things that the ACNP does – you see ACNP Bristol-Myers Squibb travel grants etc. and the names of different companies supporting teaching day and other activities. But it's upfront and we really want to be independent. I don't know what it really means to be in the pocket of the pharmaceutical industry at the level at which I think ECNP is. Does that mean that if I go in as a scientist or a clinician and I listen to the presentation it might be biased? Well, that's one of the things it means and I think in some instances it certainly is. I believe that one of the problems that a person has in an ECNP meeting is that they don't have the kind of safeguards that we have here. If you come and give a talk at the ACNP and you're going to talk on some product, I'm going to find out if you've ever gotten any money from them because of requirements for disclosure. ECNP doesn't have that and I think that's a problem.

I think the same thing is true with the CINP to a lesser degree. But that's an expensive organisation – the Congresses are expensive to run. The Glasgow Congress has an industry panel, I hear, and everybody sits around the table and knows what Mr Lilly has given and what SKB has given and what they are getting. The whole thing, I hear, is very above board. Generally we're moving toward more disclosure. But I don't know what the CINP can do that the ECNP doesn't do. As Alec Coppen once said, and I think it's true, you have to appreciate that these meetings are not just for information exchange, they're for culturally broadening scientists – letting them see another part of the world. Maybe the CINP will reach a point where it should never go to Europe and have a meeting there. But its 1998, 2000 and 2004 Congresses are there. Like every other organisation, except the ACNP, up to now it's been a good old boys' organisation – if you're in, you're in and if you're not you aren't. I think they may try to get the bylaws changed before the next election so that it will be competitive. It gets very difficult for an international organisation because on Council you've got to have somebody from here and somebody from there – on a popular vote you might get the Americans voting as a block and we have more members than all the other countries.

CINP, the World Federation and WPA are all different but they all tangle with the same problem – how do you deal with all the different loyalties that cut across continents and countries and still provide good science? I guess they at least deliver enough entertainment, enough culture to satisfy the people who say they were coming for science. The nice thing about the ACNP is that all you really have to worry about is the science and the people who come here have all been everywhere anyway. There are a lot of stars here like our current President, Charlie Nemeroff, and if you're a rising star you don't continue to rise if you hide your light under a bushel. Like the old song says, when you're hot you're hot and you've got to take advantage of it. So I push him to jump into every game he can. Back in the early 1980s and the late 1970s Fridolin Sulser was hot and he was telling me once about how he had to travel so much – I said, Fridolin if it bothers you, so much to travel, just say no. He said, 'Oakley, if you say no once, they may not ask you again.'

Can we chase your interest in the history of psychopharmacology?

I got interested in the history of the ACNP about three years ago. I started the procedure of video-taping all of our big names because I realised that people were getting old – the people who were in at the beginning. I wanted to start taping them to get it down ... and some of them I think we need to tape again and again. I've also had the idea, beginning with this meeting, to try to tape people at the height of their career as well as when they get to be 60 or 70. I'm going to do it by trying to get tapes on all Council members and officers as they come on Council – Dan Weinberger, for instance, now and again in 30 years' time.

I got involved in the CINP history book because Tom Ban has been doing this kind of thing and he needed someone to help him make it happen. I did it at my own expense since there were no CINP funds. We had lots of fun meeting and going over it all and I was up in Toronto to meet with Tom and Frank Berger and Heinz Lehmann and Ned Shorter, the University of Toronto historian of psychiatry. Over lunch, I became convinced that we had to do more to salvage everything for an archive – even what may seem silly material and old stories. Heinz was saying the reason ACNP started to meet in Puerto Rico way back in the beginning was because it was cold as hell in Washington and Eastern Airlines had a special that made it so cheap to come that they couldn't not come. That started the whole tradition of having the meetings in Puerto Rico.

I think people like Frank Ayd need to be interviewed at length. He is probably the most under-rated person in the whole field. He was involved from the beginning of the CINP as well as the ACNP and on top of that you know he must be one of the world's best Catholics. He was very much involved in the Vatican and he was was able to get the Vatican Pontifical Council to sign on with the Decade of the Brain. He talks about stories with his kids at the Second Vatican Council back in 1962 or whatever, and the priest next to their room in the Vatican didn't like cats and so his kids would go out and bring in cats off the street and put them in his room. He raised hell about it – of course he's the current Pope. That's the kind of thing that gives flesh to the skeleton of the history. To hear Frank Berger talk about how he got out of Czechoslovakia – I think the Germans came in one day and he left the next day, taking only his camera with him. When Heinz Lehmann got his degree in Berlin the people said, we will send your degree once you go to North America and get a job – when you have a job then we'll send you your degree. I'm afraid all of that's going to be lost if we don't just tape everything.

I was talking last night to Len Cook. I said, Len you've got to send all your stuff to the archives. He said, 'Well, I'll go through it.' I said, 'Don't go through it. Everybody wants to go through it but I don't want you to go through it – just send everything. How do you know what historians are going to think is important?' So he says he has all the original correspondence back from when he was with SKF back in the early 1950s. He's saved all of this stuff – he's a pack-rat. He said, 'I've wanted to throw it out many times and then said well, I'll wait.' I said, 'Don't throw it out. I want you to send it in.' I talked to Joel Elkes but he's got rid of it here and there. That's what I'm worried about. Everybody does it – you purge. But I think an awful lot of history is going to come out from the comments you get back when you send an article into *Neuropsychopharmacology*, when the editor writes back and says, 'David, this is ridiculous. That correspondence I think is going to be important. How do people see this particular topic and this finding? How about pink sheets on your grants? – that's the kind of stuff that I think is important and I think needs to be salvaged before it gets lost forever.

So at this meeting, the history task-force is going to meet and I'm sure decide to do a history of the ACNP. That will make a major contribution. I think we need to go back and ask, for instance, what was it like two years before Morruzzi and Magoun wrote *The Waking Brain*. Unfortunately I don't have anymore the physiological psychology book that I had then but I still remember a CIBA symposium volume on behaviour and brain mechanisms – one of the early ones, probably in the late 1950s. I remember Larry Stein got a copy and he and I kept stealing it back and forth because we only had one copy. That opened up a whole universe for us and others. I remember arguing in the early 1960s with people on the pharmacology faculty at Pittsburgh about neurotransmitters – some of whom didn't even believe in neurotransmitters.

In Vanderbilt, the medical school decided they wanted an archive but they made a policy decision they only wanted in their archives material from world-famous faculty and so they haven't sent out a general invitation. They didn't even send anything to Allen Bass, who's an emeritus. When they finally needed his office, I was talking to Fridolin, who was saying that he was helping Allen and Sarah his wife pick up all of his stuff and put it into boxes and take it home. I said, 'What are they going to do with it?' and he said that Sarah said, 'Probably throw it out.' So I told him not to do that but to put it into the psychopharmacology archive. He started teaching in the late 1930s at Syracuse and he still has his original hand-written notes from then. Well, I think that's important to see how somebody thought about the issues then.

We need to have as much as we can of everything and if we end up filling barn after barn so much the better because at some point somebody will wander through the barn and begin to pick out things. I think it's been a fascinating era and area to be in. I just wish that I had more time and energy and money to put into it but I've got so many irons in the fire. I will continue in this role as Secretary and history collector as long as ACNP will have me and I want them and can do the job. It's given me an opportunity to interact with people that I would never have interacted with having come out of a non-medical, non-physiological, non-biological tradition. I really think that the brain is the last frontier and that we are going to have more fun, particularly finding out how the brain and behaviour, the psyche, the endocrine system and the immune system mesh together.

The foundation of the British Association for Psychopharmacology

Reading the Clinical Journal in 1974, it seems as though some of the first meetings of the BAP were recorded. Have those recordings survived?

Not that I know of. Some acquaintance of one of us asked if he could record it but when he found we didn't have any money to pay him – that was the last we ever heard of him.

Pity about that. It would have been nice to have some record. What do you remember of the foundation of the BAP?

To begin with, George Beaumont's description as far as it goes is pretty accurate. From my point of view I first conceived an idea of forming a British Association of some kind or other because at that time I had a grant from the US National Institute for Mental Health (NIMH). I had that for 12 years to do psychotropic drug trials in general practice because they couldn't do it in the USA. It was written into the grant that I should attend two meetings a year, one of which was the American College of Neuropsychopharmacology (ACNP), which was held usually in Puerto Rico in December.

Now as a result of going to those meetings I learnt quite a bit about the ACNP and how it was set up. At that time, they hadn't been going for very long, I think only about 4 years, and they were rather concerned because they had one pharmaceutical company sponsorship, I think it was Geigy, and they were really dependent on the one company for money. So they decided it wouldn't do and they established a corporate membership, which meant that any pharmaceutical company could pay, I think it was $1000, and that entitled one of their staff to attend the ACNP meetings. There had been a lot of dissension over this – a lot of people felt they were too dependent on the pharmaceutical industry so when we were discussing setting up the BAP we had this very much in mind. This is quite important, as you will see given what ultimately happened.

Well, I first was thinking about this at the CINP meeting in Prague and I mentioned it to Alec Coppen. This, as far as I was concerned, was the first, if you like, discussion of the idea with anybody else and he agreed it was a jolly good idea and let's go ahead with it. Well, as so often happens nothing was done until the next CINP meeting which was held in Copenhagen. Now in the meantime I had become very friendly with Anthony Horden, who was then a consultant psychiatrist at King's, and he came to that meeting. He hadn't been to one before. I took him as my guest and he was rather horrified to find that the bulk of the meeting was concerned with basic research and that there was very little clinical material. So that also we had in mind when we came to discuss the BAP again. After that meeting I got together with Anthony Horden – we were really the originators of it – and we discussed it and I thought, well we must go ahead and do something about it.

So we had these two important facts in mind. Firstly we would be rather wary of what arrangement we might have with the pharmaceutical industry, and secondly we wanted it to be a clinical association, and those two facts led to a lot of the problems we had. Anyway, to cut it short, I in fact composed the letter outlining the intention to form a British Academy of Psychopharmacology. I approached various other people and of course they were notable as being clinicians but with one obvious exception and that was Malcolm Lader. How we missed him I don't know. Well, this of course upset the basic scientists, particularly Philip Bradley, who was a very good friend of mine actually. I remember at one meeting, I think it was at the Paris CINP, he came over shaking his head and looking dolefully at me saying, 'David, what have you done, what have you done?' He said, 'I wouldn't have minded if you called it (it was called the Academy in those days) the Academy of Clinical Psychopharmacology.' Of course, he had a good point there. Anyway he got together with Malcolm Lader and with various other basic science people and they were threatening to set up a rival organisation. Well, as it happened a long acrimonious correspondence went on between Max Hamilton and Philip Bradley. At one time they were hardly speaking to one another. However, it all got smoothed out and we realised this error and so of course we opened the doors to the basic scientists and also to anyone who had an interest in psychopharmacology.

Can I go back and ask you more about the other people whose names are on the letter and how they came to be there? Sidney Brandon, from an alphabetical point of view, was the first. Did you have reasons for this particular group?

Yes, it was alphabetical. Anthony Hordern and myself drew up the list. We thought they were people who would be interested in the idea of setting it up. They were people we knew personally, who were perhaps fairly eminent in the field of psychopharmacology and doing research in psychopharmacology.

As regards eminence in the field, one of the curious things about the foundation of the BAP, and a flavour that comes through when one talks to the people involved in the start, is that well, yes, you picked the people like Alec Coppen who were doing the work and who were well known but on the other hand they weren't at Oxford, Cambridge or the Maudsley – they weren't part of the established centres, as it were. This seems somewhat strange. Any ideas?

There was no particular reason. It was just people we knew who we thought would be keen on the idea and would co-operate and in fact that's what happened.

Do you think there's anything about psychopharmacology that means that it is something that can often happen better outside the established centres of excellence?

No, we didn't have any ideas like that at all. The people we chose were just people we thought would support the establishment of a psychopharmacology organisation. We didn't want the organisation to be a society because we felt other countries all had colleges but we couldn't call it a college because of the Royal Colleges. There was a precedent in America with the Academy of Psychosomatic Medicine, so we went for that but clearly to the British ear that didn't sound very well and that name soon changed. Fortunately we didn't have to change the initials. It was still BAP.

How useful was it to have Max Hamilton on board?

Oh, he was absolutely invaluable because his name was very important. You couldn't possibly have founded something like this without including him and he was very, very good in the early days. He was very good in controlling meetings. The inaugural meeting was noisy.

Do you want to go into that in a bit more detail? There were a few meetings between the first one in June and then the two meetings on 22 and 23 November.

Yes, my memory of the initial opening meeting is perhaps not all that clear but there was a lot of dissension at that meeting. Firstly from some basic scientists there, obviously because they hadn't been included, but also from representatives from the pharmaceutical industry. They took great exception because in the founding letter that was published I had said something about relations with the pharmaceutical industry and their argument was that they were psychopharmacologists like any of the rest of us. They argued that we were discriminating against them. But of course the reason for that was this background that had happened at the ACNP. But all of those things got smoothed out. Max Hamilton in fact smoothed it all over and everything then was set up I think to most people's satisfaction. Philip Bradley was brought into it.

later on they were all brought in ...

I don't know if they were all brought in at that meeting because at that meeting we only had a Steering Committee – we weren't a formally elected Council at that time. It was at a later meeting where we actually had an election – and I remember thinking, I was sitting up on the platform with Max Hamilton, and I said, well, all this effort I've put in and perhaps now I won't get elected. But I was and I think George Beaumont was elected assistant secretary. We had two secretaries originally, a principal secretary and an assistant secretary. We then set up various sub-committees, the most important of which was the programme committee, and the programme committee appointed their own meeting's secretary. Well, as time went on it was clear that the meeting's secretary was really the most important person because he would be responsible for the whole programme of what we did but in point of fact that person wasn't actually an elected officer.

Anyway we set out with Max Hamilton, as Chairman and President and I was the secretary. I in fact had arranged most of the early meetings, including the first clinical meeting we ever had at the Royal Society of Medicine – on Stress and the Heart. I got various contributors to come and speak at that meeting. I remember very vividly Max Hamilton insisting that the membership fee should be £10 and in those days a lot of people felt that was too high but he said, 'No, if we put it at that level then we won't have to increase it.' I don't think it was increased for about 10 years, which again was showing his very good common sense. Merton Sandler became involved at a very early stage and he organised a meeting which clearly was mainly concerned with the laboratory side of things.

In terms of office in those days you spent 3 years on Council then you went off for a year and if you were re-elected back you could be, but you had to go off for a year. Except of course for the immediate Past President. The President served 2 years and then became immediate Past President and there was also a Vice-President who was the President-elect. But of course the problem was that we had all started together and were due to go off together after a 3-year period and there was not enough continuity and that was when I think the 'disastrous RSM meeting', referred to by George Beaumont, occurred.

I didn't know about a disastrous RSM meeting.

I don't know what happened. They didn't get any advertising and it floundered rather. It was after that that Merton Sandler became President. He was the third or fourth President. At that point, I believe, George Beaumont was the programme secretary. He was absolutely invaluable to the Association because he drafted the Constitution and that was a major contribution.

It was he who drew up the Constitution rather than Max Hamilton?

No, it was George Beaumont but he only served a year I think as programme secretary and he then resigned. I remember Merton Sandler phoning me and saying, look we haven't got a programme secretary; could you come back as programme secretary? I agreed to do this. Although I had been very much involved in the foundation, this was really the period that I enjoyed the most because I was organising all the meetings. It was really what I had wanted to do from the word go. And I think we never looked back after that. But it was Merton Sandler who pulled it all together. He knew everybody.

We then had a routine summer meeting which would be held two out of three outside London and two other meetings which were 1-day meetings, one in the spring and one in the autumn. Merton arranged for us to hold those meetings at the Royal Society, which is really a much nicer place than the Royal Society of Medicine. And he gave me really a very free hand. I organised a meeting at Exeter University and three of the BAP monograph meetings.

Some of our early publications were through Raven Press, again because of Merton Sandler. When Oxford turned them down, he said, why don't you go to Raven? *Stress and the Heart*, written 13 years ago, is still selling. It badly needs a third edition but I haven't the time to do it. Then there were another two that came from organised symposia. These were all half-day symposia which are not enough for a proper book. So I invited extra contributors from outside to cover the whole subject. So, as I say I was then very much involved in the management of the meetings. One was in Aberystwyth – I always remember that one.

Aberystwyth? Who did you expect to go?

Well, it was a very well-attended meeting. There were over 100 people there. That was Philip Bradley's suggestion. I think he was President. He suggested Aberystwyth. Nobody knew anything about it and I remember going on a trip to see what facilities there were and they were good, so the meeting was set up. I think it was on a Monday, Tuesday and Wednesday. But what nobody told me and I didn't find out, there was no train service there on a Sunday so how people got there I have no idea. I know somebody actually hired a helicopter and flew in by helicopter. We had 10 pharmaceutical companies and they paid £250 each to exhibit, which paid for the meeting – dinner and everything. That was what I used to do for the annual meetings. For the 1-day meetings in the spring and the autumn, I would approach one company but never the same one twice in a row and ask, 'Would you sponsor this meeting?' and that paid for those meetings too. So, we started off on really a good financial basis and I think it's gone from strength to strength.

The other thing was was that nobody realised that Aberystwyth was 'dry' on a Sunday. However, other means were found of circumventing that and the meeting went extremely well. Another one in Exeter also went extremely well and the third one I did I think was the one in Birmingham which had already been more or less set up by Merton and Phillip Bradley, and I never had very much to do with that.

When it came to the end of my 3-year term and they asked me if I'd like to be the Treasurer, I didn't want to very much – I had other interests by then. So I really dropped out of things from thereon. I used to go to the meetings, but over the years I've tended to attend less and less. Just like the CINP, they tended to get dominated by the basic scientists. I'm afraid this is the tendency – clinicians unfortunately have responsibilities to their patients and can't always get to meetings. Basic scientists it seems are always able to. And I think that is a pity. So over the years I've tended to be less and less involved with the BAP.

Why was Merton Sandler so important? Do you want to expand on that a bit more?

Yes, he was responsible for re-galvanising it. I've found that this happens with so many organisations, with societies and so on. The initial enthusiasm is usually carried on – in this case only for the first 3 years because all the founding members were on the Council for that time. When they go off there is a hiatus for a period and that is a very dangerous period because the organisation can founder completely. I think that we were in danger of doing that. But Merton really took the reins. He's a very good delegator and I think he was really responsible for inspiring people. He didn't actually do a great deal unless it was necessary. If somebody was supposed to do something and didn't do it then he would do it himself. He would prefer to delegate but he chose the right people to delegate to. And he was invaluable if you were stuck for speakers. I knew clinical speakers but didn't know basic science speakers but he just knows everybody in his own sphere or not. So I think that was really a turning point and I don't know what would have happened if ...

Knowing Merton I'm sure he brought a certain humour to the proceedings. For a long time during the 1980s the BAP was a fun group and it has always seemed to me that a great deal of that stemmed from Merton.

Oh yes it was. But that was how we had started. We used to have our Council meetings, I think once a month when we were setting it up, at the RSM – we had a private room there. I used to arrange the food and I went along and saw the catering manager and asked if he could improve on the standard buffet – so we always had cold duck and we used to sit around then, help ourselves and eat while we were talking and there was a very good feeling – everybody was full of enthusiasm. As the group broke up it didn't always continue. Anthony Horden had really been responsible with me in setting it up but lost interest and went off to Australia.

As you say, you went to the BAP meeting this year and it was very much basic scientists. Why do you think that is, because clearly the primary use of psychotropic drugs is in general practice? What can be done to bring this element of psychopharmacology back on board? – at the moment the only GPs involved are yourself and George Beaumont.

Exactly, and you will find that I put this in the original objectives that we would envisage our membership would consist of basic scientists, psychiatrists, psychologists and various other categories. General practitioners were also in fact included. Many years after one of the popular journals phoned me up and said they were looking at this and wondered what the contribution of the GP was – how many GP members did we actually get? The answer was we didn't get any, other than George Beaumont and myself.

   The reason for that? Well, GPs are very busy for one thing. They don't have the time to come to meetings and of course psychopharmacology is only a small part of their work and there is a certain lack of realisation of its importance; in particular, in relation to the affective disorders. I find even now I'll get patients referred to me with depression and they say I went to my GP and he told me just to shake it off and refused to give drug treatment. So clearly there is a need, I think, for better education for general practitioners particularly in the area of depression. Anthony Hordern used to say that suicide is the mortality of depression and he was right.

What can be done about the lack of GP involvement?

I don't know what the present constitution of the Council is or what is recommended but in one of the early minutes you will probably see that it was decided that there should be an equal representation between basic and clinical branches and also that the presidency should alternate between a clinician one year and a basic scientist the next. I would have thought a GP could be brought in in some way like this. I am not sure whether the presidency still alternates like that or not.

It has done, but that caused some fuss when it came to Philip Bradley's turn to take over the presidency.

Yes, it did. It was the only time when we had an alternative candidate and an election. The arrangement had been that we would recommend a candidate. I remember it very well because if there were counter-nominations they had to be in 3 weeks before the actual meeting when the election would be made. There very seldom were but on that occasion Merton certainly was one. Philip Bradley was the nominee of Council and Merton must have been nominated by somebody else but they always got on very well with each other. I'm not really quite sure why an election happened at all.

One more meeting that you were actually involved in generated a great deal of fuss – that was the Guernsey meeting.

The Guernsey meeting – yes well, I was surprised to read what George Beaumont had written about that meeting. To begin with it wasn't the first meeting that was held abroad. One had been held in Paris a year or two before – Mike Trimble was the secretary then; it was a joint meeting with a French organisation. There was a comment that it was too expensive for people to go but I was puzzled by that because I went to the meeting and I thought it was a jolly good meeting. It was very well attended, the hotel was full and some people had to stay outside.

The issue there was that the basic people were saying well, it's all very well drug companies taking clinical people to plush venues but basic scientists won't be able to be involved if that's the way things go.

I'm not sure that is the case. Maybe it was then but I don't know. I wasn't officially involved at that stage but from my point of view I appreciated that meeting very much because they made Max Hamilton and myself honorary members for life, which is the highest honour the Association can give. We were the first two British – I think they made people from abroad and there were about 10 honorary members and we were the first two British clinicians to be made honorary members. So I enjoyed the meeting very much but also I helped organise a symposium – something to do with sex.

Sex was a very unusual thing to organise meetings about 10–15 years ago.

Yes that's true, but there you are. It's an important subject.

Well yes, clearly, but George in his interview was saying that when he began to get these reports about clomipramine and made something of them, the company weren't keen for him to discuss it in public.

No, quite. These days I'm sure they would be but I also remember one of the spring or autumn meetings at which we had Patricia Gillen speaking. She was working at the Maudsley, which had a sex clinic in those days which she ran. Some of the slides she showed didn't leave anything to the imagination. And I always remember this meeting was held at the Royal Society, and she was up on the stage and I was chairing it and the lights were half down and she had one of these slides up showing some esoteric position and Max Hamilton came in and sort of peered round, blinking a bit and looking at the screen – he was absolutely transfixed. So, as I say, they were rather fun the meetings in those days.

Taking you back to the RSM meetings, some of the other themes that appeared to come up were the issues of why are we having this group? – the argument that if you're interested in pharmacology you should join the British Pharmacological Society and if you're interested in biochemistry you should join the Biochemical Society and so on. Do you want to comment on that? The idea that this wouldn't be a proper scientific organisation – it would be a mongrel organisation.

There were very good precedents for us setting it up. There was an American College, there was the International College which had been going for some considerable time. There were Czech, Scandinavian, German and there was even a Turkish College. So other countries were setting up organisations in this particular discipline and of course the main precedent was the CINP itself which had been going for about 10 years or more. So clearly if there was an international organisation devoted to this speciality and other countries have national organisations it was about time we joined the bandwagon and indeed we should be in the forefront of developing this very important speciality. This was our feeling so I don't think those objections ever came to very much. They certainly didn't impress us.

What about the feelings of exclusion on the part of the basic scientists? – in a sense they had their own organisation – the Brain Research Group, so the impetus to form a BAP wouldn't have been there in a sense.

Oh no – and they were well catered for by the CINP. So no, there was little impetus from that direction. Initially, it was purely clinicians. I myself was involved in clinical work and I didn't realise how much relevant basic science work was being done – and of course there were very important contributions. However, sometimes the clinical implications of some of the work, that is when I could understand it, escapes me.

So do you think the BAP has lost its way? For instance, should there be more prescribers, especially perhaps GPs, because after all it is GPs who actually prescribe these drugs more than anyone else and actually these days they also do more clinical trials on psychotropic drugs than anyone else.

This is very very true. As I say, I was involved in this at a very early stage, even before George Beaumont. In 1958 in fact I set up the General Practitioner Research Group, which I've described in *The Practitioner*, which also carried many of our early trial reports. At that time I had an arrangement with *The Practitioner* – WAR Thompson ran it from this lovely office in Bentinck Street which had a circular lift. I hadn't seen a circular lift before, and I think it was owned by the *Financial Times* at that time. We had a regular slot in *The Practitioner* which was called General Practitioner Clinical Trials section. In every month's issue we had one or two of our trial reports and that went on for many years.

Why were you so keen to get involved in that area so early? Clinical trials really only began in the late 1950s so it was very early to be talking about a clinical trials group.

I'll tell you how it started. I was in general practice but I never really cared much about general practice – I had gone into it for a living. But as I continued I became more and more interested in the use of drugs and when I saw an advertisement from Menley and James, which was a drug company in those days – it was later taken over by SmithKline & French – for a part-time General Practice Advisor, I applied. Now the reason for that was that they were just bringing in oral penicillin preparations in a mixture form for children. The main use of oral penicillin was for children but they had a great problem disguising the taste of it. It's not much good having a preparation if a child spits it out. And so they wanted a general practitioner advisor. I tried out lots of preparations in my own practice and that extended then to other drugs. I even got my first trip to the States under their auspices. I remember travelling on a wonderful plane called a StratoCruiser which had four propellers and it took 12 hours coming back, which was faster than going out, and it was all first class. It had two decks with a bar down below and then you slept in what is now the luggage rack.

Anyway Kenneth Carter their medical director transferred to Ames, and I followed him although of course they were mainly into urine testing strips. They didn't have many drugs. I was their part-time advisor for quite a while – it involved 1 day a week, that's all, but after a while I felt, well how on earth can I branch out of this? So I conceived the idea that the limits on what I could do were that I didn't see enough patients to do a proper trial. So I felt, well let's get a few people together and then approach several firms. I wrote around to old friends, most of whom I had known at Guy's. I got a nucleus of 12 and I then approached four companies. Of the companies I chose two large ones and two small ones; the two small ones didn't have a medical director but they were glad of advice as well. I think Ciba was one, Pfizer was one and one of the two small ones was Bengue. They are probably no longer in existence but they had a number of products as well as a well-known balsam. The other one was Camden Chemicals, who made lithium. Anyway they all came in and immediately started giving us all sorts of drugs to try out. Of course in those days there were no regulations about at all. It was just a matter of handing it out to the patients – here's the latest thing! We didn't really think about side-effects.

Were these all drugs or just psychotropic drugs?

No, all drugs. I was still in general practice then. My interest in psychotropic drugs came about shortly after this. Kenneth Carter was a good friend, who although I think he disapproved of my leaving Ames, when I had a trip to the

States, phoned me up. He said: 'By the way, I was talking to some people down in Washington and they are very interested in the idea of your general practitioner research group; Jonathan Cole of the Psychopharmacology Research Service is interested. I was telling him about your work with general practitioners and he said, 'If you'd like to go and see him they'll pay your flight from New York and your expenses there.' I'd never seen Washington and thought it was a good chance to see it. I didn't have a particular interest in psychopharmacology then. But I remember this meeting clearly. I remember people like Mitch Balter, who was one of the people present, and as the meeting went on somebody said, 'Now when you apply for one of our grants, here is what you should do.' I remember feeling quite amazed at the idea but I thought, 'That's a jolly good idea' and so I did ...

This was when?

It would be around about the early 1960s because the group hadn't been going all that long. So, anyway I applied for one of these grants and I got it. In those days they had a lot of money to give grants in psychiatry and they didn't know quite what to do with it – at least that's what I was told. And somebody else said, when I asked why Jonathan Cole chose me, that 'Well, he's a guy who plays hunches and you were one of his hunches.' I think the main reason was that it was quite impossible to do any drug trial in the States with general practitioners. They just weren't interested. They all earn so much money anyway, so they felt, well here's someone doing them. It was a wonderful 12 years I had. I was the only foreign grant holder. The original organisation was the ECDEU, Early Clinical Drug Evaluation Unit, which is now the NCDEU. Each year there was a meeting and that consisted of all the investigators who had grants and we numbered 24. And I was the only one other than Lehmann and Ban from Canada who was not American. It was very nice. We used to get together once a year, initially in Washington but it moved to Key Biscayne, which was even better. Those were my two meetings, ECDEU at the end of May and ACNP in Puerto Rico in December – who could wish for anything better than that? They were lovely meetings because they were relatively small, particularly the NCDEU. I got very friendly with all the American investigators and this was very pleasant.

Who were the key people in the US at this point?

George Simpson, who worked with Nate Kline, Jonathan Cole and then his successor at NIMH, Jerry Levine, as well as Mitch Balter, Martin Katz and Ronnie Lipman. There were a number of people involved who had played a part in developing rating scales such as Al Raskin and Lino Covi at Johns Hopkins, Leo Hollister in LA and John Overall from Houston who put together the BPRS. There was William Zung of the Zung self rating scale and of course Donald Klein, Karl Rickels and Ronald Fieve. There was Heinz Lehman and Tom Ban from Montreal. There was always a strong representation from psychologists. In America psychologists were doing all the ratings – Richard Wittenborn from Rutgers I remember ...

What do you mean, they were doing all the ratings?

They were actually rating patients. These were often done by psychologists and they would do a lot of the design of clinical trials and virtually all the statistical analysis so there was a very strong influence from PhDs but no influence at all from basic scientists. It was always clinical and I think ACNP was the same, certainly in my time. There was very little, if any, basic science in it which is probably another thing which influenced my interest to model BAP on the ACNP example.

So it was under Jonathan Cole's influence that you moved from just being a GP in a general drugs group to being a GP interested in psychotropic drugs.

Yes, that started my interest and as I got more and more involved, of course I became fascinated by it and our General Practitioner Research Group, which by that time had grown – at one time I had 500 GPs all over the country doing clinical trials.

An organisational feat that! How did you manage it?

It was, and it was all run by myself with one secretary but she was very good. There were no computers in those days, no calculators even. I remember getting an early statistical calculator which was invaluable but it cost a fortune. I think it was just methodology really. Everything was done with pre-printed letters or my secretary would call up the GPs. But anyway I then formed a subsection of the General Practitioner Research Group which was the Psychopharmacology Research Group and that consisted of members who had a particular interest to do psychotropic drug trials. Now of course they became more and more expert as time went on, but at that time we didn't have meetings or anything else. It would have been impossible with that number.

On that point, were you using any inter-rater reliability assessments and all that?

No. We just presented the rating scales to the investigators and said, fill them in. I have to give George Beaumont credit there for starting protocol meetings and having video tapes and really checking inter-rater reliability. No, we just muddled on – which was really what everybody else was doing. Even in the States they weren't doing inter-rater reliability. It all came later.

Again my aim was to do everything as easily as possible. We had a punch card but because I really didn't want to waste time and money on printing punch cards they used to be mimeographed. There were no photocopiers in those days but I had a local agency who could produce these – on foolscap sheets. I remember Jon Cole saying at one meeting, 'Dr Wheatley uses the largest punch card I have ever seen.' The answers to the questions were put against a punched hole so all the investigator had to do was make a mark – they didn't have to write very much at all. And so that was what we used. Then of course you needed to collect very little data in those days. If we needed more data, we used more than one card but then analysis became more difficult. But by that time pharmaceutical companies were tending to do their own analysis of the data although I have always tried wherever possible to do my own analysis.

Now of course clinical trials aren't just run by the companies but they are run by the companies in various different parts of the world, so no one owns them in a way I guess you owned your trials.

Exactly, and a lot of companies tend to only pay lip service to the pharmaceutical associations' guidelines, particularly the section that companies should encourage publication even of negative results, while reserving the right to ask the investigator to discuss their report with them or something like that. The last time I was involved in this way there was a little dissension over a study, a few years back. That was a multi-centre study. My group contributed 150 patients to this trial, which was an appreciable contribution. When it came to an end, I had done my own analysis and written my own report which I always sent to the company, so if they had any objection to it they would come back to me. And they came back and said, 'Well, we've decided not to go ahead with the drug because we had an adverse report from one hospital but certainly go ahead and publish what you like.' So I went ahead and published it but meanwhile they had a re-think on this and without really consulting me at all, had written up all the results, putting my name on as a co-author on something I hadn't then seen. Then my report appeared in print and they were annoyed about this, saying well we didn't know you had actually submitted it – you should have let us see the final version. But they had seen my report and I said my submission to a journal was based on that report. They have a habit of changing the text, which I don't like – I'm not going to have my English changed around into phraseology which I would never use. Someone, I can't remember who it was, said that I was a disgrace, I had let my colleagues down and this, that and the other. But they didn't have a leg to stand on because I had, in fact, strictly observed everything that was in the contract.

But that was the last time I did it because now one's only such a small cog. We're doing a trial on Alzheimer's disease here – an enormous, multi-national study. I enjoy doing it because even though it's double blind, I think the drug is working and I think I can pick up patients who are responding. But the documentation is vast for just one patient. There are other trials I am doing here – they're on antidepressants and a hypnotic coming up. These are just bread and butter although I hate filling in all these forms. I enjoy doing things like Hamilton Ratings but I sometimes find the monitoring visits somewhat tedious. Anyway I appreciate if you're going to do clinical trials you have to do this. But I try to keep individual research going particularly in the psychopharmacology of sleep. I was the first, in this country, to publish reports on the clinical use of both zopiclone and zolpidem. Zopiclone was in the *British Journal of Psychiatry* and I presented zolpidem at one of the NCDEU meetings.

I'm trying to do further work on sleep. At the moment I'm particularly interested in sleep in patients with HIV. I've been studying HIV patients for the last 6 years, at an AIDS Centre in Crouch End. I've got no support for this one whatsoever. What I want to do is some polysomnography on these patients and now through the good offices of Chris Idzikowski I have a loan of an Oxford portable machine and he's doing the analysis free of charge. We plan to do them on half a dozen cases and it looks promising – we are doing our fourth one on Tuesday. My only expense is to pay the technician – she has to come over from Wimbledon. I've tried to get a grant and I've been promised one but it hasn't materialised. I'll pay for that out of my own pocket because I make enough out of the other trials to indulge my hobby, if you like.

What are you hoping to show?

A very good question. I'm particularly interested in sleep staging and especially deep sleep because there is no doubt deep sleep is a stage of sleep in which changes take place in the body, whether they are concerned with repair or what is less clear but it is certainly a very essential part of sleep. This clearly raises the question of what drugs might be helpful, because you don't want to use the benzodiazepines, which increase sleep by increasing the light stages, in somebody who is already immuno-compromised.

But to advocate anything what you've got to show in the first place is that people with HIV in fact have sleep problems – that's been done. We've studied a group of 45 HIV-positive patients and 45 matched controls, matched for age within 5-year limits and sex, because they are mostly male – there are three females out of that group. And in fact clinically, using a simple clinical scale asking how they've slept there is greater impairment of sleep in patients with HIV and much greater in fact if they've actually got AIDS. So the next step is to do sleep EEGs and see how this correlates clinically. And as I say, we've done three patients and the results so far have been interesting.

The problem is to try and get funding. I tried to get an NIMH grant. At that time I had no access to AIDS patients here because I didn't know about Crouch End and obviously all the big centres have got their own programmes and they're not interested in somebody who's got no experience with AIDS. But I got in touch with David Sheahan in Tampa who is Professor of Psychiatry there and he was very interested, and it occurred to me that perhaps they would have AIDS patients and he said, 'Yes we do but nobody wants to know them – come over here and treat as many as you like and people will say thank you very much.' So I went over there a few times and in fact I still have a work permit to work there. And we put in a grant application, or rather I did. Because of the possibility of plagiarism, I had to disguise the main objectives and make it much more general and inevitably it got turned down.

Listening to you talk, what I am struck by is the fact that quite a few of those who were involved, in the early days – this has come through in a number of interviews – had such a range of interests. These days psychopharmacologists, like everyone else, are often forced to be one-issue people, whereas you're clearly not a one-issue person.

No. I'm interested in ideas and I pursue my ideas. What I am hoping is that if these EEG traces do show that HIV patients who are having sleep problems have a deep sleep problem then it will be an inducement to try and get some financial support. If I could set up a sleep laboratory here, then we could buy our own machine which would be the main expense.

The other thing that interests me is that you are very entrepreneurial. Why have you broken the mould so often?

I don't know. I have always liked to do something different. That's just the way I am. I think I've never been one to go along with the herd. I like to do my own thing. I like to do it, if you like, with advice from other people but not really at the behest of other people. The beauty of the grant that I had from NIMH was that they gave me an open brief. They said, David, you do whatever you like, we'd just like you to tell us what comes out of it. They would send me money and I would say, 'We'll do this trial.'

I was interested at one time in the use of tranquillisers and coronary heart disease – this was before benzodiazepines came under a cloud and we did some double-blind studies to compare diazepam with a placebo added to standard cardiac therapy and I just did it. Someone would make a suggestion and say, look this might be an idea, but there was no veto over it which was what I liked about it. Of course in the early days there were no ethical committees although towards the end of the 12 years I had to set up an ethical committee and use them.

That was, I guess, in order for the data to be used for regulatory purposes ?

Not under the grant. Nothing to do with regulations – that was the job of the pharmaceutical companies. I was just doing research. I obviously needed to get supplies of drugs from companies so the 2 things might be combined but ...

So you weren't so much only doing trials on new agents as doing interesting trials on anything that was in the field?

Yes. For instance, Arthur Prange wrote a couple of articles on thyroid hormone potentiation of tricyclics. He was a very good friend of mine. He was very keen to get confirmation and he asked me if I could do a study with my GPs, which I did. Now in order to do that I had to get triiodothyronine from Glaxo I think. I remember writing to Glaxo asking, could you supply me with this, and in those days if you asked for something like that from a company they would do it out of good will. And they wrote back and said, well – they obviously didn't want to do it you see – and they said well, we can supply you with placebos but you'll have to pay for them. So I said, oh that's all right, I have funds to pay, which I did. They never in fact charged me, so they did supply me. That was one study which I did. The benzodiazepines after heart attacks was another but in the end I couldn't pursue that, which was a great pity because the clouds started to descend on the benzos.

You've raised a number of issues there to do with how things have changed in recent years in terms of pharmaceutical companies and the way they interact with researchers. They have necessarily become much more bureaucratic because of the CSM, the FDA and all the regulations of various sorts – has the weight of regulation begun to poison the goose that laid the golden egg? Even if they wish to be, companies are not as able to be as freely co-operative as they once were.

No, they can't and it's a problem clinically. There's been an enormous change and I think it's gone too far the other way really, because now the complexity of drug trials and all the checks and so on really make for inaccuracy. The documentation of this trial I'm doing with Alzheimer's is pedantic. An initial interview with the patient takes about 5 hours and they are also seen by a psychologist and then by a general physician – in other words about a day, and we each have a volume to fill in. If I make any alterations, the alterations must be initialled with the date even if I have just written a 7 and changed it to an 8. That won't do – it's got to be crossed out and re-written. The other thing is that some of the sections have a space for comments but comments have to be written in capital letters because they are going outside the country for analysis and maybe they can't read my handwriting. This is the sort of totally unnecessary workload that is being put on clinicians and it's bound to interfere with your clinical judgements.

In my view it's defeating the purpose of the exercise and quite unnecessary. Really what I think pharmaceutical companies should be doing, if they really want accuracy, is take all this tedious drudgery away from the skilled clinical investigator, who should be giving much more attention to the assessments he is making because clearly in conditions like Alzheimer's, for example, the assessments depend very much on your clinical impressions.

To an extent we are becoming deskilled then. What you are saying is that the companies want to standardise things so much, there will be no room for the creative clinical impressions that have proved so important in the past.

Exactly. In other words they are trying to make a precision machine out of what still remains an inexact science.

One more name which comes up in the clinical trial area was Linford Rees. Reading round and having had the opportunity to talk to him it seems that in the late 1950s or thereabouts, as I say, clinical trials were new around that point, there were only a few people who really understood them in psychiatry in this country, such as Max Hamilton and Linford Rees. But he never became so heavily involved in the BAP.

Yes, I'm not quite sure why not. He was a great friend of Anthony Horden and Anthony was a great admirer of his and may I think have mentioned his name as the first president but perhaps he declined because he was very busy at the time. I would look upon him as a sort of a diplomat. He was a wonderful diplomat as well as being a very good clinician.

What about the MRC trials?

Oh yes, well the one I think of is the one which purported to show that there was just a tranquillising effect to antidepressants. That was something which I thought we would try and duplicate in one of our early trials. Edward Hare was the guy who was involved in that. He was then editor of the *British Journal of Psychiatry*.

Yes, I had actually forgotten about that, because the early editors of the British Journal of Psychiatry, Slater and Hare, while biologically oriented really have not been drug oriented.

No, that's very true. I remember what we did. I wanted to find out whether it might just be a sedative effect so what I did was to look at the number of trials we had done and look at the proportions of patients who complained of sedation and then compare the outcome with the drugs and see whether those who were sedated got better quicker. I think that was published in the *British Journal of Psychiatry*.

Another suggestion of the NIMH was that we should look upon doctors' attitudes and that gave me one of the very few papers which I got into *The Lancet*. We classified doctors as to whether their attitude to each individual patient was optimistic, indifferent or pessimistic as to whether they were going to respond to a particular drug. Now this is compounded obviously in the case of a particular patient of what one knows about the patient and whether they ever respond to anything and also there's the belief about whether the drug is effective or not. The patient would be assessed in the same manner.

In anxiety there was a very clear-cut distinction from depression. In anxiety expectations of treatment made a big difference. Optimistic doctor/patient relationships did much better than pessimistic ones but in depression you didn't get that relationship at all. At that time a lot of people were saying, well you can treat depressed patients as well with psychotherapies as with drugs. But this study pretty well demonstrated that, in general practice anyway, the attitude of the doctor wouldn't make any difference. Anxiety yes, depression no. So that was something we did with NIMH which had been suggested by them. They did come up with some very good ideas sometimes but it was up to me whether I liked their idea. I found that a very nice way to work.

Stress is another area you've been one of the first into, which has again become very fashionable. Did you anticipate it becoming fashionable again?

Yes indeed. When I became interested in it, I was a bit disconcerted at the sort of people who were practising 'stress therapy' of various kinds. They often seemed to be people without any qualifications at all. And I felt there was a need to put it on a more scientific basis. I suppose my interest started with that book *Stress and the Heart* in 1977. I was interested then in the effects on the heart because cardiology has been my second love, if you like, after psychiatry and it was my first love until I met psychiatry, or psychopharmacology. So I did have that interest in the effect of the mind on the heart and then I felt, well what do you mean by stress? I had asked Hans Selye to write the opening chapters of the book. I used to go and see all my authors so I went to see Selye when he was alive and ...

What was he like?

He was a funny little man, sitting in this great high-back chair. You'd go down this great corridor with signed pictures of Winston Churchill, De Gaulle and every world leader who had been to see him or sent congratulations to him. He was very pleasant and said, yes of course he would write an introduction, which was great. But there again I read his books and I wasn't really awfully clear about the clinical implications of a lot of his work. I think I felt there was a need to try and define exactly what stress is and how we measure it and to set up a stress clinic.

Malcolm Lader has been a very good friend indeed to me. When I tried to set up a stress clinic in order to do this, I tried a number of hospitals. I had tried Guy's and Charing Cross and the initial reaction was always very poor. I think Malcolm Lader was my last resort and Malcolm said, what a good idea, let's go and talk to the Dean, and so it was set up at the Maudsley.

Then I had to devise an instrument to measure stress. After a lot of thinking I decided there were nine areas which I would try to measure, including social habits, such as smoking, drinking, use of drugs, caffeine-containing drinks, then social relationships, which include personal relationships, stress at work, stress in the home. Then came life events, things that have happened in the past which are still causing stress in the present. Then I had a section on sexual stresses which was concerned with aspects of sex, especially libido and whether the individual is satisfied with it, whether they felt they were over-sexed or under-sexed in relation to their partner. That and different physical aspects, such as anorgasmia in a woman, premature ejaculation and so on, and then the psychological aspects of the actual techniques of love making. People are only too pleased to talk about this – very very frankly too. Then there is masturbation and feelings of guilt over masturbation. The other areas covered are psychiatric disorders, a section on sleep, a section on menstrual stress for women, the peculiar stresses of old age and inevitably a section on stress and the heart. You've got measurements there – you can measure the heart rate, blood pressure and see if they change when hopefully you relieve the stress problem.

Each of the individual items is scored on defined scales so that you can make a score on each. I just called it the stress profile to begin with but then I thought, well I might as well be known for something, so I called it the Wheatley Stress Profile (Wheatley, 1993). It has generated quite a lot of interest. I think the main finding when I studied 300 patients at the Maudsley was the very high incidence of depression as a sequela of long continuing chronic stress – stress that could not be avoided such as a person you hated at work but you couldn't do anything about it because you daren't lose your job. One woman, she came in and she was 87 and she said, the trouble is my husband – I can't make up my mind whether to leave him or not. I said, well how long has this being going on? And she said oh, ever since we got married. I think in the end she did decide to leave him and she did leave. Depression is important because it is something you can treat, because the more depressed a person becomes the less able they are to cope with their stress problems and antide-pressant treatment really is very very effective. The minute you can relieve their depression then they say I don't know why I put up with this all this time, I'm going to divorce my wife or whatever the problem might have been, or I'm going to change my job.

So, that was how I started the clinic and this went very well and I got quite a few publications. In particular I did a study with Dr Ji Jianlin in China. There is also a hospital in America where they use it. I shall be presenting a paper on that at the World Stress Congress in Washington in October. It has been trans-lated into Spanish and into Japanese.

The issue of stress leads on to the question of the minor tranquillisers and your book The Anxiolytic Jungle. Do you want to comment on the impact of all those controversies on psychopharmacology generally?

Well, I'm not going to speculate on that one. I have my own ideas as to what may be behind all the fuss. Just we might say this, that a kind of climate has been created in this country which has made people very suspicious. Obviously we had to pay heed to the question of dependence but the way things have developed has made life very very difficult. When I first started the clinic I was prescribing tranquillisers but I very quickly found out that there was a lot of resistance from patients and I very quickly had to stop it.

So what do you give them? They're not all depressed. I have patients with panic disorder, for example, obsessive-compulsive disorder and just gener-alised anxiety. In some cases propranolol helps – that was another early study I did – it can sometimes help the panic attacks for musicians and so on. So what do you use? There isn't anything. I don't know whether there are any non-benzodiazepine tranquillisers in the pipeline. I think there is a need for them, there's no question about it. I personally will go on prescribing benzodi-azepines because according to the main expert Malcolm Lader, it's only 20% of people who are likely to become dependent. It means that 80% won't. But you need long-term treatment; short-term treatment, say confined to 4 weeks, is not much good really. And since benzodiazepines don't cause any other major side-effects it's only dependence that's a problem – any evidence from over-dosage shows that suicide is very doubtful, compared with other drugs.

What would happen, do you think, if we had a blood test that would pick out the people, who would be likely to become dependent?

It would be an absolute godsend. The restraining factors are the medico-legal implications of it. You're scared to. And I very quickly stopped doing it at the Maudsley.

Related to this issue is the growing involvment of the media and the law had come in psy-chopharmacology. Up until the benzodiazepine saga, psychopharmacology was just some-thing for clinicians and basic scientists but now there are a lot of other stakeholders.

Well, I think it's part of the whole change of attitude generally towards the medical profession. We live in a era of doubt and uncertainty, whereas when I started in practice you were the authority figure and nobody would ever think to question any opinions that a doctor made or any drug. If you gave a drug, the side-effects had no publicity even if they were appreciated. It was thalidomide that really blew the lid on it. People certainly realised then that drugs can be dangerous and clearly that's a theme of great attraction to the media, who have been dining out on it ever since.

I quite often now get people who are severely depressed to whom I give an explanation of the biochemical cause of depression, exactly what the antidepressant drug does – it's not a tranquilliser, you won't become hooked on it – it corrects a chemical abnormality. A bit simplistic maybe but they do work provided the patient continues taking them but I still get this 'I don't want to take any drugs.' I shrug my shoulders and say, 'Well, what else is there?' Usually people do come back and they take them and they get better. So unfortunately the controversy over tranquillisers and benzodiazepines in particular has clouded I think the whole area of psychotropic drugs being prescribed, in that people think that anything psychotropic is going to produce dependence or addiction, or that in some way the drugs are 'taking over their minds'.

This is partly responsible but it's part of the general, I think, increased awareness of the public that medicine is not as perfect as we once thought it was, that some illnesses cannot be cured and that some drugs produce serious side-effects, which was glossed over before even when it was actually known. And the media want sensationalism – anything so mundane as the number of depressed patients who are saved from suicide is not of interest. But the one patient who takes an overdose and has a cardiac arrest – it immediately has to be somebody's fault. Whose fault? It must have been a negligent doctor or it's the medical profession itself or of course the pharmaceutical industry. And then there is this enormous growth of paramedical procedures and fringe medicine and so on – you can't really blame the general public if they are not getting relief from standard medical treatment. They need to get relief, there's no good telling them there's no scientific basis for homeopathy, they will just try anything. And unfortunately some people seem to make claims which we in the medical profession would be wary of making.

Picking up the issue of the industry – when you wrote the letter proposing the establishment of the BAP, as you say there was concern to have a policy as regards the industry. It seems to me that in the UK, perhaps more than in Europe and more than in US, we've been very wary of the industry. Why is this?

That is very very true. I think it all stems from the thalidomide affair. This was a shock, not only to the general public but certainly to the practising clinical profession too. I think up to then we had complete faith in any new drug that came along and serious side-effects were not reported or they were not associated with the drugs and I would certainly say that for any new drug that came along, the very fact that it had been marketed meant that it was safe. I took many things myself but since then I'm much more wary about taking things. I think an education after all has happened about drugs and their effects and their disadvantages as well as their advantages, and that's progress.

It's just that you can progress too far sometimes, I think, without weighing up the other side of the picture – the other side of the picture clearly being the morbidity or even the mortality caused by the illness itself. This emphasises the role of the doctor as the person who has to make that decision – whether the treatment I'm using now will do my patient more harm than the illness if I leave it untreated and I often quote that when I'm talking about sleep and sleep disorders – because some of the adverse effects of chronic insomnia are far worse than any possible problem you might produce with a benzodiazepine.

Can I chase further the question of the responsibility of the BAP to educate the public? It seems to me that there's something about educating public perception of risk that we're falling down on – we're leaving the public to be influenced by programmes on TV or whatever.

I couldn't agree more. It was felt, in the early days, that by holding our meetings and generally improving standards we were in a sense informing the public. But these days that is certainly something that we could turn our attention to. We could organise an open meeting, to which the public could come. Now there's a very good precedent for this which is the Edinburgh Science Festival, which is now in its 4th or 5th year. This is open to anybody who wants to go – they run the whole range of meetings concerned with science and it goes on for 2 weeks and there are all sorts of exhibitions and so on. The public pays to come in but a very modest entrance fee, £1 or £2 per session. I've been involved in the last two. The first one was a session on stress and it was packed to overflowing and there was enormous interest from the public. There were the speakers, who were able to answer any questions on the spot, and if they had more publicity and perhaps a publication on it, it would be even more helpful. Last year I did two, one on depression and one on sleep, and again both meetings were sold out and people had to be turned away. The topics had such general interest and one was able to put them in simple language and convey some of the problems involved. So there's undoubtedly a demand for knowledge from the general public but it needs to be well informed. It can only come from the experts.

Select bibliography
See Wheatley D, Healy D (1994). The foundation of the British Association for Psychopharmacology. *Journal of Psychopharmacology*, **8**, 268–278.
See also Healy D (1996). The history of british psychopharmacology. In *150 Years of British Psychiatry* Vol 2 (Freeman H, Berrios G, eds). Athlone Press, pp 61–88.
See also interview with Merton Sandler in *The Psychopharmacologists* Vol 1 and Ian Stolerman in this volume.

21 Ian Stolerman

Behavioural pharmacology

One of my criteria has been to interview people over the age of 60, which you are clearly not, but with your interest in history Ian and your role in the foundation of groups like the BAP and EBPS and background in behavioural pharmacology I was keen to chase both you and Joe Brady.

Joe could provide you with an interesting, very lively perspective from the other side of the Atlantic. His coverage in several areas would approximate to mine but would perhaps tend to emphasise the tradition of radical behaviourism to a greater extent. While I have a lot of sympathy with that approach, which has influenced much that I have done, I cannot claim to be a true believer in all the implications.

So how did you move into the area?

How did I get started? I developed an interest in the psychological effects of drugs during the course of my undergraduate studies for a pharmacy degree in the London School of Pharmacy (the Square). It gave an opportunity for interested people to take quite an extensive pharmacology option and to do half of their final year of studies exclusively in pharmacology. One of the areas that I liked best by then was the psychological effects of drugs. I think one reason I liked it was that there wasn't a huge amount of information to get one's head around. I also had a long-standing but entirely amateur interest in psychology since school days and I suppose if I hadn't done a pharmacy degree, I would probably have done something in the psychological sphere and perhaps ended up looking at drugs anyway.

One of the things that struck me when you were talking a few moments ago was the relationship between psychopharmacology and behavioural pharmacology and how the meaning of these terms has changed over the years. When I began as a postgraduate student with Hannah Steinberg, in 1964, I understood psychopharmacology to mean the study of the psychological effects of drugs. Only when I browsed through your first volume of interviews did I realise that some psychiatrists apparently thought the term was restricted to the use of drugs in psychiatry. Extraordinary! As the years went by the most common meaning of the term changed very substantially, I think, to mean the study of drugs with psychological effects by all available methods, ranging from the psychosocial right through the spectrum down to molecular biology. I find the notion that a boundary can be drawn at any particular point, such as between neuropharmacology and psychopharmacology, to be indefensible and unquestionably damaging to everyone involved if it had been accepted. And the study of the psychological effects did not have a single all-embracing unique term. Behavioural pharmacology has a slightly different and limiting connotation emphasising behavioural approaches to psychology. There isn't as far as I know a term that will cover the whole gamut of psychological studies as pertaining to drug action. So when one has a journal called *Behavioural Pharmacology*, it's already seen by many people as a statement of a theoretical position in favour of radical behaviourism, whereas I believe it is the intention that it should in fact cover as wide a range as possible of work within the psychological domain.

So I developed this interest in psychopharmacology which was encouraged by several pharmacologists at the Square, like Michael Rand, Bill Bowman and Geoffrey West. The tracks of my career and Mike Rand's have crossed subsequently. At that time he was a lecturer and influential in pushing me towards psychopharmacology and encouraged me to contact Hannah Steinberg. Mike worked on nicotine at that time. He had a PhD student, Michael Clark (now a senior scientist at SmithKline Beecham), whose thesis was on nicotine and my first contact really with the nicotine area was serving as a subject in one of Michael Clark's experiments, which was something to do with the knee-jerk reflex and the effects of nicotine thereon; as I didn't smoke, I can only suppose in retrospect that I must have been some type of control subject. Many years after that, subsequent to completion of my PhD, I got into nicotine research and eventually resumed contact with Rand and Clark. In fact, Clark and I were co-supervisors of Max Mirza, an MRC Collaborative Student who completed his studies on nicotine recently.

Around 1965, thinking back about what very roughly the state of knowledge was, as far as I can recall there were a handful of substances that were discussed as potential neurotransmitters in the brain and really there was not that much known about the central actions of even these substances. So at that time the notion of relating behavioural effects of drugs to neurotransmitter systems was really quite a distant prospect. Of course a lot of people were attempting to do so but given that one hardly knew any neurotransmitters in the brain, it seemed to me rather futile to base one's whole effort upon trying to relate some particular behavioural effects to a substance when one did not really know whether it served a useful or important purpose in the CNS at all. I think that was one of the things – one of the factors – that shall we say encouraged me to focus on purely behavioural studies for a long time. There were, maybe fortunately, more ambitious people who felt they could do otherwise but at that stage behavioural methods for the evaluation of drug effects were also relatively primitive – most of the techniques that are widely used now were just really getting off the ground.

Which ones?

If we think particularly about the drug dependence area, there were a handful of publications on drug self-administration by the mid 1960s. It looked interesting but there were no standardised procedures. Although there was a lot of potential, there hadn't been a great deal done other than showing that the phenomenon could occur with some of the classic drugs of dependence. Drug discrimination was a mysterious phenomenon that had been demonstrated but what its practical significance or utility as an assay might be was really obscure to most of us. Studies of tolerance to behavioural effects were held back by the lack of recognition that the environmental context in which drugs were given chronically was a critical determinant of outcome – the key study of Schuster and colleagues came in 1964. It was a period of exploration of a wide variety of psychological behavioural methods and approaches to find out which ones were sensitive to drugs and which could be used for demonstrating clear and substantial dose-related effects of substances, effects that were of biological and not only statistical significance. Quite a lot of time in my PhD was spent just on trying to get an effect of a drug; now if I have a PhD student who spends a year or two just trying to get an effect of the substance being studied, I worry about whether I have set unreasonable goals.

At that time I think that much of the field was really exploring possible approaches. Looking at maze learning methods, operant conditioning approaches, locomotor activity, what we now call ethopharmacology – all of those areas existed but in a rather rudimentary form and it wasn't very clear as to how each one of them might develop.

Who were the people in the field at the time? Roger Russell, Hannah Steinberg, Michael Chance.

They were among the most prominent people. In addition, Philip Bradley and his associates such as Brian Key had done notable work on the psychological effects of drugs in the early days in the early 1960s, as well as doing the neurophysiological work for which they became best known. So they had a nucleus of interdisciplinary research there. Philip never did give up that interest in having behavioural studies in parallel with the more cellular work that he was involved with and that led into my move to his unit in 1974. Chance, also of course in Birmingham, did some of the early important studies on drugs and social behaviour. It was an approach that I was never personally involved with and I suppose the main reason was the difficulty of recording in an automatic manner many of the phenomena and also because I did not really fully comprehend the theoretical structure of the approach. In the same early period, Bradshaw and Szabadi were active in Manchester, Derek Blackman in Nottingham, and of course the nucleus of the Cambridge group was forming. Trevor Robbins and I put together a partial history of the early years of psychopharmacology in Britain although it appeared only in the EBPS newsletter (Robbins and Stolerman, 1990).

Can I pick up on a point there? When psychopharmacology began during the 1960s, people were in very distinct groups. There were the neurochemists, neurophysiologists, behavioural pharmacologists and then the clinical people. In recent years the trend has been toward people working on common problems and becoming neuroscientists. But what you are describing seems to me almost the opposite – a field that is splintering to some extent.

I don't believe the field is splintering. Some people seem to stir up issues by emphasizing lines between, for example, basic and clinical psychopharmacology. Such an attitude harks back to the 1960s. I recall during the early days within the Department of Pharmacology where I studied there was a neuropharmacology group who were assaying concentrations and turnover of monoamines, but those of us who were doing behavioural research never spent any time in those laboratories. We learnt nothing of significance about the neurochemical techniques other than what came out at departmental seminars, and the notion of collaborative research was something that was pretty alien to the prevailing ethos. The neuropharmacologists didn't spend much time in our laboratories. It was very separate lines of work. It was a missed opportunity although I do not think we were unusual in missing it. There were some real scientific difficulties too. Neurochemical work with the methods of the time, such as looking at whole brain concentration of transmitters for example, showed effects of the common psychoactive drugs at doses that were maybe ten times larger than those that produced behavioural effects. That tended to put us off from seeing that there would be a lot of scope for collaboration. Of course that changed fairly quickly. In retrospect, it seems that neurochemistry was refining some of its methodology, just as was behavioural pharmacology as we mentioned earlier, and it was not until at least the mid-1970s that the potential of interdisciplinary studies was realisable. For many years there has been a tremendous amount of encouragement to people to do interdisciplinary collaborations. I fully support this but I think it is also important that we don't go overboard and say that only work of an interdisciplinary nature is necessary or desirable because then we will see fewer advances within the capabilities of individual disciplines.

Can we go back to University College and how you then moved to Birmingham?

During the time I was with Hannah I was influenced to a large extent by research that was carried out in the United States in behavioural pharmacology. There seems to be a different historical line here since many feel that clinical psychopharmacology developed earlier in Europe than in the USA, but this was not true for basic behavioural pharmacology. One reason was that the size of the endeavour there was larger. Another reason was that I had become attracted towards operant conditioning as a method within behavioural pharmacology and that was something that was developing much more in the United States than it was in Britain at that time – though it has to be noted that one of the outstanding exponents of the approach was Peter Dews who, of course, had come from England.

What can you tell me about Peter Dews?

Less than you would like! Peter had left England before I became involved in the area and I did not meet him until about 1982. He was a pharmacologist who wanted to study behavioural effects of drugs who did a certain amount of work in Cambridge and in fact gave an entertaining after-dinner lecture on all of that background at the EBPS meeting in Italy this year. Now, Peter wanted to have a way of quantifying psychological behaviour effects of drugs objectively and as they actually happened – moment by moment, perhaps rather analogous to the way that pharmacological data could be recorded with a kymograph. The available methods didn't meet those criteria. When he visited Skinner's laboratory at Harvard, he was entranced by cumulative recorders drawing out real time records of animal behaviour and of course it emerged that this type of behaviour was sensitive to a wide variety of psychoactive drugs and various types of selectivity were demonstrable. But it is interesting to note that it was very much this criterion of sensitivity – being able to measure the effect – that seemed to have driven Peter that way rather than a particular psychological orientation or theoretical approach. His work did have an enormous impact but it was a delayed impact. His early papers appeared in the early 1950s but it was really in the 1960s that the impact became apparent, when activity in psychopharmacology as a whole was expanding rapidly. Anyway, somewhat to Hannah's disappointment I think, I was very interested in that. I remember Hannah very clearly telling me at one point that the concerns of operant conditioning were not what she considered psychopharmacology was all about. Obviously I disagreed to the extent that I thought it could be an extremely important part.

What did you understand her position then to be in contrast to the way you were developing?

Hannah was very good at cutting through dogma and seeing where the substitution of jargon for real ideas was taking place. I think that was part of why she was rightly critical of some of the more optimistic claims that were made on behalf of radical behaviourism in psychopharmacology, although one does have to say that similarly optimistic excessive claims were made on behalf of other approaches as well. It certainly seemed to be an era where people were saying one approach could be the way to go rather than seeing as we do now that putting different aspects together into a three-dimensional model is much more important.

I think also that very much in our minds at that time was the view taken by some of the radical behaviourists to the effect that the expression of subjective states was something that we perhaps shouldn't be concerned with. Fewer people take that view now but at that time it was something that I think bothered a lot of people. The concept of the organism as a black box with stimuli going in and responses coming out with not very much attention to what was going on in between either in cognitive terms or neuropharmacological terms was a major limitation to thinking. Many people derived their ideas while thinking in non-behavioural terms even if ultimately the results could be explained in a less mentalistic manner, without hypothetical intervening constructs.

That having been said, when I did go off to the United States it was partly for these wonderful scientific reasons but it also seemed to be a good practical move. The BTA (Been-to-America) degree was thought to be of some value and the whole experience was very appealing. And it proved to be a very good experience. I joined Murray Jarvik's group. It was a curious group that he had built up at the Albert Einstein College of Medicine in the Bronx. He was best known for work on drug effects on learning and memory. He had the idea that one could use drugs as tools to differentiate between processes involved in different aspects and stages of learning. That doesn't sound very remarkable now but in the early 1960s it was notable. By the time I was interested in going there, which was around 1969, he had quite a big programme of that sort of work. I wanted to join in but such experience was very much in demand and Murray didn't have any posts available in that area. But he did have something for work on nicotine, which was a line of work for which he was not so widely known at that time. He had published just one or two papers and an excellent book chapter which was very influential.

So when I was offered the opportunity to go to work on nicotine I realised that I would also be able to do something on drugs, learning and memory. When I actually joined Murray's group I found that in fact nearly everybody who had arrived there to do work on nicotine had come because they really wanted to do work on learning and memory; as a result, few of them had actually done any serious work on nicotine which was then highly unfashionable as a research topic in psychopharmacology. It was not universally seen as a drug of course ...

Although so many people wanted to do learning and memory work with drugs, by that time it had already become apparent that the simple notion that one could take the agents available then and dissect stages of learning and memory was not really working. Murray Jarvik's group had tested in two or three procedures in rodents and in primates a vast array of the available substances and almost none of them had any selective effects on memory. Of course any drug would disrupt the performance of the tasks but they had terrible difficulty in finding anything that had any selective effects. I think scopolamine and cannabis ingredients were about the only ones at that time and of course they were detrimental. So that programme seemed to me to be nowhere near as exciting as it looked from the outside; the nicotine area was just in its early stages and beginning to open up, although whether that would actually happen was not apparent to me at the time.

It took me a while to realise that I was one of very few people who had been appointed there to work on nicotine and had actually taken the task seriously. Stan Glick had done some before and that had been very important in leading into my studies. What we did was to take the techniques that I had learnt in London with Hannah, both for animal psychopharmacology and for human research, and modify those for carrying out experiments on nicotine. Somewhat to my surprise it actually worked quite well during that first year. We did obtain publishable results and it marked the beginning of a very long and happy friendship with Murray Jarvik, who acquired some confidence in these lines of work quite quickly. It took about six months I suppose before he saw me as being a worthwhile person to have there instead of another troublesome postdoc, and after that he was immensely supportive.

Who actually was he? Where did he come from?

What I would like to record is the marvellous experience I had in Murray's group. He was full of ideas, very creative in approach, although these were often rather impractically ambitious. On the other hand, I was very cautious, not a risk-taker (and I feel I have often suffered as a result), so perhaps between the two of us we functioned as a balanced unit. I was particularly taken by the the gentle and kindly way in which Murray directed his group.

What was interesting about the background at that time was that the Pharmacology Department at the Albert Einstein College of Medicine in New York was one which had been very strong in psychopharmacology and drug dependence research. Murray had developed this idea of nicotine at a time when it was extremely unfashionable and there was almost no grant support for it. The reasoning there as far as I could see – to simplify it a little bit – was the world seemed to be divided into two types of people. There were those who *knew* for certain that smoking was nothing to do with drug action and that it was something that was entirely rewarded by the various types of psychological phenomena associated with smoke, the act of smoking, the taste, the smells, the sensations, the visual things and various combinations of these and that it had nothing to do with nicotine and therefore there was no point in funding nicotine research. That was half the world. The rest of the people *knew* that nicotine was an old drug, and indeed it was first discovered in the 19th century, but they thought there was nothing more that needed to be found out about this substance and one should work with newer and more selective substances. That line of thinking was often extended to the conclusion that there were not any nicotine receptors in the brain anyway, so the psychopharmacology of nicotine didn't really matter! So for completely conflicting, diametrically opposed reasons, there was very little to encourage anyone to work in that area.

I believe that when Murray Jarvik did obtain his first grant, which was from the American Cancer Society for nicotine research, it was a very controversial project for them to support. The project did eventually get off the ground and he did ultimately find some people to work on it although there weren't very many in those early days. We faced a certain amount of scorn. When I said I was going to work on nicotine, one of my colleagues in the opiate area suggested that I should not waste my time on that 'rubbish'; it was not really a proper legitimate type of thing for a psychopharmacologist to do at all. Now it looks as if the evidence that smoking is drug-taking and produces dependence will be among the most influential of outcomes from psychopharmacological research. It impacts upon the 30–40% of the population who have been smokers, upon non-smokers who finally obtained some basic rights regarding the air they breathe, and of course upon the tobacco industry.

It proved to be a very rewarding experience personally, developing into a lasting friendship with Murray and working in the group because of many people I contacted there. There can be no doubt that it was as close to an idyllic work experience as I have encountered and that applies especially to the last two years after I had moved with Murray to the University of California at Los Angeles. I was able to meet numerous psychopharmacologists in North America at a time when I knew of their work but hadn't been able to put faces to it. I think in retrospect that one of the things that surprised me most was that a lot of people whose innovative and prolific publications were known to me were postdoctoral researchers or at early stages in their careers. I had assumed that because of their notable series of publications, they would be senior people with well-established groups but that wasn't so. It was also clear that they had a similar perception of the activities that we had carried out in London, particularly the work that Channi Kumar and I were involved with.

Channi Kumar – do you want to talk about the work you did with him?

The University College Group was in fact cooperative with Birkbeck College, where Daphne Joyce and Arthur Summerfield were located. It was spread across psychology in Birkbeck and pharmacology and psychology in University College. There was a diverse range of activities that were to a substantial extent supported by grants from the US National Institute of Mental Health. The development of that group was greatly facilitated by that foreign support. I think at that time American National Institutes did actually have a policy of seeding research in other countries. When I ultimately came to the Institute of Psychiatry, more than 15 years later, support from the National Institute on Drug Abuse, another agency of the United States Public Health Service, played a very large role in the development of my group's activities although our core funding has always been from the British Medical Research Council.

While at University College, if we go back to that momentarily, I shared an office with Channi Kumar, who was also doing a PhD at that time. We spent more time talking, instead of working, than we usually have the opportunity to do now. It proved to be beneficial because, together with Hannah, we did embark on a series of studies on the oral self-administration of opiates and other drugs at a time when self-administration research was just becoming an active area. I suppose we were dreadfully arrogant because we felt that with 150 or so rats we could solve the major problems in the drug dependence area within the next 3–5 years. We certainly thought we could do a lot more than we did ultimately achieve. In the long run it was the method rather than the specific results that had the greatest impact. At the time we were actually hesitant to even publish the method as such because we thought it was not new enough – there had been some oral self-administration before. But it did mark the beginning of a collaboration and friendship with Channi that has persisted right through my career.

What's his background?

Channi did medicine and psychology before joining us. He had a very different experience from mine. It was complementary and it was very stimulating to have him there because of his formal training in medicine and psychology, which I of course did not have. But what was curious was that we did not have as far as I can remember a communication problem which I have often seen in subsequent years when trying to work on projects with people who are not in my discipline – a neurochemist or maybe a molecular biologist or a neuro-physiologist; they often find it very difficult to understand my language and I suppose I find it difficult to understand their language sometimes as well. So there is a communication problem. We didn't have that problem although our training was very different and so that made the collaboration much more enjoyable although I don't know whether it made it ultimately more successful.

The other influence in University College in those days was Malcolm Lader, who was a Postdoctoral Fellow in the same department and I was a subject in some of his experiments too. Malcolm did provide some useful comments on the studies with morphine although we never did get him very near to a rat. Ultimately it was Malcolm and Channi who were responsible for getting me to come to the Institute of Psychiatry.

But in between I had joined the staff of the MRC in the Neuropharmacology Unit in Birmingham – that was in 1974. It was already a unit that was at a fairly mature stage of development. I think it had been running for at least 10 years and longer if one considers the period of time before it was formally a unit but was still quite a major activity. It was an opportunity to develop behavioural research within the general framework of the unit with a very considerable degree of freedom. Although the unit had a defined programme, I was not constrained very much. I told the Director, Philip Bradley, what sort of things I thought would be appropriate if I came and he agreed, and I was just starting to carry it out when the MRC initiated procedures for closing down the unit. That took several years to actually occur – I was in Birmingham until 1980 by which time MRC had awarded both me and to most of the senior staff of the unit long-term appointments stretching on beyond the agreed closure date. Therefore, much of the work that we did there, with some degree of success, was done with a unit that was formally dead in a sense. That was when I first became involved with drug discrimination and taste aversion research, methods that have played a major role in much of what I did subsequently.

What were you doing there?

Drug discrimination was one of a number of methods we tried in relation to a particular series of experiments that I was doing on cocaine. We tried various ways of examining the effects of this substance and I suppose it would be fair to say that after we ran the first two animals on drug discrimination we (Glen

D'Mello and I) were seduced by the power of the technique and by what I thought was a wide range of things that could be done with it, in an efficient and economical way with interesting possible relevance to what was tradition-ally dangerous territory for behavioural pharmacologists. By dangerous terri-tory I mean subjective phenomena evoked by drugs. Arguably, drug discrimi-nation is one of the ways of getting at objective correlates of subjective states induced by substances. But it wasn't only that, it was also the precision and the reliability of the method, as I saw it then without being aware of perhaps some of the difficulties that would emerge later – notably the difficulties of inter-preting intermediate or partial generalisation effects. This made it appear very attractive. It turned out to be a sensible or a fortunate move because that method formed the basis for our proposals for nicotine research that were ulti-mately approved by the MRC around 1980, and led into the work that I have been doing in the institute ever since, both with nicotine and on the discrim-ination of abused drug mixtures.

For the non-behavioural pharmacologist are there any implications of the drug discrimi-nation work? Clearly, if animals can do all this, humans can too. Could the methods for working on animals be applied to humans as well and would this offer anything to the field of testing cognitive function in healthy volunteers using drug probes, which has been left relatively undeveloped in recent years?

Well, it is interesting that you should say that because one of the things that we have done here in recent years is to maintain a comprehensive database of drug discrimination research as a service to the field – although it began as some-thing for our own purposes. In that database one can search for the number of publications using human subjects, which I am now doing, and we will see how many it actually generates. Interestingly, precisely 100 publications in human subjects on discriminative stimulus effects of drugs. So work has cer-tainly been happening in humans as well as animals.

Is it feeding into therapy in any way or into other aspects of cognitive psychology?

It is being utilised in several areas. It is one of many methods used in drug devel-opment for characterising the effects of novel compounds and in helping to identify compounds with unusual profiles of effect. So part of the success of the field has been its widespread use within the pharmaceutical industry as part of that process. A second area is in relation to drug dependence where, perhaps to put it in a very plain way, people who misuse or become dependent upon drugs learn about the effects of the drugs as a result of consuming them. They learn to recognise the drugs in some populations of users with more precision than one would might expect. Drug discrimination, when carried out in a formal way regardless of whether it be in animals or in humans, is a way of teaching the sub-jects of those experiments about the effects of drugs. Then they report to us what they have learned. To the extent that the identification of particular drug effects is based upon the changes in the internal state of the organism that they bring about, it is linked to subjective changes.

Perhaps that could be put better by saying (as others did before me) that what are described as subjective changes are learned discriminative responses using language to describe phenomena in the same way that a subject trained to discriminate drugs will typically use one type of motor response rather than another. A verbal report is using language instead of motor responses to describe internal states. I think there is a very close homology of process there, although that is something which is rarely explored in a specific way because it is extremely difficult to know how to distinguish that type of interpretation from one which takes a very strict stimulus–response view and does not say anything about the intervening events.

There is another angle, which is that discriminative effects of drugs may be part of the process whereby drugs prime or induce bouts of drug-taking behaviour – there may be an important relationship to do with drug dependence which has yet to be fully elucidated.

During the Birmingham period the whole issue about the foundation of the BAP began to emerge?

This blew up almost immediately upon my arrival in Phillip Bradley's unit in 1974, where at a very early stage we had learned about the development of the psychopharmacology association or academy in Britain. For the reasons I have detailed in a letter in the *Journal of Psychopharmacology* (Stolerman, 1995), we were not happy about the way this was occurring. The idea of an association was something that many people welcomed. Of hundreds of people who were contacted about this at the time I can only recall one person who actually said that he thought there should not be a society because there were enough societies already and there was no need for one in psychopharmacology.

Your letter outlines how the debate evolved before the RSM meeting, how you had to in a sense threaten people with the idea of a letter to Nature. But having got to the RSM meeting how did you view how things went there?

Well, when we had the great debate on this at the RSM, which was very skilfully chaired by Max Hamilton, the issues were certainly brought out very clearly. I don't think there was much coming together of minds or that either side gave very much ground there.

On one issue that did concern you they did give ground – the issue of closed membership.

That was subsequently. The result of that meeting was that the governing body of the association, the BAP, was broadened to include a wider range of people and the membership was not restricted in the way it was originally intended but I don't think those things were actually agreed at that open meeting. The open meeting was really to let everybody air their views and for us to try to get a broader representation. We did succeed in getting a broader representation in the Council although we actually lost the vote that was taken at the meeting. It was a rather complicated affair in which amendments to the resolution that we put forward were proposed which had the effect of negating it. The amendments were voted upon first and accepted, so by the time the meeting came round to voting upon our resolution it had already been voted out. I suppose I was rather naive with regard to the conduct of such meetings so it was a learning experience.

I thought we had lost that round but we did ultimately achieve the intended effect, although it took much longer than we had hoped. There was a lot of bad feeling that persisted for a long time, which was unfortunate, but in the circumstances I think that if we had not taken a very firm line nothing at all would have happened because the founding group were not really convinced by our arguments, but they were convinced by the fact that a lot of people were going to oppose it and quite likely form an alternative association. None of us would have liked to have had to do that.

Why did you feel the need to go down this road, because in a sense there would have been other groups open to you like the Brain Research Association?

Well, a lot of people who had invested a number of years in psychopharmacology research felt that this organisation claimed to represent them because it was the only one of these groups that had psychopharmacology in its title. It was distinctly different from the Brain Research Association, which at that time in London was a very informal group that used to meet in a pub to chat and have presentations over a glass of beer. This was clearly a very good way of beginning because it became a major national organisation eventually. But it wasn't covering our ground. The BAP was clearly the one in the area and it had already the most obvious sort of name or title. It was clearly purporting to represent the whole area and the prospect of just ignoring something and then starting up an alternative organisation seemed to be less satisfactory than trying to improve the one that was already coming about. There was no doubt that the people who were setting it up had put a great deal of time and effort into it. It must have been very discouraging for them to find that a group of other people were complaining about what they were doing. But because they were not really prepared to listen to our requests, initially put forward privately, it was necessary to go through this public route. I think the fact that the change was so slow, that it took so many years for this society to become the sort of the vibrant and important organisation that it ultimately did, indicates that the initial formula was not right.

Were you aware that the clinical people involved didn't really have any associations with Oxford, Cambridge or the Maudsley – it was very much a group of clinicians from the periphery as it were?

Well, that would not have bothered me much as I was in Birmingham at the time and would not have much truck with anyone who argued it needed London or Oxbridge involved. But anyone who thinks that Oxbridge was not involved seems to have forgotten Susan Iversen and the Cambridge group and David Grahame-Smith, Richard Green and others at Oxford. I don't think the people who start a society need to come from any particular prestigious organisation or part of the country but they do need to gather the support of those who do. I think that if the individuals who were starting the society had proposed to do it in a more appropriate manner, then we wouldn't have taken those steps. The argument was very much about what was being done and which areas of the subject were being represented and where it would go in the future if it had only a very small number of members. We objected to the small number of people at the start – 150 or less – on principle because it sounded like a club for having conferences in nice places rather than for developing the subject.

When do you think BAP became what it has since become? Is it since it moved to Cambridge in 1985?

I think it does approximate to that. I think it was the style and content of the meetings which happened to take place in Cambridge that was the determining factor. I didn't think they had to be in Cambridge for this to be a success. I think the representation of the full range of disciplines is more important. Initially BAP didn't do that. There were some clinical and some non-clinical disciplines represented but not the full range and that was a major problem. I think in practical terms if a group of people do wish to set up a major national organisation then they need to involve on their side as many of the major people in that area as they can rather than setting it up and then saying please join us.

Let's move to the European Behavioural Pharmacology Society (EBPS). Can you tell me what the reason for moving towards EBPS was around 1985/86?

Yes, its roots go back a little bit earlier than that. The reasoning was that studies of the psychological effects of drugs were seen by many of us as a valuable contribution both to pharmacology, basic and clinical, and also in psychology. There were quite a substantial number of people in Europe, indeed around the world, working in that area. We felt that we didn't have a regular meeting place for this community of scientists. It was scientists predominantly, rather than scientists and clinicians.

The existing national or international societies didn't entirely serve that group. In Britain we were almost the exception because by having the BAP we had an organisation that very largely met the requirement along with covering other areas of research as well. But on a broader international scale that wasn't really so. Furthermore, the perspective of EBPS was not limited to Europe. It was always the intention that this should be open to people from wherever they come but the major focus of its activity should be in Europe because in the United States there already was a Behavioral Pharmacology Society, albeit a very different group in the nature of its activities and its style. In Europe there was a need to foster the development of the subject, partly so that younger people coming into it would have a forum to present their work and to meet other people, and partly to enhance recognition of the area as a distinctive field within psychopharmacology and to help to protect it against the inevitable competitions between different approaches to studying psychoactive drugs and the brain and behaviour.

It actually grew out of a smaller European study group. Around 1979, I and others started a European group for the study of drugs as discriminative stimuli. That was a more specialised area – at that time there were very few groups doing it. In 1979, in Birmingham, we got nearly everyone in Europe who was doing that sort of work together in one room to found a study group and I think there were about 25 of us, as far as I can remember. The study group met annually for several years but they were very small, single-session evening meetings as a satellite of some other major society, usually the European Neuroscience Association. Either we had to formalise that link or we had to expand it because it wasn't really a viable activity in its original form. There was already by that time a lot of people suggesting that it be broadened to cover all of behavioural pharmacology or psychopharmacology or whatever. We resisted that because the prospect of founding a substantial new society was fairly horrific, but ultimately we did and thus the EBPS grew out of the European study group for drugs as stimuli. The early history of EBPS was outlined in an Editorial in *Psychopharmacology* (Colpaert and Stolerman, 1990).

Yourself and Francis Colpaert were the prime movers?

In the beginning of the EBPS, I became a front person for taking the first formal step which was forming a steering committee but that had been discussed at some length with several people. I wrote to about a dozen people in different European countries explaining a little about the idea about a European Society asking them to join a steering committee, with an intention of meeting a year later in London at the time of the IUPHAR Congress that took place in 1984. So we had a year in which to correspond and discuss ideas and then we had the steering committee meeting open by the fountains outside the Barbican and ...

Because there wasn't any room in the inn?

Well, we didn't have any money to pay for a room! More seriously, I thought that if people would agree to sit around under those rather uncomfortable circumstances and possibly get drenched with rain they must be sufficiently motivated to be the sort of people I would like to have on the steering committee. We formulated a plan for an inaugural meeting two years later. The steering committee of the society became essentially that group, with two or three more people brought in. We became the initiating group for the society and the most active people at that time I suppose in developing the plans for the meeting and the society were Francis and myself. The way it panned out was that Frances took on the main responsibility for the inaugural meeting and I worked on trying to set up the foundations of a society so that there would be something that would survive beyond that meeting, to make sure that two years later it wouldn't be necessary to start all over again.

The main thing I can remember doing in that period was writing large numbers of letters and making lots of telephone calls. It sounds rather glamorous when you talk about starting a society but in fact you are sitting there at a desk or at a word processor or on the telephone; it takes up a lot of time and it has its frustrating moments as well the exciting ones. But there were many other people who, although they were not quite so prominent in the society then, were extremely helpful with ideas and practical advice. I can't recollect all of them but I certainly remember Georgio Bignami being extremely encouraging and helpful. Trevor Robbins played a major role in shaping up our ideas although he wasn't really free to take a leading role at that particular point, but of course he did subsequently by getting the EBPS and BAP together in Cambridge for the 1992 meeting. I think one of the things that enabled me to get EBPS going successfully was the BAP experience. I wanted at all costs to avoid the same thing and so I tried to do what I could to involve as many different people and to provide enough opportunities for people to put their views forward so that even if ultimately they didn't prevail, nobody could say that they didn't have a chance to participate in the development.

Ultimately it turned out that we did have the opening meeting in 1986 and it was successful in that I think the 150 or so people participating was somewhat larger than we had originally anticipated. They expressed a great deal of satisfaction with the format of that meeting. I think there was a certain atmosphere of excitement and of achieving something. Delegates said that here they could see a home for themselves at last. That was very rewarding for us who had spent nearly 3 years getting to that point. So it was clearly going to proceed as a society and it turned out of course in parallel with the ECNP.

Had you known that ECNP was being started ...

At the particular time that we initiated EBPS we did not know that there was a proposal to form ECNP. I suppose if we had been aware of that, we would have communicated with whoever was founding the ECNP to see whether or not it was necessary for there to be two organisations. Yes, ECNP and EBPS started around the same time, largely unaware of each other's existence and with very different objectives. ECNP as I understand it was a union of a number of European national societies in the area and it was intended to bring those groups together for larger meetings and perhaps other purposes. Whereas EBPS was in an area where hardly any of the countries actually had a national society devoted exclusively to that field. Also, in EBPS basic science rather than clinical practice was to the fore; its meetings are devoted to the basic science of psychopharmacology, often with concern about and emphasis on potential applications, and the depth and coverage of the science are usually much greater. There is a lot there for everybody who is doing behavioural pharmacology research. It is very different in that respect and it was for that reason, and in order to have enough programme time to cover the area, the society was formed. We could for example have probably had a half-day symposium within the European Neuroscience Association meetings. We might even have been able to get a couple of sessions but that isn't enough to serve the needs of the area. We have no difficulty in filling a three-day programme with two to three parallel sessions and it would not have been possible to have that level of activity within another society, and to have had a similar degee of control of the content.

One advantage of having the breadth of ECNP and BAP is that when it comes to obtaining funds for sponsorship of meetings there is a wider pool of resources within the pharmaceutical industry from which a claim can be made. BAP can garner support through the clinical and marketing end of companies, whereas an organisation like EBPS relies upon support from the scientific research departments who have relatively small budgets for that sort of thing.

Within a group like BAP, the basic scientists will often be seen as being somewhat concerned about the input from industry and the clinical people will be seen as quite keen to have an input from industry. But taking it further, as you said there is quite a bit of funding from industry for basic science research and within a group like EBPS a significant number of the scientists are working within the industry, so is the problem not so much the industry or the funding from industry as the disease model? It seems to me to some extent that basic scientists and particularly psychologists would often take a much more dimensional view of problems and from this perspective the disease model is the problem rather than the funding from industry per se. At the ECNP programme for Venice last year things were taken to an extreme I thought and all symposia were disease oriented. When meetings are so disease oriented, the amount of science that can come in is very limited.

I don't think that that should necessarily be so because most of these diseases are studied over such a wide range of disciplines that one can see contributions from nearly all levels with varying significance depending on the particular condition. So it can be the case that disease-oriented parts of meetings can be scientifically excellent but to have the whole meeting oriented that way is sometimes a problem because one can see major scientific developments in understanding of the nature of drug actions which may go across diseases, or they may not necessarily have a very clear relevance to disease at an early stage. That takes time to come out and of course that would be lost within a programme like that of the ECNP where the application very much dominates over the science. Many contributors to your earlier volume of interviews talked about a dichotomy of disease and dimensional models but that has never seemed a major practical issue to me; it seems paradoxical that as a basic scientist I am less obsessed with such theoretical questions than many clinicians. As others said before, research is the art of the possible. It's strange that factional groupings seem to have played such a big role in the development of some societies whereas EBPS has always been a partnership between industrial and academic researchers, with a generally positive atmosphere and only occasional minor bits of tension, at least during the times I was involved and aware of the inside story.

I think that as things are at the moment ECNP has gone down the route that I have just outlined to a greater extent than any other group and it's unsettling almost.

Well, its unsettling in some ways. For societies that might have felt ECNP to be competition it has been helpful because many, many of their members don't feel very drawn towards ECNP meetings. So although originally it was very worrying because we didn't know what direction it would go, ultimately they seem to be complementary because of the focus of the ECNP being very different. Now whether or not the ECNP is serving another constituency effectively is something I don't know.

Was there something about the early 1980s that fostered the development of European institutions of this sort? Because AEP also began in this period.

I think people were thinking more about European societies than at any earlier stage because of the influence of the European Community. It was inevitable and it seemed to be a sensible parallel to the economic union and a possible way that organisations would become recognised as filling a role in Europe. If there is a growing closeness between European nations this should also be reflected in scientific activities. Of course there were previous organisations as well. The European Neuroscience Association began in the late 1970s. The European Brain and Behaviour Society was there quite a few years before that. No doubt there were others but it tended to proliferate in the 1980s and there was not a development in the science or clinical spheres across such a wide range of disciplines that would suddenly make European societies appropriate if there hadn't been a political background.

When you talk to some of the other founders of the various groups there is a sense that it was useful to pull Europe together as a counterweight to the Americans. Did you have that?

We did, because we felt that in order to get to meetings where we could get together with other behavioural pharmacologists, it was often necessary to go to the US. Many of our meetings have been extremely attractive for North American behavioural pharmacologists. In fact, at times there were more US members of this European society than there were from any single European country. We did that because we wanted as good a society as could be established. I think it's fair to say we were keen to have an international society but we wanted it based in an area that would be reasonably convenient for us. If it were wholly international a substantial proportion of the meetings would have to be in North America and that would not have served the purpose we wanted. To some extent we have succeeded because the meetings all do take place in Europe but they are also more expensive than I had originally envisaged and they seem to be getting more so as time goes by. It's getting harder to raise funds for student bursaries and support and some of the younger people are getting squeezed out.

The other thing we've realised is that the US organisations are rather different from ours. The Behavioural Pharmacology Society is a rather informal group that has smaller meetings, perhaps narrower in scope, so they serve a more specialised need and don't satisfy the need that we saw. I think that behavioural pharmacology as a discipline needs a prominent society to maintain its position with all the competing areas and I believe we do a better job in that respect. A lot of the American research in behavioural pharmacology appears at the Society for Neuroscience, for example, where it is not a big player. There are very few behavioural pharmacology symposia within that society; all of the work tends to come out in posters. So I think there is something we do which the American organisations don't have and that is one reason why they come.

Where does behavioural pharmacology stand now as compared with 1965?

I suppose one could see the mid-1960s and much of the 1970s as a period when the discipline was finding its feet and exploring its methods. During the late 1970s and 1980s it would appear to have become relatively strong both in terms of academic and industrial science and increasingly integrated with other disciplines and contributing to a whole range of problem areas.

Is this because during the 1970s and 1980s the use of animal models was very important for drug development – models like learned helplessness? The industry had signed up to the idea that we need to understand the processes involved in depression or behavioural despair but that has now been eclipsed by the molecular biological approaches.

There seems to be a cycle over periods of 10–15 years, or even longer, in which the emphasis on behavioural pharmacology in industry rises, then diminishes, and then comes up again. Because of the scientific difficulties with working with an intact complex system, there will always be a need for more elemental studies – in vitro, subcellular and molecular studies of various types – and we have seen a time when the techniques of molecular neurobiology have advanced at a tremendous rate. This has been coupled with another factor, which is the difficulty industry has had in using models of psychiatric states as a critical part of the drug development process. We all know that psychiatric states have been notably difficult to model; the fundamental features of the states are not usually known and so one has models whose validity is difficult to establish. I think a lot of the difficulty has come because inappropriate models have been utilised and conclusions have been reached which were not really ly strongly supported even by the data available for the particular models used. It is also the case that some of the best models have been in drug dependence but industry has often wished to steer clear of that area.

It's pretty tough for a team of researchers in a pharmaceutical firm to produce a novel compound that works. They may have a novel idea but can't find a compound or they may find a novel compound with no obvious application, but to get the whole thing together when you don't really know what your target receptors are is extremely difficult. When they get something that looks reasonably promising on the basis of an animal model among other data, they have to push it. If a team has nothing to offer it's going to have a very poor prospect of survival. So people are inevitably pushed toward promoting, perhaps more than they would like, the best that it has been possible to find. That means the importance of certain observations in models may become rather exaggerated. When you then go to the clinic and it doesn't work, your conclusion may be that animal models don't work; often I think what it means is that if you don't use animal models in a rigorous way, or just use ones that can be set up most easily, then you will have a problem. Approaches seem to vary markedly between different firms.

I think there will always be a need for the use of in vivo research such as behavioural pharmacology as part of the drug development process because as far as I can see we are nowhere near being able to say that a particular perturbation at the molecular level is going to produce a particular psychological effect. But to say that the behavioural analysis will itself produce for you a new compound is not realistic either; in order to identify compounds you have to know something about the receptor or enzymic target as well as the behavioural target. One without the other doesn't work. I think it's regrettable that people in one area think that their approach has all the answers. Very often one sees now the same mistakes that were familiar 20 years ago. The extent of rediscovery that is going on is becoming much more apparent. I can see this particularly in the drug dependence area where there has been a large amount of activity since the 1960s. Things that were reported in the 1960s or even earlier and put aside are coming up again now at meetings but often with a different name.

Is that because some of the literature from the 1960s is not on CD-ROM?

That is a possibility since people rely very much on the computerised databases now. But for us, getting into this area in the 1960s, the literature was relatively small – it didn't seem small at the time but the fact was that at that time one could read a much larger proportion of all the work that had been done in the area than one can now. I suppose we saw a limited number of papers before the 1950s that met search criteria, but since the 1960s there has been a huge outpouring of this work, much of which is still relevant, so for someone coming into the area now, instead of having to catch up with 10 years' work on the psychological effects of drugs as I did, they've got to catch up on 30 years of work. It's extremely difficult for someone to do that now in an exhaustive manner and as far as I can see not all groups attempt to do so, whereas we would be given hell by our supervisors if we didn't know about one particular paper – we were supposed to have read literally everything that was relevant. I suppose this is a manifestation of something that goes on in society generally – there are types of knowledge that are accessible for a certain number of years and then they are lost, sometimes for long periods of time. We really need to think about how to rectify that but it's not easy to see how to resolve it. Just having more review articles written is unlikely to solve it.

How does the position of science in society look to you now compared to 30 years ago?

We are increasingly asked to justify what we have done in terms of short-term practical and economic benefits, to put forward our major achievements, often in terms that are readily understandable by non-specialists. This can be extremely difficult to do because where there are advances in health care, to trace the multiple influences that result in that particular step forward may be very difficult. It's easy to point to a drug and say that came out of a certain laboratory but none of these things ever occur in isolation. I subscribe to the 'cathedral model' of research where major developments are seen as comprised of innumerable 'bricks' of information, any one of which may be rather insignificant in isolation but the structure as a whole would be impossible without them. Paying for the bricks is not very glamorous and that is where part of our difficulty lies. Every piece of work that goes on is based on a large amount of previous work, which may perhaps be perceived by the individual scientist in a novel way. They see something that has been missed. But to trace all the influences, including that of the unsuccessful projects, is a very complex matter. That is where our accountability is very difficult if we say that the nine out of ten projects that didn't provide a health care advance were as valuable as the one which did because they provided pointers, equally, in relation to many of the major findings in psychopharmacology, it is futile to try to allocate dominant roles to individual scientists or clinicians who would never have been able to function without the collective endeavour.

You don't see the discontinuity that may appear to be there later?

They are there because, when presenting something in a simplified manner later, you can't tell the whole story so you say, 'This is what someone discovered and isn't that great.' But it all does build on earlier knowledge, as those who produce the more significant findings are usually among the first to recognise. In the early 1970s, the development of ligand-binding methodology began with some unsuccesful experiments which nevertheless pointed the way for others to proceed. Similarly, some of the early studies on drug self-administration and drug discrimination in the late 1960s showed relatively weak effects. But those early reports of studies which were not in themselves completely successful encouraged other members of the behavioural pharmacology community to do further experiments that ultimately were successful.

Something that intrigues me is whether the potential for developing drugs that at the receptor level act with enormous specificity will be of therapeutic benefit or whether it the case that most of the conditions we will be aiming for involve multiple disturbances in parallel systems, so that it may not be possible to do very much better than we have already done by means of selective targetting of drug action. Does one need to take the approach, for example, as Janssen has done with risperidone, of producing a drug with multiple actions? But if that is the case, there is no reason why the two or more desired effects have to be effects of the same substance. Using combinations of two drugs would have the advantage of enabling relative effect magnitudes to be adjusted easily. This could be a way back towards polypharmacy, which everybody will no doubt laugh at. This general area is not very much addressed because it is not very clear how, with the methods and theories that we have, we could address the question of useful multiple actions. This has interested me because of our work to look at drug combinations.

You said your career has crossed with that Michael Rand again, after having been introduced to the area by him.

Yes, Michael was instrumental in encouraging me to work in psychopharmacology at University College and later encouraged my work on nicotine. He's worked in the nicotine area over the years and it would seem to be a nice outcome that we both ended up working in the same place. But in fact it is disturbing to find out that we seem to be in opposite camps. About two years ago, I gave a talk on the addictive nature of tobacco smoking only to hear Michael say in his summing up of the session that this was a ludicrous notion, and he then went on to question the evidence that tobacco smoke constituents have a causative role in lung cancer and heart conditions.

That incident occurred in a scientific meeting that was in part supported by a foundation whose funds came largely through the tobacco industry. There was an influence on the programming of that meeting that was subtle but pernicious, and altered its character in a manner that quite a few of us felt was unfortunate. It certainly had not been the intention of the scientific organisers of the meeting for it to go that way. In recent times researchers in the alcohol and smoking areas have become much more aware of the difficult ethical issues associated with support from the respective industries.

The whole field of substance dependence provokes extraordinary emotions. A considerable proportion of the psychiatric profession even would write substance dependence off. This isn't a disease – it's a problem of living.

This still apparently is so and I find that very puzzling. Its not something that makes sense for the psychiatric community, given a number of factors, such as the historical difficulty of the disease model for many psychiatric states and the co-morbidity between substance use and other psychiatric states which can be taken as indicating that the relationship between them is closer than traditional diagnostic categories imply.

It's paralleled by a tremendous reluctance in the past for the pharmaceutical industry to have its products associated with the treatment of dependence disorders. That is curious. Obviously it's going to be a negative if a drug itself is associated with dependence but it seems to be regarded in such a negative way that even having something that would be useful for it is dangerous – it might be seen as not being in a respectable area.

Within psychiatry, substance abuse seems to take the spot that psychiatry takes within the rest of medicine.

You are absolutely right there. And within substance dependence, research on different substances has varying degrees of respectability. At one time nicotine had very low levels of respectability, whereas now among most of the drug dependence community the research is accepted, the problems are seen as shared between the nicotine and classical areas that are mutually supporting each other. Much the same seems to apply to alcohol, at least in Britain.

One of the worrying things about psychopharmacology is the extent to which many major research groups have become involved in the dependence area. We have often said we need more research in the area but one does see more and more groups working in the field, which is ultimately going to be harmful to us as a discipline. If most of our effort is seen as counteracting problems that our agents have produced we are going to have a negative image.

The industry view is one that surprised me a lot when I first encountered it. It was the view that scientifically there may not be a unique problem in working in the area but we do not know how to market these substances because we've never had any before. It is said that nobody has ever made any money before out of developing a drug for dependence disorders. Then in Britain there is the concern about health service prescriptions. All these things tend to militate against getting companies actively involved. Yet I do sense that there is a change. We can all see from the published work of various companies that there is now a much stronger interest in various aspects of dependence.

Is the fact that naltrexone and acamprosate have just hit the market for alcohol dependence going to make a difference?

If they are a big success, yes. Certainly a precedent for success is going to be an important factor. I think it's a question of where the market will come from for the sale of the substances that is a little difficult. Not many users of illicit substances are going to pay for prescriptions, so how are they going to be treated? This has to be looked at carefully. In that respect one is much better off trying to treat something that is legal. There is not a problem divulging that one is a smoker. The difficulty there seems to be a matter of health services recognising that this is something that they need to treat. And I don't have a simple recipe for that because one does have to take some account of the cost implications if 30% and more of the population have to be treated with a new expensive product. One of the interesting models was the behavioural intervention devised by Higgins and his group in Vermont for cocaine which involved providing rewards for people who were free of the drugs when tested from time to time. But if there's a climate that sees the use of both legal and illegal drugs as something that individuals bring upon themselves, it becomes very difficult to justify any intervention at all.

Is seems to me that these attitudes have tended to obscure the fact that compared with research on schizophrenia and mood disorders, the basic sciences, both the biology and psychology, are much more advanced in the area of substance dependence.

We certainly have learned a lot about the effects and mechanisms of the drugs. Particularly it seems that the animal models for dependence are among the best validated in the psychopharmacological arena. Where we are still weak is why, with equivalent availability and equivalent early experience, experimenting with drugs in some individuals results in a major problem developing, in some cases a minor problem and in other cases nothing at all. Most of the laboratory work does not easily solve this because if we want to work with a model of dependence we want one in which typically every subject will become dependent, which immediately bypasses that critical question.

Well, that's how I would see it, which makes it more surprising the area has remained …

Outside the mainstream. Yes, but I don't think that's got anything to do with the amount of information and progress in the area, it's about the perception of the area by the public and the rest of the profession. It's about application of a double standard where treatments for drug dependence are seen as failures if their effects are less than permanent, instead of recognition that it is a chronic, relapsing disorder; there is no objection if someone has to have a second course of antibiotic treatment, so why should there be a problem with repeated treatments in drug abuse? It is, sadly, still to do with moralistic judgements, and a real difficulty that many have in identifying with the predicament of a drug abuser.

Select Bibliography

Goldberg SR, Stolerman IP, eds (1986). *Behavioral Analysis of Drug Dependence*. Academic Press, New York.

Kumar R, Steinberg H, Stolerman IP (1968). Inducing a preference for morphine in rats without premedication. *Nature*, **218**, 564–565.

Robbins TW, Stolerman IP (1990). A brief history of British psychopharmacology. *European Behavioural Pharmacology Society Newsletter*, No. 5, 2–6.

Stolerman IP, Colpaert FC (1990). Editorial: The European Behavioural Pharmacology Society. *Psychopharmacology*, **101**, 289–291.

Stolerman IP (1992). Drugs of abuse: behavioural principles, methods and terms. *Trends in Pharmacological Sciences*, **13**, 170–176.

Stolerman IP (1995). Origins of the British Association for Psychopharmacology. *Journal of Psychopharmacology*, **9**, 287–288.

Stolerman IP, Shoaib M (1991). The neurobiology of tobacco addiction. *Trends in Pharmacological Sciences*, **12**, 467–473.

Stolerman IP, Goldfarb T, Fink R, Jarvik ME (1973). Influencing cigarette smoking with nicotine antagonists. *Psychopharmacologia*, **28**, 247–259.

Wonnacott S, Russell MAH, Stolerman IP, eds (1990). *Nicotine Psychopharmacology: Molecular, Cellular and Behavioural Aspects*. Oxford University Press, Oxford.

Measurement and organisation in psychopharmacology

Can we begin with how you came into psychiatry and why you moved into the area of measurement so early in your career?

I only studied medicine to become a psychiatrist actually. One of my colleagues from the high school had the same idea but when he came to the psychiatric department as a student he called me and said, no it was not really what he wanted, and he is now a dermatologist. But I always had the idea and so when I finished my examinations in 1969, I came directly to the Psychochemistry Institute in Copenhagen under Professor Rafaelseon. Actually at the same time the clinical professor of the department of psychiatry, Villars Lunn, wanted me to measure a more philosophical subject, namely the experience of time in depressive patients. So I went into two areas of research at the same time. The first area, one was to measure the experience of time in depressed patients and there I needed some standardisation about what is a depression, endogenous versus non-endogenous, and on severity because the literature on this subject indicated that altered time experience may be a measure of severity rather than diagnosis.

The second area was that Ole Rafaelseon, at that time in the Psychochemistry Institute, wanted to look at the effect of cannabis – this was in 1969. This research project was delayed because we decided to use as experimental subjects males in the military but the Minister of Defence did not think he could allow that because of a fear at that time that cannabis could perhaps cause long-term damage. Another Minister finally said that we could use conscientious objectors The Minister of Domestic Affairs under whom the Civil Defence belonged was very eager to obtain knowledge of the effect of cannabis on car driving. He gave us permission to study 10 young men. So we made a small study on the acute effect of tetrahydrocannabinol on driving. We had at that time what we thought was a measurement of the blood level so it was a study to measure which blood level would be dangerous for car driving.

Now because of my interest in time experience, which is also of interest with cannabis, I combined these areas of research. At this time I picked up the Hamilton Scale and Beck's Depression Inventory so I used those two scales and did a validation study. In the cannabis study I introduced the experience of time as one of the extra psychological dimensions apart from car driving behaviour in a car simulator – the cannabis part has been published in *Nature* and *Science*. We used cannabis as a cake but in a US study they smoked it. They found no effect on car driving but the content of THC in our batch was tested one year after and there was still the same amount but in the US study there was no active principle left. We showed, compared to alcohol, that if you went up to an equivalent level in the blood (to one per thousand) the subject could not comply with the instructions and so on. I also described that in cannabis intoxication you can have a feeling as if time has lost dimension but if you ask for an objective estimate it was also impaired. In the depressed patient it was more a subjective feeling. They could estimate time intervals as well as others objectively but they had the feeling that time passed slowly. In the cannabis study I realised that to measure the clinical experience under cannabis intoxication you need to have the same scale. Some scales measured positive well-being, others negative, and it was difficult to compare scales. So it was because of this I went into psychometrics and scale construction. In Denmark clinical psychologists in the 1960s and 1970s were against the use of questionnaires or rating scales. They used in their daily practice the Rorschach test and Murray's Thematic Apperception Test. However, both these tests have very low reliability and no validity in depressive disorders. Danish psychiatrists had no experience either with rating scales. I am really self-taught.

In the depression study I asked two of the best clinicians in the department to make a 15-minute interview with the patient and give a mark from 0 – no depression – to 10 – the most severe depression. They had never seen the Hamilton Scale and it was an unstructured interview. Half of the patients they interviewed together and the other half one of them did first and the other in another room later. With the Hamilton Scale I got two Hamilton raters to do the same – they saw the patients at different locations but at the same time of the day in the morning. And then the patient filled out the Beck Scale. There were only 24 patients at baseline; Four weeks later Ole Rafaelsen asked me to stop the investigation to evaluate if such scales had any meaning in clinical research. Just like the psychologists, he was very sceptical. Although the number of patients was rather small I had the advantage compared to other such studies that the inter-rater reliability both of the global depression scale and of the Hamilton Scale was high. When I correlated the scales with the global ratings I realised how difficult it is to interpret the coefficients because they are so dependent on the dispersion. Thus, one single outlier patient could change the coefficient dramatically but I found some methods that compensate for that. I also found out that with the Hamilton Scale when you come up to what experienced psychiatrists will call a score of 5 or 6 on the global scale from 0 to 10 you will score 22 on the Hamilton but when the experienced psychiatrists go up to a 9 on the global the Hamilton only goes up 25. So I looked for which items the experienced psychiatrist had used and I came down to six items. At that time Max Hamilton said to me, 'The best scale for your information is not my own scale, it is the Cronholm–Ottoson scale.' This was designed by these two Swedish psychiatrists who looked at change in depression symptoms during ECT and so I looked up their scale and added some of their items on psychomotor retardation to the ones I already had and that is where the Bech Depression Scale came from.

This was the same year that Montgomery and Asberg came out with their scale and essentially there is not much difference between the two scales in principle. But as Rafaelseon, who now was convinced that the future of clinical psychiatry was in rating scales, told me, 'Per Bech, you have to go around the world to sell your scale. There is a lot of politics in such a scale.' But I refused and did not do that at that time. So I still think it is a good scale but it has not been used as much as it could have been – the Hamilton Scale is still the one people refer to. So in summary, in the beginning I went into how to measure things in my cannabis work and in depression and then later I took the same approach to mania and anxiety and personality issues. Scaling problems became my passion in clinical research.

When the Hamilton Scale came out first, people were not happy with the idea that you would reduce the richness of clinical reality to this kind of scale. Max Hamilton, when asked about this, said that there was some truth to this but that very often the rich clinical reality is not actually assessed all that well whereas at least if people use a scale you can be sure that certain things that should be asked will be asked. But scales like this do introduce a standardisation into psychiatry which is possibly like the standardisation that was introduced into the manufacture of motor cars – it has its good and its bad points. What do you think?

My scale and the Montgomery–Asberg Scale along with the Hamilton were picked up in the 1970s and then came DSM-III. Now most psychiatrists agree to have around 10 symptoms defining, for example, depression. So even in diagnostic systems, the development has been to screen for some symptoms – around 10 – and then you say if there are five or six, you have a diagnosis. So I think that this kind of standardisation had even gone into the diagnostic systems. The only difference is that with the scales you can measure improvement but I think that essentially we train young psychiatrists to look at the same universe of items for depression and I think that standardisation in outcome measurements will be the next thing. Just as with cars you need them to be reliable, so for quality of care you need some kind of standardisation. Outcome is, of course, the most crucial variable in therapy and we have developed the major depression scale both in a DSM-IV and ICD-10 version.

But of course, it is common now to ask what is happening to the field of psychiatry. People seem to want something else – a more comprehensive view of a person. This is where the quality of life comes into the field – this offers a more holistic view of the person and measures both what is positive and negative, whereas the Hamilton Scale of course goes only for the negative symptoms of depression. Actually I always say to young doctors coming to my clinic, in principle psychiatry is a very easy thing. We have such a small number of disorders – depression, anxiety, mania, schizophrenia, dementia and one or two others. Essentially in the daily clinic when we have our strategies for treatment, it is really a small number of dimensions we work from. But coming to the individual depressed patient we need to know more about the patient to give them the best treatment – which comes back to the clinical arts of medicine. But in the emergency department there are only a few things we need to make a diagnosis and there has to be some structure in such situations. I also know a lot of family doctors who like to have the Hamilton on their tables just to screen for depression.

Can I ask you about Ole Rafaelsen? Quite a few people that I have interviewed have referred to him. Can you tell me a bit more about who he was, where he came from and what you think was important about him in the scheme of things?

He was originally on his way to a career in internal medicine. His scientific papers were on diabetes. At that time the University of Aarhus was the best place in Denmark for studying diabetes. He had to supplement his clinical education with psychiatry and he worked with Erik Strömgren and Mogens Schou in Risskov and here he became very interested in lithium, which actually before the development of insulin was used for diabetes in Vienna. He had the idea that from a genetic point of view you could either have diabetes or manic-depressive illness. He tried to push people to look at how many patients have both diabetes and manic-depressive illness but he was not an epidemiologist. He was really an internist in medicine who wanted to come closer to the brain. I worked with him there at the beginning of the 1970s, doing lumbar punctures and things like that to measure serotonin but I said that even for that we have to measure the severity of the condition and improve our diagnoses. When he finally accepted this and saw that the work he had been doing wouldn't lead to a Nobel Prize, he became more concerned about scales and it was then that he invited Max Hamilton to our clinic.

Rafaelsen's own psychiatric activities in neuropsychiatry were rather limited. Every time he went to an international meeting and heard that you should measure this or that metabolite in cerebrospinal fluid, he came back and said we should try to measure it. But we had, however, often difficulty in replicating others findings. We were more among those who could not replicate others' work. There was no new thinking – it was more a case of trying to test others' hypotheses. He was in a sense an old medical internist. He wanted to measure electrolytes, things in the CSF. But lithium has so many different actions and nobody knew what was the most relevant – he thought it was only a matter of time but it was not so and he never had a breakthrough paper people can refer to, and his institute is no longer there. But he was a great chairman of meetings and he was a stern man when it came to criticising our manuscripts, which pushed us younger people on. Above all, he created a group of young biological psychiatrists around him in the late 1970s, among them, apart from myself, Bolwig, Hemmingsen, Kragh-Sörensen, Rosenberg and Vestergaard. They are today all of them important professors of psychiatry in Denmark.

When you were working in the manic-depressive area did you have much contact with Mogens Schou?

Unfortunately not, partly because Ole Rafaelsen in a way belonged to a generation between Mogens Schou and myself. Already in 1953 Mogens Schou and Strömgren made the first placebo-controlled trial in clinical psychopharmacology that showed the superiority of lithium in the acute therapy of mania. Schou and Strömgren shifted the weight of Danish psychiatry towards biological psychiatry and persuaded such bright medical doctors as Ole Rafaelsen to go into psychiatry. Rafaelsen, then, as I just mentioned, in the 1970s inspired my own generation to continue the Danish tradition in biological psychiatry.

Concerning the use of lithium in Denmark some interesting differences emerged when Rafaelsen moved from Aarhus to Copenhagen. Thus, Rafaelsen felt that lithium carbonate was the best lithium salt whereas Mogens Schou thought it was lithium citrate. In other words, in Aarhus, lithium citrate is used most often and in Copenhagen we use lithium carbonate – which is funny in such a small country.

Then in the mid-1970s there came some cases from Aarhus of people who were intoxicated with lithium with kidney problems. Mogens Schou was very concerned about whether he had to stop all lithium treatment. He approached Ole Rafaelsen and they tried to look at it together. They found out that it was not the case and indeed that they could go down to a lower level of lithium daily. At that time we advised a dose of over 0.80 nmol/l lithium in the blood but now we use 0.50 and don't see any problems.

In 1976 I published a paper which I had actually started on two years before one summer when Rafaelsen was away. There was a secretary there doing nothing, so I said to her, let us go through all records in this hospital from when the first patient received lithium. The inclusion criterion was that patients should have had lithium for at least two years. The first patient who took lithium in Copenhagen was on 23 December 1959. I was able to find close to 80 patients and I made up a questionnaire about whether they thought it had had some effect on their illness – one of my colleagues was also interested in weight gain and compliance. I was actually interested in personality – I wanted to replicate the findings of Carlo Perris that unipolars are more neurotic than bipolars. When Rafaelsen came back and the secretary had told him about all the things we had done, he said to me, don't start such projects without permission. At that time we had no ethical committees and anyway such an investigation could be carried out within an interval equal to the period of latency to get approvals from ethical committees. Two days later he came to me and pointed out that I had found that in the so-called lithium clinic only 59% received lithium, which was one of the results of my small study. This made him very happy because it indicated that we used drugs other than lithium – so it was not a lithium clinic it was a mood clinic. This was at the time when there was some question, as I just mentioned, whether treatment with lithium should be stopped.

The next point was that of those who had been treated for so many years with lithium, only 35% received lithium alone. Some patients with a greater tendency to mania had a small dose of haloperidol with it while for those with a tendency to depression, at that time we used amitriyptyline, which was Rafaelsen's favourite among the tricyclics. We published my small study as a modern management study of lithium use. Eighty per cent of the patients felt that they were helped by lithium. Those who had stopped had done so mostly because of weight gain. Poul Baastrup, who collaborated with Mogens Schou when lithium was introduced, called me when he read the paper we had published in *Acta Scandinavica* and said that in his clinic much more than 35% received lithium alone but 5 years later he called me again and said, when he had checked it; even less than 35% received lithium alone. I think that this is still the case – in a few patients it is used as the only drug and it is of some help but often it is not enough on its own. But that kind of study of course was not what Ole Rafaelsen meant for his Psychochemistry Institute. For my part I moved more and more towards such clinical outcome studies. In 1980, we created what we called the Danish University Antidepressant Group (DUAG).

Yes. Can I ask you about who actually created that and why?

The main person was Lars Gram. He had been working in the Psycho-chemistry Institute but he went over to clinical pharmacology and he is now a professor in Odense in clinical pharmacology. He went to Pittsburgh and worked there for some years mainly on plasma levels of tricyclic antidepressants with Ellen Frank and David Kupfer, in the late 1970s. When he came back he became professor in Odense. In the late 1970s with Lars Gram, Niels Reisby and I did two studies – one on the plasma level effects of imipramine and the other on chlorimipramine, and showed that, if you used six items of the Hamilton Scale as outcome measures six weeks later, the more imipramine there was in the blood the more you lowered the Hamilton Scale score. If you used the whole Hamilton Scale some side-effects also were measured. I actually made a hypothesis which was published in 1981 essentially about the Hamilton Scale and the Newcastle Scale, using this as an indicator for external validity, that the more endogenous the disorder the more clear-cut this plasma level effect relationship. In another study we showed that 225 mg of imipramine was equivalent to 150mg of clomipramine.

Then came the Lundbeck drug citalopram – the first SSRI synthesised in 1971 – and it was discussed whether we should try to compare that to clomipramine as the standard. I was working still with Rafaelsen in 1980 when DUAG was established. Lars Gram at the Department of Psychiatry in Odense was chairman and leading centre. Niels Reisby was then Professor of Psychiatry in Aarhus after Erik Strömgren. In 1981 I went to Frederiksborg General Hospital, which was in the northern area of greater Copenhagen, while Rafaelsen's Department at Rigshospitalet was in the middle of Copenhagen. So DUAG originally had four departments which, however, have been extended over the years.

The first trial with citalopram versus clomipramine was published in 1986; the second with paroxetine versus clomipramine was published in 1990. Both studies showed that clomipramine was superior to the two SSRIs. Both protocols were drafted by the DUAG committee, who for instance required that we used fixed doses of the drugs because for plasma level–effect trials fixed doses are the most appropriate. Our third DUAG study was moclobemide versus clomipramine, which was published in 1993. Again clomipramine was found most effective.

The protocols of the trials were drafted by DUAG as mentioned, but they were monitored by the drug companies, following Good Clinical Practice. However, our latest, still unpublished DUAG study was monitored by DUAG itself, thereby showing a rather clear independence to the drug companies. The background for the fourth DUAG study was actually my wish to compare clomipramine with mianserin as well as with their combination. Organon was willing to support this study. During the discussion in the DUAG committee the dose of clomipramine in this combination study was problematic and a dose–response study with clomipramine was then suggested. Ciba-Geigy was interested in such a study, which was lacking in the literature. This fourth study with dose-finding of clomipramine has now been finished but not published.

One of the interesting thing that came out of all of those trials was that Clomipramine seemed to be more potent than anything else. Do you think that is true? All sorts of people have argued why the results of these studies are wrong.

It must have been around 1987–1988 when the results of our second DUAG study emerged confirming the citalopram study that I asked Lundbeck, Duphar (fluvoxamine) and Lilly (fluoxetine) to do a meta-analysis of all controlled trials with these drugs, against placebo and tricyclics. This idea was accepted by the drug companies. In my letter to these companies I have asked only to use the first 17 items of the Hamilton Scale, including my own factor of melancholia (core symptoms of depression), the sleep and anxiety factor. Among the outcome criteria I asked for a 50% reduction of the 17-item Hamilton Scale from baseline to endpoint which I equalled to a moderate to excellent improvement on the Clinical Global Improvement Scale. To my surprise no difference between citalopram or fluvoxamine and tricyclics was found in such a meta-analysis. With Dr Cialdella from the Department of Pharmacology in Lyon, France, I re-evaluated the citalopram data using an intention to treat approach. Again no difference between citalopram and tricyclics emerged.

However, if in the citalopram data you select only pure inpatients you will find two trials, the DUAG study with clomipramine and a Belgian study with maprotiline. Both trials favoured the older drugs. Hospitalisation seems to be the most important predictor for showing superiority of tricyclics over SSRIs. Hospitalisation in the 1980s meant therapy-resistant patients. It is my conviction that clomipramine is superior to amitriptyline, which again is superior to imipramine in therapy-resistant depressions.

Of course, ECT is the most powerful treatment of therapy-resistant depression. In a study which has just been published in *Acta Psychiatrica Scandinavica* we have in a randomised way combined ECT with imipramine, paroxetine and placebo. During acute therapy the imipramine–ECT combination was slightly but statistically significantly better than the other combinations. However, in the six month follow-up period after the last ECT, paroxetine was better to prevent relapse. Thus, only 12% relapse on paroxetine, 30% on imipramine and 65% on placebo.

From my experience with patients who have participated in the DUAG trials most of them have preferred the SSRIs in the long-term prophylactic treatment.

But in the full-blown depression treated in hospitals combination therapy is important. We have just finished a study with fluoxetine 20 mg daily plus 30 mg mianserin daily compared to fluoxetine 20 mg daily plus a placebo. The results have confirmed the superiority of the combination therapy.

Finally, I can add that one of my PhD students – Kurt Stage – has compared the DUAG inpatients with trials carried out in Denmark in the same period on outpatients using the same rating scales as DUAG. The item analysis showed that inpatients scored higher on depressed mood and sleep. Patients who end up in hospitals don't sleep and their family feel that it is difficult to control the patient day and night. Benzodiazepines don't work in this case – most of the DUAG patients have received oxazepam. However, clomipramine and mianserin in combination, or ECT works in these patients.

Looking at the work that was done by DUAG, a lot of people all over the world have been impressed at the independence of the work and they say that the psychiatric profession should be doing more studies of this kind – studies that are not driven by the marketing requirements of the pharmaceutical industry. How come you have been able to do it, when others haven't?

The secret of DUAG in my view has been that the committee covered persons who had worked together beforehand – Lars Gram, Ole Rafaelsen, Niels Reisby, Per Kragh-Sørensen, Per Vestergaard and myself. We covered also different aspects: pharmacokinetics, pharmacodynamics, psychometrics, clinical experience. Our relation to the drug companies was scientifically good. The first two drugs are developed by Danish companies – Lundbeck and Ferrosan. Moreover, Roche with moclobemide and Ciba-Geigy in the case of clomipramine had excellent medical research units in Copenhagen. During the trials, from 1980 to 1994, we had monthly rating sessions to maintain a high inter-rater reliability of the Hamilton and Newcastle scales for the participating research psychiatrists. Many people think that this training had a high impact on our research finding, i.e. the ability to differentiate between treatments. In this regard, Professor Zitman from the Netherlands published in 1990 a paper showing that no two research centres could be found in his survey where exactly the same version of the Hamilton Scale was used. Max Hamilton, himself, did not accept the American version used by the drug companies but he did accept the DUAG version in 1986.

DUAG is not doing a fifth trial on the acute therapy of inpatients. Over the many years with trials in which many patients did not respond adequately the departments have had difficulties to recruit patients, if not in a combination therapy. In the future DUAG will perform long-term trials.

You have also constructed rating scales for mania, social dysfunction and more recently for aggressive behaviour. Do you want to comment on any of those in particular?

The mania one came first. When I started with Rafaelsen in the institute we could not find a good scale for mania. I asked Hamilton and he said that very few patients in Leeds became manic so I created this one. We had a meeting that Hamilton participated in and he corrected some of the items and then we published it as the Bech–Rafaelsen Mania Scale (BRMAS). It is still the most used rating scale in the pharmacological research of mania. In a recent issue of *Psychopharmacology*, Post and his group at NIMH in Bethesda have published a meta-analysis of anticonvulsant therapy in mania which covers the period 1978 to 1991. Of the specific mania scales BRMAS is the most used but the BPRS (Brief Psychiatric Rating Scale) was most often used for general psychopathology.

It is interesting that BPRS has more items on aggression than the specific mania scale. Aggression is an important dimension in a manic state. When the drug company Duphar from the Netherlands contacted me for developing a specific aggression scale I was prepared because the BRMAS was limited in this respect. Duphar had produced eltoprazine, which was considered to have a specific action on aggression. I asked some of the experts in Europe both in aggression and in rating scales to join me. After some meetings we set up the European Rating Aggression Group (ERAG) and developed the Social Dysfunction and Aggression Scale (SDAS). It was published in 1992.

I have been very happy with this publication because we were able to illustrate the different statistical models for measuring the internal validity of a rating scale. When I first introduced the Rasch analysis into psychiatry in the late 1970s nobody really understood the model. However, most psychiatrists know what correlation coefficients are and most scale developers, including Max Hamilton, have clearly been influenced by Spearman's common factor theory when measuring the construct validity of their depression scales. It has always been my approach not to rely on coefficients as used in factor analysis, because they are too sensitive to sample selection. My approach has been to have an a priori theory, namely the coherence of items in terms of their hierarchical tapping of information along a dimension of severity of depression. Loevinger's or Mokken's coefficient of homogeneity is in my opinion the coefficient most close to latent trait analysis. In our 1992 publication of the aggression scale I asked my statistician, Peter Allerup, to make a latent trait analysis analogue to Mokken's coefficient of homogeneity. Our article illustrated very nicely the parallel thinking in Mokken's coefficient and latent structure analysis.

If I can go back for a moment to our ECT study I would like to give another example of latent structure analysis. In the post-ECT phase we measured the relapse of depression with the Hamilton and the Melancholia scales. In other words, this study gave us the opportunity to measure how depression develops symptomatically. We found that there was the same structure, essentially, as when patients improve during treatment. Hence, anxiety and depressive symptoms came first and then the retardation elements. Guilt and suicide came with those who developed a more severe picture. Cognitive changes came relatively early and introversion or lack of contact was one of the first things when the patients started to relapse. Because paroxetine was best to prevent relapse after ECT we now have the hypothesis that if you give an SSRI continually you can control the anxiety and depressive symptoms and if you can do that you will not get the more severe symptoms.

The hierarchical structure of the aggression scales shows that passive aggression is lowest in the hierarchy of symptoms whereas active aggression has the highest place in the hierarchy. Patients with active aggression have shown signs of passive aggression before their outbursts.

Well, there is an interesting point here. In a sense we are very focused on disease entities but of course there is no such thing as aggressive disease. Arguably, however, what we use the treatments for is aggression and many of our treatments are more effective at controlling aggression than curing diseases.

You are certainly right. Duphar with the eltoprazine drug was not asking for a new disease, but rather a scale measuring the target symptoms of aggression. It was Freyhan who in 1959 stated that the effectiveness of a neuroleptic drug must be measured in terms of its ability to improve the target symptoms. It does not make much sense to relate drug evaluation to diagnostic entities or other generic variables which ignore individual symptomatology. I was happy to have met Freyhan several times in Switzerland at the symposia Professor Kielholz held.

And if we were to say we're in the business of controlling aggression it would be the end of the psychiatric profession. We have to say we are treating diseases.

Psychiatric patients have either too much outward directed aggression or too much inward aggression, if by aggression we mean hostility or social dysfunction. In the US the word aggression has a positive value, meaning something energetic or dynamic. Our aggression scale, therefore, had to be called social dysfunction and aggression scale (SDAS). The target symptoms of most of our psychopharmacological treatment is to control outward aggression with neuroleptic drugs and inward aggression with antidepressive drugs. We are still not at the end of the psychiatric hospital profession, although it is difficult now to treat depressed patients in hospitals – in the UK even more difficult than in Scandinavia. I think.

On the rating area, you have also moved into the area of self-rating.

Yes. I used self ratings initially because I was interested in the experience of time in depressed patients when they completed the Beck Depression Scale.

Our data showed that when patients were carefully informed they were able to use this scale. My psychometric analysis focused on a subscale rather similar to that Aaron Beck has published. However, the full scale is most often used. In our plasma level-effect trials with imipramine and clomipramine I realised that when the Beck Scale was handed to the patient by the nurses without any information the scale was more often empty than completed. I think Malcolm Lader has said that questionnaires can be intrusive to the clinical process, distracting for the patient and orthogonal to clinical impressions. In our DUAG studies we didn't use self-rating scales. It is very interesting that when the clinical trials with the SSRIs were planned in the late 1970s or beginning of the 1980s self-rating scales were often excluded. I have noticed in one of my papers on meta-analysis of the SSRIs that patients seem to prefer the tricyclics to the SSRIs on the Beck or Zung self-rating scales.

In 1982 I visited Aaron Beck in Philadelphia and followed a one-week course in cognitive therapy. It was the year after my thesis on the Hamilton and Beck scales was published, at which Max Hamilton was one of the discussants. During my discussions with Aaron Beck I asked him about the difference of depressive 'symptoms' as measured by his Inventory and 'automatic thoughts' as measured within the negative triad of depression. He gave me no real answer. I still find that the 'negative automatic thoughts' and the 'depressive symptoms' belong to the same construct. When the depressed patient has recovered both the symptoms and the automatic thoughts disappear. Although I received a diploma in cognitive therapy I prefer drug treatment for major depression, both in the acute phase and in the maintenance phase.

Another thing I could not really explain was why Aaron Beck tried to minimise the work of George Kelly on repertory grid. They are both constructivists – they belong to the philosophical school saying that we individually make our own models or constructs of the world because the modern world is too complex for us to experience in toto. Kelly used the term 'constructs' while Beck tried to use the term 'schemas' for these emotional and cognitive models. Thus, 'automatic thoughts' are the depressed person's negative model of his or her world. Beck told me that these constructs are cognitions, hence the term cognitive therapy, although he preferred the word emotions.

In 1986 people told me again and again, 'You must know how to measure quality of life because you have been working with distress scales like the Beck Depression Inventory, Goldberg's General Health Questionnaire, the Zung scales, etc.' Then I realised that the questionnaires were all measuring the dimension of ill-being versus well-being. At that time quality of life was accepted as a measure of subjective well-being even in such journals as the *New England Journal of Medicine*. Questionnaires completed by the patients themselves were therefore considered an appropriate measure.

I was influenced especially by the study done by Jachuck and coworkers from Newcastle on the effect of hypotensive drugs on quality of life in patients with mild to moderate hypertension. The results of this study showed that while all the treating doctors found that the quality of life of their patients had increased during the trial, only half of the patients agreed in the question-naires, and only in one case the relatives of a patient found an increase in qual-ity of life of the patient.

We tried to replicate this study from Newcastle, but did it only to some extent. During the discussions with patients and their relatives I realised the limitations of standard questionnaires. What was important to one patient might not have any importance for another patient. In this situation George Kelly's repertory grid is very useful. It is essentially a way to develop a scale for each individual patient.

So then we did a study with a beta-blocking agent, which Ciba-Geigy thought had an antianxiety effect. It was a study on generalised anxiety disor-der compared with placebo and flupenthixol in a small dose. We had a psy-chologist who wanted to use a repertory grid technique but Ciba-Geigy were not keen because the psychologist needed so much time at baseline and they thought it would interfere with the drug treatment. So it was decided that after six weeks or when they dropped out the psychologist should make the reper-tory grid and some of the elements would be 'How were you before treat-ment?', 'How are you today?' and 'How do you wish to be?'

Lundbeck had recommended 2 mg of flupenthixol, which may have been too much – in Denmark we usually use 0.5 to 1 mg. Anyway the result was that on the Hamilton Anxiety Scale flupenthixol was the best for symptom reduc-tion but no patient in this group had a better quality of life. In the placebo group which had the worst effect on anxiety symptoms 30% had a better qual-ity of life. And in the beta-blocking group, which was a little bit worse on the symptomatic side, 60% had a better quality of life on this repertory grid. This was not captured by the the Hospital Anxiety Depression scale or the GHQ, which we also used.

We were impressed with this and since then we have tried to make a com-puter version because it takes a long time with pen and paper. There are use-ful things we can do with a computer model. In the repertory grid, you have components made from the same questions we always ask and patients can add their own important things and from this you do a factor analysis on each patient. Now if you have a computer you can press a button and in 10 seconds you have the factor analysis and a factor score. It has taken us two years to get this working. It was too comprehensive at first and had to be trimmed down because today you must not take more than half an hour – if it takes more than that nobody will use it. Even there we cannot use this in general practice because family doctors want something that takes 5 minutes.

Can we do outcomes research of that kind? If you go back to 1956 when the drugs were introduced and the question of rating scales first came up, Nate Kline said that all these rating scales are like the rabbit in the hat trick. You put the rabbit in the hat and you pull it out and everybody is impressed but in actual fact because of the particular rating scale that you have used you have really created the outcome that you want. What he was say-

ing is that the only outcomes that count are if people actually leave hospital or if they move from the back wards to the front wards. What do you think?

First of all, when the two most educated psychiatrists, who performed the global severity ratings in my very first study on the Hamilton Scale, had finished the study they told me that these ratings often correlated very closely to the patients' move from the back wards to the front wards. Now, 20 years later, we have in our country no back versus front wards. The few we have left are mixed! The Hamilton and global ratings are in my view very realistic 'bedside' instruments.

Secondly, I would like to emphasise that Nate Kline, among the MAO-I discoverers, like Roland Kuhn who was behind the discovery of imipramine had the feeling that the discovery of the antidepressants was purely clinical, without controlled trials, without placebos, without statistics. However, Kuhn has admitted that he tried in the years from 1956 to 1962 to convince other psychiatrists of the antidepressant effect of imipramine, but without success. It was with the introduction of the Hamilton Scale that people first became convinced of the outcome. Max Hamilton has stated that rating scales are not really suitable for exploring a new field of knowledge. Their construction requires much practical experience and an appropriate body of theory – in a sense they are an end-product.

Is what you are saying in one sense that it is one thing to use rating scales to map how people get well and that is what we have been doing but in actual fact it is probably more important to map how or why they are not getting well – turn the problem around in the opposite direction?

That's right, because in the daily routine those who do not get well will disappear but they will turn up in some other place. It is time, I think, to use the knowledge we have gained outside the so called randomised clinical trial.

Can I switch to another trial that you were involved in where I would be interested to hear your views, because what we have been talking about in the area of quality of life and in the area of aggression or social dysfunction is very different it seems to me from the alprazolam studies of panic disorder which were very focused on a disease entity – they were very Kraepelinian. You were one of the centres for that and there was afterwards all the controversy that blew up between Klerman and Marks. How do you read all of that?

Well, first of all I received data from the whole sample in Copenhagen and I was asked to look at the SCL-90 because in the first draft of the outcome of this study it was said that it correlated relatively well with the Hamilton scale so they didn't need to go into it. I said I would be very happy to look at it because I always liked the scale. I have actually been in contact with Frank in Baltimore who with Parloff created it. Actually, professor Frank gave me permission to publish the original 41-item version in my book on rating scales. It was actually the first scale to measure the outcome of psychotherapy in the

1950s in Baltimore. They said if we cannot demonstrate and document an effect of psychotherapy we have to stop doing it ...

In the 1950s?

Yes, it was a very bright study, the first study of SCL-41 (later becoming SCL-90) by Parloff, Kelman and Frank. They looked for something else better than symptoms as outcome measures of psychotherapy but they could not find any better language to communicate emotions in their anxiety disorder patients, so they called it a discomfort symptom scale. Parloff later became the leader of group therapy at the National Institute. Kelman became Professor in Social Ethics at Harvard and he has published on compliance and the 'crimes of obedience'. Frank is now Emeritus Professor in Baltimore and is perhaps best known for his best-seller *Persuasion and Healing*.

In the cross-national panic study the factor analysis of the SCL-90 identified the original discomfort factor as the first, then came the phobia factor, and as the third factor the panic factor. My conclusion was that the discomfort factor should be considered most important when comparing imipramine, alprazolam and placebo.

Discomfort means what?

Discomfort was changed to demoralisation when Frank published his first edition of *Persuasion and Healing*. In this book he defines demoralisation as the state of candidates for psychotherapy, whatever their diagnostic label. It is essentially a coping with illness behaviour, very much analogous to neuroticism according to Eysenck. The discomfort factor had no single anxiety item, but several depression items. I often equate neuroticism and dysthymia, which are indicators of quality of life. Most studies do not find anxiety as an indicator of quality of life. Personally, I always look for depressive symptoms in patients with anxiety disorder.

Klerman more or less said that he was in the business of using the panic disorder studies to internationalise DSM-III and the Kraepelinian view. Is that how you read it at the time? He saw it as a means to spread the use of DSM-III because you would all have to get together and you would use DSM-III criteria.

Klerman was not very interested in the SCL-90 findings, he was more interested in the DSM-III criteria of panic disorder. In my own analysis I excluded the alprazolam arm and focused on imipramine versus placebo differences. I found that Klerman focused on alprazolam as a unique drug for panic disorder. However, as a chronic disorder I prefer antidepressants for panic. At the bottom it is the Kraepelinian, medical approach.

It seems to be that he was perhaps not too concerned about showing that alprazolam was the only treatment for this condition but he wanted to sell the condition and with the condition the idea of DSM-III and with that a Kraepelinian view. Perhaps he wanted to sell it most-

ly back home to the Americans. How do you read the articles in the British Journal of
Psychiatry which took 4 years to publish, and with them was this amazing correspondence.

To be honest it was too political for me. Scientifically I could not see the problem actually, to be honest. It should also be emphasised that Freud and not
Kraepelin described panic disorder a century ago, when he separated anxiety
disorders from the American concept of neurasthenia. But I agree with
Klerman that affective disorders are biological disorders. The neurologists
have been very successful in grabbing Alzheimer's dementia and Parkinson's
disease. We should, perhaps, consider hanging onto Kraepelin's depression and
Bleuler's schizophrenia.

You were the original mover behind ECNP. How did that come about?

It happened that I was secretary for the Scandinavian Society of
Psychopharmacology – I had some years before replaced the Danish pharmacologist Erik Jacobsen, the father of disulfiram, in the committee. When it
had its 25th anniversary in 1984, I thought that one way to celebrate it could
be that during our annual meeting we might have a symposium, where I
invited the chairman for the different European countries to tell us how psychopharmacology was going in their country. So I invited, I think, Michael
Trimble and Max Hamilton from the UK and Mendlewicz from Belgium,
Professor Hippius from Germany, Ballus from Spain, Gottfries from Sweden,
Gastpar from Switzerland and so on. We had a nice symposium and then
lunch afterwards when it was discussed whether we in Europe should come
more closely together. They liked the setting in Copenhagen – all the annual
meetings in Scandinavia always take place in Copenhagen. So I said, I have
done this for many years and it would be easy for me to arrange a preliminary
meeting the next year. This was agreed around the table. We set up a small
working group of those who had attended. I called the companies and said
that we were in a situation where we wanted to have a meeting based in
Copenhagen about a European Society in Psychopharmacology. They asked
me, 'Why? There are already so many associations.' I said that from my own
point of view I see that perhaps we could harmonise standards in clinical trials in Europe so that we are not only looking for what the FDA says in the US.
They thought this was a good idea and actually I relatively easily raised
monies so I could invite 400 people and pay their cost for coming to
Copenhagen, which is where we had the first meeting. Max Hamilton was
one of the most active in this. He was very clear about how to set up a new
organisation – he had all the rules and things for that. The first official meeting was in Brussels in 1987 but I think we can say that the first meeting really was in Copenhagen in May 1985.

You say that one of the things that you were interested in was to get some standardisation of
clinical trials methods in Europe. There appears to have been something about the early
1980s because the AEP and the European Behavioural Pharmacological Society also began

then. Was there something about the early 1980s that led to the formation of European institutions?

AEP was founded at least without my knowledge the same year as ECNP. However, Professor Pichot has recently told me that the very first initiative was made in 1983 when he organised with Peter Berner the WPA congress in Vienna. There was some tension when it was clear that both AEP and ECNP were well-established associations, especially concerning sponsorship from the drug companies. It was decided that ECNP should organise their congress every odd year (1985, 87, 89 etc.) and AEP every even year. However, ECNP has later changed to yearly meetings.

Then, I think it was in 1989, I asked the committee why we shouldn't go back to our original idea about standardisation because in my opinion we now had a more political society and were looking for nice places to organise the next congress in a more ordinary or traditional way, but why couldn't we also focus on other things? There was a discussion in the general executive committee. I at the time had a small sub-committee drawn up on a Scandinavian model – in the Scandinavian Society of Psychopharmacology, we have a subgroup called UKU where we have made a side-effects scale; it is a committee for clinical trials and they receive 10% of the income for making their investigations. So I said couldn't I receive some percentage of our money and create this kind of role in Europe? But the executive committee said that I should try to raise the money myself. I said I would do it but it was the same companies I would approach. Anyway I organised a meeting in 1990 in Strasbourg, which was very successful, which was for persons working in the industry in the clinical trial area, trying to set up a dialogue so that they could exchange their knowledge and discuss what problems there were having. It was a very small closed meeting and it later became an independent group because they wanted it to be so. So we still have these small meetings but they aren't part of ECNP.

So did ECNP evolve in a different kind of way to what you had expected or hoped?

One could say that, yes. I had hoped that we could have had more of an influence on giving guidelines etc. Perhaps it was naive from my point of view because the whole thing is of course governed by FDA and in the end things have to be approved in the US and the other big countries.

But surely if there were a sufficiently strong European voice on clinical trial methods the FDA will pay heed.

This was what I hoped. At the first meeting in Strasbourg one of the main subjects was quality of life in clinical trials and we had invited representatives from the FDA precisely to be sure that we had a dialogue in the hope that a strong organisation in Europe could be more influential. But ECNP seemed to develop as another society for congresses ...

I thought the programme at the ECNP meeting in Venice in 1995 was very surprising. There was very little either clinical science or basic science – it was all focused on disease entities like Social Phobia or OCD or Panic Disorder. This AEP meeting in contrast shows, I would have thought, a much broader base.

I left ECNP democratically after 8 years and went actively into AEP. From 1993 to 1994 I was President of AEP and organised in September 1994 the AEP Congress in Copenhagen. I think it was the breakthrough of AEP. This year's joint meeting held with the Royal College in London has been a boost and with Norman Sartorius being the President after Angst I think all this is good.

Related to the question of what happened at the ECNP programme last year I suspect is something that came up at a recent CINP Members meeting in Melbourne where the debate got very acrimonious. It was said from the floor – and I think most people there probably felt the speaker from the floor had ECNP in mind – that CINP and several of the larger psychopharmacology associations appeared to be run like some of the old European Royal Houses once were; they seem to be in the control of a few people and you wondered to what end they are being run. Does that ring true?

Yes, certainly I think that is right as I see it myself.

You mentioned the UKU side-effects scale – how did the UKU side-effects scale actually come about?

The Director at that time for the Health Authorities in Sweden could not understand why in their file for reported side-effects there was nearly nothing – it was as if psychotropic drugs when they were used in Sweden had no side-effects. He asked whether it was because doctors didn't know what side-effects were or they accepted a lot of side-effects because that was the daily reality. So UKU consisted of a member from each of the Nordic countries – I was the Danish member – and we were invited by the Health Authority to look at side-effects. We decided to make a scale like the Hamilton Scale. For instance, I invited the Danish expert in sexual dysfunctions to give me some ideas – at that time we could only do that in Denmark. We asked Jes Gerlach for side-effects of neuroleptic drugs etc. Then during our annual meetings we had discussions and then we did a study where we said that all clinics in Nordic countries should use it in their departments for a month for all patients with schizophrenia – we had 2000 patients. Then we did a small inter-rater reliability study. Later I also did a small scale for the serotonin syndrome. I am no longer in the UKU for democratic reasons but I think it has been a good thing to do this.

I think it helped to put the whole area on the map.

Yes, I still receive letters from people wanting to use it and it has been translated into other languages. It was not perfect but it was a starting point.

One of the unusual things I guess about what you just referred to is that as a group the Scandinavian countries seem to be able to co-ordinate. There is no way that you could tell all the people here in the UK to all use this scale in their clinics. You wouldn't be able to get people to act in concert in that way. How come you guys have been able to?

It was in the years when an older generation of psychiatrists were still in place – Lingjærde in Norway and Dencker in Sweden. The Scandinavian society started in 1959 – it is one of the oldest. The German society may be even older. We used to meet every year. During the period that I was secretary I received some letters from well-established elder psychiatrists in Denmark saying either that they feel now that there is too much industrial influence on the meetings or the meetings have turned too much toward the basic sciences and have become less clinically relevant. I think we did what we did at a time when we still had a lot of clinicians. I think this is declining unfortunately. The members are much more pure pharmacologists; they are not daily acting psychiatrists. But at that time we had access to active psychiatrists around the Nordic countries, who came every year to the meetings and we could report back. So I think today it doesn't work as well.

What were your relationships with Lundbeck like? I know they helped start the Scandinavian Society in 1959 and they helped support ECNP ...

Well, ECNP not so much, to my knowledge. It was actually the three Swiss companies in Basle who were most active in ECNP as I remember it. In the Scandinavian Society our UKU meetings were held for many years in the auditorium in Lundbeck. PV Pedersen, who was behind most of the Lundbeck drugs, was a prominent member from industry. He was a real gentleman. When UKU was originally constructed it was arranged so that the industry could send protocols to be discussed but because there was a Lundbeck influence of course nobody did – why should they have another company etc.? So Lundbeck has been very active in the Nordic countries but less so today. The change came about in the mid-1980s.

Now I know you are also interested in the concept of hypomelancholia, which has always been an interest of mine – the idea that there might be a milder form of biological/vital depression which perhaps people don't even know that they have. Can you explain to me how you came to the idea? A few different people have written on the same kind of concept but it has never taken off, possibly because it is not clear that this is something that needs to be treated.

Yes, I am actually giving a lecture today about what I call positive melancholia. We know that of people in society who have a depression, only half of them seek help in the family doctor setting. So we have the Defeat Depression Campaign at the moment and next year in Denmark we have a Year of the Brain and I am chairman of the depression group and one of our goals is to draw attention to the fact that there are untreated depressed persons. I have speculated why those people do not go to their doctor; is it because it is part of being human that to experience some kind of depression in the long run gives a better quality of life, so to speak ? You know Kay Jamison, who has published a book on her own experience of manic-depressive illness, says that it is so that you have the insanity as the negative things and then some kind of enthusiasm as part of the positive melancholia.

I have looked at the various philosophers from this point of view – although not systematically. I started with David Hume, who in his young years had depression and he actually had letters to his doctor which described the English malady. From that I looked at William James, TS Elliot, Albert Camus and others who have had depressions, who all say that a depression leads one to speculate about whether life is worth living. So it prompts them to look at their life in a new way and it also gives them some excuse for loneliness, and it cannot have been too bad for their creative part to be alone for some periods. William James had what was called the American disease and every time he had this problem he went to Europe for three or six months to England and Germany. So this took him out of the daily routine and enabled him to speculate a little bit about new ideas. Henry James, his brother, in his novels often touches on the hours between 5 and 8 in the afternoon where he said you can know that in those hours you can move from a light depression into perhaps even a small degree of mania. He described those hours as eternity in which he could look into things in a special way. Everyone who is familiar with depression knows that the morning is a little bit worse and that in the evening you come out of it – in this situation you can have a more intense experience of presence, you are more intent to describe things around you

One of the implications of that, though, is that it might be a mistake to treat this condition.

That's right. My conclusion is that perhaps the right people go to their doctors and those who don't go shouldn't go. I don't know how exact the calculations are but we are often told that half don't go. Also there is the issue that we don't know what may happen when you start treatment – one of the problems can be causing rapid cycling and I have difficulties with these cases – I don't know what to do actually. Many people in the Copenhagen area refer patients to me and most of the time it goes OK, but in this case nobody likes to treat them and when they come to me I don't know what to do – even with lithium, and I have never seen a good effect of antiepileptics in these cases. I also use thyroid extracts, T3 and T4, but that is not an answer. I have been trying risperidone lately. Now and then I speculate whether it is all the previous treatments which have triggered the problem.

Another group that is awkward to know what to do about it is the group of recurrent brief depressions described by Angst.

I have not seen many of these myself. In a Danish study on Parkinson's disease and depression we started with citalopram and placebo firstly in which one of my psychiatrists would go around and interview using the Hamilton. When the relatives' neurologist had some video tapes and could see how to do it, they wanted to do it themselves and then they produced some video tapes for me. I could see that some of those patients could tell that two days ago they had had a depressive episode but it took only one or two days. The study didn't show any effect of citalopram on this and I know there have been two studies – one fluoxetine and one paroxetine – where no effect has been shown on primarily recurrent brief depression.

Is that because it's a different kind of condition?

Well, I had also been interested in depression in schizophrenia – whether it is again a mental part of the neuroleptic-induced Parkinson's syndrome with more fluctuating recurrent brief depressive episodes. That is another thing we are trying to do now in my department because we are moving more into schizophrenia. Recurrent brief depression is not a thing I see very much. It is interesting we had Spitzer in Copenhagen to a meeting and he was a little bit sceptical about the nature of this disorder – it's not in DSM-IV.

How has the field changed in the last 30-odd years since you began? Periodically you get the view that psychiatrists are doomed to extinction, they are going to be replaced by clinical neuroscientists and psychologists or a combination of those two.

Especially during the last decade I have experienced that a good psychiatrist should be able to work both as a clinical neuroscientist and as a clinical psychologist. The development of the selective and safer antidepressants and antipsychotics needs the neuroscientist's knowledge of the mechanism of action of such drugs and this is helping the patients and their family doctors to treat the major mental disorders. At the same time psychiatrists have to know about coping strategies both in the minor and major mental disorders, which include stress factors and quality of life, i.e. the work in clinical psychology. Only the psychiatrist is able to cover this holistic approach. Otherwise, we are back to the old dualism between brain (neuroscience) and mind (psychology).

It seems that Danish psychiatry, in contrast to other European countries, e.g. France and the Netherlands, is mainly based on biological psychiatry.

Yes. When Rafaelsen in 1974 was offered a new Chair as Professor in Psychiatry he wanted it to be in biological psychiatry like Herman van Praag or Julien Mendlewicz. However, the University of Copenhagen would not accept such a title because it was the Danish approach in general that psychiatry was biological and therefore the term biological psychiatry was considered a truism. He then became Professor of Psychopharmacology.

In Denmark we have had very few psychoanalysts compared to other European countries. The most influential was Vanggaard, who never became a professor but who worked in the same department of psychiatry as Rafaelsen. They respected each other. Vanggaard was always aware of the limitation of psychoanalysis and used antidepressants in the treatment of major depression. He was, for instance, the first to introduce into Denmark the combination of MAO-Is and TCAs using isocarboxacide and amitriptyline. In monotherapy with TCAs he preferred clomipramine because of its broad spectrum of efficacy including OCD.

All research-active departments of psychiatry in Denmark have been working in psychopharmacology and related areas. Strömgren, the most famous Danish psychiatrist this century was, however, not only a psychopharmacologist but also an epidemiologist who established the Danish Central Psychiatric

Register which now is chaired very successfully by Povl Munk-Jørgensen. He also initiated the national and international family, twin and adoption studies which have been continued so successfully by Fini Schulsinger and Aksel Bertelsen. We have already mentioned Rafaelsen and the generation of clinical psychiatrists he inspired. In this context I should also mention Annette Gjerris. Lars Gram, who is Professor of Clinical Pharmacology, is the father of pharmacokinetics and has inspired the next generation, most eminently Kim Brøsen. I should also mention the psychopharmacological research group at Sct. Hans Hospital in Roskilde. The first generation included Faurby and Munkvad. The second generation includes such names as Rasmus Fog, who has looked at the role of dopamine in schizophrenia, and Jes Gerlach, who especially works with tardive dyskinesia. The idea that psychiatry basically is biological has guided clinical research in Denmark in this century. It may explain the scientifically relatively high level and standard of Danish psychiatrists.

Select bibliography
Bech P, Gram LF, Dein E, Jacobsen O, Vitger J, Bolwig TG (1975). Quantitative rating of depressive states. *Acta Psychiatrica Scandinavica*, **51**, 42–50.

Bech P (1975). Depression: Influence on time estimation and time experience. *Acta Psychiatrica Scandinavica*, **51**, 42–50.

Bech P, Rafaelsen OJ, Kramp P, Bolwig TG (1978). The mania rating scale: scale construction and inter-observer agreement. *Neuropharmacology*, **17**, 430–431

Jachuck SJ, Brierly H, Jachuck S, Willcox PM (1982). The effect of hypotensive drugs on the quality of life. *Journal of the Royal College of General Practitioners*, **32**, 103–105.

Scandinavian Association of Psychopharmacology 1959–1984. Nord Psykiatr. Tidsskr. Supplement 10 (1984) vol 38.

Bech P (1985). European College of Neuropsychopharmacology. *Pharmacopsychiatry*, **19**, 1.

Danish University Antidepressant Group (1986). Citalopram: clinical effect profile in comparison with clomipramine. A controlled multicentre study. *Psychopharmacology*, **90**, 131–138.

Lingjaerde O, Ahlfors UG, Bech P, Dencker SJ, Elgen K (1987). The UKU side effect rating scale. *Acta Psychiatrica Scandinavica*, **76**, Supplement 334.

DUAG (1990). Paroxetine. A selective serotonin reuptake inhibitor showing better tolerance but weaker antidepressant effect than clomipramine in a controlled multicenter study. *Journal of Affective Disorders*, **18**, 289–299.

Frimodt-Møller J, Loldrup Poulsen D, Kornerup HJ, Bech P (1991). Quality of life, side effects and efficacy of lisinopril compared wtih metoprolol in patients with mild to moderate essential hypertension. *Journal of Human Hypertension*, **5**, 215–221.

European Rating of Aggression Group (ERAG) (1992). Social dysfunction and aggression scale (SDAS-21) in generalized agression and in aggressive attacks: A validity and reliability study. *International Journal of Methods in Psychiatric Research*, **2**, 15–29.

Lauritzen L, Clemmensen L, Klysner R, Loldrup D, Lunde M, Schaumburg E, Waarst S, Bech P (1992). Combined treatment with imipramine and mianserin. A controlled pilot study. *Pharmacopsychiatry*, **4**, 182–186

Bech P, Allerup P, Maier W, Albus M, Lavori P, Ayuso JL (1992). The Hamilton Scales and the Hopkins Symptom Checklist (SCL-90). A cross-national validity study in patients with panic disorders. *British Journal of Psychiatry*, **160**, 206–211.

Thunedborg K, Allerup P, Bech P, Joyce CRB (1993). Development of the Repertory Grid for measurement of individual quality of life in clinical trials. *International Journal of Methods in Psychiatric Research*, **3**, 48–58.

Bech P (1993). *Rating scales for psychopathology, health status, and quality of life. A compendium in accordance to DSM-III-R and WHO systems*. Springer, Berlin.

Bech P (1996). *The Bech, Hamilton and Zung Scales for Mood Disorders*. Second Edition. Springer, Berlin.

Lauritzen L, Odgaard K, Clemmesen L, Lunde M, Örström J, Black C, Bech P (1996). Relapse prevention by means of paroxetine in ECT-treated patients with major depression: a comparison with imipramine and placebo in medium-term continuation therapy. *Acta Psychiatrica Scandanavica*, **94**, 241–251.

23 Myrna Weissman

Gerald Klerman and psychopharmacotherapy

Gerry's first contribution came with the Psychopharmacology Service Center study of chlorpromazine in the early 1960s.

I did not know Gerry then so this is not first hand. I heard some of it when he died at his eulogies. Gerry was trained at New York University and then he went to Harvard for his residency. The psychoanalytic movement was very strong there then and he was trained as a psychoanalyst. He got an official certificate but he never completed his second analytic case so he wasn't considered a bona fide analyst but he certainly had extensive analytic training which in those days was very lengthy. He was intrigued with the ideas of psychoanalysis but he was intrigued with ideas in general. He finished his residency around the time of the Korean War and he opted to go into NIMH to do his military service. In those days it was called the 'yellow' berets. He was assigned to work with Jonathan Cole, Chief at the Psychopharmacology Service Center at NIMH. Jonathan Cole was beginning the first multi-centre study of phenothiazines in schizophrenia to establish if they worked in different settings and with different schizophrenic patients.

It was Gerry's job to help organise the study. It was a natural fit. He was fantastic at administration and very interested in seeing that it was done well. He helped in the training of the interviewers at the different sites and establishing reliability. He was also involved in developing some of the assessments, especially the measures of social functioning. He felt that it would not be a great outcome if the symptoms of schizophrenia, the thought disorder and hallucinations, were relieved but the patient was sitting home contemplating the wall and was not working. He had the idea of quality of life as an outcome very early on. He worked with a young social worker, Eva Deykin, and they developed social adjustment scales for schizophrenia which dealt with normal behaviours from brushing your teeth and dressing yourself, to going to a job.

After that he was invited to come back to Harvard to take a position in psychopharmacology and clinical psychiatry. There he linked up with Al DiMascio PhD, who was a young psychologist, also interested in clinical trials. They did a number of studies. They were not just testing drugs – they tried to answer psychoanalytic questions using research designs. Gerry was very committed to the idea that you could test most things if you could define them. For example, there was a theory that depression was 'hostility turned inward'. He tested it. He measured hostility in depressed patients before they had medication and then afterwards and concluded that depressed patients were hostile and irritable during the height of their symptoms but that this was part of the symptomatology generally and hostility diminished with recovery and thus depression was not hostility turned inward.

Can I take you onto the work with Gene Paykel on life events because that did two things – it led on to interpersonal therapy (IPT) and it also helped break down the idea that there were two forms of depression: an endogenous unprecipitated form and a neurotic form that was a consequence of adversity.

Gerry was invited to come to Yale in 1965 by Fritz Redlich, who was one of the most prominent psychiatrists in the United States at that time. Fritz was a force and an intellect, he was involved in the community mental health centre movement and he was the Chairman of the Yale department at the time. In the following year the Mental Health Center was opened and Gerry was soon after appointed its Head.

Gene Paykel was a resident in England at the time and he came to see Gerry in 1966 planning the next phase of his career. It was clear that both of them were interested in the maintenance treatment of depression. At that time treatment approaches during the acute phase of depression were clear but Gerry was interested in how long the treatment should be continued, whether continuation treatment varied by particular subtypes and also what the effect was of psychological treatment. He felt that psychosocial treatment should be part of any maintenance study because patients were receiving it anyway in clinical practice. The standard treatment for depression in clinical practice was psychotherapy. In fact there was a discrepancy between the treatment studies in depression which were on medication and the practice which was psychotherapy. The only psychotherapies which had been tested, and even then on small samples, were behavioural treatments and they were not used by psychiatrists – they were used by clinical psychologists who did not use medication. There was a real discordance in the whole field between the data and the practice.

Gene and Gerry designed the research protocol and Gene was offered a position by Gerry at Yale and they applied for an NIMH grant. First they wanted to estimate and describe the characteristics of depressed patients, so they surveyed all facilities treating depressed patients in the New Haven area. They were not community surveys but they collected data from hundreds of patients. As part of the survey they studied the nature of depression including life events, subtypes and medical history. The first papers on life events came from this survey. They looked at whether endogenous patients had life events and of course showed that they did. They showed that, as expected, hospitalised patients were more severely ill than non-hospitalised but didn't differ on the various subtypes of depression then in vogue – for instance endogenous or neurotic. They also showed that the endogenous depressions that were presumed to come 'out of the blue' had as many life events as the neurotic depressions.

The original maintenance treatment study was designed with group therapy. The reason was they had experienced group therapy staff and they felt this was most efficient for the emerging community mental health centres. They wanted the treatment tested but it should be feasible to be used in practice for a large number of patients if it turned out to be efficacious. The NIMH study section approved the grant but they decided that group therapy was not easy to study. In point of fact patients were not getting group therapy in practice, they were getting individual therapy.

This was when I came on the picture. It was 1967. I was just out of school. We had just moved to Yale. I had four small children and I was looking to work 2 days a week at something interesting. I was told to go see Gerry Klerman, I would like him and like his ideas and he would be fun to work with. I went to see Gene Paykel first and we got on very well and he had me see Gerry. Gerry and Gene were willing to agree with my two days a week condition. In those days there was a shortage of social workers and especially ones interested in research, and although I knew very little about psychotherapy or social work they hired me to help with the study, which would now have the psychotherapy delivered by social workers, until they found a senior social worker to be in charge of the psychotherapy.

Once a week, here and now, as opposed to looking in depth at the past?

No, the psychotherapy was just called high contact when I came on the picture – high versus low contact. Gerry may have had these ideas in his head but that wasn't explicit in the grant. It was going to be once a week versus assessments monthly. I remember the first day I came to work. There was Gene and Gerry and research assistants. My babysitter didn't turn up so my 18-month-old was there too. I called Gerry in the morning and said, I can't come to work, I don't have any help. He said, bring Jonathan. So I arrived at the first meeting, an interesting discussion about life events. The data were showing that there were more life events in depression before the onset of depressive symptoms compared to controls, but the events were just a laundry list and the question was how to categorise them. I remember Gerry saying it should be exits and entrances because exits would be more relevant to depression. They talked about factor analysis and cluster analysis. It was absolutely marvellous. I had never been in discussions that were so interesting about a field that I knew very little about.

I worked with Gerry and Gene. Gerry was always into generating challenges. My first assignment was 'design the psychotherapy'. I had almost no experience and so what I did was to try to go back to first principles. He had said to me, we know what amitriptyline will be like in Boston and we know it is the same in Boston and New Haven – we have to have the same assurance with psychotherapy. Thinking from first principles, therefore, the first hurdle was dose. The second should be the kind of people we hire so that psychotherapy is given in the same quality, and the third, the hard part, was to figure out the content that made sense for depressed patients. What did I know from social work training? That's where the 'here-and-now' focus came – that you don't want to undo people more by delving into past experiences that might be upsetting – you help them deal with things in the present. Gerry gave me some papers he had written. One in particular which was written with Eva Deykin was on 'The Empty Nest – Psychosocial Aspects of Conflict between Depressed Women and Their Grown Children' and another one was on the interpersonal dynamics of hospitalised depressed patients' home visits. The point that he made was that depressed patients' symptoms could be exacerbated by what was going on in their interpersonal environment. In one of the studies they looked at patient symptoms changed when the family visited and there was a dispute; they found that the symptoms returned. So although he believed that depression was a biological disorder, he saw the interpersonal context as very important to the onset and recurrence of symptoms, which made a lot of sense when I was trying to design the psychotherapy.

I remember first developing a ten page description of 'dos and don'ts' – you don't regress, there's no transference, no dream analysis etc. I tried to rule out the most obvious things it shouldn't be, hoping that what it would be would evolve as we got cases. I worked closely with Gerry on this. He was marvellous at taking what I was doing, conceptualising it and taking it to the next step. Gene at this stage was involved with the life events and in designing and managing the drug side of the study. Brig Prusoff was also hired at this point as the statistician. She was also just out of school but while inexperienced she was very smart and welcomed the challenge.

At this stage the study had one site but Gerry had had the experience of collaborations and he felt that two sites would accelerate the work. So he submitted another grant with Al Di Mascio at Harvard. The NIMH committee requested a site visit to Boston. It was Gene's, Brig's and my first site visit. It was a heady experience to be reviewed by the NIMH but we got funded and we were up and running. They never hired the senior social worker who was supposed to develop and run the psychotherapy between the two sites. During the time both sites were going we had developed the first iteration of the psychotherapy, high contact – later to become IPT.

Soon after that I was assigned a second major task by Gerry, which was to design the outcome measure for the psychotherapy. He said, design a social adjustment scale for depression because that will be a major outcome. That was a challenge because I didn't have any background in social theory, sociology or psychodynamics – but this may have been helpful. I decided to see what had been done. I collected all the scales and I remember coming to work one day with a report which I called 'all you ever wanted to know about social adjustment scales'. That review later turned out to the paper called 'The Assessment of Social Adjustment' which was used in part as an ACNP summary of relevant outcome measures for psychopharmacology trials and was later published in the *Archives of General Psychiatry*.

What was clear was that there were two types of social adjustment scales. There were the ones designed to assess schizophrenics, which was work that Gerry had done at NIMH but the level of functioning assessed was too low for depression – we really didn't need to ask depressed patients whether they were brushing their teeth or bathing. The second were scales that had been developed by psychologists to assess college students in university settings and they asked a lot of questions about sex and dating. They were relevant but they still didn't assess important areas for depressed patients, who were mostly women in their thirties and forties with families and children. Gene had met Barry Gurland, who was developing the SSIAM. Barry's scale was good, certainly better than what was available, but it didn't have a scoring system, it was somewhat complicated and it didn't have measures for parental functioning. We invited him to come to Yale and talk about his work. We were impressed but in the end we started to work on our own social adjustment scale. We came up with something that seemed to make sense. It had social roles in it. The idea of conceptualising roles as instrumental and affective was Gerry's – he had had a training in sociology.

Finally we had the first draft of the Social Adjustment Scale (SAS). Then he said to me, 'Now you have to validate it.' I remember asking, 'What does that mean?' He said you go out and get a group of non-depressed people and see if you can discriminate. Well, that is very interesting, I said, where am I going to get a group of non-depressed people and he said, 'Go talk to Jerry Myers.' Jerry Myers was a distinguished medical sociologist at Yale who had worked with Redlich and Hollingshead and had been doing studies of impairment in the community. He gave us some ideas about how to get a sample using the normal neighbour method – you select a depressed patient and then choose a neighbour ten blocks away, send an interviewer out to make sure they didn't have a psychiatric disorder and if they didn't we would interview them using the Social Adjustment Scale. We had a sampling method for who to approach if subject 1 was ill etc. and this method gave us a matched control. The result turned out to be the book *The Depressed Woman*, which I wrote with Gene Paykel, published by the University of Chicago Press.

By the time the book was finished we had some data from the maintenance study. When the study began I hired two senior experienced social workers to do the clinical work. Gerry and I and the two of them would meet once a week and discuss cases. That process helped us to refine IPT, which we developed through this iterative process. In 1970, Gerry left to be Professor at Harvard and run their new mental health centre. Gene returned to London in 1971. I went to graduate school at Yale. I would have been happy to work on that team for the rest of my life because it was so interesting. I wasn't thinking of a career but I said if I want to continue the work I'd better learn how to do it myself, because both Gerry and Gene had left, so I went to Yale to study epidemiology.

I still continued working with Gerry on the studies. The grant was transferred to Harvard with Gerry as the PI subcontracted to Yale. We started to analyse the data working with Gerry, Brig Prusoff and Gene in London. Gerry didn't think psychotherapy would show an effect. There was no reason to think it would show an effect – there had never been a positive psychotherapy study but there also had not been many studies. But, he said, if we show an effect it will be on social functioning..

Was this the Parloff–Frank idea that drugs act on the symptoms of depression and psychotherapy acts on the social adjustment?

It could have been. Gerry was very impressed with Parloff and Frank. He thought that behaviour therapy, cognitive therapy and IPT had some differences, so he wasn't convinced about the non-specificity argument. He had an open mind. Some time later when we had got further on in IPT he showed me a type-written manual that Beck had done and he said, 'We need a manual, like Beck is doing. You've got to specify the therapy. It can't just be a black box, you can't just say be supportive. You've gotta say what you do to be supportive. I want scripts, I want examples. I want somebody to be able to pick it up and be able to figure out what to do and what to do next.' I said, 'Oh you mean strategies' and he said, 'Right, not theories but strategies and scripts.' So we wrote the manual and as the therapists were bringing in patients we wrote the scripts. I didn't see patients because I wasn't experienced enough and he said we would have to have experienced clinicians because we wanted a bias in favour of an effect, so that they can't say 5 years from now that you didn't find an effect because you didn't have experienced therapists. He really had no ideologic bent on this. He just wanted accurate, unbiased results based on a good design – he and Gene spent hours on the design.

It was around that time that he wrote the paper on psychiatric ideologies, and what comes through from this is that he had no prior commitments to a particular area.

Yes. He wanted to know what the data showed and ensure it was analysed correctly. He said you can have any hypothesis you want as long as the hypothesis came first. If it came afterwards you had to be clear that it was posthoc. That was what was so much fun. You felt that you were exploring and that it wasn't to prove a point. He expected psychotherapy not to work but he said we have to be sure that we're measuring what we think we are supposed to work on. He did say that psychotherapy wasn't going to make you sleep better but it should help you take care of your children and get along with your spouse better. At one of the eulogies for him, I quoted from the Osheroff case where Gerry was called a foe of psychotherapy and then I quoted from elsewhere where he was called a foe of pharmacotherapy. You really didn't know which way he wanted the study to come out, except that he wanted it to be a good study and considered a landmark. He said if it angered both groups it would probably be good. We were outsiders in the department, which was then strongly psychoanalytic. They couldn't care less about what we were doing. We were off in a little house outside the department.

When did you become aware that IPT was working?

When we analysed the data. The first thing we did was to look at relapse rate – that was the hypothesis in our grant – and there we showed very clearly that drugs had an effect on reducing relapse rate and psychotherapy didn't. Gerry was also way ahead of his time on this – he had said before we did the analysis that we had to define relapse. This was years before more recent efforts. Then we looked at social functioning and there we showed that there was an effect of psychotherapy on social functioning. That was what we had hypothesised. When we looked at the combined drug and therapy group, we showed that in the combined group you would get the best effect because the drugs worked on symptoms and therapy on social functioning.

Then he said we had to do a follow-up, so we did 6 and 12-month and 4-year follow-ups and that was my dissertation. They wouldn't let the *Depressed Woman* book, which I though was more interesting, be my dissertation because I began it before graduate school. But I did learn a great deal about follow-up studies from doing the dissertation.

Gerry felt that we could get a stronger psychotherapy effect with a different design. In the maintenance study the patients had to first respond to medication. Therefore we should go back and see if there was an effect of psychotherapy on acute treatment. By that time Gerry was in Boston and so it was a Harvard–Yale collaboration. He designed the acute treatment before he left for Boston and he was the PI. He subcontracted the acute treatment study to us at Yale and we carried it out with regular meetings of the team in Sturbridge, Mass – about halfway between Boston and New Haven. We completed the acute treatment study in the mid-1970s. The data paralleled the maintenance study to some extent but the effects were somewhat stronger, showing that drugs worked faster than IPT but by the end the effects of drugs and IPT were equal and the combination was the most efficacious. This study went easily. We firmed up the methods of IPT, got more cases and wrote the IPT book from it.

Had High Contact become IPT at this point?

The book was published in 1984. We started working on it after 1974 when we had two trials showing efficacy. People were very interested in our approach and we were distributing a xeroxed manual which was fairly big at that point. We started to look for a contract – it was between John Wiley and Basic Books and we went with Basic Books because Jane Isay was working for them. By that time we had a couple of chapters that described our concept of the interpersonal approach to depression and when we got a contract we started to write the book. I invited Bruce Rounsaville and Eve Chevron to join us because they were therapists on the IPT acute treatment study and they provided us with all the clinical material and the scripts. Gerry provided the theoretical underpinning and I orchestrated the whole thing and made sure the work was done and that it made sense as a whole. That book is still selling and I have a contract now to revise it working with John Markowitz, who was one of Gerry's students at Cornell. Now of course there are many adaptations of IPT and many more trials and that will all be in the new book.

IPT is now part of the APA guidelines for the treatment of depression in primary care. The official guidelines all came several months after Gerry's death. He would not have anticipated it. He would have been amused and alarmed that IPT was getting this much attention because during his lifetime it didn't get that much attention. There were many more behavioural and cognitive therapists and they were much more active than we were. One of the reasons we weren't active and one of the reasons we held back the book was because Gerry said until we had shown that IPT worked outside its own home-grown place we shouldn't go out and proselytise people. But by that time the Kupfer–Frank and NIMH studies were coming and it looked like it really did work beyond Harvard and Yale. On the other hand, we really didn't want to set up training programmes ourselves as it would have taken time away from research.

The reason it has gotten the attention I think is because in fact in clinical practice this is what is mostly done – a supportive here-and-now therapy. It takes more training for a psychiatrist or a social worker to learn cognitive or behavioural approaches because these differ more from what they actually do.

Around 1969 and partly because he was perceived as being acceptable to the social side of psychiatry, Gerry got involved in the NIMH Psychobiology of Depression Program. Two things came out of that, it seems to me. First this was the occasion for him to coin the term neo-Kraepelinian. Now while people think of the neo-Kraepelinian school as being Eli Robins and Sam Guze, it seems to me that it took a certain political input from Gerry to get that bandwagon rolling

The Williamsburg meeting organised by NIMH in 1969 was a key meeting. That's where these notions that the classification of depression should be based on empirical evidence were presented. Gerry had been working on these ideas for at least 10 years – trying to have an empirical basis for some of the old concepts in psychiatry. He liked the idea of collaborations and he had already completed the Yale hospital survey and used the data for studying different subtypes of depression. He was also very impressed with Eli Robins and Sam Guze and their paper on how to validate a diagnosis. He said that's what we need to do for depression. However, he was not chosen to do the work because he was 'perceived to be acceptable to the social side of psychiatry'. He organised a group of investigators in five centres from Harvard, St Louis, Columbia, Rush in Chicago and Iowa and NIMH. He and Marty Katz and several others then wrote a grant and submitted it to NIMH to study the psychobiology of depression that would have two components – a set of biological and a set of psychopathological, clinical and epidemiological validators.

He was the person who brought Bob Spitzer in on this.

Yes, and in fact the SADS came out of this. Bob had been working on the PFF and PSE diagnostic assessment with Jean Endicott at New York State Psychiatric Institute. Marty Katz, who was in charge of the Branch at NIMH, said that they needed to have a structured diagnostic interview and he invited Bob and Jean to join the group. Eli Robins and Sam Guze's idea was that you had to have precise definitions and for this you needed a way of getting precise symptom data and that became the Schedule for Affective Disorders and Schizophrenia – the SADS.

One of Gerry's great strengths was that if he had an idea he could pick talented people to get the work done or sometimes he would take ideas that other people had and reformulate it into a broader perspective. For example, the application of life events to psychiatry originated in 100 Park Street. Gene then took it up and ran with it and he did a fantastic job. The same was true with social functioning. It was Gerry's idea to assess social functioning but he was happy to have me carry it forward. He could fertilise new ideas or reframe old ones.

There's a story with the SADS which might be of some interest. I finished my PhD at Yale in 1974. By that time Gerry was at Harvard. I was working with Jerry Myers. Gene had started the collaboration with Jerry but he had left. Jerry Myers was going into the field to do the third wave of the New Haven survey on impairment which he had begun with Hollingshead and Redlich. He asked me if I would like to work with him. We were going to look at depressive symptoms – the CESD had become available. We got the grant for the study but I was dissatisfied. I knew that there were no rates of psychiatric disorder in the community – there were rates of unhappiness or of impairment etc. There had been the mid-town Manhattan study which showed that 87% of New Yorkers were impaired – it was called Manhattan madness. So even if we used the CESD, which measured depressive symptoms, this was not the same as assessing clinical depression – you wouldn't put people with symptoms on a tricyclic without knowing their diagnosis. I also wanted to know the rates of panic and GAD etc. I had heard about the SADS from Gerry so I convinced Jerry Myers to include it in the survey. It would be good to know the data on diagnosis and it wouldn't hurt his study, so he said fine. We would never have been funded to do a SADS study because the conventional wisdom was that you couldn't make diagnoses in the community – people wouldn't answer the questions. I called up Bob and Jean and asked them whether I could change their instrument, the SADS, which covered a 5-year period, so that it would cover lifetime. They said they'd be happy for me to use it but they'd mind if I did it – they'd do it. I convinced Jerry Myers to hold up the study 6 months while they finished the SADS. They would send me pieces of it as they got it finished and we would try them out.

The New Haven study became the first study to look at psychiatric diagnoses in the community, using the same criteria as you would use in psychopharmacology trials and clinical studies. That study had only 511 people but it was the first community-based rates of major depression, panic etc. Gerry had been appointed by President Carter to be Head of the Alcohol, Drug Abuse and Mental Health Administration. The President's Commission on Mental Health with Rosalyn Carter had been formed. Califano was Secretary of Health, Education and Welfare and he said if we are going to meet needs, he wanted to know how many people have needs. Gerry asked me for the data on diagnosis from the New Haven survey and I was sending him the data as we were getting it out, which he then handed to Califano, showing what the rates of the disorder were and how many people who had disorders were getting treatment. After that the whole mood of the Commission was that we needed to do an epidemiologic study and the people who said you couldn't do it could be argued with because we had done it. That set the stage for the ECA and then of course now the CIDI and the national co-morbidity study. These methods have been adopted all over the world.

The fact that he brought in people like Bob Spitzer and they produced the RDC, which was the prototype of DSM-III, meant that by the time Bob Spitzer was hired to do DSM-III in essence a lot of the work had been done

A lot of the thinking but not the work and much of the work that had been done had been done by Bob and Jean and later Janet Williams. Bob did a phenomenal job. He also took the position as well that you could define quite precisely the symptoms and that you had to have some consensus from the field as to what symptoms should count and that there should be an empirical basis for making those decisions. Some of that empirical basis came from the ECA and the psychobiology studies.

In the five-centre study, the idea was to follow Guze and Robins' ideas on validating a diagnosis. To do this they included family history, longitudinal and biological validators and it began with precise diagnoses. Jan Fawcett, Bob Hirschfeld, Marty Keller, Jean Endicott, Sam Guze, Nancy Andreason, Ted Reich, Bob Cloninger and others worked on this study which brought depression to the forefront. It provided a lot of information not only on subtypes of depression but also on its clinical course. There is now a whole background of information on depression, which we now take for granted, but which was really not known when we started out.

Coming back to RDC and DSM-III, while Bob Spitzer was clearly the co-ordinator of the whole thing, when there was a debate at the APA in 1982 or thereabouts about the merits or otherwise of DSM-III, as well as Bob Spitzer, Gerry was up there arguing the case. Really he did as much if not more than anyone else to push it – how important was it to him?

I thought it was very important to him. Not because it was truth but because it provided a hypothesis for empirical testing. He felt it would need to be revised. But at least the script was out there in public and people can challenge it. It was not just an intellectual debate, you could actually do studies and test out hypotheses. Again he wasn't looking for truth, he was applying scientific methods so you could find out what was more likely to be correct than not correct. But the DSM-III was Bob Spitzer's, he did it with passion and great intellect. I think DSM-IIIR came too soon. People were just absorbing III. As an epidemiologist it was a pain in the neck having to switch criteria. Since these things aren't truth, they're constructs that allow you to get towards what might be more true than not true, I think it was too soon to change it.

How close was the relationship between Gerry and Bob?

On a working basis, Gerry worked more with Jean Endicott than Bob because she ran the Columbia site of the psychobiology study. I wouldn't give Gerry the credit for doing DSM-III, I would give him credit for pushing the concept of an empirical basis to diagnosis and precise definition using methods proposed by Guze and Robins.

Coming to the President's Commission, a few things stemmed from that period. One was the ECA and another was the NIMH comparative studies of IPT, cognitive therapy and imipramine – what was his role in getting that off the ground in terms of work behind the scenes to make sure it happened?

He had become the head of the Alcohol, Drug Abuse and Mental Health Administration (ADAMHA) and the President's Commission was set up under Carter to look at the unmet needs in this country for people with mental illness. So in his position he had a major role on the President's Commission and he supported the notion of epidemiological studies to establish baseline data. He had also been very keen on comparative treatment studies to be done. There was already evidence for the efficacy of cognitive therapy and that IPT worked and considerable evidence for the efficacy of psychotropic drugs in the treatment of depression. So it was important to figure out what worked on whom and what didn't work and also to replicate findings. Gerry was a consultant to the NIMH on these issues before he went to ADAMHA and was advising on the design of the multi-centre study. But once he became head of ADAMHA, he could not influence the study and he dropped out of any decision making or consulting role.

How did he take to his period in government?

Gerry considered the period in Washington the height of his career. He loved it. He was very proud of the fact that he initiated a very strong WHO–NIMH collaboration, aimed at harmonising DSM and ICD. I was in the room when the ideas for the development of a common assessment instrument, which became the CIDI, took hold. It was in Paris at Pichot's hospital, the Salpêtrière. In the room were Bob Spitzer, John Wing, Lee Robins, Gerry, myself and some others. Gerry brought us together because he thought it was ridiculous to have international wars over the two classification systems, and besides it was important to know what the disorders were in different countries and whether they were stable and consistent across cultures.

The discussion was that we needed a common instrument because the Europeans couldn't be expected to adopt DSM-III or the Americans to take ICD but that there ought to be a way of cross-walking the results of studies. In fact if you looked at the components of the disorders, the symptoms, they weren't that different. So Gerry got John Wing and Lee Robins to agree that they would put the PSE and the DIS together into an assessment instrument that would be able to generate ICD and DSM. From that effort the Composite International Diagnostic Instrument was developed – the CIDI.

Gerry was asked to stay on at ADAMHA and he agreed to stay until the election but he had no intention of leaving academia and of being a permanent government employee. After the election in November, he left in December. The outcome of these collaborations he had set up, ten years later, was ICD-

10, which is very much closer to DSM-IV and vice versa. This was helped by Norman Sartorius, who was head of the Mental Health Directorate of WHO – he and Gerry were close and respected each other. The combination of this effort and the fact that the younger generation was involved with the cross-national treatment study which he directed using DSM really helped bring the international community closer together.

He had a role in implementing the recommendations of the President's Commission on Mental Health, which led to a Bill.

Yes, the commission report submitted to Carter in 1978 stressed a number of things – greater attention to the needs of the poor, greater support for research, support for clinical training, better third party financing of mental health care and increased attention to epidemiology and prevention. The team assembed to implement the recommendations were Califano, the Secretary of State, Don Kennedy who was head of the FDA, Gerry as head of ADAMHA and Herb Pardes who was recruited by Gerry to direct NIMH. Gerry led a government task-force which submitted a draft Bill which was accepted by the administration in spring of 1979 and presented to Congress on 15 May 1979 with a special message of support from the President. After much debate the Mental Health System Act was signed in September 1980. While the Reagan administration dismantled much of the Bill, certain parts of it remained, such as increased support for research, increased focus on epidemiology and prevention and a greater coming together of advocacy groups and citizens' groups which remains even to this day.

You mentioned that he really had the intention to pull people together – because this is what he writes in the arguments with Isaac Marks over the alprazolam studies. Some people might see that as post hoc rationalisation.

That's ridiculous. Now its obvious, but you have to remember he did all this work before ICD-10 and DSM-IV. He started the WHO–NIMH collaboration in 1977. People often don't recognise what he did because he would do something and then move onto something else. He loved the ideas and the chase. He was not a self-promoter. He got restless after the initial ideas took hold and were on their way to being worked out.

Can I take the alprazolam studies and the concept of panic disorder? When did Gerry get interested in panic disorder and why? Were the Upjohn studies a vehicle to run a large multi-centre, multinational study which might show that DSM-III could be used outside the US?

One of the major outcomes of the alprazolam studies was that it created a generation of young investigators thoughout the world who had used DSM-III and who could talk to each other in the same language. A major outcome for me was that this generation of young investigators, some of whom did epidemiological work, made it easy for me to get access to form the Cross-National Epidemiologic Group. The drug study was a minor outcome although it was very interesting in its own right.

Gerry had always been interested in anxiety – some of his early papers were on the relationship between anxiety and depression. He also had a great deal of respect for Don Klein. Don, in his APPA presidential address and in his book *Anxiety Disorder Reconceptualised*, revived the notion of panic disorder which had been very well described by Freud and forgotten. There had also been studies from the Washington University group on the biological basis for panic – studies on CO_2 precipitation of panic had begun to come out from there. Gerry was impressed with that symposium. The ECA study also provided data on the epidemiology of panic disorder and our family study showed that panic disorder plus depression had the highest familial loading. I didn't have a sample of panic, only probands, so we didn't know whether this was because they had two disorders or whether there was something special about panic disorder. So we were all getting more interested in panic disorder and then alprazolam came out. When you have a treatment for a disorder it becomes more interesting and more visible.

How much did he feel or worry that panic disorder was something that Upjohn were just using to market a drug?

I can't speak for Upjohn but the data on panic was available before Upjohn's study. Don Klein's work was there way before Upjohn and alprazolam. And there had been the studies at Mass General by Jim Ballenger and David Sheehan which had showed that patients with panic disorder responded differently to treatment than patients with GAD. Gerry had worked with both of those men at Harvard. He felt panic disorder was a real entity. I don't know what Upjohn's thinking was. They felt they had a drug which worked for panic where the other benzodiazepines didn't. So there was family data, there was epidemiological data and there was some psychopharmalogical data suggesting that panic disorder was different from the other anxiety disorders. It was interesting, that was his thinking.

I actually introduced Gerry to Jim Coleman from Upjohn when Gerry returned from Washington to Boston. I was at Yale and Boris Astrachan, who was head of the Connecticut Mental Health Center, asked me to meet with the Upjohn people, who were interested in running clinical trials in depression. I was running the depression clinic at Yale but we had a study going and could not undertake another one then so I told them they should talk to Gerry Klerman. Gerry was interested at the time in designing a drugs and psychotherapy study to follow up the NIMH collaborative study. The data on the efficacy of alprazolam in panic was coming out and Upjohn said they were interested in running a multi-site study and invited Gerry to run it. Gerry laid down the conditions – there had to be joint training, inter-rater reliability, monitoring and a quality assurance team, and Jim agreed and that's how they set up the studies.

First they brought a number of investigators together from the United States, Canada and Mexico. Then they decided to broaden it to Europe. They had a meeting in Key Biscayne. Giovanni Cassano, Sir Martin Roth, Max Hamilton, Don Klein and others were there to discuss the concept of panic.

There was a lot of debate. The Germans said panic didn't exist and a lot of the Europeans felt it was a figment of the imagination of Upjohn to sell alprazolam. Gerry got Upjohn to fund studies to see whether if using DSM-III criteria it did exist in European clinics. I remember Wolfgang Maier MD from Germany, who did one of these studies coming to the World Psychiatric Association meeting in Vienna in 1984, reporting the survey result. He had found panic disorder in non-psychiatric clinics. Because of the whole history of abuse of psychiatric patients in Nazi Germany, patients didn't go to psychiatric clinics unless they were really sick and people with panic disorder would be seen in non-psychiatric clinics. Although some of the older generation had been sceptical, now they had data.

I was part of the international quality assurance team and we saw patients with panic disorder in many different countries. It was the same disorder. Cultural context might be a bit different but I saw the same syndrome in Rio de Janeiro, Cali Columbia, Madrid, Barcelona, Toronto, Montreal, Paris and Pisa. It was the same panic. That's why my genetic studies are on panic disorder and not on depression – the epidemiology of panic is much more consistent across countries – the prevalence, the risk factors, the age of onset are similar and the family studies show enormously high familial loading – seven-fold – which is much higher than in depression, which is only two- to three-fold.

Gerry did not analyse the alprazolam data. His job was to organise the sites and to see that the psychiatrists were trained and that the quality assurance was done. We visited each site twice and that was very important to ensure that the same patients were being entered at each site. He also convened the meetings so that the data could be presented, so for Gerry it was a lot of fun.

Until the end when the controversies blew up with Isaac Marks – that can't have been much fun ...

That wasn't fun but Gerry knew where that came from. Isaac had a very strong ideological bent. If alprazolam didn't work it wasn't going to be any skin off Gerry's teeth because the major work for him was defining the psychopathology of panic working with a group of investigators, which was very intellectually interesting. If the drug was efficacious, that was nice, you like to have a positive study but it wasn't going to change his career.

I was so glad that many of the things that were said were said after he died. A book came out by Peter Breggin, *Toxic Psychiatry*, in which he said that Gerry got $1 million from Upjohn for doing this study. I wish that were true. He was paid as a consultant but it was a relatively modest sum and the study took a lot of his time and energy. Gerry was not very motivated by money. And because he was paid as a consultant he could not do the study, so there was no site at Cornell and he didn't analyse the data.

What about the correspondence with Isaac in the British Journal of Psychiatry?

Gerry died on 3 April 1992. He went into the hospital the day before with a high fever. When he was going in he said to me, 'Take a look at the letter on my desk, it's my response to Isaac Marks' critique of our study.' It had been looked at by all the investigators and he said, 'See what you think, I was going to send it on.' He died the next day. When I came back from the hospital I looked at the letter and I looked at his response. Marks' comments on the cross-national study were inaccurate. I said, I'm not going to let the record stand on that, this letter has to go out clarifying Marks' inaccuracies. I sent the letter around to all the cross-national investigators for their final approval. Then after I had their signatures, I sent it to Hugh Freeman, the editor of the *British Journal of Psychiatry*. It was published but it was published with only Gerry's name. I had everybody's signature there and I felt it had less impact with only Gerry's signature – a letter from a dead man.

Is there a sense in which Gerry and Isaac were very similar people? They had both partic-ipated in the development of therapies – therapies which were the opposite to the corporate therapies such as analysis or even cognitive therapy. These were therapies that were easy to do, almost easy enough for people to do for themselves and as such very available. They were both interested in evidence-based medicine before it was fashionable to be interested in this. Both were forceful people who tended to appeal to the data.

Personality-wise they were different. I don't think Gerry was an ideologue. For him it wasn't either drugs or psychotherapy. He thought it was great that both could work because people respond to different things. Also Gerry had spent more of his career testing psychopharmacological drugs and in encouraging studies of combined treatment. Isaac will have to speak for himself but I believe that he has more of a bent on psychotherapy. Gerry didn't develop a training programme for his psychotherapy and it's only now that IPT training programmes are coming out of a groundswell. He wasn't out to proselytise people to do IPT. He was interested in it as an intellectual activity.

He was good at the apt phrase but the apt one here was 'pharmacological Calvinism'.

That was a great phrase – 'anything that made you feel good must be bad'. He said that this persisted today with the under-prescribing of drugs. But he was keen for both psychotherapy and pharmacotherapy to be utilised – he just thought treatment had to be tested. He always felt that there should have been a psychoanalytic study. He was very disappointed about the claims made for psychoanalysis because they hadn't been tested, it was not that he was against psychoanalysis.

That leads nicely into the Osheroff case. How did he get involved in the case?

He was invited to be an expert witness for Osheroff and so he reviewed the material. He was often asked to be an expert witness but he didn't do it every time he was asked because he was a busy man. When he read the case, he was appalled. This man had lost his wife, his children and his practice. He had been hospitalised for so many months without effective treatment and it was so clear from the records that he had an agitated depression. His feet were bleeding from pacing up and down so much. This history is a matter of public record.

He felt it was a very important case and from that case he developed the idea of the patient's right to effective treatment. The evidence was strong that drugs work for psychotic and agitated depression and that psychotherapy alone was not the treatment of choice. Drugs and psychotherapy would be good. Gerry never advocated not using psychotherapy.

There was a funny story which he told me about the case. He was being cross-examined by the defence's lawyers and he was asked to talk about what was the right treatment for Osheroff. He stated that the patient should have been on medication and when in fact he was transferred and put on medication he did well. Then the lawyer asked him, 'What about the writings of Weissman, who said that psychotherapy works as well as medication and found no difference between the treatments, in her study?' He smiled and he said, 'If you read Weissman's papers you'll see that she also shows that for delusional psychotic depression psychotherapy alone was worse than placebo.' The lawyers had not done the homework or they would have seen that Gerry and I had published these papers together or that we were married. Osheroff came to Gerry's funeral and I met him there – I had never met him before. He was very grateful to Gerry. I tried to locate him afterwards but I couldn't find him.

After the case there was such a barrage against Gerry. There were the letters from Alan Stone. He was the most eloquently negative and of course he was a lawyer. That case in fact has made the legal journals and textbooks. Gerry's son Daniel, a lawyer and historian, pointed them out to us when he was a student.

Well, there was a correspondence in the American Journal of Psychiatry with Alan Stone which is absolutely fascinating. Gerry was clearly in favour of guidelines, the regulation of psychotherapy and the need for evidence-based medicine etc. before these things were fashionable.

Oh yes, he would love what's going on now except he wouldn't have liked managed care because it takes the control away from the physician using his best clinical judgement. He died before the guidelines came out recommending IPT. He would have been surprised at that.

Did the exchanges with Alan Stone become heated? One of the things Michael Shepherd says Gerry said to him just before he died was that he had felt he was out there on his own and he felt let down to some extent by other people within the profession.

I can't say that. I think he liked the opportunity to debate the issues. He loved the intellectual duelling and he didn't take it personally but I think he felt that some of the things that were said about him were totally unfair, that he was against psychotherapy for instance when he had developed a psychotherapy. He felt that was unfair and personal. But he felt he was on stronger ground than anyone attacking him who were basing their position on their opinion whereas he had data.

Was there any animosity to him for saying things like there was a need for guidelines, which can be seen to be restrictive?

Sure, there was hostility. He respected Alan Stone but he just thought he was wrong. I'm sure he didn't like it but he couldn't resist the challenge and he wouldn't back down on what he thought was right. He did it because he believed in what he said and he believed it was in the best interest of patient care. He always kept a small patient practice because he liked treating patients and he felt it kept him in touch with where things were.

What about the area of the regulation of psychotherapy, which he was one of the first to raise?

Yes. He spent a lot of time in the Hastings Institute. It was a think-tank that was interested in medical ethical issues. Will Galin was there and Perry London and Sisella Bok, who wrote on ethics. So they had quite a heady time talking about issues. Perry London, who has since died, was also interested in the ethics of psychotherapy. Perry was a psychologist who did behaviour therapy and wrote textbooks on it. The two of them wrote a paper on whether there should be an FDA for psychotherapy. They felt that psychotherapy wasn't regulated as to how many trials you needed and what kind of trials you needed before you could make claims for efficacy. It wasn't regulated as to who could do it, what credentials they should have etc. They weren't against psychotherapy but they felt that this was not a good situation for patient care and they were concerned about the ethical issues involved in uncontrolled psychotherapy. The Osheroff case fit in with his notions about the ethical issues in treatment – the importance of what is effective etc. He was way ahead of his time.

You could make the argument that we shouldn't have an FDA for drug treatment – that it forces a certain corporatism on the field by raising the hurdles over which people have to jump. He raises this issue himself when he asks who should regulate the field.

He thought it should be an independent body, that the profession should regulate itself.

But if you go down that route you end up forcing a corporate development because you have to have people organised to provide the proof – I would think that you necessarily end with a situation where some group like clinical psychology will take on cognitive therapy and because they make the investment in it they push the product whereas other groups like IPT or behaviour therapy may not do so well even though the evidence for them may be better because there isn't a comparable group to push it.

At the moment there isn't a product in psychotherapy that some corporation is selling. This could change because some of these medical information companies are taking on the psychotherapies as part of their disease management. Corporate means 'for profit' but these things don't have to be set up for profit. An FDA for therapy could be set up not for profit but so that people get efficacious treatment. I don't think it's simple but I don't thing it's undoable.

There's a problem with psychotherapy as I see it. Psychotherapy is a cottage industry. There is no industry taking the testing of it through successive stages. Most psychotherapies get put on the market before they are ready – in a way that would be like taking a drug from Phase I studies and putting it straight onto the market. It should be tried in out different situations and there should be studies to find the right dose and then it should be tried against placebo. By the time a drug gets to market we know a lot about it. Psychotherapies don't work that way because no one is funding Phase I and II studies. The NIMH collaborative studies and the Kupfer–Frank studies were what you might call Phase IV studies. Gerry did discuss this at the Scientific Board of NIMH, just before his death, and there is a mechanism now for getting small amounts of money for Phase I and II studies in psychotherapy.

The first time I became aware of your work was in the early 1980s and the piece that comes to mind is a chapter from Psychopharmacology: The Second Generation of Progress, I think, where you had a piece that at the one time seemed a strange combination of the blindingly obvious and the utterly revolutionary – in essence it was making the case for a combination of psychotherapy and pharmacotherapy. This seemed obvious – perhaps more so from a European perspective – but in American terms was clearly revolutionary in that there was a tradition of just not mixing the different modalities of therapy. What kind of feedback did you get on that?

That was the one that had the quote from the Revd Baxter in the 17th century that in the treatment of melancholia you need psychic and physic. I was so unimportant a figure then – when I wrote the chapter in the 1970s I was still in graduate school, so I could just be ignored. But I was honoured to be invited to present it at the ACNP.

IPT differs from cognitive therapy in making an explicit space for the biological aspects of depression and therefore making it possible to consider using both together. While Aaron Beck and John Rush originally maybe made some accommodation clinical psychology has since taken CBT up and the focus has been very heavily on the abnormalities of logical thinking, and how could a drug undo that?

Well, I was in graduate school studying chronic disease epidemiology and this was a very compatible way of thinking. If you take diseases like hypertension, rheumatoid arthritis or cardiovascular disease, they are caused by many things. They are all biological but by changing the environment you can have a great impact on the course of the disorder if not its onset – for example, weight reduction may cure hypertension. I was trained to think about depression that way.

When Gerry asked me to design a psychotherapy, I was the perfect person to do it because I was uninformed and curious. If he had chosen somebody who was knowledgeable, then he might have had trouble because they would have had older psychodynamic concepts and he would have had to fight with them. I tried to think through what made sense regardless of theory. It was totally common sense and data driven based on our emerging data on life events, social impairment and depression. I had seen some cases of depression. But I did not feel any need to take on giants or make a need or a reputation. It was very much against the times but I wasn't part of those times in the sense that I was not a psychiatrist.

What influence if any did Michael Shepherd have on all this? He apparently met Gerry as early as 1960 when planning the MRC trial and he was also into psychiatric epidemiology.

Well, the UK led in psychiatric epidemiology. In America we didn't think you could make diagnoses in the community. The closest thing we had was this behavioural or psychosocial epidemiology. The leaders in the field were all English. There was John Wing, who developed the Present State Examination, Norman Kreitman in Edinburgh and Michael Shepherd. These were giants in the field.

Have you ever felt that the ECA studies made the market for the pharmaceutical industry? You showed how common depression was in the community and how common conditions like OCD and panic disorder were and the industry could use the ECA data wonderfully to sell their compounds.

That was not the intent. I think this study helped everybody. It made psychiatry more rational, it helped the planning of services. It helped the pharmaceutical industry – well, sure they're part of the world as well. I don't think it helped them more. It helped nosology and provided an understanding of rates, age of onset and risks. Before that cardiovascular disease had an epidemiological base but psychiatry didn't. I'm sure that some of what came out will be revised but it changed the way we think of disorders. One of the major changes was the recognition that most of these disorders begin very early – they are not disorders that begin in the menopause or the elderly. They may occur then but they begin young. So it focused attention on the field of child psychiatry.

Should we be treating children when they begin to get depressed first with antidepressants or IPT?

Well, there are no strong data. Children and adolescents have been excluded from clinical trials. Drug companies haven't wanted to get involved because the wisdom was that these disorders didn't occur in childhood. Kim Puig-Antich at Columbia then was one of the superstars here. He was out of the loop. He came over here from Spain and began studying children in the 1970s. He developed the Kiddy-SADS (K-SADS) and he did biological, neuroendocrine, sleep, family and longitudinal studies and his question was, is depression in children and adolescents the same as in adults? When he left Columbia in the 1980s and I arrived, he said to me, you can have my kids if you can find them. I have been following his children and we now have 75% of them – over 300 of them – depressed children now grown up. At present the data confirm that depression does occur in children and that it is impairing. We also know who is at risk – the children of depressed parents are at high risk – it's a three-fold increased risk. What do you do with them? The FDA has recently required studies to be done if a drug is going to be used in a population. Because of this treatment studies will increase in younger samples. The data we have for psychotherapy in children are patchy. David Brent had a study using cognitive therapy and Peter Lewinsohn has done a study of group therapy in depressed adolescents and Laura Mufson in my group has been studying IPT in depressed adolescents and there are a few other studies ongoing. That's your database, the rest is all impressions. It would be nice to have an acceleration of studies in this area.

The whole childhood area seems to bring out the psychiatric ideologies that Gerry mentioned in his 1969 article. In the childhood area there is the feeling that psychotherapy is ethically the only proper thing to be doing.

I think that's changing. It's certainly changed with hyperactivity. We also know there is early-onset bipolar disorder. I think it will change if the studies being done now on children and adolescents are positive. If they are not positive, it shouldn't change. If they aren't positive, the question then is, do these drugs not work in children and adolescents because they aren't really depressed? Our data suggest that prepubertal-onset depression may be different from postpubertal onset depression but we'll have to wait for the answers. Another question is, do these drugs not work because you have to have a certain maturation before they can be effective? We don't have the answers but if you want to do preventive interventions it should be done with younger populations – by the time you get to someone in their thirties who've had three or four episodes of depression you're dealing with someone who has a lot of co-morbidity and social morbidity which you might have prevented if they had been treated earlier. You don't know but these are good questions and this would be a very responsible way to spend research money. Gerry in fact pointed out the early age of onset of depression way before it became fashionable to study it.

A number of people have referred to the fact that Gerry kept on chasing ideas even when he was in a wheelchair and on dialysis.

He was incredible. He travelled on dialysis all over the world. I could write the Michelin guide to dialysis units – Greece, Tokyo, Switzerland, Germany, England, Italy three times. His secretary Marlene Carlson helped to set up the dialysis when he was going to a meeting. It was high anxiety because you didn't know if they would speak English or if the records had arrived. This was his life and if he had to give it up it would have been the end, so you just did it. He worked up to the day he died because he really loved what he was doing. His colleagues all over the world helped him when he travelled – Bob Hirschfeld, Marty Keller, Jan Fawcett and Sir Martin Roth in England.

Mention of Martin Roth reminds me that he had a phobic-anxiety depersonalisation concept before panic disorder which was very much the same thing as panic disorder – did he ever feel trumped by the fact that in one sense he just didn't market his concept as well?

I don't know what he felt. He was ahead of his time. He participated in many of the subsequent international meetings on panic. When Don presented the idea at the APPA, the field was more developed, there were epidemiological data coming out, there were more treatments.

Anything to do with the fact that panic disorder was just a more catchy term?

That's true but the time wasn't ready for it. There wasn't much you could do about it. By the time Don talked about it, you could try it out in different flavours – epidemiology, family studies and the technologies were there to decide what was right or not. In the 1960s the technologies hadn't evolved.

But Gerry was amazing the way he kept on working. Dialysis is pretty rough. It doesn't allow you much quality of life. It's not much quality, it's just life, especially if you have diabetes as well. He wrote the letter responding to Isaac Marks the day before he died. The year after he died he had something like three books and seven papers come out. He's been publishing up until this year. These are papers he was working on with younger colleagues that they have been finishing up. I showed one of them, Mark Olfson, the first draft of this piece and he commented that the manuscript didn't capture Gerry's sense of humour, that working with Gerry was fun. He had an appreciation of the absurdity in most disputes and a great enjoyment of life. Young people particularly liked to work with him because he would listen to their ideas and could pick out what was important. I think 1997 will be the end of his publications. Bob Michels kidded me that Gerry was the most published author at Cornell two years after he died. I spent three years after he died at memorials and awards for him.

Select bibliography
Cole JO, Goldberg SC, Klerman GL (1964). Phenothiazine treatment in acute schizophrenia. *Archives of General Psychiatry*, **10**, 246–261.

Armor DJ, Klerman GL (1968). Psychiatric treatment orientations and professional ideology. *Journal of Health and Social Behaviour*, **9**, 243–255.

Paykel ES, Myers J, Dienelt M, Klerman GL, Lindenthal JJ, Pepper M. Life events and depression: a controlled study. *Archives of General Psychiatry*, **21**, 753–760.

Klerman GL (1972). Psychotropic hedonism vs. pharmacological Calvinism. *Hastings Center Report*, **2**, 1–3.

Klerman GL, DiMascio A, Weissman MM, Prusoff B, Paykel ES (1974). Treatment of depression by drugs and psychotherapy. *American Journal of Psychiatry*, **131**, 186–191.

Weissman MM, Klerman GL, Paykel ES, Prusoff BA, Hanson B (1974). Treatment effects on the social adjustment of depressed patients. *Archives of General Psychiatry*, **30**, 771–778.

DiMascio A, Weissman MM, Prusoff BA, Neu C, Zwilling M, Klerman GL (1979). Differential symptom reduction by drugs and psychotherapy in acute depression. *Archives of General Psychiatry*, **36**, 1450–1456.

Weissman MM, Prusoff BA, DiMascio A, Neu C, Goklaney M, Klerman GL (1979). The efficacy of drugs and psychotherapy in treatment of acute depressive episodes. *American Journal of Psychiatry*, **136**, 555–558.

London P, Klerman GL (1982). Evaluating psychotherapy. *American Journal of Psychiatry*, **139**, 709–717.

Klerman GL, Vaillant G, Spitzer RL, Michels R. (1984). A debate on DSM-III: the advantages of DSM-III. *American Journal of Psychiatry*, **141**, 539–542.

Klerman GL, Weissman MM, Rounsaville BJ, Chevron ES (1984). *Interpersonal Psychotherapy of Depression*. Basic books, New York.

Klerman GL (1990). The psychiatric patient's right to effective treatment: Implications of Osheroff vs. Chesnut Lodge. *American Journal of Psychiatry*, **147**, 409–418.

Klerman GL (1991). Comments on the Klerman–Stone Debate on Osheroff vs. Chesnut Lodge. Letter to the Editor. *American Journal of Psychiatry*, **148**, 139–150.

Marketing the evidence

Behaviour therapy, with which you have been very closely associated, now seems a very practical thing and it is hard to see how anyone could find anything wrong with it. But when it was introduced first in the 1960s, it caused considerable controversy. Clearly the analysts were not happy about it but many others weren't either. Many Catholics were unhappy – for example when I was planning to go to university the Department of Psychology in University College, Dublin, which was very clerically dominated, taught a metaphysics-oriented psychology degree while the corresponding Department in Trinity College, Dublin, which was the Protestant College, was very learning theory oriented. I was dissuaded from going to Trinity College on the basis that it would not be proper to go to a university that taught materialist teachings of that sort. Pierre Pichot has said that there were considerable problems also over in France. Can I ask you to give me some feel for how the scene looked when you entered the field?

I was not in right at the beginning. By the time I came Hans Eysenck saw behaviour therapy as a role for psychologists although Joe Wolpe was not a psychologist – he was an MD – not a psychiatrist either. As regards earlier developments, Leonard in Germany was a psychiatrist as was an even earlier forebear, Janet. It is interesting how psychologists tried to take over the field – with some success because even now it is thought of as more a psychologist's domain than a psychiatrist's, although in fact only a tiny minority of clinical psychologists practise behaviour therapy. The greatest opposition came from psychodynamic analysts who perceived a conflict between the approaches. Whether one perceives a conflict or not depends upon whether one regards the glass as half full or half empty. In 1967 I wrote an article with Michael Gelder on common grounds between the two approaches for which we got many hundreds of reprint requests. There was enormous interest in the shared field. In 1970 I wrote an article about the integration of psychotherapy. It never happened. Why it never happened is not easy to say.

The idea that Janet was a forerunner of modern behaviour therapy is an arresting one.

His work on OCD was seminal and he adumbrated the idea of exposure and response prevention.

Whatever the controversies behaviour therapy very quickly established itself as possibly the premier therapy for OCD and phobic disorders. If we focus on OCD for a moment, in the early to mid-1970s Ciba-Geigy of course began to push clomipramine for OCD and this seemed to put you in a position of conflict with them.

No single therapy has a monopoly. Where different treatments work together why not use them both? There was some evidence for synergy in a proportion of OCDs and a proportion of phobias so I don't see a conflict.

OK but on the other hand you did two trials – one published in 1980 and then one later again in 1987/88 – where you were claiming that exposure therapy was superior to clomipramine.

Yes, but there were certain cases where clomipramine was necessary as an addition. So I am not saying it has no use, just that it is not the first line – except in cases who have co-morbid depression.

Fine, but in many respects your disputes with Ciba seemed something of a dress rehearsal almost for the conflict over the role of alprazolam in the management of panic disorders and phobias.

I would see that in a different light. I can't see much role for alprazolam or other benzodiazepines whereas I can see a role for antidepressants in OCD and other anxiety disorders.

Do you think clomipramine is working as an antidepressant in OCD or could it be that drugs active on the 5HT system act as an anxiolytic in a weakly neuroleptic sense?

It is hard to say. The mantra is repeated time and again that SSRI drugs are antiobsessive and that their effect doesn't correlate with the amount of depression at the start of treatment. Often this is true but the people who write this forget that usually they exclude patients below a certain threshold of depression so that they don't have a large enough range of mood to really test the issue. There is no doubt that various antidepressants, not only clomipramine, can have an effect in non-depressed patients. But there is equally no doubt that the effect is far greater in the presence of depression.

Do you think that the drugs that act on the 5HT system in this way, including clomipramine, have more effect on OCD than the other antidepressants that are not particularly active on the 5HT system?

I have seen a review by John Greist suggesting that clomipramine has more of an effect than any of the other SSRIs but I have not evaluated this in any detail.

Let me just move the focus to a further aspect of clomipramine and the SSRIs and OCD that comes through again in the panic disorder story, which is that Ciba-Geigy and now, with the four SSRIs that have been licensed for OCD, there are about five different companies who have an interest in pushing OCD as an indication. Now it isn't that they have done the work which has led to us now recognising that OCD is much more common than we thought it was 10–15 years ago but somehow they seem to have made the market. We do now recognise it much more commonly than we did – in a sense it seems that the companies have the ability to market the evidence, as well as they market the actual compounds.

'Market the evidence' is a good phrase. I was lecturing to a big symposium on OCD at the APA in Washington, DC about 10 years ago and presented some of the evidence for behaviour therapy. Much to my embarrassment, at question time a psychiatrist of Indian origin got up and spoke to this vast concourse of about 600 people. He said, 'I don't know what all the fuss is about how common OCD is. We have known about OCD for many years. Professor Marks has done all this work with OCD for decades so what is the big deal about how common OCD is?' He was making a point about the marketing of evidence by drug companies.

It has always seemed to be that you have had an interest to produce low-cost treatments – cheap enough to give away to people in one sense. You have been in the business of trying to encourage people to treat themselves with treatments that have been shown to work, which is just the opposite to what the pharmaceutical industry does. And in a sense it seems to me that your strategy, while obviously in one sense the correct one, is doomed in that you won't be generating the profits needed to give treatment away. In the real world it seems that you can't give things away.

Well, there are hundreds of therapists in this country giving behaviour therapy for OCD. Not nearly enough. We need a thousand or two. But behaviour therapy is widespread in this country. It is also widespread in France, with psychiatrists being the main behaviour therapists there. But it has not spread widely in other countries – that's true. The hope is that with the introduction of information technology, we will have a package that is marketable and inexpensive. Until somebody can market it, it is not lubricated for dissemination. The marketed product need not be horrendously expensive.

It seems to me with all of these things you've got to hypnotise the public to some extent – not just the consuming public but the prescribers, the people who decide what the treatment is going to be. They have to be hypnotised by having the regular meetings, the symposia, the company people calling round reminding them to use the product.

Have you heard of Triumph Over Phobia? This is now an England-wide network of 13 self-help groups, self-exposure groups, run by lay people who are usually ex-phobics or ex-OCDs who teach other sufferers how to become ex-sufferers. They have expanded from 8 to 13 in the last year and are about to go to 15 in the next few months. On 29 February I opened the first TOP help group in Australia. So there are initiatives for spreading this treatment, some of which by-pass the professionals – although this doesn't mean that we can do without the professionals. I imagine many sufferers would want to have professionals as well. So I am sanguine that on a 20-year time-span the development of self-help methods including computers will spread this form of treatment more widely than before.

Behaviour therapy is compatible with the use of antidepressant medication for those who need it. The difference between me and the drug companies is that the drug companies would like to see every patient on drugs and I say only about 30% need to have medication for this problem (when there is co-morbid low mood) and then usually only for 6–12 months. Very few need it for years.

Will the public tend to assume that what costs more must be best?

In that case one could make the computerised packages more expensive. But the patient doesn't pay much for medication on the NHS. So it depends ... many patients hate drugs. Perhaps I tend to get referred more of those who dislike drugs.

Can I take you back to the mid-1970s when you ran the first trial with exposure therapy compared to clomipramine. As I understand it your thoughts at the time were that it would be unethical to run a straightforward drug versus placebo study.

Well, we already had data about the efficacy of exposure therapy and the obvious question was how it compared with clomipramine, for which great claims were being made.

Do you think the claims being made then were inordinate?

Our findings were that in the depressed sub-sample it worked well temporarily, as long as the clomipramine was continued, and in the non-depressed sample we could no effect. The results we have had since then and my review of other people's work point in the same direction over the last 15 years – namely that antidepressant medication is much less specific than used to be thought. To call it antiobsessive or antiphobic or anti-this or anti-that is wrong – it's probably much more broad spectrum in its effect. You may well be dealing with antecedent problems of which the OCD is an expression. But it is a good marketing ploy to call it antiobsessive and of course it fulfils FDA requirements.

What role did the FDA play in all this?

Enormous. The FDA is more likely to approve a new drug if a compound has data that the drug is useful for a particular syndrome. So the pharmaceutical companies jump to that tune. If it is granted a drug indication, a company is made. There is much less mileage for a broader indication; it boosts sales less if one says the drug has a broad-spectrum effect, yet I think that is what the data suggest.

We are caught then in a bind because the FDA are doing what they are doing in order to improve risk–benefit ratios – they want to make sure people have a disease before they undergo the risks of therapy so that the benefits that they are likely to get will be substantial enough to justify the risks they are taking. To say that these pills are tonics, which is not far from what I believe, doesn't seem to meet the needs of the times in one sense.

Tonics is not quite right. I would say that whatever mood disturbance represents – and we don't really know – I would say that that is a very specific indication. But the FDA doesn't work by problems, it works by diseases. This is an issue for medicine as a whole. In fact medicine is much more problem driven than we are taught – problem driven rather than disease driven.

I guess one of the hallmarks of behaviour therapy is that it is not disease driven, it is disability driven. Is there a difference between a problem and a disability?

Disability tends to mean work or social problems in this country, which is one aspect of the problem. But think of the work of Lawrence Reed in the early 1970s, who was a physician in the USA – he was problem driven. But his excellent method of problem-oriented records in medicine did not gain wide acceptance.

Has it not taken off?

If it has I have not heard of it. He is still a voice in the wilderness, undeservedly I think. In 1982, I was looking at his work with fascination wondering why everybody didn't take it on. I suppose the answer is it needs a certain dedication and the average doctor isn't interested. Maybe it's more time consuming. Also it was problem-oriented records without ratings. If we understood why that didn't take off we would understand better why audits of clinical outcomes are so rare.

Any thoughts?

Well, turkeys don't vote for Christmas do they?

This comes back to your quoting George Bernard Shaw that every profession is a conspiracy against the laity ...

Of course, it's self evident isn't it? We all have our guilds and they perform a necessary function. If we didn't have this conspiracy there would be far lower salaries and if we were on far lower salaries we might have far less able people coming in, etc. etc. It's a double-edged sword. If you want good people you have to select, pay and give them decent conditions. On the other hand it is in the interest of the public to be even handed to everybody, so there is a tension there.

Which cannot actually be resolved ...

Hence the term tension. That is why we need controls over the professions. And we need controls over the lay people too, if you think of what happened with the anti-psychiatry movement. Anti-psychiatry in itself does harm and the writings of people who are anti-pharmaceutical can become too strident and mislead sufferers. So it is hard to get a decent balance.

To move on from OCD to the alprazolam story. Could you tell me how you see that having evolved?

Well, I suppose there were two driving engines for it – psychiatry and the pharmaceutical industry. Don Klein and other psychiatrists formed one engine – looking for a biological role for psychiatry and a panic button located in the brain which is thought to mean this is a brain disease – what you have to do is hit the button with a specific antipanic drug. Then Upjohn as a marketing ploy said we can hit the panic button with alprazolam and so they supported diagnostic conferences for DSM-III and so on. When I expressed considerable scepticism in 1983 about the validity of 'panic disorder' that was the last of the diagnostic conferences I was invited to. They didn't want opposing voices.

When one member of my team running the alprazolam study with me started to question the concept of panic disorder, the scientific adviser to Upjohn tried to get me to fire him.

Gerry Klerman.

The very same. We had endless battles because we didn't accept the basic philosophy. When they approached me to run the London–Toronto study I said, why are you bothering – you're going to lose, and they said, well that's your opinion. Somebody had to test it out. So we accepted the money to run the study.

There was an endless series of conflicts, with Upjohn wanting to do this and us wanting to do that and uneasy compromises being arrived at. When we asked for the data on which rested the importance of panic the result was a scream of fury at me from Gerry Klerman in the lobby of a Washington Hotel: 'Give the money back to the company' he yelled when I asked him for the evidence. That was his answer.

Can I chase this a bit further because it seems to me that Klerman and yourself have many things in common in some respects? He is also a man who developed a therapy – interpersonal therapy. One that is focused on problems and disabilities rather than a disease entity as such. One that is simple enough to give away to the public almost – which was actually devised for social workers at first. And again just as you, before evidence-based medicine became the bandwagon that it now is, wrote articles on public health policy asking why medicine does not follow the evidence that behaviour therapy works for instance, in the same way Klerman took up cudgels in the Osheroff case, saying really oughtn't we to be following the evidence?

Interpersonal therapy did not take off despite his espousal, although it is beginning to take off more now that it is being pushed on a commercial basis. But we have to realise that we don't know what is common between interpersonal and cognitive and behaviour therapies. Nobody has tested just a straight problem-oriented therapy although I received an article today from Neil Jacobson suggesting that it is the behavioural activation component of CBT that may be the most important. We need far more such dismantling studies.

I have always thought that one of the interesting things is that you rarely get the various different therapy modalities being tested against each other. Is the reason why we don't get these because the clinical psychologists are in the business of trying to make cognitive therapy look reasonably complex so that you need 2 or 3 years training to be able to deliver quality therapy – they don't want CPNs doing it?

There are both cock-ups and conspiracies everywhere, and a lack of money, a lack of research funds. It is not easy to get money to do dismantling studies these days.

Isn't there a vested interest almost against doing them because you are probably going to come out of it with some very simple components being active in their own right? So simple that you could give them away and then we would all be out of business.

Well, lithium is a very cheap medication and yet it is marketed with some profit, and Woolworths have managed to stay in business selling some very cheap things. So you can make lots of money out of cheap things when your market expands. Transistor radios have huge sales. On the other hand, perfumes and diamonds have their price maintained at an artificially high level – it depends upon which market you are aiming at. I would like to aim at the mass one, so that we can help all sufferers who want help.

But to come back, the reason to profile Klerman was to wonder whether the two of you were not similar in some respects, and did this fuel what ended up being an acrimonious situation?

No, I think acrimony came because my unit questioned the accuracy of the model that panic was a purely 'biological' problem. We know that panic is an unreliable symptom to rate. We know that it occurs across syndromes. And we know there is no relation between panic symptoms and alprazolam's action and that there is a dependency issue.

In fact the first acrimony with Gerry had nothing to do with alprazolam. It was at a WHO meeting in Copenhagen in the early 1980s. I asked a question about Briquet's syndrome, about the validity of the diagnosis and its implications, and suddenly he exploded. Much to my surprise because we had been very good friends until then. He had written letters to me saying how much he admired my work and wanted me to stay in his home and he and his first wife stayed with us etc. then suddenly ... I suppose it was this – if one dared to question the model this was taken personally, not just on panic but on the overarching importance of diagnostic classifications and categories.

His contribution to interpersonal therapy with Myrna Weissman was one of the most important things he did. And he was responsible for getting the epidemiological catchment area study off the ground and to some extent for getting the NIMH collaborative study of depression started.

He was also one of the people responsible for the nine-hospital study of chlorpromazine – the one which was published in 1965, Goldberg, Klerman and Cole.

Yes, Gerry was one of the foremost psychiatrists in the States over the last century. When he became Upjohn's scientific adviser, he was too close to the scene to see what was problematic about what Upjohn was sponsoring. And Upjohn made huge amounts of money. It was a brilliant marketing ploy to use panic criteria to make huge amounts of money but it had nothing to do with scientific reality or helping patients.

What happened when you wrote into Archives critiquing the first set of alprazolam studies? As I understand it there was a letter which took 15 months to appear, then only appeared shorn of some of its essential details.

Eleven psychiatrists from six countries helped draft this letter and we sent it off. I got it right back saying this is unacceptable. I phoned the secretary to find out what was unacceptable and was told that (a) the margins were the wrong size and that (b) the signatures were not all on one page – from six different countries. Danny was always rude in the way he wrote to me perhaps because I said to him about his publication in 1988 of all those alprazolam studies that they were very uncritical. When I told him that he said, 'Just you remember that I was on the selection committee that got you selected for the Stanford think-thank.' That was his response. He was always rude. I could never get a paper into his journal, *Archives of General Psychiatry*, from 1983 onwards. There were endless problems. They would all automatically go to Don Klein or someone like-minded for refereeing. But this is not just true for the *Archives*. In general anything that bucks a paradigm gets a hard time.

Eventually Danny did accept the letter, rather to my surprise because it was a quite damning letter. Then when I got the copy editor's corrections, I noticed the letter was shorn of its accompanying table showing that with one method of analysis alprazolam had absolutely no significant effect, whereas with another method alprazolam had some effect. So it depended on which method of analysis was used whether alprazolam had any action at all. I got an acerbic letter back from him saying he had never sent the table. I know I had sent it. I sent it to him again immediately. He replied, oh there isn't time now, it's too late. And the letter appeared five months later without the table. So that's the kind of thing that went on. I was told by one of the referees of one of the main 1988 papers in the *Archives* that Danny had written to him saying, 'We would like your quick opinion about this because we very much want to publish this article about alprazolam.'

Are you saying that his judgement was compromised?

I can only tell you what I know. I believe he was a consultant to Upjohn.

Was your London–Toronto study first submitted to Archives as well?

It was sent to the *New England Journal of Medicine* and they took twice as long as usual to send an opinion. They only sent me an opinion after I had faxed and phoned them. Finally I got trivial criticisms that did not address any of the substantive issues. They rejected it, so then I phoned up and spoke to the person who was handling it, saying, 'I think we can meet all these criticisms quite easily. I wonder, would you be willing to have another look at it?' 'Sure, sure.' I sent the revision along and exactly the same thing happened again – twice as long as usual – six weeks is the usual turnaround; this was over three months with still no answer to many phone calls. Finally they rejected it again, this time with a different set of trivial comments.

Why do you suppose the New England Journal was so hostile?

Presumably their referees were sold on the panic/alprazolam paradigm. So then I decided that I can't educate American psychiatry or American medicine against its wishes and sent it to the *British Journal of Psychiatry*. It was accepted with almost no change.

But with the most amazing correspondence.

Subsequently yes. Upjohn solicited a committee to do a hatchet job on this. In fact David Spiegel, whose name appears first on it, is still a good friend of mine. He is a fervent believer in the virtues of alprazolam. Some people received fees for participating in this exercise. It led to an interesting correspondence which attracted a lot of attention. All sorts of people wrote to me saying how wonderful it was and at conferences they congratulated me. People like a good fight perhaps, whatever the issue. Then there was this Upjohn conference in Geneva.

That was around 1989. It appeared in the Journal of Psychiatric Research supplement to 1990. Wasn't there an exchange between yourself and Gerry there – a few of those who were there have mentioned it?

It was in 1990. The conference was a superb propaganda exercise by Upjohn. They even had the gall to display above the podium what looked suspiciously like a United Nations or WHO emblem for this meeting on 10 years of panic. Lew Judd and other top people gave papers on the concept of panic and alprazolam's value for it. Although the London–Toronto study was the most controlled of all the studies, it was sidelined, marginalised to be presented to only a quarter of the audience in an afternoon session rather than a plenary morning session. But word had got round because of our abstract. The audience in our small room crowded into the aisles and overflowed into the corridor trying to listen to the presentations by Richard Swinson and me.

A Greek newspaper man said, 'Ah, at last we have got somebody honest.' And he published something in an Athens newspaper. A local Upjohn representative there contacted him and tried to rubbish our work to undo the damage we had done.

There was an exchange with Gerry months before the Geneva meeting at an investigators' meeting in New York in Gerry's office in Cornell. The first results had come through, analysed by Upjohn not by us. And the first comment made as we had the results in front of us came from Matig Mavisakalian, who said well, this shows that behaviour therapy is doing much better than alprazolam. It was as if nobody heard it. Gerry said, 'You must present these results at the CINP in Puerto Rico in December.' I asked him, why do you want to present the results to the CINP? He said, 'Why shouldn't we?' I said, 'Because they don't show alprazolam up very well, do they?' He said, 'What do you mean, what do you mean!' In other words the figures were there but he could not take them in. Nobody could take them in because it was against the paradigm. And of course we weren't invited to the CINP.

We had already been invited to Geneva by then. In Geneva, Gerry was telling me about his flying from one renal dialysis machine in New York to another in Geneva and about his recent marriage to Myrna and how the children had responded well – it was as though we were friends back again in the 1970s. Then suddenly it was like a switch being thrown and he started shouting at me,

'I never want to speak to you again!' That was that. I tried to mollify him but he just wouldn't have it. Perhaps his terrible illness exacerbated his irascibility.

About a year later I saw him for the last time at a meeting on the Eastern seaboard. I saw him having breakfast in the hotel and went up and chatted to him. We spoke about family issues and then other things. He was always fascinating, even though he had blind spots. That was the last time I spoke to him but then we had our exchange of letters in the *British Journal of Psychiatry*.

Myrna Weissman told me that my last critique of his letter, in which I pointed out that his reply to us had not dealt with any of the salient objections we had raised, reached his office the day he died. Myrna was extremely upset by this and wouldn't shake my hand when I tried to give her my condolences at a conference, where we were on the same platform. She took our critique of his work very personally. I can understand this in the light of the circumstances.

It is difficult to get an unpopular message home. First biological psychiatry took over American psychiatry using its diagnostic system and Gerry played a big part in this. The other was that Upjohn used this view to market their compound. Both were extremely successful. From the point of view of their aims, their strategy worked brilliantly but whether patients benefited is another thing entirely.

Panic disorder as a concept has maybe temporarily taken the field. Do you have a feel for how temporary this is likely to be?

Who knows? ICD-10 articulates an alternative view of panic. Whether in time that will prevail is difficult to know. There are many criticisms of DSM classifications. There has been an excellent article on American diagnostic imperialism by Richard U'ren that he had difficulty publishing. Gambling and insomnia and many other problems all become disorders and therefore susceptible to psychiatric ministrations and therefore reimbursable etc. Recently came a bid for 'shopping disorder' to be recognised.

There are two or three points there. Is part of the reaction that you got not from Klerman as such but from US psychiatry more generally down to the fact that in quite a few of the health schemes over in the States psychiatrists won't be reimbursed for anything other than actually prescribing?

Oh yes, absolutely. Not only that but prescribing by a doctor of course. There was a fine controlled study in Burlington, Ontario in the late 1970s by David Sackett showing that nurse practitioners cared for primary care populations as well as did GPs. Eventually the work ended because nurses' care was not reimbursable and that rule was not changed.

Similarly in the 1970s there was the Lobene project in Massachusetts showing that dental hygienists actually did better work than did dentists in drilling, filling etc. The dental hygienists had one year's training, the dentists had five years' training. The net result of that was the closure of the dental hygienists training course. So the term 'conspiracy against the laity' becomes meaningful with such events. I am sure we could get many such stories, and that when we get companies producing profitable computer self-care programs similar things will happen.

Will progress require the overthrow of Kraepelin or at least the version of Kraepelinism that Gerry Klerman, Eli Robbins and others set up in the 1970s? This Kraepelin has almost become an idol that one can't question.

Who knows? Michael Shepherd's last paper on Kraepelin in the *British Journal of Psychiatry* was excellent. We obviously have to have classifications. The trouble comes when it becomes a fetish, when reimbursements are linked to it. Classification simply as a means of communication is fine. But when one can't survive financially unless one squeezes patients into unrealistic boxes then all kinds of problems result.

Talking about your approach to therapeutics, social phobia would appear to be the next battleground.

It's underway. This is much the same as for OCD and for agoraphobia. It is a time-worn, simple and successful strategy. Find a disease, make it out to be something that hasn't been recognised until now, remind everyone how common it is, then claim you have a drug for it.

And it looks like it will work again?

What's worked before could well work again.

Where did the concept of social phobia come from? you're generally cited as being its originator.

It came out of my work with Michael Gelder in the mid-1960s.

Does the social phobia story bring out some of the positive aspects of the process in that you could argue that while we may end up with social phobia being vastly over-recognised in the near future, it has been markedly under-recognised it seems to me up until now.

Well, that is true of all the anxiety disorders. The ECA, Munich and Zurich studies have shown that over half the identified cases haven't been treated for their condition – that is clear – but whether treatment with medication is the right answer is moot. Behaviour therapy is effective.

To come back on that for a minute. I know you're involved in a collaborative venture with Pfizer at the moment. Are you selling out to the industry on this one?

If they are willing to promote computerised effective self-treatment of OCD, that's wonderful. Full marks for their prescience.

The outcome of the whole thing will be computer methods which they will own and market?

No. Dr Greist, Dr Baer and I own it but hopefully Pfizer will market it. If they don't we will. The pilot results in 64 patients in the UK–US studies show that the results are about as good as those on medication. And so an eight-site controlled transatlantic study is being launched soon by Pfizer. That is a unique situation.

The outcomes of the pilot studies are sufficiently encouraging to go ahead with controlled trials. Obviously we can't cure everybody. But I am fairly sure we will help a lot of people to some extent at reasonable cost and without medication side-effects.

Can you give me some indication of where the idea of delivering therapy by computer came from? Who had the idea and when?

There was Weitzenbaum's Eliza program decades ago. John Greist in 1977 suggested that I try computerising exposure therapy for phobias. I did and it worked. John's computerised CBT for depression worked too.

Coming to evidence-based-medicine. As I hinted earlier you were talking that kind of language before it became the fashionable thing it now is. But again is this one of the things that the pharmaceutical industry are going to turn to their own advantage in that they have the means of produce the data more readily than anyone else has?

The evidence for behaviour therapy is better than for most drugs and there is a simple means of producing that evidence; with the advent of computerised audit we have a great way of developing a clearing-house of clinical outcomes with a quick turnover time. This would not be a prerogative of drug companies alone. It would help clinical trials of all kinds of medication, of psychological treatments and other interventions to be done more efficiently. Evidence-based medicine can be a healthy movement as long as it doesn't become a fetish.

But it will become one, won't it?

It's a danger. But there is nothing new in what we have discussed today. I understand there was a controlled study of scurvy in the 18th century that showed very clearly that sailors would not die if you gave them citrus juice but thereafter it took 50 years before the British Navy regularly gave the limeys their ration of lime juice So there is nothing new in the present slowness to apply evidence-based medicine.

But it seems to me that the evidence about a drug it is going to be applied much more quickly because the industry will see to it that people are aware of it.

There are all kinds of inertias once a paradigm, an ethos, takes hold. Take smoking – in the early 1960s the first reports of its association with lung cancer came out and the retreat from smoking has only just begun. There are many reasons for this – in the case of tobacco there was addiction and money and a lot of other things besides – which affect whatever we do. The conservatism of our profession is good in some ways and bad in others. You don't want to go veering off in new directions every year. We have to be careful that each time we see a new drug it is not used as a panacea. But you don't sell a drug widely by saying it's got limited usefulness.

No, but what has happened which will probably come as a shock to a great number of the public is that while the campaigns were waged through the media about the horrors of benzodiazepines and the pharmaceutical industry was probably perceived by many people to have been rolled back, in actual fact the 1980s and the early 1990s were the time when the neuroses have been medicalised. Panic disorder, OCD and now social phobia have been made disease entities. It has all happened seemingly without the media being aware about what has happened. You would have thought that the benzodiazepine controversies would have sensitised them but this has gone beneath the radar completely.

There is a tension all the time, isn't there, between those against and those for and the pharmaceutical industry spends billions of pounds on advertising.

Is there the other element, though, that in the approaches that you take quite apart from the fact that you don't have billions of pounds to advertise you are offering people hard work whereas something like Prozac offers a remake?

Sure, but empowering the patient is the flavour of the decade.

Provided it doesn't require too much work?

It depends on the patient. Some love it and some hate it. Patients' demands for information will grow. Patients in this country are too passive. They don't ask their doctors for enough information and we are not trained to give information. Medical schools should pay far more attention to the dissemination of information to individual patients and to society as a whole.

Yes, and to the ability to assess risks and especially relative risks from treatments which we don't do at all.

If I have just been paid to attend a conference on a lovely island in the Mediterranean or Caribbean then I will think of the sponsoring company's drug whenever I reach for my prescription pad. When companies start to market computer self-care packages and send doctors on lovely holidays then the doctors will think of those packages for treatment, which is no healthier a way to practise medicine. I am told the same thing happens with prostheses such as hip replacements. So that is always the tension. Perhaps companies that don't oversell are less likely to survive.

This is the point I have been trying to make to you the whole way through – in a sense you aren't oriented toward an oversell ...

Sure. The great epidemiologist from Oxford, Richard Doll, didn't oversell the connection of smoking to disease. The evidence has to speak for itself and it takes time to affect policy. Duelling was a major source of mortality in French aristocratic males in the 17th century but when Louis XIV outlawed it it took a generation for it to die out.

Why have you ended up being a person who has been keen to give things way as opposed to becoming a consultant to Upjohn or whatever?

It is much more important to try and find effective treatments that help the people in the long run. In the very long run that is what will become accepted. There will be many mistakes along the route.

I trained in medicine in Cape Town, South Africa in the 1950s, when there was very much a British tradition at that stage. Epidemiological evidence was very important. Once you look at epidemiological evidence, you have to look at the mass market – that is what epidemiology is largely about. And that is the way I was taught. If you work in a children's hospital where one wing has black patients and the other wing has white patients and the white wing has the rare diseases of metabolism and other odd things and the black one has mass misery with kwashiorkor and gastroenteritis and other diseases of poverty, it soon becomes obvious that what is needed is a remedy on a mass scale and you can't fix things just on the ward.

And is that what has been the formative influence?

For me, yes. We took it for granted that one went for treatments that are easily delivered and inexpensive.

What about the Institute of Psychiatry when you came in the 1960s? It has always had a certain scepticism about drug treatments. It hasn't seen them as the great breakthrough that they have been seen as elsewhere. As Aubrey Lewis put it, if we had to choose between the rehab units we have and the new drugs the drugs would have to go.

That's interesting. Some current colleagues are gung-ho on drugs. That's more recent but epidemiology was very important in the training of psychiatrists in the 1960s as well and that had an influence. Aubrey Lewis' attitude to drugs did not influence me. I have always accepted that drugs have a role. I was taught that too. And I was amazed at the way drugs could change psychological events.

Amazed in the sense of almost dualistically not actually expecting that drugs could change psychological events?

No, I mean it makes absolute sense. When someone paranoid felt that the commies were after him last week and he has a bit of chlorpromazine and then this week they're no longer after him, that is quite an exciting change.

Who else has been a formative influence?

The most formative influences have been mainly philosophers of science, Thomas Kuhn, Carl Hempel, Karl Jaspers, because they taught how to evaluate evidence and Paul Meehl looked at clinical versus statistical prediction. People who taught me to evaluate evidence are the ones I'm particularly grateful to and those who taught me experimental design – Bob Cawley, Bob Maxwell the statistician, Felix Post who taught me phenomenology and Bob Hobson who taught me aspects of psychotherapy. They were very formative for me.

Is there anyone who has been working with you who has been particularly helpful?

John Greist and Lee Baer have a great effect on me – wonderful colleagues. Richard Swinson has been enormously helpful and I could not have done such a careful study as our London–Toronto trial without someone as good as he is who shares a similar philosophy. He has published several studies about home treatment, telephone treatment, and how rarely behaviour therapy is given, and he will be joining us in the computer treatment trial.

In the early 1970s Jack Rachman, Ray Hodgson and I had a seminal collaboration. I have mentioned Bob Cawley and Michael Gelder and I had a very fruitful partnership with John Bancroft and Adolph Tobena from Barcelona, who is a neuropharmacologist and psychiatrist. He influenced me greatly as did Randy Nesse on evolutionary theory …

How do you see things going from here? Are we wedded till death do us part to the disease model? – the FDA seems to be. But increasingly the companies, for instance, are being encouraged to consider selling the drugs over the counter. Now if the H2 blockers can go OTC, surely the SSRIs could to. In which case would the companies stop selling the medical model or at least the bacteriological model for a psychiatric disorder and sell something more dimensional?

Another change is influencing pharmaceutical companies. Several are becoming disease management companies rather than just pharmaceutical companies. This may be partly a response to what you have just described. Another influence might be the move to managed care – it might drive them in that direction. This is a healthy move. It makes them less vulnerable to failure if they are less wedded to the success of a single product. And the patient gets a better deal and a broader-spectrum approach. I can think of at least three major companies doing this on both sides of the Atlantic and this is why we are being funded by a drug company. Another drug company here has funded a computerised audit for general medical diseases. Another company also wants to apply this in general medicine. I think this is useful but of course the audit will need to be audited. As soon as money depends on results people are going to be tempted to massage those results. Few people pay more tax than they need to and few earn less than they need to.

Prescription rights. Do you think it is one of the areas of medical power. Could this be dismantled?

You were saying that OTC is getting more common. I can't see everything becoming OTC. That would probably be undesirable. I would give prescription rights to some nurses and some psychologists who have been trained – another turkey voting for Christmas.

Has Hans Eysenck been any influence to you as such, because quite apart from his learning theory work there is also a drug postulate to it, which is that drug treatment should be able to shift you along an introversion–extroversion axis and it may well be that drugs, like the SSRIs, are actually doing something like that rather than treating a disease.

That has never been an influence on me.

Another reason to bring him into it again is he wrote his famous piece around 1952 on the evaluation of psychotherapy and he followed it about 2 years ago with an article in Behaviour Research and Therapy reviewing the state of affairs 40 years later, concluding that there is no science on earth that can overcome ideology.

That is probably true. A difficulty is that many call science what they believe in yet what others believe is 'ideology'. In fact the truth may be more subtle.

Does cognitive therapy qualify as part of behaviour therapy as you understand it? Are the cognitive therapists just finding other ways to expose people unbeknownst to themselves?

Exposure is not part of cognitive treatment for depression. It is a problem-oriented method. That leads to the question: is it the problem-oriented method, is it the breaking things down into manageable bits, or is it the activation component? Good dismantling studies are very important to do. It is too early to be sure what is useful. Neil Jacobson has just done one RCT finding that behavioural activation alone reduces depression as much as does full CBT. There will be others in time because it is obvious that we have to answer these questions.

Could the pharmaceutical industry support them, because presumably the only way they are going to market another antidepressant would be as part of an integrated management package. You know drug therapy plus activation, if it came out, would be a very sellable package.

John Greist, Lee Baer and I in fact are producing a computer-aided treatment for depression, which is now being pilot tested. Once a psychotherapy method is computerised it is much easier to add and subtract components and deliver them precisely. We have designed our system in such a way that we can add or subtract these components. So we hope to do dismantling studies in time to come if we can generate enough revenue to pay for them.

You are perhaps better placed than anyone else to comment on the tension between psychology and psychiatry. Clinical psychology seems to be growing partly on the back of cognitive therapy. Perhaps in the beginning there was behaviour therapy but it's moved on now to cognitive therapy ...

There is a clash between the two professions, two conspiracies against the laity. I don't think it is resolvable. There is also a clash between nursing and medicine. These things are to be expected and have to be contained.

Will neuroscience feed into all this at some point?

Brain and mind are coming together. The dualist position has been undermined by neuro-imaging. Neuro-imaging has played no role so far in developing treatments but it is of great interest when one can show an area lighting up that behaviour therapy can change just like drugs do, which you'd expect. This is obvious common sense. There are many exciting areas. We have a long way to go before imaging tells us anything about aetiology. You know the story about the scientist and the lamppost ...

Yes, I heard it from Don Klein first – ironical in a sense that you should both cite it.[1]

Select bibliography

Klerman GL (1988). Overview of the cross-national collaborative panic study. *Archives of General Psychiatry*, **45**, 407–412 et seq.

Marks IM, De Albuquerque A, Cotteaux J, Gentil V, Greist J, Hand I, Liberman RJ, Relvas JS, Tobean A, Tyrer P, Wittchen HU (1989). The efficacy of alprazolam in panic-disorder and agoraphobia: a critique of recent reports. *Archives of General Psychiatry* 46, 670–672.

Klerman GL, Ballenger JC, Burrows GD, Dupont RL, Notes R, Pecknold JC, Rifkind QA, Ruben RT, Swinson RP (1989). In reply to Marks et al. *Archives of General Psychiatry*, **46**, 670–672.

Klerman GL et al (1992). Drug treatment of panic disorder: comparative efficacy of alprazolam, imipramine and placebo. Cross National Collaborative Panic Study second phase Investigators. *British Journal of Psychiatry*, **160**, 191–202.

Marks I, Griest J, Basoglu M, Noshirvani H, O'Sullivan G (1992). Comment on the second phase of the Cross National Collaborative Panic Study. *British Journal of Psychiatry*, **160**, 202–205.

Klerman GL (1992). Drug treatment of panic disorder. Reply to Comment by Marks and Associates. *British Journal of Psychiatry*, **161**, 465–471.

Marks IM, Swinson RP, Basoglu M, Cuch K, Noshirvani H, O'Sullivan G, Lelliott ET, Kirby M, MacNamee G, Sengun S, Wickwire K (1993). Alprazolam and exposure alone and combined in panic disorder with agoraphobia. A controlled study in London and Toronto. *British Journal of Psychiatry*, **162**, 776–787.

Spiegel DA, Roth M, Weissman M, Lavori P, Gorman J, Rush J, Ballenger J. Comment on the London/Toronto study of alprazolam in exposure in panic disorder with agoraphobia. *British Journal of Psychiatry*, **162**, 788–789.

Marks IM, Swinson RP, Basoglu M, Noshirvani H, Cuch K, O'Sullivan G, Lelliott PT (1993). Reply to Comment on London/Toronto Study. *British Journal of Psychiatry* **162**, 790–794.

Marks IM, Basoglu M, Nohirvani H, Greist J, Swinson RP, O'Sullivan G (1993). Drug treatment of panic disorder. Further comment. *British Journal of Psychiatry*, **162**, 795–796.

Beaumont G, Healy D (1993). The place of clomipramine in the development of psychopharmacology. *Journal of Psychopharmacology*, **7**, 383–393.

Marks IM, Stern RS, Mawson D, Cobb J, MacDonald R (1980). Chlomipramine and exposure for obsessive compulsive rituals. *British Journal of Psychiatry*, **136**, 1–25.

Marks IM, Basoglu M (1989). Obsessive compulsive rituals. *British Journal of Psychiatry*, **154**, 650–658.

[1]Klein DF (1996). Reaction patterns to psychotropic drugs and the discovery of panic disorder. *The Psychopharmacologists*, Vol I, pp 329–352.

Marks IM, O'Sullivan G (1988). Drugs and psychological treatments for agoraphobia/panic and obsessive compulsive disorders: a review. *British Journal of Psychiatry*, **153**, 650–658.

Marks I M (1989). The gap between research and policy in mental health care. *Journal of the Royal Society of Medicine*, **82**, 514–517.

25 Vagn Pedersen and Klaus Bøgesø

Drug hunting

How did you each come into the industry?

VP. My basic training is in pharmacy. After I had completed it and had been in the army for a few years, I did pharmacology and it seemed quite natural that I should go into the industry rather than into pharmacy. There was also a question of money. So my idea was to go into the industry, which I did. I was in pharmacology here for 11 years when I was asked would I move into development, which I did.

KB. I'm a chemical engineer from 1969. I was due to go into national service but chose to go into the civil defence. After ten months because I was a chemical engineer I got a position at the Royal Danish School of Pharmacy with the Civil Defence. I was in a laboratory analysing mustard gas taken up from the North Sea and so on. But also I was involved in a number of research projects on anticholinergics, one of which involved derivatives of the phenothiazines. I was very happy with this because I loved organic chemistry and organic synthesis and that was what I wanted to do. One day a person came with an advertisement, a clip out of a newspaper, that Lundbeck was looking for an organic chemist. I applied for the job, not knowing anything about what Lundbeck was. At the job interview with PVP it turned out to be an advantage to have worked with phenothiazines because these compounds and the thioxanthenes were a speciality at Lundbeck – which I didn't know of then. I had never been very much aware of the pharmaceutical industry but I got the job.

Where did the Lundbeck Company come from?

VP. Well, it's a 100% Danish company. It was founded by Hans Lundbeck in August 1915. It was purely a trading company in the beginning – they did not sell drugs. In the 1920s he started to collaborate with a Mr Eduard Goldschmidt, who was involved in the distribution of medicines in Denmark. He had a licensing arrangement with some German companies and he was allowed to bring some products with him to his new company. But there was no production facility then. That began in the 1930s.

The Lundbeck company today is owned 100% by the Lundbeck Foundation. In late 1967 Mrs Lundbeck, the widow of the founder, gave the

Foundation all of her shares, just before she died. In December 1967 the Foundation bought the remaining shares that were owned by the Goldschmidt family, which was about 45% of them. We are not on the stockmarket and there are no shareholders, except for the chairman of the foundation who holds all shares. At the annual general meeting he is always asked by the chairman of that meeting, 'Does the shareholder have any comment?' The purpose of the Foundation of course is to run the Lundbeck company but they also support research and other philanthropic activities. Some of the donations to research are larger than the Nobel Prize, for instance.

PV Petersen, who was heavily involved in introducing the company to the psychotropic area, was almost Mr Lundbeck at one point it seems. He was an almost legendary figure whom everyone I have talked to speaks highly of. Who was he?

VP. PV was a chemical engineer who started here in 1943. It was his second company. He had been in KVK – Kemisk Vørk Kaege – for a few months and then he joined Lundbeck. He was the one who started medicinal chemistry in Lundbeck and then later with Dr Møller-Nielsen, pharmacological research. He was first head of medicinal chemistry but later on he was appointed Director of Research and Vice-President of the company and then even later President and member of the Board of Directors.

When I joined the company, everyone knew him. He joined all the research meetings and was really the one who gave us the inspiration to try and find new drugs. He was also the one who started the research with the thioxanthenes.

When he started in 1943 the company was working with sulphonamides. Sulfametizole was actually the first Lundbeck development. This was done by Mr Hübner and some of his colleagues before PV Petersen came. Then PV was involved in planning the chemical production of that because that was very primitive when he joined the company. He was the only chemist when he joined. But later he became just as involved with pharmacology. Mrs Moller, a laboratory technician, for a while was the Department of Pharmacology. One of the pharmacologists from the Institute of Pharmacology in the University of Copenhagen was a consultant. This was quite impressive for a chemical engineer who had no background in pharmacology, he just did it.

Where did his interest in the CNS come from?

VP. I think the invention of chlorpromazine really impressed him. He wanted, it seems, to find a better drug or a drug which caused less side-effects.

KB. We had ketobemidon and became involved in pain research after the war. In fact PVP was made a lieutenant in the Danish army and provided with a uniform by the Ministry of Defence in order to go to Germany, where chemists from the Allied countries were allowed to penetrate into the German pharmaceutical industry – to look at the IG Farben Industrie patents. He actually found the synthesis of ketobemidon – the patents were open for use – and he brought it back. So pain research was of some interest to him. He put up animal models for testing pain and he made many derivatives of ketobemidon. This was before the thioxanthenes but it was CNS.

VP. Yes, narcotic analgesics are clearly CNS products but I do not know if this was the beginning of his CNS interest. I asked Dr Møller Nielsen, who knew him from 1956, and he could not answer this question either.

What kind of a man was he?

VP. I was interviewed by PV Petersen and Møller-Nielsen. I really got the impression that he was the man that everybody considered was the leader. He was very friendly. Never tough but he could motivate people. From the very first day, he came and worked with us himself. I was very impressed by him.

KB. He was a very impressive man. He was tall and with a deep very characteristic voice, which you could hear from a long distance. So there was a lot of power coming out of him. I think his heart really lay in the research. He was not a typical executive. Even though he was research director and Niels Lassen was head of the Chemistry Department he participated in all the meetings about chemistry. He loved discussing chemistry and he tried to get into the laboratory from time to time. All the chemists really liked him because he was always interested in what you were doing.

He was always called PV or PVP but what did the P and the V stand for?

VP. Poul Viggo Petersen. He got a stroke at the party for his retirement and he was paralysed and lay immobile until he died more than a year later.

Møller-Nielsen's is the other name that features on all the early papers. Who was he?

VP. He qualified as a vet initially in Copenhagen in 1948. Then he went to Michigan and later Wisconsin where he did a Master of Science thesis on mink. From that he came back to the Department of Pharmacology in Lundbeck in 1956. Dr Kopff, a German pharmacologist, was the head of the department for the first few years. Then Dr Møller-Nielsen became the head in 1958. He left the company after 24 years to go breeding laboratory animals in Jutland. He was also inspiring but a different type, quieter and a more thoughtful type and a rather short man. They complemented each other.

There weren't any medical people then, were there? They liaised with clinicians from the hospitals – Jorgen Ravn and others.

VP. That's true. They had a close collaboration with psychiatrists from the big hospitals in Denmark first of all, later in Scandinavia and of course recently everywhere else.

Psychiatry and psychotropic drugs seem to have had more respect in Denmark and Scandinavia than almost anywhere else. There seems, in particular, to be something of a contrast between Holland and Denmark in this regard. I'm not aware of any vituperative anti-psychiatry movement here. Herman van Praag would say that the problems in Holland stem from a certain Calvinism ...

VP. Well, the Danish Church is not Calvinistic. I think we have always been more practical and we have a tradition in psychiatry. Psychiatry is highly estimated in Denmark, more so than in the UK. We have had big figures here in

Denmark – Erik Strömgen, Mogens Schou, Ole Rafaelsen and the Saint Hans Research Institute, which had a research department started by Ib Munkvad. He and Randrup were the ones who put forward the amphetamine model of psychosis. They knew that amphetamine could induce a psychosis very similar to schizophrenia and then developed animal models using amphetamine and the antagonism of amphetamine-induced stereotyped behaviours. We had a very close collaboration with them. Then there was Arbild Faurbye, who first described tardive dyskinesia.

Coming to the thioxanthenes – in a sense they were a very logical development, simply substituting a carbon with a double bond for a nitrogen in the phenothiazine ring structure in an effort to produce fewer side-effects. Tell me about chlorprothixene.

VP. It's still used. In some countries, for instance Denmark and Germany, it is used quite a lot because it induces so few extrapyramidal side-effects. Our colleagues in pharmacology have now made a modern receptor profile of chlorprothixene which differs only a little bit from clozapine.

KB. It's interesting in perspective that the old drugs are 'mixed' compounds with actions on many receptors, although of course that wasn't known when they were discovered. Then came the tendency to remove side-effects by looking for selective drugs and many companies developed selective D-2 antagonists – at least they believed they were selective. But when clozapine came in focus again after it had been withdrawn and more and more receptors were cloned and identified it became clear that the mixed profiles had a potential and chlorprothixene also has a mixed profile. It's one of those with a relatively good ratio between serotonin and dopamine, which might be the reason why it has relatively few side-effects.

In Denmark it's called by the trade name Truxal, which comes from a Danish magician called Truxa. His trick was that he and his wife would read people's minds. He would stand in the audience and his wife was on the stage and he would pick something out of the pocket of someone in the audience and she would have to say what it was. This kind of name has become almost modern again – x and z are now in fashion for drug names.

Right from the first article by Jørgen Ravn there are these hints about chlorprothixene that it had antidepressant effects, which is very interesting given how the story developed later with flupenthixol. Is there something about this group of compounds?

VP. It seems as if they have a certain mood-elevating effect – I don't know if we should call it an antidepressant effect. But it's quite clear that there are fewer shall we say post-psychotic depressions in patients treated long term with the thioxanthenes than with fluphenazine, for instance. There are quite a few studies which have shown that, and we have never seen other antipsychotics coming out superior to the thioxanthenes in this regard. We haven't done any big studies with chlorprothixene but as you say the older studies do suggest it has an antidepressant effect. Flupenthixol is not an uptake inhibitor, that's for sure, but the first metabolite of chlorprothixene shares some properties of antidepressants, although I don't know whether that has any clinical relevance.

Part of the reason for asking is because chlorprothixene is a very similar compound to amitriptyline – same side chain, just a small difference in the ring structure and in some ways amitriptyline is somewhere on the spectrum between a drug with a pure effect on mood and an antipsychotic.

KB. Well, imipramine and chlorpromazine share comparable similarities and imipramine is an analogue, in a sense, of chlorpromazine. The rationale to produce amitriptyline followed the same logic – it was a similar analogue of chlorprothixene. But the six-membered central ring structures are normally not uptake inhibitors, whereas the corresponding compounds with a seven-membered ring are.

One of the other interesting points here is that both Roche and Merck were in the business of making the exact same two compounds at the same point in time. Can you take me through what happened?

KB. Well, the reason that several companies could end up with the same compounds is that at that time you had process patents solely, which meant that if you could find another way to produce a compound which the other hadn't covered in their patents you could have a patent position too. That is exactly what happened in the case of amitriptyline. There are several different chemical routes to the compound. I don't know if the idea to make this compound came at exactly the same time and then the companies found different routes or if one heard about it from the other, but as I've just said when you know imipramine it's an obvious change to make.

From a purely medicinal chemistry point of view, now when we have computers and pharmacophore models of the receptors, I would say that it is not at all obvious to 'the modern eye' that the thioxanthenes would be dopamine antagonists. A medicinal chemist looking at these compounds today would not be so sure but back then they apparently thought that there was a very high probability that these drugs would work too. It was only many years later that we could show that they fit into the same D-2 pharmacophore as the other neuroleptics.

As regards chlorprothixene, Lundbeck filed a patent application in 1958. Merck had a patent issued in the USA in May of 1960 but it could have also been filed in 1958. Roche's patent was published in mid-1959. This means that all three companies probably filed patent applications at about the same time but Lundbeck had not seen any applications from the other companies when we filed ours.

As regards amitriptyline, Roche has three patents with priority from 1958. These are compound patents in a few countries where this was possible at the time and process patents in all other countries. They filed process patents in the period 1959 to 1962. Lundbeck has a process patent with priority from 12 October 1960 and a later patent from 1962. Roche acknowledged that Lundbeck had an independent process and in the USA Merck's patent had priority over Roche's. We made a licence agreement with Roche in 1961, which respected another agreement between Roche and Merck. We made our own pharmacological and toxicological studies but 'exchanged certain information' with Roche, sending them a report in 1961, and they helped us with 10 kg of the compound in June of 1961. So I think it is fair to say that chemists at all three companies got the same idea at the same time and all three companies were able to make a business of their discoveries in the years after.

VP. It was strange though that imipramine was the first tricyclic antidepressant and amitriptyline was the second but amitriptyline was by far the bigger one.

As these things go, it's often the compound that is second in the group that does best and also between Merck and Roche there was a lot of marketing clout behind amitriptyline.

VP. I think there were also clinical reasons. There's no doubt that amitriptyline has a much stronger anxiolytic effect than imipramine. This might be the reason why it became so popular although the side-effect profile is certainly no better than imipramine's.

Even though Roche and Merck ended up at war with each other over amitriptyline and even in the courts about it, in some sense the atmosphere feels as though it were more gentlemanly then, is this right?

KB. It's my clear impression that the competition has become much more intense. You can see it on the number of developments and patents that we file. In the years 1970 through to 1987 we filed about one patent a year. The research was different, we made a lot of derivatives of the thioxanthenes. It was like there was a gentleman's agreement that you didn't interfere with other people's invention areas. So in terms of patents, we normally didn't file a patent until we had a compound that we actually put into development but nowadays you know that everything can be stolen so you simply cannot wait to file a patent. From a principle point of view you wait as long as possible to give yourself scope on the development side but you cannot wait that long anymore and once you file the clock starts ticking.

VP. Also 25 years ago compared to now there were differencs as far as the promotional activities of the the different companies were concerned. We promoted and other companies promoted our products but we never mentioned the products of other companies. Now today you can find some nasty things being said about a competitor's products. That was unheard of 25 years ago.

On the question of derivatives, whether the thioxanthenes or citalopram, once you had one or two compounds why on earth make more?

KB. Well, the project was to eliminate side-effects. When I started Truxal, Fluanxol and Sordinol were all made. While they have differences, all three compounds were typical antipsychotics with extrapyramidal side-effects. So when I came I got the story, 'We have these compounds but they have side-effects and we have to get rid of these.' How did you do that in the 1970s? – only by making systematic variations in the compounds you already had. You must remember we didn't have receptor binding models. All the testing was on in vivo models – mice and rat models. We made a broad screening of every compound we made using reserpine ptosis and apomorphine gnawing for antidepressant effects and methylphenidate antagonism for antipsychotic effects. The induction of catalepsy was and still is used as a measure of the liability to produce neurological side-effects. We also tested for analgesic and anticonvulsant effects. And we did all of that for every compound. For the antipsychotics it was the ratio between anti-stereotypy effects, methylphenidate antagonism, and catalepsy production we were interested in and we tried to improve this ratio. And so we made hundreds of thioxanthenes but we didn't find what we were after – instead we found another thing.

We found some very, very potent compounds. In this work we started to put in fluorine atoms in the molecules and at a certain position in the ring structure this gave us some very potent and longer-acting compounds. Potency was very much the in thing; people liked potent compounds. They were thrilled when we made piflutixol, which was one of the most potent dopamine antagonists ever made. That compound was put into development together with teflutixol, which had a better profile as regards side-effects. Finally we had a very long-acting compound Lu 13-135 but this was given up because about that time we discovered another group of compounds with a completely new chemical structure – the phenylindanes, which we have been working with ever since. Out of that came sertindole and it was then we let the thioxanthenes go.

So how did you find the phenylindanes?

KB. We found them because we had an anti-inflammatory project. These anti-inflammatory compounds were amines and all other anti-inflammatory compounds at that time were organic acid derivatives. At that time the prostaglandin story was not known for these anti-inflammatory compounds and we had the naive thought that because they were basic rather than acidic they would give fewer gastrointestinal problems. They were active in our tests of anti-inflammatory activity and we made some ring-closed derivatives of these compounds simply by connecting the side chain to the aromate. This gave us these indanes, which had some anti-inflammatory effects too but not in the final test model – the adjuvant arthritis model. But because we had this broad screening programme it was found that one of these derivatives inhibited methylphenidate-induced stereotypy and in this way we discovered this new class of antipsychotics. Of course then we started to make hundreds of them and we have since made 600–700 of them. These compounds have the problem that there are four stereoisomers every time you make a new compound and it was difficult to separate the optical isomers. So we made some analogues where we removed the stereochemistry and one of these analogues was sertindole.

It would be fair to say that what first attracted our interest with these compounds was the very potent $5HT_2$ antagonism, which in fact some of the old thioxanthenes also had. It's funny that several companies had the same idea at the same time. Janssen had a lot of $5HT_2$ compounds which ended up in risperidone.

Can you recall the day that you found that this new compound had an effect on the methylphenidate model?

KB. No, but I can remember another day. Because we had a trifluoromethyl group in the thioxanthenes I always wanted to make the same substituent in these compounds, but it turned out to be extremely difficult and it took me more than a year to solve that problem. When we had the compound finally I said to Vibeke Christensen, 'Here is the compound – this is the compound.' It was called 18012, like the Tchaikovsky overture, and when it was tested I remember Vibeke running down the corridor saying it was indeed extremely potent. The problem with the first indanes was that they were not very potent and potency was a god at that time. Remember, we had just had piflutixol, which was a thousand times more potent that these compounds.

You've taken piflutixol Vagn, haven't you?

VP. Yes, and I was heavily sedated after a single 1 mg dose – I slept for about 15 hours. I have also tried teflutixol, which gave me akathisia. We made a one or two week Phase I study and we were the healthy volunteers. I got akathisia, which was very unpleasant. So we discovered that it could cause extrapyramidal side-effects – if akathisia is extrapyramidal.

KB. Piflutixol was so potent that one of our techicians, Peter Bregnedal, who is still here and who made the compound, got very sedated, before we knew from the animal experiments that it was so potent, simply from a little dust which he must have had. He couldn't wake up the next morning so we had to fetch him.

VP. He was also a member of the Lundbeck badminton club and he had made piflutixol on the Monday and he was so sleepy that he had to stay at home on the Tuesday and the Wednesday. On the Friday we had the annual party in the badminton club in the canteen. I was sitting at his side and we just had a glass of white wine and he drank half of it and we had to order a taxi to take him home. Alcohol, you see, potentiated the sedative effects of piflutixol.

In those days it was fairly routine for company employees to be the healthy volunteers but that doesn't happen now does it?

VP. No, it does not any longer. I think that's fair enough. It changed in the early 1980s. Ethical committees won't approve a protocol like this because if you are a company employee there could be the suspicion that you are under pressure.

I can see that but is there a drawback in that if you have had the compound yourself you have a much better understanding of what you are dealing with – as with you and the akathisia, Vagn?

VP. Yes, I realised what it was and I didn't know it was so unpleasant. Although it was a mild akathisia you couldn't watch TV, you couldn't do your work. As soon as you could find an opportunity to leave your office you did so. With piflutixol the problem was sedation. I got 1 mg and I didn't come to work the day after. I slept until midday and I couldn't drive the car.

After producing amitriptyline, Lundbeck produced nortriptyline which I suppose was an obvious step but then you produced melitracen. What was that?

KB. Its also a tricyclic but just to contradict what I said earlier, now you had a dimethylated six-membered ring in the middle and still it was an uptake inhibitor – a rather selective noradrenaline uptake inhibitor but it has a strong anticholinergic effect and so the side-effects profile of melitracen was the same as that of imipramine.

Talking about selective uptake inhibitors raises the question of citalopram. How did that come about?

KB. In fact melitracen was the key. It was made in the early 1960s and after that they were making derivatives of melitracen in the laboratory. They wanted to make a trifluoromethyl substituted derivative. But when they made the reaction in the way they used to make melitracen, they got a compound which they first thought was the right compound but after the analysis it became clear it couldn't be. They spent quite some time trying to find out what it was. It turned out to be the first phenylphthalane derivative. Melitracen, everyone knew, was a noradrenaline reuptake inhibitor – now if you make a wrong reaction in the laboratory and get a completely different compound what is the chance that this compound will also be a noradrenaline reuptake inhibitor? Probably one in a million. But it turned out that this compound and close derivatives were extremely potent and selective noradrenaline reuptake inhibitors. So in a serendipitous way they had discovered a completely new group of noradrenaline reuptake inhibitors.

The compounds that came into focus then were talopram and its sulphur analogue talsupram and both these compounds went into clinical trials. PV in the beginning was quite enthusiastic about these compounds but they were very stimulating and there were some suicide attempts. There always are with antidepressants but he was afraid that they were too stimulating.

In what sense – they interfered with sleep?

VP. No, this was a hypothesis that was put forward in the 1970s but this has not been supported. In the papers put forward by Lizzie Stromgren, who was the psychiatrist who worked on them, they speak of an activating effect rather than an antidepressant effect and that is the reason we left off.

KB. Talopram was discovered in 1965. Then in 1967, there was the work of Carlsson which was published in 1969, who suggested that noradrenaline was involved in activation and 5HT in mood elevation. Arvid has been here a few times and he put forward the idea of going for a 5HT reuptake inhibitor, so when I started in 1971 I was presented with talopram and two derivatives which were dual uptake inhibitors and I was told we should try to produce a selective serotonin reuptake inhibitor. We made 55 compounds before we had it – citalopram. Until a few months ago it was still something of a mystery why two structurally very close derivatives such as talopram and citalopram have such different pharmacological profiles – being one of the most selective noradrenaline and serotonin reuptake inhibitors respectively. But now we have a pharmacophore model upon which we have based a hypothesis about what this is due to. You know Eli Lilly have the same story because they also made a selective noradrenaline reuptake inhibitor, nisoxetine, and by making a very small change in that they got fluoxetine. We think we can explain that now.

So there you are. It's very few medicinal chemists that see one of their compounds come on the market. I've told you how I came into Lundbeck. Very soon after I joined I was caught by the excitement of not just making new compounds but having them tested and having a result. That's the suspense of being a medicinal chemist – a drug-hunter, as someone has called it. I've always seen myself as a drug-hunter. It's always exciting. You always feel that the next compound is the compound.

But if very few people ever see a compound get through to the market, it must be a very frustrating job?

KB. Yes, that's the paradox but in the meantime you have the synthetic challenges. You wish to make this and that molecule but it's not always very easy to do it. So you are always occupied with these synthetic problems and every time you succeed in making the molecule you want to make you have a success as a chemist. Then from time to time you get lead compounds which go into further development but most of them of course don't make it. Lundbeck, however, has very good statistics. You will very often see in journals that one in 10 000 compounds becomes a drug. We haven't yet made 10 000 compounds in Lundbeck but from 1958 to 1965 we got seven molecules onto the market and now we have citalopram and sertindole and others in clinical development, so that's more like one in 1000.

There are a lot of differences between the SSRIs?

KB. Yes, but only from a simple two-dimensional point of view. Two years ago I realised that nobody had actually made conformational studies or what we call pharmacophore models. Look at it as a lock and key model where all the drugs are keys and the receptor is the lock. When you don't know the lock, what you can do is compare all the keys and prepare a common key using all the shapes that have a sufficiently low steric energy. We have done that with all the serotonin reuptake inhibitors and found a very accurate pharmacophore model and from this you can see that they all fit nicely into the pharmacophore. But these tools were not available in the 1970s and it's strange that so many companies succeeded in making so many selective compounds in such a short time. We made it, Astra did with zimelidine, which was the first but was withdrawn from the market and Rhône-Poulenc had indalpine but it was also withdrawn. Then later came fluoxetine, fluvoxamine and a little later paroxetine from Ferrosan and later again sertraline from Pfizer.

You say you can see why they are all active on the 5HT uptake site but they are never-theless structurally diverse. Would you not expect there to be some differences in their behavioural profiles? Are you aware of any feedback from clinical use as to differences? – there seems to be some data particularly from use in the elderly and for aggession that there are differences as well as from behavioural models in animals.

KB. Well, on the uptake site they are similar but in recent years the number of serotonin receptors has risen from five to 17 and there are now five dopamine receptors not counting the isoforms of some of the receptors. Nobody has made the complete receptor profile of the 5HT reuptake inhibitors. So I would not be surprised, I would predict actually that differences on other serotonin receptors will be there and this might explain why psychiatrists say they are different.

VP. Clinically the selective serotonin reuptake inhibitors are rather similar but there seem to be certain differences. Especially in the elderly, citalopram seems to differ somewhat from the others but it's difficult getting an explanation from clinicians that we can work with.

Is there a problem here these days particularly with the antidepressants? In the old days a psychiatrist using a new antidepressant would maybe see a few hundred depressed patients a year and he or she could build up an impression of the differences between drugs but these days depression is treated by GPs who may be just as good observers but they haven't the time to pursue their observations systematically.

I think there was a problem but today there are increasingly close collaborations between general practitioners and psychiatrists and high-quality research in depression is being done by GPs – in the Scandinavian countries anyway and so far as I know also in the UK.

Lundbeck is one of the few companies who have both an antidepressant and an antipsychotic. Is this in any way linked to the fact that in recent years you have opted to go down the CNS route more exclusively than before?

KB. The CNS has always been our major research area but in 1988 the strategy was changed to be only CNS. The size of the company dictated it. After Erik Sprunk-Jansen became the director he made the analysis that it didn't make sense for a company of this size to also be involved in antibiotics and a little involved in cancer research. It's very obvious these days in research you have have a detailed knowledge of the therapeutic areas you are in – from basic research to marketing. Previously you could in-license compounds from other therapeutic areas but this isn't a good strategy anymore. In CNS we have real expertise and we could see that there was enough to do just in the CNS area. But making that decision you are bound to continue research with both antipsychotics and antidepressants. If your turnover is dependent on just these two areas you cannot allow yourself to leave these research areas because if you do you are out of business when the next generation comes.

Lundbeck, at least in Europe, have almost been the experts in the intramuscular preparations of the antipsychotics. How did that come about?

VP. Flupenthixol was not the first depot – fluphenazine decanoate from Squibb was the first. I think that gave us the inspiration to develop flupenthixol decanoate, which we did successfully. We had seen from the literature that there were some problems with the stability of fluphenazine decanoate. It had been published that there was an early peak some hours after the intramuscular injection of the formulation which was due to a content of free fluphenazine base formed by hydrolysis of the decanoate. As far as I can remember our idea was to find an oil which could be almost completely free of water in order to get a better stability. We chose a thin vegetable oil which is based on coconut oil. This has another advantage over sesame oil – at least in Scandinavia – even when it is cold it is still a fluid whereas sesame oil becomes something like butter if it is stored in the fridge. I remember we compared flupenthixol decanoate with pipotiazine undecylenate in a double-blind study carried out in the north of Norway and we couldn't maintain the blind because the district nurses and psychiatrists kept their drugs in the boot of their cars and pipotiazine but not flupenthixol became extremely difficult to inject.

Zuclopenthixol decanoate came later and now we also have the acetate of zuclopenthixol, Acuphase. The idea for this was given to us by one of the psychiatrists at the Saint Hans, Lars Kirk. He came to us and said we have a problem with the severely disturbed patients who are admitted to our wards – they don't like to take their medication and both they and we hate to have to give them regular injections which is necessary sometimes, two three or four times a day, so why don't you develop a formulation with a duration of effect of a few days? We made a lot of different things but ended up with the acetic acid ester of zuclopenthixol, which is the most powerful of our antipsychotics. The clinical development was very quick and it became very popular and it's quite clear that the duration of effect is about right. Its seems that this really is an advantage – perhaps a bigger advantage than we had expected. The patient gets fewer injections and it gives personnel on the ward time for some other clinical work. Unfortunately Lars Kirk had retired by the time this became available so he has not been involved in it further.

KB. At the start it was not clear that this would be possible. It's kind of logical that going from a long ester to a short ester should result in a shorter duration of action but that's in a way a very primitive point of view so it was nice that it worked out. Nobody else has really done the same thing. We actually made haloperidol acetate also and discovered that Janssen hadn't patented this compound.

The intramuscular forms are hugely useful practically and once you see how useful any possible ethical objections melt away, but it's often occurred to me that if depots hadn't existed and you proposed to make one today there would be a lot of agonised debate about the ethics of treating people against their will for a month. Were there any human rights type issues put forward in the early days?

VP. We were very careful in the beginning. All psychiatrists in the beginning gave a half dose first and watched the patient for any adverse reactions because, as you say, once you give the injection there is no going back. I think this test dose has disappeared now but initially they were a little bit scared and we recommended the half dose.

Why is there such a huge variation in the use of depots from country to country, with extensive use in the UK for instance and very little use in the US?

VP. This question is very difficult to answer. I have heard an American psychiatrist say that if they suggested giving a depot because of bad compliance on the patient's part and they are relapsing frequently, he more or less needs signed informed consent to do it. But John Kane, from New York, has said to me that depots will ultimately be used much more in the US. As you said, they are not used much at the moment – there are only two on the market: fluphenazine and haloperidol.

Why is flupenthixol not in the US?

VP. Because we don't have a US branch and there hasn't been a licence agreement that has functioned. It's on the market in Canada and in most Latin American countries. But we were a very small company when this was being developed and it was not easy to find a licence partner. We were more or less focused on the Nordic and a few other countries. In the 1960s, Europe and the Far East was enough – you could make a living there. It's no longer enough. Now we always look for a licence partner in the US and Japan, which is what we have with sertindole.

Are Danish psychiatrists like US psychiatrists? Do they prescribe home products preferentially?

VP. Well, if you look at citalopram it's number one in a number of European countries – Denmark but also Sweden, Finland, Austria and Switzerland. In Sweden it's between 50 and 60% of the antidepressant market.

In the past I have used the 'antidepressant effects' of flupenthixol as an example of very clever marketing but I wonder if I have had this wrong. As you will no doubt tell me there are a large number of studies which bear out this antidepressant profile but also, as I've hinted above, there seems to be something about the thioxanthene nucleus which has right from the start pointed to something of a profile in between the classical neuroleptics and antidepressants. How did the possible antidepressant effects of flupenthixol come into focus?

Well, Lars Sonne reported a few years after the launch of oral flupenthixol in Denmark that he had treated more than 500 depressed patients with low doses of flupenthixol and he was convinced that it was an extremely good antidepressant. We were very surprised because we had expected that flupenthixol would be the most selective antischizophrenic drug that had been developed by the company. Later, a number of publications appeared supporting the use of low-dose flupenthixol in the treatment of mild to moderate and severe depression in general practice. In low doses it is almost completely devoid of adverse effects.

After you distinguished the isomers of flupenthixol, in the mid-1970s there was the Johnstone and Crow study in the UK, where they showed that the z isomer was the active one. For one moment there seemed to be the implication that they had almost proven the dopamine hypothesis of schizophrenia whereas in fact what they had done can retrospectively be seen to have demonstrated the dopamine hypothesis of neuroleptic action, but it was an exciting piece of research. How did it look from your point of view?

VP. Yes, we made the formulations. We were interested in the trial because we thought it would be interesting to have it confirmed that the clinically active isomer was the one that worked on the dopamine system.

There were other pieces of science you chased, which raises the question of how much a drug company is in the business of chasing scientific leads rather than drug development issues. One of these other studies was a study on the possible prophylactic effects of flupenthixol in depression after the early studies showing that it had an antidepressant effect.

VP. Yes, there was a pilot study by Kielholz and Poldinger who had treated a small group of 30 to 40 patients over one year with flupenthixol – a group of patients who may have been non-compliant with lithium normally because they said they couldn't treat them with lithium – but anyway they noticed that flupenthixol had a certain antidepressant effect and we discussed a prophylactic study with a group of psychiatrists. Mogen Schou was the co-ordinator. It was an interesting study but flupenthixol did not, in that study, have a prophylactic effect but in a small group of bipolars it seemed to have a mania-protective effect.

How does the future look in the CNS area?

KB. If you are speaking about antidepressants and antipsychotics you have to ask what is the unmet need. For every group of drugs you have two to four generations. The first drug is a breakthrough but it's not the ideal drug from the point of view of either side-effects or efficacy. The next generations come nearer to the ideal drug. In some areas we are there: the ACE inhibitors for hypertension, I think, probably cannot be much improved on.

In terms of the antipsychotics or antidepressants how close are we to that? It's too early to tell with the new generation of antipsychotics. In a few years after there have been controlled trials for treatment resistance, negative symptoms and other areas we will see what is left – how much it is likely that we can improve on what we have. In the antidepressant field everybody is talking about the onset of action and efficacy as the two remaining areas. That's what the competition is about now and of course we are competing.

There have been the claims for the combination of pindolol and the SSRIs where it was believed that there might be a faster onset of action. Now it seems that this might have to do with different patient populations – that the so-called fast onset is related to higher efficacy in some drug-resistant populations but is not seen in a population where there is no drug resistant patients. I think onset of action and efficacy is probably very closely linked together. Pindolol is also a very dirty drug and a lot of companies are looking into what aspect of it counts. I am not convinced that anyone will make a faster onset of action drug but I think we might make a more effective antidepressant or an antidepressant that is more effective for a particular population. Is depression one illness?

Probably not, but surely from a marketing point of view it has to be kept as one illness. What about the idea that the SSRIs are not as potent as some of the older antidepressants in terms of getting the severely depressed person well but that perhaps they are more pro-phylactic than the older drugs?

VP. I think there is evidence that they have a good prophylactic action and that they are very well tolerated during long-term treatment, which is very important for compliance.

Coming back to the antipsychotics we have a phrase in Britain which is that you can't teach your granny to suck eggs, but I wonder whether that isn't just what you guys are doing with the new compounds. When clozapine was introduced there were all these marvellous stories about producing miraculous effects, but listening to the people who prescribed it one of the things you find is that the patient formerly was on perhaps 300 mg of fluphenazine i.m. weekly, along maybe with an oral neuroleptic and an anticholinergic and maybe even an antidepressant and all this was stopped in favour of a relatively low dose of clozapine as monotherapy. Now both you and Lilly have brought out drugs and you're almost insisting that the dose can only be what in the old days would have been a very low dose. Are you teaching us to suck eggs in the sense that you're saying that all these clinician grannies have got the dose of these drugs very badly wrong for a long time?

VP. Yes, but there is a difference between clinical development today and clinical development 20 years ago. In the case of haloperidol 30 years ago, Janssen didn't make a dose finding study; we didn't either with ours but today it's a requirement. Today you must estimate the optimal dose and the minimum effective dose so there is a scientific basis to our dose recommendations. John Kane said when he saw the results of our studies against haloperidol where we used 12, 16 and 20 mg of sertindole against 4, 8 and 16 mg of haloperidol and the 4 mg of haloperidol was as good as 20 mg that we're only finding out now what the proper dose of haloperidol is. But it's not just that we are not poisoning people anymore, because sertindole in those studies was in a number of respects better than even low-dose haloperidol.

I suppose that a longer clinical development time has its good and its bad points. In 1959 as I understand it chlorprothixene went from first clinical testing to launch in a matter of weeks. Jorgen Ravn's first use was in early November 1958, his report to the company was in December, the licence was granted in January and the drug was launched in March. The comparable period for sertindole must have been much much longer.

VP. Yes, about 5 years – which these days is something like a world record. But it's strange nevertheless that the products developed during the 1950s and 1960s were very safe products.

But to come back to the question of dosage, the megadose philosophy has almost disappeared because there was no evidence that there was any better effect when you gave flupenthixol for instance in 200 mg doses rather than 10 mg doses per day. The most I ever heard of being given was 1000 mg daily of flupenthixol. It was by some clinicians in Norway who phoned and asked what I thought about doubling the dose – giving it b.d. The strange thing about it apparently was the girl involved didn't have any side-effects.

What will happen in the case of the smaller group of patients who need immobilisation – who need chemical restraints?

VP. You will need a product with a strong sedative effect. Perhaps use the old drugs. I heard a paper by Robin McCreadie in Melbourne who suggested that zuclopenthixol acetate had become almost standard therapy in the acute phase in the UK and that he felt this would remain the case for some time to come.

What about the figures in Danish psychiatry – Erik Stromgren?

VP. He collaborated with us on the noradrenaline reuptake inhibitors. His wife Lizzie Stromgren was the principal investigator on the talsupram studies, for instance. He got the PV Petersen Prize, which is now called the Lundbeck Foundation Prize. It was instituted the year that PV retired. It is quite a big prize. It is given out every year, Stromgren got it, Arvid Carlsson got it, Gottfries got it. It alternates between clinicians and basic scientists.

We have had a close collaboration with Ib Munkvad and his colleagues at the Saint Hans but he has retired now. Per Bech and Jess Gerlach have advised us on many of our clinical studies. Rasmus Fog was another person. He is now the medical director of the Sct Hans Hospital. Some years ago he put forward a hypothesis that Mozart suffered from Gilles de la Tourette syndrome but there are many colleagues of his who disagree with this.

KB. We had a very close collaboration with Arvid Carlsson on the basic sciences side. No one else has had quite as big an impact as he has. Otherwise in medicinal chemistry we have more or less been working with our own type of compounds. The biggest inspiration in medicinal chemistry terms has been the Janssen company because they are a highly respected company – both as a competitor but also a company we respect very much for their research.

VP. In the early 1970s Dr Møller-Nielsen and I were invited by Janssen to his company to see it and how they had computerised their screening results. They were very open minded. That would never happen today. Paul Janssen himself showed us around.

Chasing the history of the SSRIs, another Danish Company comes into the frame – Ferrosan, who made femoxetine and later paroxetine. Can you tell me something about them and what happened to them?

Ferrosan was mainly a CNS company and the head of pharmacology there was Buus-Lassen. However, they were bought by Novo-Nordisk and Buus-Lassen left and started Neuro Search together with key scientists from Ferrosan. Last year Novo-Nordisk abandoned CNS research completely but Neuro Search, where Buus-Lassen is the chief executive, lives on selling CNS projects to larger companies.

Where is the field going now?

KB. Today we are moving into combinatorial chemistry. It cannot be used for everything – it is a supplementary technique but this, combined with identification of disease-relevant genes and new drug targets, means that I see the coming years as most challenging. These genes, for instance, might identify what is responsible for onset of action of antidepressants. So the quality of the research group will be important, the cleverness and the enthusiasm and the possibilities of working with biotechnological companies. The winners may not be the very big companies, it will be the people who manage through the jungle of opportunities, who choose the right things and who have some luck. Citalopram and sertindole came about by serendipity or what is sometimes today called pseudo-serendipity. Both examples you could just have walked by. The chemist who makes a compound that is not the one he wants could just dismiss that compound and try to get back to his original goal. I'm sure the 'prepared mind' will play an even bigger role in future.

We had a visitor from a company called Gene-Logic recently who are able to screen for these turn-on and turn-off genes – they can show hundreds of genes turned on and off when you give an anti-inflammatory compound. How do you go forward from there? I am sure serendipity will play a role, that the unexpected will happen. In all my time as a medicinal chemist I have looked at relatively simple structure–activity relationships such as effect in methylphenidate antagonism, catalepsy or on a limited receptor profile but now we have so many results for each compound and what are the efficacy profiles? It's already now known that many of the neuroleptics which we have been calling antagonists for so long are not antagonists – they are everything between a full agonist and full inverse agonist on every single receptor they work on. We need to map out these efficacy profiles and then we will see that they are different. Then we will see differences between the ten derivatives of sertindole which look quite similar today. That's my picture of the future – very exciting but also very demanding. The people who just leave it to the machines will be the losers.

If it isn't going to be left to the machines, what will it take?

KB. It will take discussions about strategies for selecting the compounds. In psychopharmacology it's not just affinity for one target. In many other diseases this will do – a selective ACE inhibitor, a selective H-1 antagonist along with one indication and one model such as lowering the blood pressure and you are there. Here you are playing on so many things. It will be what you believe in. It will be important to make a clever evaluation of the strategies you will have to pursue.

But where will these strategies come from? Once upon a time you could talk to clinical people but now do any of them have the same kind of feel for what the issues are? Knowledge wasn't so specialised on either side before, there were more people who knew everything.

KB. Clinical people are still very important. They are the ones who will define the unmet needs – what are the clinical differences between the compounds.

A colleague of mine, Tom McMonagle, has come up with a term that seems appropriate for the new antipsychotics – he calls them cocktail compounds. Previously when the idea was to have highly selective compounds with one target action, everything else was seen as side-effects, but now that you have more than one target action built into each compound, it's as though the one compound contains a cocktail of active principles whereas previously the idea of treatment cocktails implied that you were giving more than one drug. But isn't there a natural limit to how many actions you can build into one compound ?

KB. It's not us that build in the actions, the actions are there. Incidentally we have never pursued an antipsychotic with selective actions, except for a D-1 antagonist which we did not succeed with. Otherwise we have looked at both dopamine and serotonin antagonism, just like Janssen. As more and more receptors were cloned we found that our compounds were beginning to look more and more like cocktails, as you call them. So they are already built in and our job is to understand which receptors are important and which are not and what is the right cocktail. Our job would not be to build in, rather it is to take out the things you don't need. For instance, sertindole is an alpha-1 antagonist; now there are some indications that alpha-1 antagonism can be important for lowering extrapyramidal side-effects but it can also lower blood pressure. If we take it out we need to design compounds that do everything else except that and that can be a difficult task for the medicinal chemist.

In addition to our antidepressants and antipsychotics we have a muscarinic receptor M-1 partial agonist/M-2 antagonist in clinical development for Alzheimer's disease. We also have compounds for epilepsy, Parkinson's disease and a sigma-2 ligand for anxiety.

The whole area of anxiolysis has been very tricky since the benzodiazepines. This will have to be quite a different therapeutic principle.

KB. It is. The first idea about sigma compounds was that they would be antipsychotic because haloperidol was the first ligand used to identify the sigma site. But then by serendipity we discovered sigma ligands. We put up a binding assay for sigma compounds and in a project for $5HT_{1A}$ compounds we found some very potent and selective compounds for the sigma receptor. When it was established that there were two sigma receptors, we found that our compounds were sigma-2 selective, which is unique because no other sigma-2 selective compounds were known. We put it into various behavioural models and found a very potent effect on certain anxious behaviours. If it is effective in the clinic it will be a very different kind of compound.

Select bibliography

Ravn J (1970). The story of the thioxanthenes. In *Discoveries in Biological Psychiatry* (Ayd FJ, ed). Blackwell/Lippincott, Philadelphia.

Approaching rationality?

How did you start in the area?

I started as a chemist and oddly enough I've ended up in exactly the same field I started in. I did a PhD on alpha-adrenoceptor antagonists, as they then were. We didn't know about alpha-2A, 2B, 2C, and presynaptic control of catecholamine release was still to be described. That was from 1962 to 1965, which seems an awfully long time ago now. I went to the University of Hull, which had a chemistry department that was well known for its pioneering research in liquid crystal chemistry. I did a PhD in chemistry and pharmacology because Reckitt & Colman was still a very active pharmaceutical company in those days and they were just down the road.

Then I did a postdoc in the US with Alfred Burger. He was an Austrian who emigrated to the US in 1929 and worked initially for a government organisation located in the University of Virginia. When the Drug Addiction Laboratory moved to Bethesda he stayed on at the university and became Professor there eventually. He invented the concept of medicinal chemistry.

Which is what?

The study of the design of drugs, looking at what structural features are important for a particular type of biological activity and trying to predict biological activities from chemical structure. In a nutshell, it's the relationship between the chemical structure and biological activity and trying to manipulate the structure to modify and further refine biological activity. It used to be called pharmaceutical chemistry and chemical pharmacology but the phrase that was eventually settled on was medicinal chemistry. When he and Arnold Beckett founded the first journal in the field in 1959, it was called the *Journal of Medicinal and Pharmaceutical Chemistry*. This was renamed the *Journal of Medicinal Chemistry* in 1963, which is now the major journal in this area. It is now published by the American Chemical Society, so it's still perceived as part of chemistry rather than part of biology. Burger was the founding editor and he remained editor for 12 years. In the 1950s and 1960s, he was the doyen of medicinal chemistry worldwide. In 1951, he wrote one of the first and now the standard textbook, *Burger's Medicinal Chemistry*. This is the equivalent of *Gray's*

Anatomy. Other people write it now, of course, but although he is now over 90, he's still active reviewing books, refereeing papers, writing occasional articles. He still has a very good mind. In those days, in 1965, if you wanted to work in medicinal chemistry he was the person to go and work for.

Structure–activity relationships were a big thing in the 1960s at CINP meetings etc. but today you only hear about $5HT_2$ receptors and alpha-2 receptors – people like me would never hear about the actual structures.

They still are a big thing. If you go to medicinal chemistry meetings or chemical meetings you will certainly hear about the structures. I think the accent in psychopharmacology meetings is much more on the functional end. But, using much more sophisticated technology than in the past, people are still trying to relate structure to function. These days we have the ability to model complex structures like proteins and to manipulate their structures on the computer screen. Modern medicinal chemistry is very much about visualising the structure of an enzyme perhaps and finding the active site and then searching databanks for molecules that will fit that active site and then going away and making those molecules or their analogues. But the basic idea is still to relate structure to function.

Peter Waldemeier suggests that there's only so far that you can go.[1] Chemists can optimise for one or two things but once you get into optimising for three things there's problems and because of that chemists don't like the dirty drugs, they like the clean, the specific and maybe they're making a mistake.

It's degrees of complexity of course. It's easy, as Peter said, to identify and manipulate the structural features that will determine one or two biological factors but as you move on to three or four, the interactions between them become more complex. It's fairly easy these days to sit down and design a serotonin reuptake inhibitor but we don't need another. What you really need is the innovative leap in concepts. If somebody were to say depression is due to some change in glucocorticoid receptors, for example – the chemist is the servant of the biology in this instance – the chemist will come up with any number of possible structures. But somebody has to have that innovative idea that this is the target we are going for. The first lead is what you want to find.

If you have got an unusual target for which there are no known active compounds you have to find a lead compound which has some sort of activity. There are large-scale technologies such as combinatorial chemistry, which are very heavily touted these days as the answer to the maiden's prayer, to identify a substance which is active at a certain level in your biological assay. People thought it would be the death of traditional medicinal chemistry but of course all that these very capital-intensive programmes do is identify a compound with some activity. That is not your drug. Having found it, you have to do tra-

---

[1] See Waldmeier P in *The Psychopharmacologists*, Vol I.

ditional medicinal chemistry to modify that compound to the drug that you want. So medicinal chemistry as it was in the past still exists, although it's been overtaken in the screening stage by these very highly sophisticated techniques.

So you went to Virginia. What was Burger like?

I went to Virginia for 2 years. He was really nice, hospitable, very slight in build, a very sharp mind, highly interested in the arts, especially music. When I went he must have been nearly 60, so he was nearing the end of his academic career. It was a very interesting lab. The University of Virginia is an old traditional southern university. It looked like a scene from *Gone with the Wind* with marble columns and town houses. The town of Charlottesville, in those days, was 35,000 people and when the university was in it was 50,000. The students were very elegantly dressed. These days it's a modern university with a top academic hospital and a very fine law school. Charlottesville is a much bigger town although it still has the same charm as it did in 1965. The Chemistry and Pharmacology Departments were housed in an extremely ancient building. You'd come in at night and the cockroaches would dash away. The facilities were not exactly the best. When I went back 2 years ago it was unrecognisable because there were new buildings, new equipment, everything. But in my day it was still very much a traditional, very old lab, of the sort you would associate with Britain.

Surely this was the kind of man the industry would have been supporting.

Yes, they did. He had a very long standing relationship with SmithKline & French to the extent that my first year was financed by a fellowship from SK&F working on sympathomimetic agents. He had quite a number of advisorships with pharmaceutical companies but his main research support money came from SK&F in those days. Because of his contacts within the pharmaceutical industry in the US, he could place his students. There is a sort of Burger's old students group now in the American pharmaceutical industry – so his influence is much greater than it might seem.

This doesn't only apply to Burger. Certain individuals with a good reputation attract students or postdocs and if it is well accepted by the industry that these father figures are good trainers of people, they can get their students placed everywhere, so they have a much greater influence all over the industry than it would seem at first sight. Burger is a fine example but you can think also of people like this in the UK. A lot of people will go and work with Sir James Black, for example. He's that kind of figure because he has worked in the industry before. He has got good contacts. He is a famous figure and he was responsible for sub-classifying two or three of the major receptor families, beta receptors and histamine receptors, for example.

Was Burger responsible for any receptors?

Well, he was responsible for the whole science of medicinal chemistry as I've said. And also tranylcypromine is Burger's drug. He synthesised it in the 1950s and later of course it was an SK&F drug. It came onto the market round about 1960. He was interested in cyclopropane chemistry and this was just one of the things he made.

I've thought for a while that tranylcypromine is one of the most interesting compounds around. Have we dismissed it as an MAOI? In actual fact in extremely low doses it inhibits monoamine oxidase completely but this isn't enough to get some people well who at a higher dose do get well. So between that and isoniazid, which has been shown to be antidepressant but is not a monoamine oxidase inhibitor at all, have we been too synaptocentric, calling these things monoamine oxidase inhibitors, and thinking because of that that we know what they are?

I think that drugs tend to get labelled and people forget that they have a spectrum of effects. We always try and classify things. But by grouping disparate drugs together you often forget that drugs like tranylcypromine can be something entirely different from an ordinary monoamine oxidase inhibitor. This is also the case with the group of SSRIs now and the group of double action antidepressants and within these there are individual drugs with a very diverse pharmacology and action. I like tranylcypromine although it has fallen out of favour. It was never used very widely but its a very good drug. It has almost a psycho-stimulant action. The original chemical publication was in the *Journal of Medicinal Chemistry* in the early 1960s and its still on world markets.

There was another famous drug that emerged from Burger's research activities, in my second year in Charlottesville. It was the heyday of the Vietnam War and I was drafted because I was on an immigrant visa. I was called by the draft board and classified 1A for immediate shipment to Vietnam but my wife just happened to be pregnant and I was re-classified to 3A. Fortunately I avoided it. But anyway in my second year, because of the Vietnamese War they had a lot of falciparum malaria resistant to the then standard drug chloroquine. So the US Army instituted research at the Walter Reed Hospital and were pouring large funds into chemical and microbiology labs to develop new antimalarials. We worked on a series of compounds, one of which became mefloquine, which is now the standard one-shot prophylactic. Our publication came out in 1968 in the *Journal of Medicinal Chemistry*. Mefloquine is the one that's causing all the problems with psychotic reactions that you've read about in the press. It's been on 'Watchdog' and other programmes. It was financed by the US Army within a World Health Organization context but they had to have a company to market it, which was Roche. So it's not a bad record to get two major drugs out.

You worked on alpha receptors – before they became alpha-1 and 2 ?

Ahlquist had already suggested in 1948 that there were possibly two types of adrenoceptors (alpha and beta) but it was not until 1973 that Delbarre and Schmitt proposed a subdivision into alpha-1 and alpha-2. Presynaptic control of catecholamine release was absolutely unknown. That was a 1970s concept. Sol Langer really invented presynaptic regulation. His first major paper about presynaptic regulation via auto-receptors appeared in 1973. In 1965 there were simply alpha receptors but now of course we have alpha-1 and alpha-2, sub-families, hetero-receptors and we have all these complicated interdependencies of neurones which rely on one neurotransmitter for their main actions but are also influenced by other neurotransmitters. In the context of depression also, noradrenaline and serotonin have lots of interactions with each other in the brain.

After Virginia, what did you do? How did you end up in the industry?

After returning to Britain I worked for 7 years in the Chemical Defence Establishment in Porton Down on hallucinogens and dopamine agonists. I had quite a nice research line in hallucinogens. We did a lot of original work looking at structure–activity relationships of hallucinogens, and published the definitive paper on the ecstasy type molecules in 1974. The military worldwide, especially in the US, were interested in the dangers of hallucinogens being used to incapacitate soldiers in the field. Countermeasures were required, including antidotes. To design antidotes you needed an awfully good understanding of what hallucinogens were and what they did in biological terms. Now we realise that 5HT receptors are involved in the actions of many of them. This period included my first contact with Brian Leonard, then an earnest young pharmacologist at ICI.[2] He visited Porton Down and we discovered a mutual interest in psychopharmacology after his lecture. I supplied him with a number of compounds for his research work. Unfortunately, and we still joke about it today, he failed to acknowledge my contribution in his subsequent publication. Nevertheless, an inauspicious start was the basis for a friendship which has lasted.

The other strong interest was dopamine as a result of the military's interest in emetic agents. I did a lot of work on dopamine agonists. I got associated with all the Parkinson groups and worked a lot with Brenda Costall in her early days in Bradford, with Leon Goldberg in Chicago and David Marsden and Peter Jenner in London. I collaborated with Geoff Woodruff who was then in Southampton and also with Les Iversen and Alan Horne in Cambridge. With that group we worked on what has now become the D1 receptor. We didn't know in 1973 that there was a D1 and D2 receptor but the structure–activity relationships of the compounds that I provided them with were so strange that when you look back you can see that it was two receptors we were dealing with.

That work was all going very nicely but my wife and I got fed up living in England and we wanted a change. Adis Press, which was then called the Australasian Drug Information Service, offered me an interesting position and transported us to Auckland. But we didn't take to life in New Zealand – it was too far away, too isolated. After a while we decided we were Europeans and we wanted to come back. In New Zealand you were always treated as an immigrant, whereas we didn't feel we had emigrated; it was merely another

---

[2]See Leonard B in *The Psychopharmacologists*, Vol I.

job and a step in one's career. Anyway I wrote to many friends in industry and academia, one of whom, David Savage, who died a few years ago, worked for Organon in Scotland. I had met him at a medicinal chemistry congress years ago in Lyon, when I lost my baggage and he lent me a shaver and so we had known each other a long time. He passed my letter on to Organon International and after a few negotiations and interviews in Australia and Holland they offered me a position. So we came back in 1977. I had several other job offers but this was the most interesting position which was to ultimately manage worldwide CNS R&D. They were just about to change their research structure to therapeutic area programmes so I suppose my application arrived at the right time. Life is about being in the right place at the right time.

Mianserin, historically I've always thought, has been one of the most important psychotropic drugs. It links back to drugs like cyproheptadine. It catalysed a change to a receptor mode of thinking within psychopharmacology yet, just like tranylcypromine in a sense, it cannot be pigeon-holed in terms of its receptor profile and of course difficulties surrounding its use provoked one of the most important regulatory debates in recent years. You joined Organon soon after the mianserin story started, didn't you?

I joined Organon in March 1977, by which time the drug was on the major markets. It was already becoming well established, particularly in places like the UK, where it had been introduced in 1974/75. It was first synthesised in 1966 as an attempt to make a better antiallergic drug. The chemist, Wim van den Berg, tried to combine the structure of an antiserotonergic drug – cyproheptadine – with an antihistamine – phenbenzamine – and succeeded quite well. It began life, in fact, as an antiallergy drug. It was tested in asthma, in migraine, and it is effective there. Patients in the first hospital study for asthma felt reasonably happy on the drug, more happy than they should have done, and astute clinicians realised perhaps this might represent a psychotropic effect. So the drug was subsequently investigated for antidepressant activity.

Where did the EEG profiling come into the story?

Pharmaco-EEG was just beginning as a technique for detecting the activity of drugs and it was used to look at mianserin, which displayed the same sort of EEG profile as an antidepressant, like amitriptyline. That helped in deciding that it could be antidepressant. In fact, Itil, the Turkish-American guy who did that work, I believe, tried to claim the credit for having discovered mianserin, but I think the psychotropic properties were already evident. But this happy coming together of some scientific evidence and a bit of astute clinical observation pushed the drug forward at the time. Subsequently we have used pharmaco-EEG for profiling our potential psychotropics. Max Fink was our adviser for many years and he suggested that ORG 3770, which is now mirtazapine, had an antidepressant profile. We have also developed an extensive rat EEG system for preclinical evaluation.

So it was about 1970/71 when it began to switch over to being an antidepressant?

The company had a 50th Jubilee in 1973 because Organon was founded in 1923 and they desperately wanted to have a new drug registered, launched and preferably something which was outside the company's normal insulin-relat-ed, steroid-related activities, so a CNS drug they thought was great. They had a symposium in 1973 to celebrate the 50th Anniversary of the company, focusing on mianserin. It was a bit early I think. There might have been a bit of pressure to get everything ready for this symposium and I think the data were a bit deficient at that time – although the data were subsequently quite sufficient for gaining registration in the UK and in places like Switzerland and Germany.

What went wrong in the US?

The US is an interesting story. I think the file as it existed in the mid-1970s as used in Europe was insufficient for the different conditions in the US. The studies that had been done, by today's norms, you would not regard as of very high standard and the FDA even in the 1970s was quite exacting in its demands. A clinical trials programme had been initiated by Akzona, which was the American arm of Akzo, the parent company. Organon Inc. operated virtually totally independently in those days of Organon International as it was in Oss. They took their own decisions, although they obviously consulted Organon International. They were relatively inexperienced in psychopharmacology and they put themselves in the hands of Donald Klein, then and now a very dis-tinguished psychopharmacologist, who advised them on a set of investigators including John Feighner and Tom Ban. They started a series of studies which included amitriptyline control without placebo in seriously depressed patients, the sort we would still take into trials today. It's a shame it wasn't placebo con-trolled as we would do today. It was amitriptyline controlled because Klein advised that mianserin was perceived in America and in some parts of Europe as a sedative anxiolytic rather than a hard-core antidepressant and that it would be quite difficult to demonstrate the drug was better than placebo.

He suggested a special placebo-controlled study to test the hypothesis that antidepressants would be effective in endogenomorphic depression and not in chronic dysphoria or disappointment reactions. In a way this had a good sci-entific rationale but it was inappropriate for registration of a new antidepres-sant for major depressive disorder. He designed a study where people entered with Hamilton's between 4 and 18. We now know, and I think we knew then, that between 12 and 18 is the most difficult group in which to demonstrate placebo, antidepressant differences and it is almost in principle impossible between 4 and 12. It was a nice hypothesis to be tested from the psychophar-macological point of view but it was inappropriate for a new antidepressant. Donald Klein felt at the time that he would still be able to convince the FDA that mianserin should be registered for the treatment of minor depressive disorders as they were then. We disagreed. The study was subsequently published in 1985 in *Neuropsychobiology*, with the amitriptyline study appearing a year earlier in the same journal.

When the parent company, Organon International, took over responsibility from Akzona in 1981, it was realised that the file being generated in the US was not appropriate for the registration they hoped to get for the drug as a major antidepressant. Subsequently new studies were started and completed, some of which have been published, very fine up-to-date studies – placebo as well as active control, big groups of patients – the sort of thing we would really do today for any modern antidepressant and mianserin turned out to be very effective in these studies. If we had not had mirtazapine coming along at the same time, we probably would have filed an NDA for mianserin in the late 1980s or early 1990s.

So we ended up with the oddity that a drug which was the best-selling antidepressant in quite a few European countries wasn't registered for the US market at all.

I think it had a very unfortunate history in the US. If Organon Inc had got the studies right in the early 1980s, I think you would have seen mianserin as a major drug in the US market. As it turned out, trazodone, which in my opinion is an inferior drug even though it is an anxiolytic sedative type of antidepressant like mianserin, was the first new non-tricyclic antidepressant in the US. When you look at the new drugs that are coming out, they are all better than trazodone but trazodone made a great splash in the US, because it was simply the first that was different. Mianserin could have been that first one. So US psychiatrists don't know the profile of mianserin or the concept of alpha-2 antagonism, which may be advantageous for mirtazapine.

One of the things that mianserin partly did was to help catalyse the change to a receptor view of things – partly perhaps because it came at the right time, partly because it had no effects on reuptake or on monoamine oxidase.

Up until then people had focused on noradrenaline and serotonin – we still do, I think we are stuck in a time-warp really. It all comes from the fact that all our new antidepressants and all our thinking about depression is based on the old work about reserpine and catecholamines and we can't get out of this vicious circle we're in. I am sure one day we'll come up with an antidepressant and it will have nothing to do with noradrenaline and serotonin. But until mianserin, people thought in terms of uptake and monoamine oxidase inhibition. Mianserin was the first drug where people had to think about a receptor approach – still focusing on presynaptic events but on release mechanisms in a totally different manner than uptake. This ushered in an era where people focused more on receptor-selective events. I think drugs like venlafaxine and milnacipran are the 'Last of the Mohicans' in terms of the uptake inhibitors.

While it helped to change things and to usher in the alpha-2 and 5HT receptors and all that, do you think we have become too much synaptocentric? We think because we know *this drug blocks alpha-2 and 5HT$_2$ receptors for instance, that we know what it does. But mianserin in one sense is another of these drugs that tear up the receptor copy book when you hear that the Japanese are using it for delirium – you would never predict that thinking about it just in terms of receptors.*

Oh, course it has a lot of pharmacology attached to it – it's an antihistamine, it interacts with various serotonin receptors. If it's any one thing it's probably an anti-serotonin agent. Multiple pharmacology can lead to multiple potential uses.

Is there a difference between it and cyproheptadine – which for my money is another of the worm-holes in the psychotropic firmament, which if followed can lead to a totally different universe?

As I've said, part of its structure was based on cyproheptadine, so the essential structural elements of cyproheptadine are in the molecule and, like cyproheptadine, mianserin was often used for increasing appetite in people who are seriously underweight. This is a common property of what we now know as 5HT$_{2C}$ antagonists. It looks as though the 5HT$_{2C}$ receptor is involved in the control of appetite and weight – 5HT$_{2C}$ agonists would be fine antiobesity agents and may be responsible for the anorexic effects of the SSRIs. In those days of course we just knew about serotonin receptors, we didn't know about sub-classification. That's another thing that has happened in the last 15 years which has really got the whole antidepressant receptor-specific approach off the ground as people are now looking at drugs which will interact specifically with sub-sets of receptors.

Well, that raises a point that was made by Claude de Montigny in a plenary lecture at this meeting when he made the claim that we have left serendipity behind and we're into the rational design of treatments, but are we?

I still think it is very much serendipitous. I think most drug companies these days run programmes where they identify target mechanisms that they are interested in – it may be a receptor or an enzyme. Then they scan millions of compounds because people are now using combinatorial chemistry where you synthesise very small amounts of very large numbers of compounds and you have a high-throughput robotised screen that goes 24 hours a day, 7 days a week. Companies build up huge databanks of millions of compounds in this way, but they've identified before that a target mechanism. So in one sense it is much more rational, but that target mechanism is based on current knowledge. In depression you might do it for, say, a certain type of serotonin receptor. To make that quantum leap to a totally different mechanism you have to take something quite unknown, which might not have any connection with depression, and screen the compounds past this. That then is a form of serendipity because you don't really know what you are in for – whether it's going to work in depression or something else.

The ability to screen very large numbers of compounds means there is a lot of structural diversity but narrowing down to one target means there is a risk that you are going to miss some of the old chance findings where pharmacologists in the lab were working with a group of compounds and found something quite unexpected. That chance has been lessened by modern drug screening techniques. Combinatorial chemistry has been likened to the search for the same needles in even bigger haystacks.

Does the capacity to design things so easily leave you increasingly vulnerable to the claims-makers in the field? For example, two or three years ago there were big claims made for the D4 receptor in schizophrenia, made by one of the senior figures in the field. This looked good for a while and at least one large company went out and did trials on a D4 receptor antagonist, showing if anything it made schizophrenia worse. The field is repeatedly assailed by this sort of claim. Are you likely to get de-railed even quicker because these days you can go on to test these claims out because of your ability to design drugs as readily as you now can.

I think psychopharmacology, like most fields in medicine, has always been subject to and will still be the subject of speculation and claims – there are fashionable areas of research. If claims are made by the appropriate person of high reputation, they will be followed and believed and drug companies will actually go out and design compounds which have the requisite specific properties. Often these things take you down a blind alley. I think the finest example in recent years has been the $5HT_3$ antagonists. A very nice concept. It all came from Gaddum's work in the 1950s on the then M-serotonin receptor. The $5HT_3$ antagonists were specifically designed to work in emesis – and they are the best thing since sliced bread for chemotherapy-induced emesis.

There was a whole series of experiments, mostly carried out by the group in Bradford of Brenda Costall, indicative of an antipsychotic effect, as well later of an antianxiety effect and an effect on cognition. And these were shown in nice animal paradigms which we all believe are predictive of antipsychotic effects or effects on cognition. Testing in the clinic has gone on for the last 8 or 10 years but one by one the indications for psychosis, anxiety and for Alzheimer's or old age memory impairment have fallen by the wayside. One has to ask oneself, does this mean that the animal paradigms we use are not very indicative or were people over-enthusiastic – did they extrapolate the animal data much further than they should? It's a very difficult point to tease out but certainly $5HT_3$ antagonists for CNS indications have been a major disappointment for Glaxo and some other companies. I think there's a lesson to be learned there. I think we shouldn't over-interpret our animal data. I think animal models of CNS diseases are very far from the situation in the human. We still don't know what most CNS diseases are in neurobiological terms and to try and reproduce in a behavioural model or even in a simple biochemical model in animals what you think might happen in schizophrenia or in depression or Alzheimer's is probably stretching the science a bit far. We have to have these models and hypotheses to test but it was a little unbelievable that the $5HT_3$ antagonists would work in every psychiatric condition known to man. Ondansetron may actually have some psychotropic effects but insufficient to justify an indication as an antipsychotic, anxiolytic or cognition enhancer.

But isn't the issue also that it was the claims of one group in essence that really made the issue?

That comes back to the point that if the group or the personality of a member of the group is so strong and influential in science they can override the objections of others and even in this case override the caution exercised by major pharmaceutical companies in their investment in a project. And the whole project sort of fuels itself. At every conference that you went to, people would talk about ondansetron in this and that indication. Then it all went very quiet as slowly the news emerged that it wasn't an effective antipsychotic or a useful anxiolytic and that it isn't very good in cognition. There was a presentation in this meeting (ECNP, 1996) by Mike Palfreyman, who was involved in this research when he was at Merrell Dow in Strasbourg – in fact it all began there with John Fozard. Anyway he admitted that of the wide range of CNS indications they might be suitable for, nothing had come out. This was a fine example of the way individuals or groups of individuals can push along an idea, which is taken up and people run with the ball for nearly 10 years.

Mianserin began running into trouble around the same time as nomifensine.

Before nomifensine. Mianserin had a long history, particularly with the British, although other countries like the Germans for example kept it under surveillance for quite a long time. The first case of agranulocytosis was reported in 1979 in the BMJ and slowly more cases began to appear. We had a number of cases in our pharmacovigilance/product surveillance – not enough to be worried about taking the drug off the market or anything. Organon was very responsible and when the first case came in the package information was changed and slowly the warnings and the precautions became stronger in the product information. I think the problem with nomifensine and Hoechst was that they were overtaken by events. They must have waited until there were sufficient cases of haemolytic anemia for it to be seen as a major problem and at that time they hardly had anything in their package information.

On the other hand, it was quite an interesting development because in the UK the CSM tried to restrict mianserin to the treatment of patients in whom anticholinergic effects were unacceptable – people with very severe reactions to tricyclics, old men with prostate problems for example and the elderly particularly with problems with tricyclic anticholinergic effects. We fought that proposal very hard at that time because we believed the risk–benefit ratio was very much in favour of the drug. I think companies should always do that if they believe they have got the benefit–risk ratio on their side – even if the drug has a major rare side-effect. You have to balance that against the relative benefits and the benefits within the class of drugs in which the compound exists. At that time, in the early 1980s, there were no SSRIs and so mianserin was in a class with nomifensin, trazodone and the tricyclics and we fought the issue on the basis that mianserin had a well-deserved reputation for safety in overdose. The same should have been done for nomifensin, which was a very useful drug especially in the elderly and quite benign in overdose.

We had very rapidly to generate data from mortality statistics of the OPCS in the UK, which every year publishes tables of causes of death including suicide. You can find out which drugs are associated with suicide and we could at the same time look at the company sales in kilograms of drug and the defined daily dosages and duration of treatment and come up with a very crude estimate of the number of deaths per million patients.

Where did the Fatal Toxicity Index come from?

Well, the Fatal Toxicity Index was John Henry's invention. He did a very fine job on looking at data both in England and Wales and Scotland – but he had access to the NHS prescription database. He combined that with exactly the same data as we did – OPCS mortality statistics – and came out with the Fatal Toxicity Index, showing that the old tricyclics were very nasty, causing about 30–50 deaths per million prescriptions, whereas a drug like mianserin was near the bottom with single-figure deaths. We were doing this, I guess, simultaneously with John as he published in 1987, while Stuart Montgomery and I had a letter to the editor of *Psychopharmacology* published in the same year. There was a remarkable consistency between his data and ours. Obviously our individual figures are different but the rank order of toxicity was identical. So we used the data in our discussions with the authorities. I think that idea of looking at the whole benefit and risk ratio and the whole pattern of what a drug is doing has become firmly embedded in the psyche now. People are not prepared to take drugs off the market for a side-effect and I think authorities have learnt their lesson that they shouldn't just focus on one side-effect but should take the whole profile of the drug into consideration within the context in which it is used.

Why was the CSM so awkward?

Well, the CSM and then the Medicines Commission didn't want to accept that you looked at the whole benefit–risk ratio. They focused entirely on the fact that mianserin produced agranulocytosis and that's dangerous per se.

Is the rate at which it actually does that much higher than for tricyclics?

I think it's probably comparable to tricyclics although getting at tricyclic data is very difficult because none of it is reported any more. Tricyclics were available long before the Dunlop Committee and yellow-card reporting and doctors are so used to the fact that they produce blood dyscrasias that they never report them anymore, but if you go back to the old literature of the 1960s there are a lot of imipramine, amitriptyline and clomipramine cases. In contrast, new drugs are particularly focused on and I think these days agranulocytosis will be reported for new drugs if it's seen. In my opinion mianserin was not very much different; there may be a slight increase compared with the tricyclics but we couldn't get that data and so we were working on our own problem and trying to relate that to the benefits of the drug in terms of overdosing. But the CSM and the Medicines Committee were very obdurate. They interpreted the law very tightly ...

Why?

I don't know. Most of the clinicians on the CSM are not psychiatrists but I don't see why any clinician cannot see the argument of balancing what is a major risk in that therapeutic class and in that particular type of patient – suicide and overdosage – within the overall profile of the compound. Balancing the benefits of a drug which was safe in overdosage against its potential danger in terms of agranulocytosis. They listened politely but they didn't accept the case. I really don't know, even to this day, why they were so obdurate about it because in the end we were so convinced about the merits of our case that we actually took the Health Authorities in the UK to the courts. At that time the British hadn't taken the European law on medicines into their legislation so potentially it could have gone on for a very long time, but we won in the High Court.

There were very expensive and long discussions in court over whether overdosage is to be considered. The British law at that time stated something along the lines that the authorities should consider 'drugs in the dose in which they are normally used'. They strictly interpreted that as meaning an overdose is a dose that is not normally used and so they could, therefore, not take the overdose argument into account. But in fact the judge ruled that you should take overdosage into account in depression. The British authorities appealed to the Court of Appeal, so we went through another very long process.

What was in it for them to appeal?

A point of principle I guess. The scientific debate, which obviously went on outside regulatory circles in psychiatric congresses and so on, had accepted the argument that suicide and overdosage fatalities are an important aspect of depression. The CSM even produced in their regular publication *Current Problems* a review of mianserin and agranulocytoses where they actually published a league table of ADR fatalities per million prescriptions for all available antidepressants and we used that data and stacked it up alongside the Cassidy and Henry generated overdose data and you could see that the total fatality index was much greater with other antidepressants. This should have convinced them because this was their own data on ADRs along with other quite independent data on overdose fatalities. Nevertheless they appealed to the Court of Appeal where they again lost and were refused permission to appeal to the House of Lords, which they intended to do. The Appeal Court judges decided enough was enough. In fact, it could well have ended up in the European Court because as I have said European law was different from the UK law at that time. It then stopped and we made a minor change in the package information which could have been achieved without all this fuss, many years before.

We have had another illustration in the company recently with third-generation oral contraceptives and venous thrombosis. Here the MCA have taken a very strange attitude – treating it as a public health hazard. OCs were restricted overnight with very little time for the company to present any evidence. It should have been dealt with like the mianserin case should have been dealt with, in my opinion, by a proper discussion and the company agreeing to make the appropriate change in the product information. With the OCs what you have had is a well-accepted risk – there has been an accepted incidence of venous thrombosis over the last 25 years. These new studies, although they demonstrated for whatever reasons, apparently a two-fold increased risk of venous thrombosis with the third as compared with the second-generation OCs, that two-fold risk was still within and below the old accepted risk. So it wasn't that there was a new enhanced risk for which immediate action must be taken. What had happened was the risks for the older drugs had gone down and the risk for the newer drugs seemed to be like the older drugs were 25 years ago. This may be a cohort effect and a prescription bias. New, young and at-risk women receive the third-generation OCs and it seems as though women may get a thrombosis when they are first exposed to a surge of oestrogen either when they are pregnant or when they first get an oral contraceptive. So the generally older women who have received second-generation OCs are in essence healthy users and are less likely to experience a thrombosis. Recent epidemiological evidence suggests that when such biases and confounders are corrected for there is no difference in risk for venous thrombosis. Furthermore, the risk for acute myocardial infarction seems to be less for third-generation OC users.

So why did this extraordinary fuss happen? – it was front page news on the newspapers in the UK. There was severe criticism about the way the MCA went about it and the interesting thing is that it's your company again.[3]

I have been heavily involved with this and it's so reminiscent of the mianserin case where actions were going to be taken of a public health nature when the data did not suggest that degree of urgency. I think the OCs are even worse than the mianserin case because here are drugs which are used by healthy volunteers in essence, whereas mianserin is a drug used by sick people. The MCA acted in a way that caused panic. Not only did women stop using third-generation OCs, they stopped using OCs altogether and there has been an increase in abortions in the UK and in other countries where it happened. The only other country which took precipitate action was Germany. In the rest of the world it has been treated in the way it should have been treated with a change in the product information.

The UK action has in fact destroyed confidence in contraception, which is a major thing to do over such a trivial business. The perception of women in Europe to oral contraception has changed. There is resistance to what is a fairly safe group of drugs, which has come about purely by the action of one Health Authority. But the discussion is still ongoing. The CPMP, the

---

[3]On Saturday 2 November, the *Guardian* newspaper in the UK reported that UK official statistics indicated a 7% rise in abortions and a 25% increase in live births for the first 3 months of 1996. Abortions in England and Wales were 2688 higher in the first quarter than in the same period in 1995.

European Authority, believe that we were right. We are still supplying data to the CPMP and one of these days there will be another discussion. A lot of distinguished epidemiologists are studying the problem and publishing data and I believe in the end we will win through. But to come back to your point about why Organon and why ... twice

And mirtazapine has now been licensed in the US, which is supposed to be the hardest arena to enter, but is still not licensed in the UK ...

I don't believe in conspiracy theories but yes, we feel again the demons may be working against us because we still haven't got a UK licence. As you say, if you talk about the countries that are usually regarded as having the most stringent regulatory authorities, the FDA in the US and the British, the Swedes and the Australians, well we are approved and on the market in the US, we introduce in Sweden in October (1996) and Australian approval is in, but we are still arguing with the British about the benefit and risk ratio.

We have had one symptomatic neutropenia which we think is possibly attributable to the drug in our clinical trial programme but we also had one with imipramine. The FDA handled it in a very sophisticated way. They accepted that this happened. It's in the labelling, in heavy type. They even quote a so-called incidence of severe neutropenia but it's obviously difficult to quote an incidence on so few patients. But they thought the drug was of sufficient value and novel with good data on efficacy that they were prepared to accept it with this risk. Indeed the FDA Psychopharmacology Advisory Committee thought that the efficacy part of the file was among the strongest that they had seen in terms of positive studies. And that has been the case in most of the European countries and Australia, but the UK and France are still being difficult about it. One of these days we will go back to talk to them when we've got much more pharmacovigilance data from Germany, for example, where it's been on the market for 4 or 5 months. There has been no symptomatic neutropenias in the 50,000 patients we have treated in the last 6 months, so the incidence is falling. Trying to explain the situation to British psychiatrists is very strange.

When the mianserin story was building up a head of steam, as I remember it some German pharmacovigilance group wrote asking 'What you going to do about it?' and you mentioned the issue of overdosage, to which they replied that they weren't interested in overdosage because suicide isn't legal. I used to tell this as a comment on German 'principles' but the MCA attitude seems even more strange.

This was Moebius and his famous Arzneimittel Telegram, a monthly newsletter that is put out in Germany, highly critical of the pharmaceutical industry usually. There is a clinical pharmacologist associated with Moebius, Schönhoffer, who is Professor in Bremen, and the two of them are part of the anti-industry group in Germany. They've popped up again in the OC business; they had a long-running campaign against Schering but we have been caught in the flak. But yes, they had a very big go at Mianserin in the 1980s with messages in their newsletter, calling upon the German authorities to take it off the market.

They wrote to us, as you have said, but to give them their due, they did accept that there was a case to be made although they maintained their point of view. The suicide point was actually made but in fact it was almost exactly the same with the CSM. It was a very fine legalistic point to argue. I think in discussions about drug safety anything of relevance to the benefits and risks of medication should be on the table to be discussed. If the law has some fine points which can be used to eliminate public discussion I think it's incumbent on a body like the CSM not to focus upon those elements. I think the company's view was that they were eliminating the discussion of a proper topic which is very relevant to the use of antidepressants.

Since 1962, regulators have been in the business of trying to persuade the industry to produce drugs which have a good risk–benefit ratio and they achieve this partly by restricting them to a disease indication. In contrast, before 1962, the drugs that people wanted weren't necessarily disease based – they wanted a tonic or pick-me-up or an anti-halitosis drug. Now if you look at what actually happens today, the OC market is not a disease-based market and its not clear that steroids for minor skin complaints or nasal inhalers for rhinitis are disease based – these seem more a discomfort market than a disease market. So drugs work but not necessarily for disease indications, which sets up a conflict with regulators taking a very purist or categorical view of things. Medical people such as Juan Lopez-Ibor or Pierre Pichot will still say we should have to make a diagnosis and that we abandon the medical model at our peril but is the industry being tied to a medical model, when this is not the way drugs are developed and it is not clear that that is what people want?

I personally think that things like homeopathy and alternative medicine should fall under the same rules as conventional pharmaceuticals. There should be the same standards of proof for any medical procedure, be it drugs or whatever. If we are obliged for a new antidepressant to prove efficacy and safety in a large body of patients, I think it's incumbent on the authorities to ask for that same evidence for what passes as a drug and is used by many people and prescribed by physicians for the same conditions. Homeopathy is not as popular, I think, in the UK as it is in Holland and Germany for example. Germans like to take natural types of medicines and in fact if you look at the depression market in Germany it's dominated by St John's wort, which probably has a very mild euphoriant effect but it's certainly not a proven antidepressant.

But is this happening partly because of the regulatory framework? For you to sell mirtazapine, you've got to sell a disease model. You have got to tell people they've got a depressive disease before they can have it. Whereas for St John's wort you don't have to do that. They don't have to go to a person like me and be evaluated by me. They can take the stuff when they want. And there is a stigma associated with all disease models. Even if you've got a tumour, you become a diseased person, a leper of some sort. Whereas the homeopathic market is a problems-of-living market – it's life we are talking about, not leprosy.

Exactly. There is stigma associated with all disease – you're different, you're stigmatised, but I think mental illness is particularly stigmatised. People can accept that a physical problem like a tumour is a disease, but to be mentally ill is unacceptable. Particularly with depression, where if you see surveys that have been done of the general public, like what do you think of depression, most people don't see it as a disease, they think it's something that you grow out of, a weakness of character, people who are just giving in to a stress. It's not seen as a serious treatable disease.

On this point, when I came to north Wales first there was still an old GP there who was using a lot of cyproheptadine – as a tonic. It's a perfect tonic – it will increase your appetite, improve your sleep and people would buy the idea of having a tonic and having it for a few months, in a way they wouldn't buy the idea of being depressed and needing an anti-depressant. Now is the regulatory framework doing this to us?

Yes. I guess there was no regulatory framework before the days of thalidomide and companies made drugs and marketed them for what they liked. In that sense I think we are in a better situation today because drugs are for diseases rather than just out there for anyone to use and you need a prescription to get the drug for your disease. But I still think mental illness presents a major problem and I think depression within mental illness is the worst example of all because it is under-diagnosed. Doctors don't recognise it. Patients don't want to admit they've got it. They often present to doctors with all sorts of other strange symptoms which they are really presenting instead of the underlying depression.

Well, if you were to ask them are you depressed, they would say no. If you were to ask them have they psychological problems, they might say yes but if you were to ask them are you a bit under the weather, would a tonic do you good, an awful lot would say 'yes'. They'd be keen to have a tonic but you can't get one these days.

Yes indeed.

Can I hop to what may be a related issue? In both Holland and Germany, to have a career in the pharmaceutical industry was a good career to have. But somewhere it seems to me in the late 1960s, perhaps associated with the 1968 events, the industry became evil and biological psychiatry in particular was a problem. Here in Holland Herman van Praag ended up being escorted by the police for his own safety.[4] What's going on?

I'm not Dutch but I think we had in Holland in those days a reaction to society like the students in Paris. There were the provos here, which was a group that was very much anti-society in general, not only anti-industry. In those days psychiatry was perceived as something evil because it was regarded as a sort of manipulation of minds. I think this was a very prevalent view, not only in Holland but in many countries. Here it was particularly strong. You can see this in the interview that you had with van Praag and yes, it got to a very serious stage where the more famous people in Dutch psychopharmacology like van Praag, like David de Wied in Utrecht, were pilloried in the press, were

---

[4]van Praag H in *The Psychopharmacologists*, Vol I.

physically intimidated and were threatened. I think psychiatry in Holland suffered for a long time. ECT, for example, which is a very useful technique and has never been out of fashion in the UK, was virtually banned here for 20 years and only now is there a resurgence of interest but it is still very much less used than in other psychiatric communities outside the Netherlands. You still have the feeling that here psychiatry is not quite respectable. There's an awful lot of psychology and of non-drug psychiatry practised. The general standard of biological psychiatry and drug therapy, I think, is less well developed because of this history of the anti-psychiatry movement, than it is in other parts of western Europe.

How is the industry perceived?

There are only two major pharmaceutical companies here – Organon and Solvay Duphar. The rest of the industry is mainly local offices of large multinationals. It's quite difficult to get young physicians to join the pharmaceutical industry in the Netherlands. The industry is regarded as a good career for young managers and scientists. Dutch universities produce a lot of good basic scientists and there's not enough jobs to absorb them so we have more than our fair share of good chemists and good biologists, but finding good physicians and psychiatrists to join the industry is very difficult. I think in Holland specialist physicians, psychiatrists, cardiologists and the like are extremely well paid. Their rewards outside the industry are more than their potential rewards within the industry, which is a quite different situation from say the UK, where relatively it's more tempting to join the industry.

Organon have recently decided to focus on two areas: gynaecology and CNS. Lundbeck have also decided to focus on the CNS only. Is this the way the companies are going – specialising on just one area?

I think it depends entirely on the size of the company, and of course on their traditional expertise and niche areas. I think companies like Roche and MSD and Glaxo can quite happily, with their size, afford to be in several therapeutic areas. A company the size of Organon, which in world terms is currently in the 30s – we move up several places each year as companies fuse above us – can't afford to be active on a broad front across all therapeutic areas. Gynaecology, of course, has been the traditional area of the company for many years. It is very much a steroid-based company. Actually we do steroid-based work in the CNS.

We have in fact four therapeutic programmes within a system of therapeutic area research. So in addition to CNS and gynaecology, there is a small vascular programme focusing on thrombosis which also does work in stroke, which has a connection with CNS, and a small innovative experimental programme in immunology. But the company has decided that because of its past strengths, it will focus on reproductive medicine and CNS. In reproductive medicine we have the OCs but also fertility drugs and hormone replacement therapy. In CNS, depression and schizophrenia, which of course are only two of the many possible diseases you could study in the CNS but a small company with the limited resources it has for R&D can't cover all of the CNS diseases.

In the last year the company has made a real commitment for going for CNS as a second leg to stand on next to reproductive medicine. The other two programmes, thrombosis and immunology, are regarded as experimental. They may become things which we would want to spend a lot more money on if they turn out promising or they may wither away. I think it's essential for companies not to become too focused. If you become too focused and the field dries out or if your innovative compounds don't come through, then you can find yourself in very serious difficulties because pharmaceutical research is such a long-winded affair that what we are doing today in the research lab will not be on the market for another 12 or 15 years. If things do foul up you've no time to catch up before the company goes bankrupt, so you always have to have a good pipeline of compounds. The job of a research director is to see across the whole company that there's a pyramid of compounds with one or two coming into registration, three or four in Phase III, six or seven in Phase II and so on down to the bottom of the pile. Within each therapeutic area, there should be a similar pipeline but for the overall research manager it doesn't matter whether they are gynaecology, CNS or vascular projects as long as that pipeline is adequately filled with new innovative compounds. As soon as you perceive that there's a gap, that's the time when you should take some action like licensing in a compound to fill the gap or co-develop a compound with another company.

It is fatal for the future of the company if you end up with a 5 or 6-year gap in your pipeline. This can happen by default. If there are very successful drugs like Tagamet or Zantac, they can become such a major part of the company sales that everything else goes to the wall for it and you can forget that behind it you have to have several projects coming through. For all the Tagamets and Zantacs, it's nice to have half a dozen smaller products in your portfolio which are selling in total as much as the major product because when a block-buster comes off patent, it's quite a serious matter. You need to maintain the revenues to fuel the research organisation you have built up on the back of your block-buster. Some companies have been successful in living on after the block-buster, others not so successful.

At the ECNP AGM yesterday you were critical of the motion to increase the membership fee. There was also a big fuss, as you know, at the CINP AGM as well this year and at the BAP AGM. What's happening? Are all these organisations hitting some kind of crisis?

I think all organisations go through periods of crisis. I don't think psychopharmacology societies are any exception, but I think we got into a position in all three organisations where we had a fossilised situation almost, a coterie of people who had been in the organisation for a long time, a self-perpetuating group. In BAP the constitutional changes proposed by council and the officers would have kept all the power with those who already had it. The meeting was dramatic. Most members objected to the proposed changes. I think the CINP is the example to which the BAP would have headed if they had changed its constitution in this way. The CINP already has a self perpetuating oligarchy. I don't like organisations where the constitution allows the current committee to appoint the next president and the officers, and so it goes on.

ECNP is now the most expensive psychopharmacology society by far, which will discourage younger psychopharmacologists from joining. Lets face it, even you and I who can afford to pay the fees, are members of more than ECNP – between other pharmacological and chemical societies and so on, it adds up to quite a large sum of money. For this organisation which, after all, had a massive balance of cash and assets, to increase the yearly fees by 25% is asking a lot. It will put off a lot of the younger people from joining, who already see it as a slightly elitest organisation.

But not elitest in the ACNP sense, which they may be aiming at, but rather elitest in the sense of owned by an in-group, which is exactly the wrong perception.

It is exactly the wrong perception. I was particularly upset at the ECNP AGM because I don't think there was a proper debate about the fees and the finances. They had made a decision and they wanted it pushed through. Both the BAP and the ECNP have used their journal as an excuse to increase the fees. I think one should have the right to be able to chose whether you want the journal as in the British Pharmacological Society. Many of us don't want journals lying on our shelves as personal subscriptions. I can see in the beginning of a new journal it's essential that the membership supports it, so a construction where-by for a short time, while the journal gets going, you are obliged to take it would be all right but I think there should be a choice once the journal is established, as *European Neuropsychopharmacology* and the *Journal of Psychopharmacology* now are.

Coming back to the point that ECNP looks owned. This translates on the ground into a feeling that the meetings are not quite right. This may reflect the constitutional issues and the fact that ECNP isn't alive in some sense. The automatic response to that is to blame the industry.

Yes, the industry has got flak at ECNP and CINP because the last few congresses of CINP and ECNP have been in the eyes of a lot of psychiatrists dominated by industry. There have been sessions which purported to be part of the scientific programme and not satellites which were dominated by industry speakers who gave the same talk in the real sessions as they did in the satellite symposia. There's a general feeling that industry has taken too big a role in the psychopharmacology associations. It's a fine line. You can't do without the industry because without us paying for exhibition space and satellite symposia, the organisation would wither away to be simply a learned society, which you don't want in fact. But there is a fine dividing line and I think Venice last year (ECNP/1995) was a good example of over-commercialisation. I think this meeting (ECNP/1996) probably got it just about right.

I think companies have to have the opportunities to have satellite symposia where they present new drugs, and exhibition space where they can pass out information. I think a situation where you separate satellite symposia from the rest of the programme where the speakers and the topics are chosen by the scientific committee is quite acceptable. But gone are the glory days when our budgets were growing. We want to see something for what we are giving to ECNP for example. I have had the same argument with ECNP about companies' educational grants to specific symposia of interest to the company. In addition to a satellite, for instance, we might want to see our money assigned to a speed of onset of antidepressant action symposium, without the company having any influence at all on the choice of speakers, Chairman or topics. This year the ECNP committee decided that they couldn't have particular symposia sponsored by an educational grant and decided on just a blanket listing in the front of the book of the companies who have sponsored. But we are not giving money to the ECNP just to support ECNP, we are giving it to support particular activities and we have to find a formula with the psychiatric organisations and societies, where the company's support can be identified as being associated with a particular activity and not just as a general grant to the organisation. ECNP, and all societies for that matter, have to find a balance between commercialism on the one hand and pure academic interest on the other. The confusions were symbolised in a sense by a fuss that happened this year at the AGM where the recipient of a prize had problems with the fact that Lilly had their logo on the plaque for what is the Lilly Prize. If it is the Lilly Prize I can't see any objection to having the Lilly logo on the plaque. If it was my company I would certainly want the Organon symbol on it.

A theme I've had for some time is that scientific concepts don't work just because they are right. There has always been the idea that they work best when they come from Harvard, Yale, Oxford or Cambridge but there's also the question of commercially viability and in addition there's the question of the friends a concept has. For instance, the Galway panic disorder study which involved Brian Leonard and Tom Fahy was one of the best pieces of research in the field but it didn't have any friends in the sense of commercial viability. They weren't working with drugs that one of the companies was going to register for panic. Neither were they working with the non-drug lobby. They produced disinterested findings but disinterested findings have no friends. And that study has vanished.

Yes, and you find people reinventing the wheel and forgetting that the study was ever done. I think it's very difficult unless you have a powerful set of friends, either on the academic side or in the industry, who will pick up the ball and run with it. The ball has been dropped with the Galway study in fact. It's best, I guess if you want a study to be well known, that you've done it with drugs which are going to be also well known.

There is an issue of friends in the whole thing. Because when mianserin ran into problems in the UK there were a few friends who were outside the industry who came on board ...

I think both academics and the industry need friends and the industry in particular needs friends in times of crisis. I think most of my job really is about creating networks, creating friends for the company who might be useful one day, people you can call upon in times of crisis, or for advice generally. With any study or drug you do need people who are going to talk spontaneously about your drug or study to their friends. It is important to be perceived by the psychiatric community as a serious and responsible company which deals properly with people and which thinks seriously about R&D in psychiatry.

Within groups like ECNP there is also that kind of networking but there was a stage, perhaps with the Venice meeting, when people were talking, almost openly, about the networks being the wrong kind of networks. From the outside, a person might think, well it was the industry to blame but the insider story was that there were networks within ECNP that the industry probably weren't too keen on either..

Yes, I think within ECNP and the other international psychiatric organisations there can be networks of people who are perceived to be manipulating events and you have to be very careful I think within organisations that you don't create such groups. The International Academy of Biomedical and Drug Research, an independent organisation which operates to organise congresses and do research, made up of current or former committee members of CINP or ECNP, is an example. I don't think it's good for science and organisations if three or four core people, however benign their motives, are in a position of being able to influence several organisations. There are enough interested scientists who would join committees if it were possible. We should never end up in a situation where a few people are always there in all the societies.

In the mid-1970s, catecholamines were where the action was in depression. Then the SSRIs came along and you heard about nothing except 5HT. The catecholamine story was dead but Organon hung on in there.

Yes. We tried other things. We had an SSRI of our own, which was killed in Phase II. Not because it wasn't effective. We had decent pilot studies to suggest it would be effective. But we had this toxicological problem common to all SSRIs, that it causes phospholipidosis in tissues of rats and dogs. It was regarded in the toxicological world in those days as a really killing effect for drug development. We stopped our programme and it also delayed fluoxetine for a number of years while they considered the problem. Now it's not perceived as a problem – it has no relevance to human toxicology. All the SSRIs do it. We were one of the first caught by it. We might have been one of the first companies with an SSRI. It was a compound from a series being worked on in our Scottish lab in Newhouse and they had certainly been working in that chemical area for quite a long time before I joined the company, since the early 1970s in fact.

But we hung in with alpha-2 agents or rather we hung in with the chemical series, shall we say, the tetracyclics, because within the group you could also find dopamine antagonists. We, in fact, have a tetracyclic, Organon 5222 – it's an SDA for schizophrenia. I was in the scientific group within my first few years in the company that selected mirtazapine as a potential anxiolytic antidepressant. Only later did we realise the very attractive extra effect it had on serotonin release. We always knew that there were alpha-2 hetero-receptors on serotonin terminals but because mianserin was equipotent as an alpha-1 and alpha-2 antagonist, we didn't realise you could have this facilitating effect on serotonin firing, via the alpha-2 adrenoreceptors on the cell bodies. So we carried on with the chemical series and out of that chemical series came other alpha-2 antagonists and other types of drugs.

In terms of the alpha-2 story, there has been a range of things that have been linked to it, like the speed of onset of effects in depression and actions in schizophrenia.

In depression, Per Bech has recently shown that mianserin accelerates the onset of action of fluoxetine. There is also nice work by Bill Potter suggesting that addition of idazoxan to fluphenazine gives an extra effect in drug-resistant schizophrenia and mianserin has long been used to augment antipsychotic therapy. Clozapine has a very strong alpha-2 effect in its profile of course. If you look at some of the newer antipsychotics coming along now, some of them have retained this alpha-2 effect and others have not. It will be interesting to compare them. What you should do of course is a study adding mirtazapine to a standard neuroleptic because not only is there evidence that you can add serotonin antagonism into dopamine antagonism in one molecule (the SDA concept) but you could also unhook them and give a normal dopamine antagonist together with a serotonin antagonist and an alpha-2 antagonist. Sulpiride and mirtazapine would be a very good combination. I think mirtazapine could find a place as add-on therapy in schizophrenia.

We come back here to the regulators because a few people have said to me that the way we need to go is in terms of rational polyprescribing. But the FDA will never license claims for this. They're just geared to deal with one drug.

They deal with one indication and one drug. It's a shame. It's left to clinicians to do these combinations in the US but it leaves them very vulnerable to litigation if something goes wrong because this is not in the listed ways of using the drug. I hope that situation never develops in the same sense in Europe.

But isn't part of the problem that the industry won't support anyone with a good hunch of this kind either, because you won't be able to get an application to the FDA out of it.

I think if there's an established basis and a reasonable market drug companies would do studies. One of the suggestions with mirtazapine is that it would be a great drug to combine with SSRIs to bring about an earlier onset of action and to eliminate typical SSRI side-effects. A lot of people take a long time to respond to SSRIs and if you had a drug which you could add to them, it could present quite a large market. We are going to do such a study, although whether we will ever pursue it to a stage where you could file a claim, that's different. What you can do is to do some studies which provide good evidence, publish those and you can on the basis of those get a small additional wording in the product information and that's probably sufficient to establish it as a technique which could be used by clinicians without any fear of them being later accused of using it for an unlicensed indication.

This situation throws up some interesting ambiguities. The rational way for Janssen to go a few years ago, after they had first produced the 5HT$_2$ antagonists, ritanserin and ketanserin, might have been to add these into depot haloperidol as a treatment for schizophrenia. This would have made perfect sense but they would never have got a separate licence for ritanserin in schizophrenia because it is not independently antipsychotic and if they had brought it out under a sleep architecture assisting or appetite stimulating label, arguably everyone using it in schizophrenia would have been using it off-licence.

Developing combination products is more difficult and expensive than single entities and modern regulators tend to frown on combinations. Take Limbitrol, for instance, where despite a large US study demonstrating the combination to be superior to the individual constituents in the treatment of depression, it is no longer available in many countries. Augmentation strategies are easier because they usually involve drugs that are already approved and not given in inflexible fixed combinations. However, lithium is the classic example of an unlicensed but well accepted augmentation therapy based upon a body of evidence that may actually be insufficient to achieve regulatory approval.

Data from a trial of mirtazapine and Prozac came through a few days ago and I understand that it almost immediately boosted your share price.

Yes. It's not as bad as in the biotech industry where shares are up and down on the basis of one drug having a result in Phase II. Analysts are very strange. They regard the pharmaceutical industry totally differently from the biotech industry. Whether we lose a compound in development doesn't affect us at all but the biotech companies go up and down depending on where products and projects are going. I think it was the way it was written up in the press release – people said, 'Well, it's better than Prozac, Prozac has a $2 billion market. Organon's ambition is to be among the top three antidepressants with this drug' ... so this was interpreted by analysts as 'Hey, they are going to get a third of $2 billion and it's better than the $2 billion drug maybe.' Akzo Nobel shares are usually very stable. They don't vary between wide margins and it's quite remarkable to see this sort of dramatic change. And on good news! It was nothing to do with gynaecology, where it was surprising how little the share price was affected by the OC crisis even though the company lost a lot of sales in the UK and Germany. And yet here we have a drug which is hardly selling anything at the moment but the share price is massively affected by just an announcement that it's better than Prozac. I think without that study, this wouldn't have happened – it would have just been another new antidepressant.

But it is interesting that all these new antidepressants are turning out to be better in the trials that have been done than the SSRIs especially in the more severe forms of depression. It has been rare in the past to find differences between two antidepressants. It's fascinating that not only mirtazapine but also venlafaxine and milnacipran have got these studies – there must be something peculiar about the new drugs, with their dual mechanism of action.

Perhaps catecholamines are important for speed of onset. It would be a nice touch if the area you did your original work in came into the frame again after being eclipsed for two decades. But these ideas about what works in depression are something that you'd imagine a department of psychiatry or even of neuroscience should be testing but they can't – they don't have the resources. Is there a sense in which companies like Organon have become the only departments that count?

Yes, in terms of the big programmes of trials needed to prove that a new drug is both safe and effective. But departments of psychiatry and neuroscience have major roles to play in teasing out new uses and new mechanisms of action. They, and not the industry, are the vehicles for innovative research into the neurobiology of psychiatric disorders. The industry will capitalise on their findings, doing what it does best – medicinal chemistry, applied pharmacology and drug development. We can also support collaborations with university departments and the biotech industry, initiatives which may eventually lead to product development.

The process of drug development you've described has been rational but empirical and maybe pragmatic rather than theory driven. I'm hoping to see Les Iversen next, who has seemed to be on the opposite side of the theory/empirical divide. How do you see his approach compared with what you think works?

I admire Les and I enjoyed our brief collaboration in the dopamine area when Alan Home was still alive and working in Cambridge. Les had a chance to put his philosophy into practice at MSD when he was the first director of their Neurosciences Centre in Harlow. Innovative research, however, does not always lead to drug development, although it can add considerably to the body of knowledge. Les was unfortunate in that a lot of fine research did not lead to new product opportunities. I believe that a judicious mix of innovative academic research and opportunistic product development is the best way to proceed, and that the industry can sometimes better achieve its aims by actively supporting outside research and incorporating the results into its drug development programmes.

Select bibliography
Aldous FAB, Barrass BC, Brewster K, Buxton DA, Green DM, Pinder RM, Rich P, Skeels M, Tutt KJ (1974). Structure–activity relationships in psychotomimetic phenylalkylamines. *Journal of Medicinal Chemistry*, **17**, 1100–1111.

Brimblecombe RW, Pinder RM (1975). *Hallucinogenic Agents*. Wright-Scientechnica, Bristol.

Costall B, Naylor RJ, Pinder RM (1974). Design of agents for stimulation of neo-striatal dopaminergic mechanisms. *Journal of Pharmacy and Pharmacology*, **26**, 753–762.

Miller RJ, Horn AS, Iversen LL, Pinder RM (1974). Effects of dopamine-like drugs on rat striatal adenyl cyclase have implications for CNS dopamine receptor topography. *Nature*, **250**, 238–241.

Pinder RM (1971). Recent advances in the chemotherapy of malaria. *Progress in Medicinal Chemistry*, **8**, 231–316.

Pinder RM (1988). The benefits and risks of antidepressant drugs. *Human Psychopharmacology*, **3**, 73–86.

See also interview with Brian Leonard in *The Psychopharmacologists* Vol I.

27 Paul Leber

Managing uncertainty

Why did you choose to become a physician?

My father had a lot to do with my choice of career, although not because he ever directly encouraged me to become a doctor. A paediatrician, he practised in the days before medicine was reimbursed at a rate to make physicians wealthy. In retrospect, little about his work-a-day way of life seems especially appealing, let alone glamorous. To the contrary, his practice was extremely busy. He worked terribly long hours, and I remember him being, more often than not, on the verge of literal physical exhaustion. Yet, his way of life brought him an abundance of respect and admiration, and, as a child, I suppose that was what most impressed me. As far back as I can remember, when anyone, be it a patient, colleague or tradesman, learned that I was my father's son, they invariably seemed compelled to tell me, in glowing terms, just how wonderful he was – competent, reliable, dedicated etc. Early on in life, I resolved, as so many others have done, to be like, even better, than my father. And so, not too surprisingly I suppose, I set out to become a physician. Once the choice was made, all that followed was derivative – going to a 'good' liberal arts college, majoring in chemistry, a 'tough' major for a pre-med, getting the grades to gain acceptance to a 'good' medical school, etc.

Then into pathology?

No, immediately after medical school my postgraduate clinical training was in internal medicine. But the story of my peripatetic medical career begins even earlier. I first wandered from the ordinary path of training while I was a medical student. Between my third and fourth years, I competed for, and was awarded, a Medical Sciences Year Fellowship in enzyme kinetics. A fore-runner of the now prevalent MD/PhD training programmes, the fellowship programme was intended to foster the development of a cadre of physician-scientists who would pursue full-time careers in academic medicine and research. It may seem somewhat odd that someone who had presumably entered medicine to become a clinician – to follow in his father's footsteps, so to speak – would take such a step, but, in light of the environment prevailing at NYU at the time, it is readily understandable.

At NYU, perhaps more than at other American medical schools at the time, the prestigious members of the faculty were known for their academic and research accomplishments, not their clinical skills or acumen. Numbered among the faculty were world-renowned luminaries in science and medicine, among them Severo Ochoa who won the Nobel Prize in biochemistry while I was a student, Lewis Thomas, Chair of the Department of Medicine, who, incidentally, although a medical essayist nonpareil, was anything but a skilled clinician, Homer Smith, the famed renal physiologist, Otto Loewi, yet another Nobel Laureate, as well as yet to be acclaimed innovators in the field of immunology such as Baruch Bennaceref. Thus, by the time I had completed my second year at NYU, my interest in clinical care had waned, replaced by hopes of a career in academic medicine and research. No doubt my 'conversion' was assisted by the discovery during my third year that, unlike my father, I had no 'calling' for the practice of clinical medicine.

In any event, based on the work I did during my fellowship on the modification of enzyme active sites, I earned an 'MD with Honours in physiology'. I enjoyed working in the lab and I gave serious thought to foregoing further clinical training and pursuing a full-time career in bench research, but I was strongly counselled by my advisors that an MD, even one with a seemingly hot hand at the bench, needed clinical skills if he was to pursue a career in academic medicine. And so, heeding their advice, I went off for clinical training in internal medicine. Following an internship in medicine at the Johns Hopkins in Baltimore, I returned to New York City, serving for a year as a resident on NYU's medical service at Bellevue Hospital. My experiences as a medical intern and resident persuaded me, however, that the day-to-day life of the medical practitioner was demanding and it would be exceedingly difficult, therefore, to be simultaneously both a good clinical internist and a productive bench investigator. That judgement is primarily responsible for my decision to train in pathology, a field in which I concluded teaching and research could more readily be pursued simultaneously.

My decision to become a pathologist proved short-sighted, however, because, I suspect, it was driven too much by reason and too little by enthusiasm for the substance of the field. Although the intellectual content of pathology is extremely interesting and basically one and the same as that of medicine, I found the day-to-day chores that constitute the actual practice of anatomical and surgical pathology only marginally tolerable. My lack of intrinsic enthusiasm for the practice of service pathology notwithstanding, I completed residency training, gained Board Certification in Anatomical and Clinical Pathology, and, subsequently held academic positions in the Pathology Departments of three medical schools. During my years as an academic pathologist, I taught – an activity that I truly enjoyed – and pursued a number of research projects in renal pathophysiology and immunopathology.

Why did you move then from pathology into psychiatry? It's an extraordinary jump.

As the years passed, I was forced to accept the fact that success in research requires more than clever ideas, hard work, and long hours at the bench.

Perhaps, if I had truly enjoyed the day-to-day practice of pathology, I might, as have so many other fledgling academics whose careers begin to stall, gradually shifted more and more from bench research to the service side of pathology. But, for me, even the thought of such a move was intolerable. And so, some 10 years out from medical school, I resolved to change course and become the clinician I had once intended to be.

Doing so by becoming a psychiatrist, albeit a seemingly extraordinary jump, as you put it, actually made considerable sense at the time. It allowed me to make a clean and complete break, to go in a single step from a field engaged entirely in the reductionistic explanation of pathophysiological mechanisms to one devoted to an understanding of the mind of man in a global and empathic way. On a more mundane and practical level, I wouldn't have made the change, if I had not also thought that I'd be a good therapist. I had the hubris to believe that I actually knew something about the field, my wife being a clinical psychologist. Perhaps more important, I thought, incorrectly it turns out, that I had had a good grasp of what psychiatrists actually did, having, during my time teaching pathology, worked with psychiatrists in efforts to help 'troubled' students 'make it through' medical school.

Where did you train?

I went to the Westchester Division of New York Hospital–Cornell from 1974 to 1977, a large private psychiatric hospital situated on a park-like campus in White Plains, New York, commonly known as Bloomingdale's. The hospital, by dint of its private nature, had a somewhat more manageable psychiatric patient mix than the typical city or state institution of the time. It also had a largely non-analytic eclectic orientation, and a clinical staff that, for the most part, shared an interest in phenomenology. In the United States, at the time, this was decidedly unusual. The hospital's unique orientation had come about in part as a result of its affiliation with Cornell, long a bastion of anti-analytic persuasion, and in part, as a result of the singular efforts of Paul McHugh who had been in charge of the Westchester division shortly before I became a resident there.

Who was Paul McHugh?

Paul McHugh, originally trained as a neurologist, is now Chief of Psychiatry at Johns Hopkins. I know him entirely by reputation, but he was largely responsible for the Jasperian–Schneiderian German English approach to psychiatry that was being taught by the Westchester division faculty when I first began there as a resident. While clearly at odds with the analytically styled training offered by most other major university-affiliated training programmes of the time, the phenomenological approach taught at Bloomingdale's provided residents with an observational 'set' and descriptive tools that I am convinced prepared them to deal with the revolution that subsequently took place in the field of psychiatry far better than analytical mumbo-jumbo being taught elsewhere.

Newly admitted patients were regularly assessed in group settings and, afterwards, faculty and residents reviewed, together, what had been observed.

Whether, for example, there was evidence, and if so, what it was, that a patient had experienced thought-broadcasting, had auditory hallucinations, or exhibited bradyphrenia. The systems of description and classification employed were at odds with those employed by the majority of the profession, however, and this proved to be somewhat of a problem.

Nonetheless, to this day, I am thankful that I had the opportunity, if only for a year or two, to observe highly competent and experienced medically oriented psychiatrists and psychologists evaluate and describe the form of the psychopathology exhibited by a wide variety and kind of acutely and chronically ill psychiatric patients. Regrettably, in the midst of my residency, the new Chair of the Department of Psychiatry at Cornell, Bob Michels, began to recruit increasing numbers of analytically trained psychiatrists to the Westchester faculty. It was not long, therefore, before the objective eclecticism that had made the residency so fascinating and instructive gave way to a pedantic orthodoxy of the most oppressive kind. What the analytically styled faculty advanced as 'training' was all too often little more than a homiletic indoctrination into the rituals of their cult. There was little, if any, tolerance for disagreement between teacher and student. Appeals to evidence and reason, even clinical training and experience deriving from sources external to the analytical system of belief, were not only deemed irrelevant, but treated as a threat to the very survival of analytical psychiatry.

Residents were expected to accept, without question or reservation, virtually every silly pronouncement of every petty analytic acolyte who had been recruited to the department. It was mind-boggling. Untestable speculations about the origins of putatively dysfunctional operations of each patient's internal object relations were the focus of virtually every supervisory session. Worse, it was not only the patient, but the resident who became the target of such gratuitous speculations. Why I might have elected to stand up and open the door for a female patient entering my office, I recall, became the focus of several hours of inquiry and speculation by one especially silly supervisor.

Did all your analytical supervisors behave that way?

No! And I'm glad you asked. First, not every supervisor who was analytically trained behaved as I have described. To the contrary, several to whom I was assigned were highly skilled and competent psychiatrists who provided invaluable advice and counsel. Moreover, one must take care to distinguish between the teacher of a subject and its value. The teachings of analytical psychiatry, while largely irrelevant to the treatment of individuals who suffer from the majority of the major psychiatric conditions, do provide invaluable insights into the motivations that drive much of human behaviour. In sum, although I found analytically styled supervision a dysphoric experience, analytical theory was not entirely without value.

Fortunately, analytically styled supervision that focused on the details of the therapeutic process had little effect on the actual medical and psychiatric care given to my patients. While supervisors held forth in analytic 'metaspeak' on matters such as projective identification and narcissistic rage, I comforted and

supported each of my patients as best I could, prescribing, when required, tricyclics, phenothiazines, lithium and benzodiazepines in accord with the recommendations of the biological psychiatric literature of the time.

I must admit that I felt somewhat vindicated, when, in the waning days of
my residency, one supervisor, a prominent analyst who had obvious difficulties in dealing with his personal ambivalence towards me, confessed that he,
along with many of the analytic faculty, found me a 'perplexing' fellow. They
could not figure out, since I did everything so 'wrong' in delivering therapy,
why all my patients had done so well.

*Had Washington University begun to have an impact by then with their neo-
Kraepelinian programme?*

Those who were among the phenomenological-oriented faculty at the
Westchester Division regularly cited the work of Sam Guze and his group at St
Louis; in fact, much of what I to this day hold true about psychiatric nosology
is put forth in the 1974 monograph, *Psychiatric Diagnosis*, that Guze co-
authored with Woodruff and Goodwin.

How did the DSM-III process look to you from where you were at?

The coming of DSM-III was anticipated with considerable enthusiasm by
those with biological and/or phenomenological orientations. DSM-III's
approach to psychiatric classification dovetailed with the research being done
by several on the faculty who had been recruited by McHugh. For them phenomenological homogeneity was a necessary first step to a nosology based on
biological homogeneity, and with that a system of psychiatric diagnosis that
could reliably predict both treatment and outcome.

Because of the influx of the analysts, there was an opportunity to witness,
up close and personal as they say, the impact of DSM-III on the struggle
between the analysts, who largely seemed to prefer a dimensional approach to
diagnosis, and the proponents of the new nosology who saw it as the way to
bring psychiatry back into the fold of medical subspecialties.

Interestingly, Bob Spitzer, who led the fight for DSM-III's adoption, was on
the faculty at Columbia, the source of many of the analysts that had just come
to Westchester. Incidentally, there is a very good and interesting account of
DSM-III's role in the transformation of American psychiatry by Mitchell
Wilson (*American Journal of Psychiatry*, **150**, 399–410, 1993). Wilson provides an
interesting political and social account of the struggle, part of which I witnessed from the perspective of a resident in training.

*In terms of DSM-III coming in, there are a few different issues involved. One was the idea
that if you had more clearly defined phenotypes we may be able to proceed further with our
research. Then there was the personality aspect to it – the politicians – people like Klerman
who were interested to push this forward. There was also the insurance industry and the
pharmaceutical/regulatory complex for whom more clearly defined entities would be useful.*

Well, those are all points made by Mitchell Wilson. I recall that he also
emphasised that some of the opposition to the dimensional diagnostic

approach reflected concerns about cost. A dimensional diagnostic system allows virtually everyone to be classified as suffering from a psychiatric disorder and this obliges government and other third-party payers to spend more than they intend on reimbursement for psychiatric services. Accordingly, such groups favoured the adoption of DSM-III because it seemed likely to reduce the prevalence of individuals carrying psychiatric diagnoses.

In any event, I hardly have a systematic understanding of the forces and interests involved. As noted earlier, the classification of psychiatric illness offered in draft versions of DSM-III were clearly attractive to what remained of Westchester's biologically oriented faculty. DSM-III was also attractive to residents like myself because it provided a basis to challenge the capricious, and often bizarre, labels applied to our patients by some of the analytical faculty. From their perspective, diagnostic classification was largely a nuisance, paper work that was required for reimbursement from third-party payers. Their attitude, given their perspective, is understandable – if all who appear receive an identical treatment in form at least, there is little, if any, need for diagnosis at the categorical level.

In any case, at the time, I was certain that a diagnostic system based on unique biological entities could be developed. I am far less convinced of that today. Indeed, the complexity that has been revealed by research in the neurosciences persuades me that nature will not be divided quite so cleanly and easily as I once hoped it would.

So, DSM-V could be quite different again from III/IV?

Perhaps, there will be a sudden break in the way we conceive of psychiatric illness in the sense that Kuhn has written about and we'll move to an entirely new system of classification. Perhaps, the neuro-anatomical basis of diagnosis, the model from which the Kraepelinian approach to psychiatric illness derives, will prove untenable. Perhaps, the field will find it more useful to define psychiatric behavioural impairments in terms of specific symptoms, signs, and phenomena that can be relieved with specific treatments. Whatever the future may hold, the current diagnostic system is not ideal. It remains little more than a set of tentatively held hypotheses in need of modification and revision. In short, I expect that the psychiatric nosology will continue to evolve as new evidence about the causes of psychiatric illness and disturbed behaviour emerge.

You also worked in the psychiatric service at Bellevue at one point.

Not for very long. Less than a year. Actually it was my experience at Bellevue that got me to the FDA. After completing my training at the Westchester Division, I obtained a position on the faculty of NYU's Department of Psychiatry. I had yet to decide precisely how I would earn a living in psychiatry, but I had some hope of working as a liaisonist on the medical service, developing a small private practice, and becoming involved, part time, in some form of clinical research. This was not to be.

Bellevue at the time was undergoing a number of changes. I had taken a position there with the understanding that I would serve as one of several attending on the residency teaching service, but I was, instead, assigned to head a unit that served as the ward that admitted patients only when the rest of the psychiatric hospital was filled to capacity. In theory , this 'overflow' condition would occur only infrequently, and I would have time, therefore, because of the unit's low census, to pursue my interests in liaison and clinical research, etc. Unfortunately, the psychiatric hospital was regularly filled to capacity, and, as a result, my unit was not only very busy, but was regularly filled with especially difficult cases.

For example, if charges against a prisoner with a psychiatric diagnosis being held in the hospital's forensic unit were suddenly dropped, the individual would be transferred to my ward. On a given morning, as a result, I might arrive to find as many as half a dozen new patients, undiagnosed, in restraints, unmedicated, awaiting evaluation and disposition. The ward had only part-time psychiatric staff assigned to it, no permanent head nurse and no established nursing team. It took me relatively little time to recognise that protests about the conditions extant were not going to affect the resources available to support the unit. Having reached that conclusion, I decided to leave Bellevue. I looked at a number of different opportunities. Among those available, a position as a 'Medical Officer' in the Division of Neuropharmacological Drug Products at FDA's Headquarters in Rockville, Maryland, was uniquely attractive.

Before moving onto the FDA, can I ask you, did your pathology training influence your outlook in psychiatry and your subsequent outlook in regulatory affairs?

Well, the notion that taxonomic diagnostic systems are authoritarian systems where people with declared positions of power say something is something because they say it – certainly pathology is rampant with that. A pathologist looking at a slide will say with great confidence but no evidence that the lymphocyte is travelling from one direction to the other in the lamina propria. There is no way to know that of course in a section of dead tissue but he feels quite confident that he can explain what he or she needs to explain that way. I think when I came to psychiatry I was struck by the fact that there was a shared similarity between the pronouncements of pathologists about tissues they knew little of but could describe fairly well and the psychiatrists looking at patients who they could describe very well but they could in no way explain what they were doing. In the course then of working for an agency where you had to assess whether or not an expert reaching a conclusion about something has a basis to reach it, not that they have an opinion – that's understood, it became obvious that sometimes experts offer opinions like the pathologist and the lymphocytes. It's that experience which has led me to become an enthusiast for experimental designs that provide the kind of evidence that would allow an expert, as we say in the language of the law, responsibly and fairly to conclude from the evidence that something is so or is not so. I distinguish that from simply associating some body of information with some conclusion and asserting there's a link. As someone who acts to make decisions in the area I would just as soon be able to say I can explain how I made my decision.

What did a medical officer in the FDA do?

FDA Medical Officers served as leaders of multi-disciplinary review teams responsible for evaluating INDs and NDAs. The job, accordingly, seemed ideally suited for someone with my background and experience in medicine, pathology and psychiatry.

At the time I joined the Division, the agency was still enmeshed in the Drug Efficacy Supplement Implementation project, known commonly as DESI. It was intended to deal with the fact that all drugs marketed in the United States in the period between 1938 and 1963 had been evaluated only for 'safety'. With the passage of the 1962 amendments to the Federal Food, Drug and Cosmetic Act, drug products could only be legally marketed if they were determined, upon assessment, to be effective in use. The DESI project was the programme under which that assessment was being conducted.

Thus, I cut my proverbial teeth as a clinical reviewer evaluating clinical trial reports put forward by sponsors to meet the DESI requirements. My task was to determine whether or not the evidence presented had been adduced in adequate and well-controlled clinical trials, and, if so, whether it provided valid support for the claims for which the DESI drug product was being marketed.

When did it hit you about the placebo controlled trial – the fact that the field at the time was using other antidepressants as a control for new compounds but the trial designs might not in actual fact be proving that either drug worked?

I had come to the FDA with no experience whatsoever in clinical trials, and little, if any, familiarity with the methods used in their analysis. I did, of course, have a clear enough understanding of the need for controls in research, but experiments of the sort I had conducted with laboratory animals did not ordinarily require randomised assignment or employ statistical assessment. The lesions I sought to induce in animals were of a kind unexpected in the inbred strains with which I worked. Accordingly, the success of any given line of investigation turned on the demonstration that a given intervention induced, in one repetition of the experiment after another, a characteristic lesion in experimental animals and not in the vehicle-treated controls.

In short, I came to the FDA with much to learn about how clinical trial data were evaluated. Aware of my near total ignorance, I began to read avidly and to seek the counsel of experts, many of whom were but a few steps from my office in the Pharmacologic and Somatic Treatments Branch of the NIMH. Several experts from academia also contributed to my education. Among the many who offered insights and counsel, none was more helpful than Bill Beaver, a physician and Professor of Pharmacology at Georgetown, who served as a consultant to the Division on analgesic drug assessment. The agency's regulations detailing the attributes of adequate and well-controlled clinical investigations (now appearing at 21 CFR 314.126) were largely a product of his work. Also of note is the fact that he had been trained by and worked with Raymond Houde, a prominent clinical pharmacologist and clinical investigator. This link is especially important because Houde and Walter Modell, another famous pharmacologist, were champions of the notion that experiments with drugs, whether conducted with animals or humans, must have 'assay sensitivity', to be interpretable.

What is meant by assay sensitivity?

An experimental trial has assay sensitivity if it can distinguish an active treatment from an inert control, and better still, can discriminate one level of the active treatment from another. Clinical trials of analgesics were regularly designed to have assay sensitivity. It made considerable sense to me that a principle that applied regularly to the assessment of analgesic drug efficacy should apply with equal force to almost every class of therapeutic drug products used in psychiatry and neurology.

Were you alone in taking this view?

Hardly. Other clinicians and scientists working at the FDA reached very similar conclusions about design and interpretation of clinical trials. Indeed, during the late 1970s and early 1980s, most of the methods and strategies now accepted as routine regulatory practice were being developed by FDA staff.

How come the field took so long to recognise the importance of assay sensitivity? They spent 20 years doing the wrong kind of trial.

I don't know if that's entirely fair. Remember, it was not until 1962 that marketed drugs in the United States had to be shown to be effective in use. Only then was serious consideration given to the question of what would constitute valid experimental evidence of a drug's efficacy in depression. Indeed, the tools for measuring the effects of drugs on the signs and symptoms of depressive illness were not widely available until the 1960s. Didn't Max Hamilton develop his scale to assess the effects of drug treatments on depression?

I don't think so. I think he had it before the first antidepressants came on stream and found to his pleasure and surprise that they seemed to fit hand in glove. In fact it did fit extremely well with the first tricyclics.

In any case, despite the theoretical justification for demanding that evidence of antidepressant efficacy turn on the showing of a difference, a policy enforcing that standard might have met far more resistance had it not been for a set of data presented in an NDA submitted in the early 1980s for an antidepressant drug product that, at the time, had already been marketed in Europe for several years.

Among the controlled studies submitted were a set of six, identically designed, three-way, parallel, controlled trials – that is, each of the six trials had both a placebo and an active control arm. Had the analyses of the results of these six trials been restricted to a comparison of the investigational drug and the active control, we would, in the fashion of the time, have reached a conclusion that the new drug was equivalent to the active control, imipramine. However, in five of these six studies, because of the placebo arm, it could be determined that neither the new drug nor imipramine had exerted any therapeutic effect whatsoever.

This set of studies demonstrated unequivocally why it was so critical for the agency to insist that studies of antidepressants be designed to rely on showing a difference to establish efficacy. The epistemological desirability of relying on the demonstration of a difference, incidentally, was recognised long before Modell and Houde described the principle in terms of 'assay sensitivity'; it was advanced as the preferred path to inference by John Stuart Mill in his writings in the 1840s on the scientific method.

Authority seems to have been a really big thing in the early days. Chatting to Michael Shepherd, who was one of the first trialists in the field with his study on reserpine in depressives, he said that no one paid any heed to the result because they had tables and figures and methods and all that and as he put it, the field was just not used to that. They were used to the expert saying 'I gave this drug and I saw such and such.'

It is not uncommon for clinicians to disparage the value of statistics. There has always been an unreasoned fear that it can be used to mislead – for example, the quote that there are lies, dammed lies, and statistics. Much is also made of the supposed distinction between clinical significance and statistical significance. That observation, however, is, more often than not, off point.

Certainly, given sufficient sample size, it is possible to declare a clinically unimportant between-treatment difference statistically significant. In such circumstances, it is not unreasonable to opine that the result, although not likely to be explained by chance, is of little importance. To claim, however, that there can be clinical without statistical significance is completely illogical. How can a difference that may reflect no more than the operation of chance be acclaimed as meaningful?

Must every probative result derive from a difference shown in placebo-controlled experiment?

No. The agency's regulations make clear that in some, very limited, circumstances active and historical controlled trials may adduce probative evidence of a drug's efficacy. To illustrate, a concurrent control for an anaesthetic that induces its effects within minutes of administration is hardly necessary; the reason is that the outcome observed is almost unimaginable in the absence of treatment.

An historical control trial, or an active controlled trial that fails to show a difference – they are much the same – provides little useful information, however, when the course of the disease involved is highly variable. In such circumstances, only a between-treatment difference can be unambiguously interpreted.

But this was extraordinarily obvious when you look back.

Perhaps, but the insight was hardly welcomed by the drug industry. By requiring sponsors to establish efficacy by the showing of a difference, we were establishing a much more demanding standard than that required elsewhere in the world.

Not only that, the imposition of the standard, logical and defensible as it may now seem, was probably viewed at the time as unfair. One of the things that industry has regularly complained about is that after they, 'in good faith', initiate a drug development programme, the FDA comes along and changes the rules. My refusal to interpret a failure to find a difference in an active control trial as evidence of efficacy is likely an example of what they have in mind.

Did the NIMH provide support for the agency's approach?

Some certainly did. I mentioned earlier that a number of individuals on the extramural side of the NIMH were quite helpful to me when I first came to the FDA; they continued to help after I became a group leader for Psychopharmacology and, subsequently, Director of the Division. Nina Schooler, Jerry Levine, Bob Prien and Alan Raskin were especially helpful in psychopharmacology and Tom Crook did much to help in the dementia area.

One of the criticisms you were potentially open to, and I am not sure how much you heard it, when you insisted on the placebo controlled trial was that it then became a means for companies to introduce an antidepressant that wasn't potentially as effective – that it could be superior to placebo but not necessarily as good as the old ones.

Well, I don't think that's a legitimate criticism at all. Commercial drug developers did not design their clinical trials to demonstrate the superiority of their new drug products to the standard treatment being used as a control, but to fail to find a difference between the treatments compared. Such designs, therefore, not only are uninterpretable vis-à-vis inferences about efficacy, but provide no information whatsoever about comparative performance.

Importantly, too, no company has ever been told that it would be unacceptable to document the effectiveness of their product by demonstrating its superiority to an established drug used as an active control. The problem with such an approach is that a study designed to show a new drug's superiority to a standard control must ordinarily be much, much larger than a placebo-controlled trial. From a sponsor's perspective, that is unattractive, especially because a finding of superiority in such a study cannot logically be advanced as evidence of superiority in general.

Thus, although the argument that new drugs should always be compared with already marketed drugs is appealing on face, it is not very practical. Moreover, those who advocate it fail to consider the difficulty of making truly valid comparisons among drug products.

In terms of fast-tracking the registration of drugs and of challenges to the placebo-controlled trial, the whole AIDS thing blew up a few years after a requirement for placebo-controlled trials were introduced and all of a sudden the ethical aspects of placebos came on the agenda again.

The AIDS epidemic has forced everyone to recognise that government programmes intended to control the quality of the drug supply impose a variety of costs and limitations. If new drugs are required to be assessed for safety and

618   The Psychopharmacologists II

efficacy prior to their marketing, individuals who seek access to them before the assessment process is complete can be claimed, at least arguably, to be adversely affected. Not unexpectedly, opponents of drug regulation make much of this libertarian point.

Opponents of drug regulation also find common cause with those who believe, as a matter of ethical doctrine, that society has no right to pursue its collective interests at the expense of its individual citizens. For those who take this view, randomisation is an anathema because it requires that individuals be assigned to treatments, not in accord with their immediate individual interests, but in regard to those of society. Indeed, their position would seem to be entirely in keeping with the tenets of the Declaration of Helsinki that hold that in experiments with medical patients, every subject, including those assigned to the control treatment, should receive the best available treatment.

While I personally find this facet of the demands of the Helsinki Declaration illogical, and, if taken literally, one that would require virtually all randomised clinical research to end once a nominally effective treatment became available, the issue is a serious one. Just who is to pay the human costs of new drug development? The issues are vexing and terribly complex. Nonetheless, I tend to believe that the placebo control serves largely as a stalking horse for those with other agendas. No one is compelled to employ a placebo control; there are alternative ways to show a difference – graded dose designs, in particular, provide a highly satisfactory alternative.

The attackers of the randomised control trial sometimes point to outcomes research. Where did all that come from, who were the key players?

I'm less familiar with the issues here; no one has yet, to my knowledge, submitted an NDA that relies upon evidence developed in an outcomes assessment database.

It could happen, of course, although I doubt it would succeed; it's hardly the kind of evidence that could meet the Act's substantial evidence requirement. I've heard some proponents of outcomes research suggest that it could be, but I find their arguments unpersuasive. Indeed, the oft cited assertion that outcomes research can, in contrast to randomised controlled trials, generate results with external validity seems to border on the paralogical. How can evidence that has no internal validity have external validity? To be clear, I am among the first to acknowledge that the external validity of the results of a typical randomised trial used to assess the efficacy of a new drug is limited, but the results are at least internally valid, and, as such, are a source of proof, in principle, that the drug has the effect claimed for it.

The randomised controlled trial is clearly a powerful means to produce evidence that things work but it's also an extremely costly means to produce evidence and the problem with all of that is that powerful interests will tend to be the only people who can produce the evidence. So you are forcing a certain corporate development on the field.

Perhaps, but there may be no alternative if society wants to have new drugs marketed that have relatively modest treatment effects. The effort required to develop a new drug with a truly substantial treatment effect would, of course, require far less effort. The reason large trials are required is the fact that sponsors are attempting to market products that have relatively modest effects relative to the degree of the variation present in the population of patients being treated. Of course, in the future, as our systems of diagnosis become more biologically homogeneous, variation will be reduced, and relatively small studies may be all that is required to show the efficacy of a new drug.

Do you think that pharmacogenetics will play a part here in due course?

Possibly, if by pharmacogenetics you mean efforts that facilitate the identification and selection of biologically homogeneous samples.

At a BAP meeting 3 years ago you said that your job is to act as a lens focusing debate.

Well, I'm not sure if the metaphor is perfect, but regulators do try to operate in a way that takes into consideration the diversity of scientific and political views extant in society. I believe I made the point that even if I wanted to advance a particular point of view, I could not succeed in doing so without the agreement and support of the physicians and scientists who serve as the agency's advisors. Anti-dementia drugs are an example where the FDA has not done what I would have preferred personally, but what those who served as our expert consultants thought best.

Well, on the dementia guidelines issue, you were saying about that at one point that really what you do is you get the field to come to a consensus but people on the outside often see it as your business to lay down the law, which is not what you are saying you do.

Actually, what we are supposed to do is very clear. The process by which the law is construed is known as notice and comment Rule making. The agency proposes a set of regulations by publishing them for comment in the Federal Register. The agency considers these comments, amends its proposal as its policy makers and legal counsel conclude is necessary, and publishes the rule in final form. Thus, the FDA is not the source of the law, but a good-faith interpreter of what Congress intended the law to do.

The Federal Food, Drug and Cosmetic Act, for example, instructs the agency to disapprove an NDA unless there is evidence, adduced in adequate and well-controlled investigations, that the drug will perform as claimed. It was the agency's task to interpret what Congress meant, but it did not create the standard.

In 1962, people moved towards encouraging the industry to develop drugs for disease entities. They wanted to move away from the idea of non-specific compounds, such as tonics.

Well, I'm not so sure of that. Among the definitions given in the Act, a drug is a substance claimed to have an effect on the structure, function or body of many. Accordingly, nothing in the Act precludes the development of tonics, per se. As a matter of practical enforcement, however, it is much easier to develop a drug for a defined disease entity, and that is why, I believe, you may have inferred what you have.

Some of the antidepressants, for instance, then could have been developed as a tonic. Has the industry made a mistake? You see at the moment we have got very bad compliance with antidepressants, it would seem. Is this because compared to compounds like St John's wort, which is a problem-of-living compound, a pick-me-up, a tonic and people say 'Yeah, I'm under stress, I need a tonic', but in contrast with the antidepressants, for you to get one you have got to be sold a disease as well?

Well, is depression a disease or a symptom? Indeed, what's a disease? In a taxonomic system it's entirely arbitrary. A homeopathic medicine, as much as any other, can be subjected to test in controlled trials. If its efficacy were established, and its safety shown, it could be legally marketed.

Sure, but would there be anything to stop someone like Bristol Myers Squibb at the moment, for instance, calling nefazodone a tonic?

Yes. We would probably argue that such a claim is potentially 'misleading', and, on those grounds, reject it. We could take such a position because the concept of a tonic is so vague that we could not write adequate directions for its use. For example, to whom and under what labelling would it be promoted?

It improves sleep, it improves appetite.

Then why not make those specific actions claims in their own right? If a treatment improves sleep, it could be marketed for the purpose, provided, of course, one can define what it means to 'improve' the sleep of someone who is sleeping normally. A claim for improving appetite might be somewhat more difficult because it is uncertain when and in whom a product stimulating appetite provides a benefit. It's difficult to assess it. Similar concerns affect claims for drugs with putative antiaggression effects.

Wouldn't it be easier to assess improved appetite or sleep or reduced aggression than to assess improvement in a disease state?

Well, improved sleep, perhaps, but even there I would have difficulty because the question is what happens if you have no change in total sleep time? What's improved sleep? If the idea was that people more often, after treatment than before, said they had improved sleep, it would still be a tough call because you wouldn't know what the effect you were you're dealing with actually was. It's rather hard to answer these kinds of questions definitively; the only way to approach them is with an open mind. The agency is not tasked to prevent sponsors from developing medications that provide meaningful benefit, but it is obliged to prevent the marketing of products that carry false and misleading claims.

I am not saying that any of this is readily nailed down. It is not always obvious where the interests of the public reside. At some point, government control over the accuracy and truth of drug product labelling can become excessive.

Coming back to the improved sleep front. Janssen some years ago had a 5HT$_2$ blocker, ritanserin, which as it turns out now, you could argue is a therapeutic principle in schiz-

ophrenia – when you add in 5HT$_2$ blockade into a D2 blockade you seem to produce something useful.

It so happens that some drugs with antipsychotic activity exhibit those two properties, but that might not be what determines their effectiveness.

But aren't we stuck with a problem here which is when they had their 5HT$_2$ blocker in the first instance, which I think was actually developed for use in schizophrenia because LSD acts on the 5HT$_2$ receptor but it turned out not to be useful as a single free standing agent for schizophrenia? Arguably added in to say Haldol decanoate it would have been extremely good but who was going to do that kind of trial?

Well, they might have, but I'm not sure of the point you make. A sponsor is always free to develop a fixed combination product. As long as the evidence adduced shows that each component makes a contribution to the efficacy of the combination, it's legitimate. Of course, if it turns out that the combination is no better than one of its components, the combination is irrational and will not be approved.

Nearly 20 years have passed since you joined the FDA in 1978. During that time you and your colleagues have had to face and resolve a variety of vexing issues affecting the fate of a number of psychotropic drugs. How do you manage? Clearly you can't possibly know enough in detail and depth on each and every medical/psychiatric and statistical issue that comes before you, or can you?

Of course, you're right, but I'm not expected to be a technical expert. To the contrary my business is to assess the quality of scientific evidence and the quality of those who assess it. In fact I often think of myself now more as an expert in what experts can and can't do and what they can reliably testify to than in the details per se. This is part of what anybody at the FDA would be doing – when my expert tells me something, are they in a position to offer me a judgement that derives from a well thought through body of evidence or fact or are they, in fact, doing no more than offering an opinion from the top of their fantasies?

I wouldn't know one form of a receptor from another and I don't really care anymore, although I certainly have gone through periods in my life when I cared vitally about allosteric hindrance and different forms of binding. Today that's a detail that is irrelevant to me although it might be very important in determining whether a drug is effective or not. It's not the level that I look at things. We recently had an interesting situation regarding antipsychotics and changes in ECG records. I listened to experts on both sides of the aisle give me very different views about what significance those changes had. That's the classic example of where you're getting involved in an area that you can't possibly know as much as the experts but you listen to them and try to decide how claim they know what they know.

Decisions about the marketing of drugs are invariably made on the incomplete and imperfect knowledge. Anyone who is involved in development and approval process must, therefore, find their own dealing with the uncertainties that affect all but the most routine regulatory decisions. I cannot claim to have found an ideal approach; indeed, I doubt that one exists. I do believe that drug regulators are paid to be sceptical about claims advanced for new drugs. Public health decisions should not be made on the basis of hopeful expectations and sanguine theories, but upon facts and findings that are robust enough to withstand careful, thorough, and thoughtful examination and challenge. Extrapolations from evidence should be reasonably circumspect where effectiveness claims are concerned and rather more liberal where drug-associated risk is involved. This asymmetric approach is sometimes characterised as being unreasonably risk averse but I am convinced that it remains, in the vast majority of instances, the preferred approach when decisions are being taken in the face of uncertainty.

Author index

Subject index

Abecarnil 341
Abortions 594
Acamprosate 496
Accutane 152
ACE inhibitors 342
Acetylcholine 188, 189, 192, 312, 356, 357, 366
Acetycholine shocks 411
ACNP, 19, 37, 135, 160, 163, 200, 205, 206, 211, 224, 297, 298, 304, 348, 428, 445, 446, 449–53, 455, 457, 464
Acuphase 572
ADHD 301, 302
Adoption Study 380–4, 390, 401, 402
Adrenoceptors 584
AEP (Association of European Psychiatrists) 491, 513, 514, 515
Affective disorders 415, 429
Agent Orange 405
Aggression 275, 620
Agitation 42, 54
Agranulocytosis 53, 55, 56, 591, 592, 593
AIDS 155, 157, 617
Akathisia 299, 300, 301, 568
Alcohol 35, 36
Alcohol, Drug Abuse and Mental Health Administration 531, 532
Allan Memorial Hospital 287
Alprazolam 247, 425, 426, 511, 512, 532, 534, 543, 547, 548, 549, 550, 551
Alzheimer's 372, 466, 469
American College of Neuropsychopharmacology, *see* ACNP
American Society of Clinical Psychopharmacology (ASCP) 298, 450
American Society for Human Genetics 380
Amitriptyline 112, 113, 173, 274, 278, 343, 565, 566, 569

Amphetamine 46, 49, 56, 78, 188, 189, 190, 192, 287, 303, 349
Amphetamine model of psychosis 564
Amyotrophic lateral sclerosis 372
Amytal 287
Anaesthesia 139, 153
Anafranil (clomipramine) 10, 11, 105, 110, 113, 114
Analgesic 135, 137, 150, 153, 161, 567
Analysts 543, 609–12
Animal models 135, 161, 492, 496
Annales School of History 317
Anthropological psychiatry 410
Antiaggressive agent 431
Anti-apomorphine 22, 26
Anticonvulsant 336, 567
Antidepressants 1, 3, 10, 11, 12, 14, 28, 30, 62, 63, 122, 123, 125, 126, 127, 128, 129, 132, 133, 134, 413–15, 417, 430, 564, 573
Antidiarrhoeals 51, 56
Antiemetic 23, 26, 50, 62, 218
Antihistamine 21, 22
Anti-parkinsonian 96
Anti-psychiatry 411, 412, 430, 598
Antipsychotic 53, 54, 59
Antisocial personality disorder 402
Anxiety 169–74
Anxiolytic 372, 373
Anzio Beachhead 136
Apomorphine gnawing 567
Archives of General Psychiatry 453, 550
Arrowsmith 378
Artists 280
Assay sensitivity 615, 626
Astra Pharmaceutical Company 110, 343, 570
Audiogenic seizures 78
Authoritarian 613
Autonomous 422

EBPS (European Behavioural
   Pharmacology Society) 475, 477, 479,
   487, 488, 489, 490
ECA 530, 531, 532, 539, 553
ECDEU 464
ECNP (European College of
   Neuropsychopharmacology) 418, 428,
   489, 490, 491, 513, 514, 515, 516, 591,
   599, 600, 601, 602
Ecstasy 585
ECT 259, 261, 411, 429
Effect size 619
Effort syndrome 169
Egyptologist 409
Einheits-psychose 98
Elective affinities 187
Electric shock therapy 121, 122, 123
Electrical transmission 352
Electroconvulsive shock 72, 73, 74, 75, 76,
   77, 78
Electronarcosis 171, 175
Electronic publishing 449
Eli Lilly 81, 82, 124, 126, 130
Eliza program 554
Eltoprazine 507, 508
Encephalopathy 279
Endocrine response 420
Endogenous depressions 62, 63, 522
Endorphin 303, 304
Enthusiasm 253
Ephedrine 18
Epidemiology 251, 525, 532, 533, 534, 538,
   539, 541, 556
EPS 299, 300
ERAG 507
Ethics of psychotherapy 537
Eugenics 399
European Behavioural Pharmacological
   Society, see EBPS
European Community 491
Evaluation 238, 248
Evidence-based medicine 548, 554
Excitatory 352, 353, 356–9, 361, 366, 368,
   369, 371, 372
Excitotoxicity 371
Expectations of treatment 470
Experimental psychiatry 190, 193, 197, 201,
   206
Explosive experts 418–22
Extinction 48
Extrapyramidal side-effects 564, 566, 568

Fatal Toxicity Index 592

FDA 110, 338, 546, 557, 587, 595, 603,
   612, 613, 615, 617, 619, 621
FDA for psychotherapy 537
Feeding 313, 314, 315
Feighner criteria 394
Ferrosan 341, 570, 577
First Glutamate Symposium 365
Fluoxetine 114, 180, 422, 505, 506, 517,
   570
   see also Prozac
Flupenthixol 274, 510, 564, 572, 573, 574,
   576
Fluphenazine 564, 572, 573, 575
Fluvoxamine 505, 570
Focal sepsis 168
Fort Sam Huston 72
Functional polymorphisms 402, 404
Fungal diseases 58

G22150 98
G22355 (imipramine) 98
GABA 328, 329, 356, 359, 362, 365, 366
Galvanic skin responses 287
Gambling 419, 552
Geigy 10, 11, 96, 97, 102, 104, 105, 106,
   107, 111, 113, 414, 417
Gene-Logic 567
General practice 251, 252, 253
General Practitioner Research Group 462,
   465
Genetic bias 384
Genetic counselling 399
Genetic discrimination 397
Genetic research 420
Genetic studies 438
Genetics of schizophrenia 381, 400, 401
Geneva 551
Gilles de la Tourette's syndrome 47, 51
Glutamate 336, 337, 352, 355–9, 361–7,
   369–72
Glutamate antagonists 361, 364
Glutamate receptors 358, 359, 365, 368,
   372, 373, 374
Glycine 364
Good Clinical Practice 57
Good Laboratory Practice 57, 58, 59
Guernsey 461
Guidelines 527, 536
Guinea-pig 266
Guinness Book of Records 409

HA-966 362, 364, 365
Haldol decanoate 44, 55